ARTERIA MAGNA, AOPTH, הָאוֹרְטִי HAORTI EX SI-
NISTRO CORDIS SINV ORIENS, ET VITALEM SPIRITVM TOTI CORPORI DEFERENS, NATVRALEMQVE CALOREM
PER CONTRACTIONEM ET DILATATIONEM TEMPERANS.

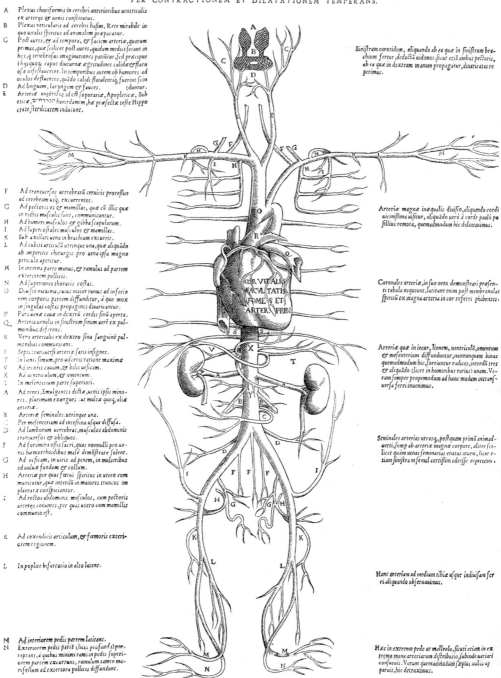

A. Plexus choriformis in cerebri anterioribus uentriculis ex arterijs & uenis constitutus.
B. Plexus reticularis ad cerebri basim, Rete mirabile in quo uitalis spiritus ad animalem praeparatur.
C. Post aures, & ad tempora, & faciem arteriae, quarum primas, quae scilicet post aures, quidam medici secant in hys, q tenebrosas imaginationes patiuntur, sed praecipue i hsjcunqz caput diuturnae aegritudines calidæ & flatu os æ infestauerint. In temporibus autem ob humores ad oculos defluentes, quãdo calidi flatulentiq, fuerint scin
D. Ad linguam, laryngem & fauces.   (duntur.
E. Arteria καρότιδεϛ id est soporariæ, Apoplecticæ, Sub eticæ, הנרדמים hanirdamm, hæ praesectæ teste Hippo crate sterilitatem inducunt.

F. Ad transuersos uertebraru ceruicis processus ad cerebrum usq; excurrentes.
G. Ad pectoris os & mamillas, quae cu illis quæ in rectis musculis sunt, communicantur.
H. Ad humeri musculos & gibba scapularum.
I. Ad supercostales musculos & mamillas.
K. Sub axillari uena in brachium excurrit.
L. Ad cubiti articulu utrinque una, quæ aliquado ab imperitis chirurgis pro uena ipsa magno periculo aperitur.
M. In interna parte manus, & ramulus ad partem exteriorem pollicis.
N. Ad superiores thoracis costas.
O. Diuisio maxima, cuius maior ramus ad inferiorem corporis partem diffunditur, à quo mox in singulas costas propagines diuaricantur.
P. Pars uenæ cauæ in dextru cordis sinu aperta.
Q. Arteria uenalis in sinistrum sinum aere ex pulmonibus deferens.
R. Vena arterialis ex dextro sinu sanguine pulmonibus communicans.
S. Septi transuersi arteriæ satis insignes.
T. In lienis simum, pro uisceris ratione maximæ.
V. Ad iecoris cauum, & bilis uesicam.
X. Ad uentriculum, & omentum.
?. In melenterium parte superiori.
A. Ad renes, Emulgentes dictæ, uenis ipsis minores, plurimum exangues :ut multæ quoq, aliæ arteriæ.
B. Arteriæ seminales:utrinque una.
C. Per mesenterium ad intestina usq; diffusa.
D. Ad lumborum uertebras, musculos abdominis transuersos & obliquos.
E. Ad foramina ossis sacri, quas nonnulli pro uenis haemorrhoidibus male demostrare solent.
G. Ad uesicam, in uiris ad penem, in mulieribus ad uuluæ fundum & collum.
H. Arteriæ per quas fœtui spiritus in utero communicatur, quæ interdu in maiores truncos im plantatæ conspiciuntur.
?. Ad rectos abdominis musculos, cum pectoris arterijs coeuntes, per quas utero cum mamillis communio est.

K. Ad coxendicis articulum, & femoris exteriorem regionem.

L. In poplite bifurcatio in alto latens.

M. Ad interiorem pedis partem latitans.
N. Exteriorem pedis parte (licet profundi) sep reptant, à quibus minimi rami in pedis superiorem partem excurrunt, ramulum tamen manifestum ad exteriore pollicis diffundunt.

CORVITALIS FACVLTATIS FOMES ET ARTER PRIN

Sinistram caroticem, aliquando ab ea quæ in sinistrum brachium fertur, deductã uidimus.sicut etiã ambas pectoris, ab ea quæ in dextram manum propagatur, diuaricatas reperimus.

Arteriæ magnæ inæqualis diuisio, aliquando cordi uicinissima uisitur, aliquando uerò è corde paulò pusillius remota, quemadmodum hic delineauimus.

Coronales arteriæ, in suo ortu demonstrari praesenti tabula nequeunt, latitant enim post membranulas spiritù ex magna arteria in cor referri phibentes.

Arteriæ quæ in iecur, lienem, uentriculu, omentum & mesenterium diffunduntur, nonnunquam binas quemadmodum hic, sortiuntur radices, interdù tres & aliquãdo (licet in hominibus rarius) unam. Verum semper propemodum ad hunc modum in transuersa ferri inuenimus.

Seminales arterias utrasq, postquam primù animaduerti, semp ab arteriæ magnæ corpore, aliter scilicet quàm uenas seminarias enatas inueni, licet etiam sinistra m semel certissim edeesse repererim.

Hanc arteriam ad medium tibiæ usque indiuisam ferri aliquando obseruauimus.

Hæc in extremo pede ac malleolo, sicuti etiam in extrema manu arteriarum distributio, subinde uariari consueuit. Verum quemadmodum sæpius nobis ap paruit, hic detraximus.

NOTATV DIGNAE ARTERIAE MAGNAE SOBOLES CENTVM ET QVADRAGINTA SEPTEM APPARENT.

The Heart and Great Arteries; in Tabulae Sex, Andreas Versalius, 1540 – by courtesy of Prof. Gaetano Thiene, Institute of Pathological Anatomy, the University of Padua.

Endothelial Dysfunctions and Vascular Disease

EDITED BY

Raffaele De Caterina, MD, PhD

Professor of Cardiology
Chair and Postgraduate School of Cardiology; "G. d'Annunzio" University – Chieti
Ospedale San Camillo de Lellis; Via C. Forlanni, 50
66100 Chieti

Director
Laboratory for Thrombosis and Vascular Research; CNR Institute of Clinical Physiology
Area della Ricerca di S. Cataldo; Via G. Moruzzi, 1
56124 Pisa
Italy

Peter Libby, MD

Mallinckrodt Professor, Harvard Medical School and Chief,
Cardiovascular Division, Brigham and Women's Hospital,
Boston, MA,
USA

FOREWORD BY
Michael A. Gimbrone Jr.

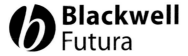

Blackwell Publishing, Inc., 350 Main Street, Malden, MA 02148-5020, USA
Blackwell Publishing Ltd, 9600 Garsington Road, Oxford OX4 2DQ, UK
Blackwell Science Asia Pty Ltd, 550 Swanston Street, Carlton, Victoria 3053, Australia

First published 2007

1   2007

ISBN: 978-1-4051-2208-5

Library of Congress Cataloging-in-Publication Data

Endothelial dysfunctions and vascular disease / edited by Raffaele De Caterina, Peter Libby; foreword by Michael A. Gibmbrone Jr.
    p. ; cm
  Includes bibliographical references.
  ISBN-13: 978-1-4051-2208-5 (hard cover)
  ISBN-10: 1-4051-2208-0 (hard cover)
1. Blood-vessels—Pathophysiology. 2. Vascular endothelium.
I. De Caterina, R., 1954– II. Libby, Peter.
[DNLM: 1. Vascular Diseases—Physiopathology. 2. Endothelium,
Vascular—Physiopathology.   WG 500 E555 2007]
RC691.4.E535 2007
616.1′93—dc22

                                                              2006020580

A catalogue record for this title is available from the British Library.

Acquisitions: Steve Korn
Development: Fiona Pattison
Set in Minion 9.5/12pt by Charon Tec Ltd (A Macmillan Company), Chennai, India
Printed and bound in Singapore by COS Printers Pte Ltd

For further information on Blackwell Publishing, visit our website:
www.blackwellfutura.com

Contents

Contributors

Mark R. Adams, MBBS, PhD, FRACP
Department of Cardiology
Royal Prince Alfred Hospital
Sydney
Australia

Masanori Aikawa, MD, PhD
Brigham and Women's Hospital
Vascular Medicine
Boston, MA
USA

Todd J. Anderson, MD, FRCPC
Department of Cardiovascular Sciences
Libin Cardiovascular Institute
University of Calgary
Calgary, AB
Canada

Mikko P.S. Ares, MD
Department of Clinical Sciences
Malmö University Hospital
Lund University
Sweden

Giuseppina Basta, DBiol
CNR Institute of Clinical Physiology
Pisa
Italy

Joshua A. Beckman, MD
The Cardiovascular Division, Brigham and Women's
    Hospital *and*
Harvard Medical School
Boston, MA
USA

Dominik Behrendt, MD
Department of Medicine
Cardiovascular Division
Brigham and Women's Hospital
Boston, MA
USA

Umberto Campia, MD
Cardiovascular Research Institute
Washington, DC
USA

David S. Celermajer, MBBS, PhD, FRACP
Department of Cardiology
Royal Prince Alfred Hospital
Sydney
Australia

Sammy Y. Chan, MD, FRCP(C)
St. Paul's Hospital
University of British Columbia
Canada

Francois Charbonneau, MSc, MD
Department of Cardiovascular Sciences
Libin Cardiovascular Institute
University of Calgary
Calgary, AB
Canada

Mark A. Creager, MD
The Cardiovascular Division, Brigham and Women's
    Hospital *and*
Harvard Medical School
Boston, MA
USA

John E. Deanfield, FRCP
Department of Cardiology
University College London
UK

Serena Del Turco, DBiol, PhD
CNR Institute of Clinical Physiology
Pisa
Italy

Wolfgang Dichtl, MD
Department of Internal Medicine
Leopold-Franzens-Universität Innsbruck
Austria

Victor J. Dzau, MD
Department of Medicine
Duke University Medical Center
Durham, NC
USA

Erling Falk, MD
Department of Cardiology and Institute of Experimental
    Clinical Research
Skejby University Hospital
Aarhus
Denmark

Marilena Formato, MD
Department of Physiological, Biochemical and Cellular
    Sciences
University of Sassari
Sassari
Italy

Peter Ganz, MD
Department of Medicine
Cardiovascular Division
Brigham and Women's Hospital
Boston, MA
USA

Yong-Jian Geng, MD, PhD
The Center for Cardiovascular Biology and Atherosclerosis
Department of Internal Medicine
University of Texas Health Science Center at Houston
    School of Medicine *and*
Stem Cells and Heart Failure Research Laboratory
Texas Heart Institute—St. Luke's Episcopal Hospital
Houston, TX
USA

Jacopo Gianetti, MD, PhD
CNR Institute of Clinical Physiology
Massa and Pisa
Italy

Michael A. Gimbrone Jr., MD
Brigham and Women's Hospital
Boston, MA
USA

Massimiliano Gnecchi, PhD
Department of Medicine
Duke University Medical Center
Durham, NC
USA

Julian P.J. Halcox, MA, MD, MRCP
Department of Cardiology
University College London
UK

Reynold Homan, PhD
Esperion Therapeutics
Division of Pfizer Global R&D
Ann Arbor, MI
USA

Scott Kinlay, MBBS
Department of Medicine
Cardiovascular Division
Brigham and Women's Hospital
Boston, MA
USA

Amir Kol, MD, PhD
Dipartimento Malattie del Cuore
A.C.O. San Filippo Neri
Rome
Italy

Deling Kong, PhD
Department of Medicine
Brigham and Women's Hospital
Harvard Medical School
Boston, MA
USA

Brian Krause, PhD
Esperion Therapeutics
    Division of Pfizer Global R&D
Ann Arbor, MI
USA

Guido Lazzerini, BSc
CNR Institute of Clinical Physiology
Pisa
Italy

Rosalinda Madonna, MD, PhD
Cardiology Division and Center of Excellence on Aging
"G. d'Annunzio" University
Chieti
Italy *and*
University of Texas
Health Science Center Medical School
Houston, TX
USA

G.B. John Mancini, MD, FRCP(C), FACC
Vancouver Hospital and Health Sciences Centre
University of British Columbia
Canada

Nikolaus Marx, MD
Cardiovascular Division
University of Ulm
Ulm
Germany

Marika Massaro, DBiol, PhD
CNR Institute of Clinical Physiology
Pisa and Lecce
Italy

Luis G. Melo, PhD
Department of Medicine
Brigham and Women's Hospital
Harvard Medical School
Boston, MA
USA

Karen S. Moulton, MD
Department of Surgery
Vascular Biology Program
Children's Hospital *and*
Cardiovascular Division
Brigham and Women's Hospital
Boston
USA

Roger Newton, PhD
Esperion Therapeutics
Division of Pfizer Global R&D
Ann Arbor, MI
USA

Jan Nilsson, MD
Department of Clinical Sciences
Malmö University Hospital
Lund University
Sweden

Alok S. Pachori, PhD
Department of Medicine
Duke University Medical Center
Durham, NC *and*
Department of Medicine
Brigham and Women's Hospital and
Harvard Medical School
Boston, MA
USA

Julio A. Panza, MD
Coronary Care Unit
Washington Hospital Center
Washington, DC
USA

Jorge Plutzky, MD
Cardiovascular Division
Brigham and Women's Hospital
Boston, MA
USA

Domenico Praticò, MD
Department of Pharmacology
University of Pennsylvania
School of Medicine
Philadelphia, PA
USA

Angelo M. Scanu, MD
Departments of Medicine and of Biochemistry and
    Molecular Biology
University of Chicago
Chicago, IL
USA

Ann Marie Schmidt, MD
Columbia University
New York, NY
USA

Tommaso Simoncini, MD, PhD
Molecular and Cellular Gynecological Endocrinology
    Laboratory (MCGEL)
Department of Reproductive Medicine and Child
    Development
Division of Obstetrics and Gynecology
University of Pisa
Pisa
Italy

Antonella Zampolli, DBiol, PhD
B-forskning
Skejby Sygehus
Brendsr´trupgaardsvej
DK-8200N Aarhus N
Denmark *and*
Scuola Superiore S. Anna
Pisa
Italy

Ouliana Ziouzenkova, PhD
Cardiovascular Division
Brigham and Women's Hospital
Boston, MA
USA

Preface

Every book has a history, this one not excepted, having emerged from intersections in professional lives of the editors. This book bears the fruits of a collaboration between the "pupil" (RDC) and the "mentor" (PL). During an extended sabbatical of the pupil in Boston in 1994, we probed together the concept that endothelial dysfunction served as a common denominator of vascular disease, with the balance between inflammation and its inhibition as a fulcrum of the regulation of the behavior of endothelial cells. As practicing cardiologists in our clinical lives, we sought to link to endothelial function the mechanisms of action of risk factors and of pharmacologic agents used to treat and prevent vascular disease. The pupil therefore authored a few reviews on the mechanism of action of risk factors and included them in a small book, published in Italian, for which the mentor wrote a preface. This book was greeted with favor from the Italian cardiologic community, and provided the nidus for the present, more ambitious endeavor, which includes updated reviews on the pathogenesis of vascular disease and on the most novel aspects of vascular biology. This enterprise was enabled by the contributions of many of our former or present collaborators and colleagues, without whose enthusiasm and engagement this work could never have seen light. We largely underestimated the devotion necessary on our own side at the beginning, but it ultimately yielded a product that we feel achieves our original goals. We are aware that we confront a continuously evolving topic, where frequent updates would be desirable – if not necessary. Yet, we believe in the value of books – such as the current one – that attempt to organize in a snapshot of time, the vast amount of literature available in a coherent and comprehensive scheme. We are aware of existing gaps, of emerging material not paid its due, and of the rapid evolution of some of the concepts highlighted within. The links between the laboratory and the clinic have never afforded more opportunity for new understanding and advances in diagnosis and treatment than today. We hope that our colleagues, vascular biologists, cardiologists, internists, and other physicians alike will find this compendium a useful guide to this most exciting time in vascular biology and medicine.

Raffaele De Caterina and Peter Libby

Foreword

Functions and dysfunctions of vascular endothelium: nature's container for blood

Recent decades have witnessed an explosion of our knowledge of the functions and dysfunctions of the vascular endothelium, nature's container for blood, and their implications for health and disease. In his classic monograph, published in 1954, entitled *Endothelium: Its Development, Morphology, Function, and Pathology* [1], Rudolf Altschul, Professor in Histology at the University of Saskatchewan, devoted a total of 124 pages to all aspects of his subject, and only 20 pages to the then known functions of endothelium – fewer than the number of chapters that comprise this compendium! Interestingly, he chose to preface his treatise with the sobering comment that "The largest number of natural deaths from a single cause in North America, and probably in many other parts of the world, is ascribed to cardiovascular diseases. . .," a statement that unfortunately is as true today as it was a half-century ago, and hence the critical challenge this timely volume addresses. He opined "While working on the problem of arteriosclerosis, I have realized not only how little I knew about endothelium, but also how much I ought to know for the proper understanding of [that disease process]." Implicit in the latter statement is an increasingly more appreciated experimental strategy in the modern biomedical sciences, namely that the natural diseases that afflict the various organs and tissues of the body provide "lens" through which to view the inner workings of normal biologic systems. The basic mechanistic insights so gained then become relevant, indeed enabling, to our ability to translate basic research knowledge into clinical applications – earlier diagnostic tests, more targeted therapies, and ultimately disease prevention.

As one peruses the table of contents of this volume, one cannot help but be impressed by the sheer bulk of new knowledge related to endothelial function/dysfunction that has been obtained through the study of diseases that affect the cardiovascular system, in particular, atherosclerosis, diabetes and the metabolic syndrome, and their classic risk factors and molecular effectors, including dyslipidemia, hyperhomocysteinemia, cytokines, and oxidative stress. However, one cannot lose sight of the simple fact that endothelium per se is a "distributed organ" whose functional properties are indeed relevant to all organ systems and vascularized tissues. Thus, the study of endothelial functions/dysfunctions is by its very nature a multidisciplinary pursuit, one well suited to the matrix organizational structure toward which the modern biologic sciences are rapidly evolving. This progression in our understanding of the endothelium has been enabled by both technological and conceptual advances, as is amply illustrated by the content of the various chapters of this volume. Initially, the fundamental "blood container function" of endothelium was appreciated in morphologic terms, through the pioneering ultrastructural studies of Palade, Karnovsky, Majno, and Cotran. Indeed, structural loss of endothelial barrier function ("leakiness") was equated with one of the fundamental signs of inflammation. A major and relatively recent conceptual advance was the realization that the endothelium is a dynamically mutable interface, whose fundamental functional properties – permselectivity, non-thrombogenic surface, selective leukocyte adhesion, paracrine, autocrine and systemic secretory activity, as well as cell replication and survival – are actively regulated through the endothelial-directed actions of various endogenous mediators (cytokines, chemokines, growth factors, survival factors). This conceptual model of "endothelial activation" encompassed a dynamic range of functional responses to a variety of inciting factors – thus setting the stage for the definition of pathophysiologic important stimuli of endothelial dysfunction. Interestingly, the term "endothelial dysfunction," often equated with the phenomenon of impaired EDRF/nitric oxide production, was first introduced in the broader context of multiple endothelial functions (in particular, the loss of blood compatibility and the stimulation of leukocyte adhesion by proinflammatory cytokines) that were susceptible to regulation/dysregulation by various biochemical/humoral stimuli [2]. Most recently, the repertoire of pathologically relevant stimuli of endothelial dysfunction has been expanded to include altered biomechanical forces, generated by the pulsatile flow of blood in certain vascular geometries that are susceptible to atherosclerotic lesion formation. In parallel with the definition of the spectrum of endothelial dysfunctions has come the delineation of the intrinsic mechanisms by which the endothelial lining maintains its functional integrity. As is explored in various chapters of this volume, these studies can provide invaluable insights relevant to the development of biomarkers and other diagnostic tools for assessing endothelial dysfunction, and ultimately perfecting endothelial-directed therapeutics designed to bolster these endogenous protective mechanisms.

What then does the future hold for our practical utilization of this rapidly expanding fund of knowledge about endothelial functions and dysfunctions?

A worthwhile, and indeed strategic, goal will continue to be the development of quantifiable indices of endothelial dysfunction – preferably linked to pathogenetic progression, and thus useful in the context of both diagnosis and therapy. A logical extension of this line of translational research will be non-invasive bioimaging techniques that can both localize spatially, and demarcate temporally, disease progression/regression. Enabled by these practical tools, one can only imagine that our appreciation for the role of endothelial functions/dysfunctions will continue to grow, and that the benefactors of this expanding wealth of knowledge will be our patients. And, hopefully as a result, in the next comprehensive volume devoted to this topic, the prevalence of cardiovascular disease will be referenced historically in the past tense.

Michael A. Gimbrone Jr., MD
Elsie T. Friedman Professor of Pathology
Harvard Medical School
Chairman, Department of Pathology
Director, Center for Excellence in Vascular Biology
Brigham and Women's Hospital
Boston, MA, USA

1   Rudolf Altschul. "*Endothelium: Its Development, Morphology, Function, and Pathology.* New York: The Macmillan Company; 1954.
2   Gimbrone Jr. MA. Endothelial dysfunction and the pathogenesis of atherosclerosis. In: Gotto A, ed. *Atherosclerosis-V, Proceedings of the Vth International Symposium on Atherosclerosis.* New York: Springer-Verlag; 1980:415–425.

Acknowledgments

This book would not have been possible without the contributions of many, whose patience, abnegation, and persistence overcame the many intervening obstacles. We are deeply grateful, in particular, to Karen E. Williams, whose expert and thoughtful editorial assistance improved each single chapter substantially and gave the present shape to this work.

Dedication

To our families, and to our coworkers – our extended families

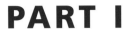

PART I

The basis of endothelial involvement in vascular diseases

CHAPTER 1

Endothelial functions and dysfunctions

Raffaele De Caterina, MD, PhD, *Marika Massaro*, DBiol, PhD, & *Peter Libby*, MD

Introduction

Key elements in the maintenance of tissue home-ostasis, blood vessels serve as the conduits of circulation, transporting nutrients and oxygen to organs and tissues, and removing destructive catabolites and xenobiotics from the blood flow.

William Harvey first described the ceaseless and circular motion of the vascular system in 1628 [1]. Using primitive microscopes, Marcello Malpighi later elucidated a network of vessels throughout the body (Table 1.1). In 1661, Malpighi described the physical separation between blood and tissues and also identified the capillaries that connect small arteries with small veins [2]. During the 1880s, von Recklinghausen determined that tunnel-like blood vessels, lined by cells, bore deeply in the tissues [3,4]. After Starling proposed the law of capillary exchanges in 1896, scientists understood the endothelium as a selective physical barrier. By the mid-20th century, Palade's electron microscopy studies of the vessel wall [5] and Gowans' description of the interaction between lymphocytes and the endothelium of post-capillary venules [6] determined an active role of the endothelium in the circulation. Since then, numerous studies have elucidated our current view of the endothelium as a dynamic, heterogeneous, and widespread organ with vital synthetic, secretory, metabolic, and immunologic functions [1,7].

We have long understood two specialized endothelial functions: gas exchange in pulmonary circulation and fenestration in hepatic and splenic circulation. Under normal homeostatic conditions, the endothelium resists vasospasm, prevents leukocyte and platelet adhesion to the vessel wall, favors fibrinolysis, combats coagulation of blood, and inhibits the proliferation of vascular smooth muscle cells (SMC) (Figure 1.1). For these reasons, we now appreciate the vascular endothelium as a dynamic and heterogeneous autocrine/paracrine organ capable of synthesizing, secreting, and metabolizing a variety of substances as well as performing vital immunologic functions. This chapter will briefly review endothelial physiology.

Dysfunctional and activated endothelium: definitions

During the last two decades, accumulating evidence has described the vascular endothelium as an active endocrine, paracrine, and autocrine organ, indispensable for the maintenance of vascular homeostasis. Such maintenance occurs by continuous monitoring by the vascular endothelium of blood-borne and locally generated stimuli and also through subsequent immediate- or long-term responses to changes in its environment [8–10]. Altered homeostasis induced by various stimuli may cause localized alterations, or "endothelial dysfunctions," of the antihemostatic properties, vascular tone, heightened leukocyte adhesion, and increased production of cytokines and growth factors [9]. The term "endothelial activation" designates a subset of endothelial dysfunction whereby changes produced by various stimuli (e.g., inflammatory cytokines) elicit new functional and molecular properties. The dramatic change of endothelial interactions with blood leukocytes occurring in

Table 1.1 This brief history of vessel anatomy and biology as well as the discovery of the endothelium outline the principal theories and discoveries leading to the current understanding of blood circulation and the endothelium as a key regulator of vascular wall functions.

Who	When	What
Greek colony in Egypt	About 250 BC	Taught that the heart was connected with two separated sets of vessel: arteries full of air and veins full of blood. It was supposed that the two trees were entirely separated [4,223].
Erasistratos	304–250 BC	First hypothesized the existence of "synastomoses" between veins and arteries [4,223].
Galen	131–201 AD	Taught that blood passed from the right to the left ventricle through invisible pores in the interventricular septum [224].
Galilei	1609	Developed an *occhiolino* or compound microscope with a convex and a concave lens.
Cesalpino	1509–1603	Maintained that the blood circulated through the whole body [4].
Harvey	1628	Discovered the circulation of the blood without the use of the microscope [225].
Malpighi	1661	With the use of a primitive microscope, described the physical separation between blood and tissues and the existence of capillaries connecting small arteries with small veins [2].
Van Leuwenhoek	1674	Improved the microscope and finely described where a small artery ends and a vein begins [226].
von Recklinghausen	1881	Showed that vessels were lined by cells [3].
Starling	1896	Described the law of "capillary exchanges" [227].
Ernest Ruska	1931	Built the first electron microscope.
Pappenheimer	1953	For the first time proposes a physical theory on capillary permeability [228].
Palade	1953	Described the ultrastructure of the blood capillaries [5].
Gowans	1959	First described the interaction between lymphocytes and the endothelium in post-capillary venules [6].
Moncada and Vane	1976	Discovered prostacyclin [229].
Furchgott and Zawadzki	1980	Postulated the existence of an endothelium-derived vascular relaxing factor (EDRF) [8].
Ignarro and Palmer	1987	Demonstrated that endothelium-derived relaxing factor is nitric oxide (NO) [38,39].

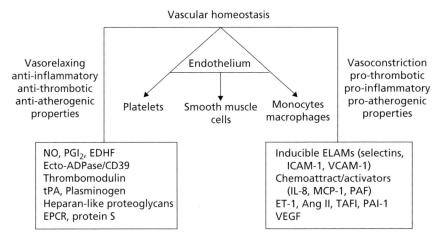

Figure 1.1 A schematic representation of the role of the endothelium in the maintenance of vascularhomeostasis. Endothelium-derived factors act in concert to appropriately control vasoconstriction, smooth muscle proliferation, thrombosis, inflammation, coagulation, and fibrinolysis. Endothelial dysfunction is defined as the loss of any of these balanced functions, with resulting pathologic consequences. NO: nitric oxide; PGI$_2$: prostacyclin; EDHF: endothelium-derived hyperpolarizing factor; EPCR: endothelial protein C receptor; ELAMs: endothelial-leukocyte adhesion molecules; ICAM-1: intercellular adhesion molecule-1; VCAM-1: Vascular cell adhesion molecule-1; IL-8: interleukin-8; MCP-1: monocyte chemoattractant protein-1; PAF: platelet-activating factor; ET-1: endothelin-1; Ang II: angiotensin II; TAFI: thrombin-activatable fibrinolysis inhibitor; PAI-1: plasminogen activator inhibitor-1; VEGF: vascular endothelial growth factor.

inflammation provides an example of endothelial activation [11].

Endothelial cell morphology

Generally of squamous morphology and usually elongated in the direction of blood flow, endothelial cells (EC) form a 0.2–4 μm-thick monolayer that lines the lumina of the entire surface of the vascular tree. Often considered the body's largest "organ," the 6 trillion cells of the endothelium cover an area of ≈5000 m² in a vessel network that develops beyond 100,000 km and weighs about 1 kg, representing about 1% of body mass [12]

The cytoskeleton determines EC shape and orientation. Flow variations result in the rearrangement of stress fibers (dense bundles of actin fibers) to localize predominantly in the periphery of the cell [13]. Stress fibers also associate with intermediate filaments rich in vimentin and tubulin, this last protein predominant in microtubules. Together, these three protein families largely maintain cell shape and orientation [13].

EC markers include angiotensin-converting enzyme (ACE); von Willebrand factor (vWF, stored in the Weibel–Palade bodies); vascular endothelial growth factor receptors (VEGFR)-1 and -2; the vascular endothelial (VE)-cadherin, platelet–EC adhesion molecule-1 (PECAM-1; CD31); P-selectin; the mucin-like molecule CD34; and E-selectin. While VE-cadherin, E-selectin, and VEGFR are entirely endothelium-specific, ACE, vWF, CD31, P-selectin, and CD34 also reside in megakaryocytes, platelets, and other predominantly hematopoietic cell types (Figure 1.2) [14].

Barrier function of the endothelium

The normal endothelium features a compact monolayer characterized by scant intercellular spaces, thus forming an active barrier between blood and the underlying tissues. Several elements, including intercellular junctions, cell-surface-binding proteins, electrostatic charges of endothelial membranes, and basement membrane composition, regulate endothelial integrity and permeability.

Transmembrane proteins linked to cytoplasmic and cytoskeletal proteins form intercellular junctions with close physical attachments between two contiguous cell membranes [15,16]. Within minutes, this highly dynamic and reversible system allows the passage of blood components into tissues. Three major intercellular junctions occur in EC: tight junctions, gap junctions, and *adherens* junctions (Figure 1.3).

Tight junction (*zonula occludens*)

Tight junctions allow very close contacts between adjacent cells. The number of tight junctions varies according to EC type, e.g., brain and large arteries contain many tight junctions, while post-capillary EC contain few or none [17]. Occludin, a transmembrane protein associated with intracellular proteins, i.e., *zonula occludens* (ZO)-1 and -2, cingulin, and RAB, member of RAS oncogene family-like 3, form tight junctions. ZO-1 likely localizes at initial cell-to-cell contacts, whereas cingulin and ZO-2 link to actin microfilaments [18,19]. Some evidence suggests that tight junctions may protect the endothelium against hemodynamic forces. Indeed, the number of tight junctions increases in cultured

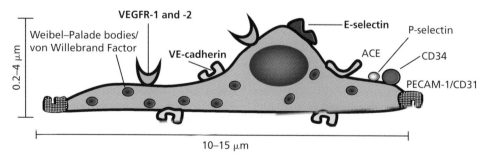

Figure 1.2 EC markers. VEGFR-1 and -2, VE-cadherin, and E-selectin (in bold) are specific for the endothelium. ACE, von Willebrand Factor (stored in the Weibel–Palade bodies), PECAM-1 (CD31), P-selectin, and the mucin-like molecule CD34 are also present in megakaryocytes, platelets, and some other predominantly hematopoietic cell types. VEGFR-1 and -2: vascular endothelial growth factors receptors-1 and -2; ACE: angiotensin-converting enzyme; vWF: von Willebrand factor; PECAM-1: platelet-EC adhesion molecule-1.

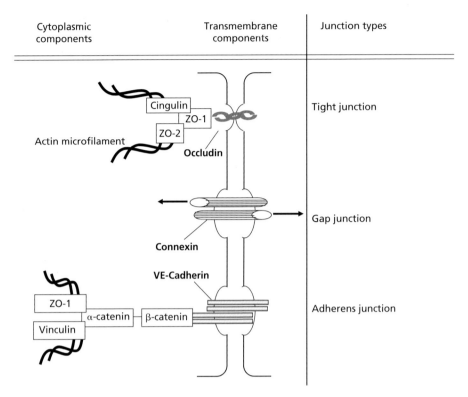

Figure 1.3 A schematic representation of the molecular organization of endothelial cell-to-cell junctions. ZO-1 and -2: zonula occludens-1 and -2; VE-cadherin: vascular endothelial-cadherin.

EC exposed to laminar shear stress [20,21], and tight junctions occur only rarely in aortic regions exposed to higher levels of shear stress [22], sites relatively spared by lipid deposition and atherosclerotic lesion formation.

Gap junction

Clusters of transmembrane channels, or gap junctions, link the cytoplasmic compartments of neighboring cells, allowing a direct exchange of ions and second messengers [23]. A gap junction channel consists of a pair of hemi-channels or connexons; each connexon contains six connexin molecules. In mammals, connexins form a multigene family comprising at least 15 members [24]. Each connexin forms channels with different properties of permeability and selective interaction with other connexin molecules. Gap junctions likely facilitate communication between EC (homotypic cell communication) and also between EC and other cell types, i.e., SMC or leukocytes (heterotypic cell communication). Some have suggested that gap

junction signaling permits and coordinates EC migration and replication during angiogenesis or injury repair [15]. Recent findings indicate differentially regulated expression of EC and SMC connexins during atherogenesis [25]. The distribution pattern of individual connexins in disparate areas of the atherosclerotic plaque suggests that these molecules may differentially regulate the cell-to-cell transfer of factors important for lesion development, a hypothesis that raises the intriguing possibility that direct cell-to-cell communication via gap junctions may contribute to the pathogenesis of atherosclerosis in humans [25,26].

Adherens junction (zonula adherens)

Transmembrane proteins termed cadherins form *adherens* junctions that allow calcium-dependent homophilic recognition, i.e., recognition between EC [13]. Adherens junctions appear essential for the organization of EC contacts [27]. *Adherens* junctions likely participate importantly in the control of cell migration, growth, and differentiation

[13,15,18]. EC express specific and non-specific cadherins [28]. Non-specific cadherins, present in disparate cell types, include N-, P-, and E-cadherin. Their role in the determination of endothelial structure remains controversial. EC specifically possess a cadherin termed VE-cadherin [13,29], the most common component of *adherens* junctions [13]. Recent studies suggest that EC associated with neovascularization express VE-cadherin in atherosclerotic lesions [30]. In particular, reduced expression of VE-cadherin within intimal neovessels coincides with an increased entry of immunocompetent cells into the intimal matrix surrounding areas of neovascularization, thus suggesting that disorganized endothelial cell-to-cell interactions within neovessels may represent a significant event in atherogenesis [30].

Regulation of endothelial permeability

An altered rate of macromolecular diffusion or transport through endothelial junctions (paracellular transport) provides the major mechanism for increased endothelial permeability in response to selected inflammatory mediators such as thrombin or histamine [16]. These inflammatory substances can increase endothelial permeability within minutes by modulating the phosphorylation of proteins involved in the organization of endothelial junctions, followed by actin–myosin contraction, a centripetal retraction of EC, and increased formation of inter-endothelial gaps [16]. Thrombin alters the normal distribution of VE-cadherin, which disappears from areas of inter-EC pore formation and sequestration at the remaining sites of cell-to-cell contact, anchored to the cytoskeleton [31]. Signal transduction mechanisms involved in EC retraction and increased endothelial permeability can vary according to stimuli, and remain largely undetermined. Recent studies show that thrombin may increase intracellular calcium levels and, by the subsequent activation of protein kinase C (PKC), mediate the phosphorylation of junctional and actin-binding proteins [32,33]. Several important EC-derived factors can also modulate endothelial permeability. For example, the inhibition of basally produced endothelial nitric oxide (NO) increases permeability across vascular endothelium [34,35]. On the other hand, higher levels of NO induced by cytokines such as tumor necrosis factor alpha

(TNF-α) also seem to mediate increased permeability [36]. Finally, mildly oxidized low-density lipoproteins (LDL), but not native LDL, may act in early atherosclerosis to increase endothelial permeability through the formation of actin stress fibers and intercellular gaps [37].

Endothelial regulation of vascular tone

We now recognize that the endothelium secretes mediators that influence vascular hemodynamics (Table 1.2). Moreover, the endothelium contributes to the regulation of blood pressure and blood flow by releasing vasodilators such as NO and prostacyclin (PGI$_2$) as well as vasoconstrictors, including endothelin (ET) and platelet-activating factor (PAF). These chemically diverse compounds usually do not reside preformed in intracellular granules; rather, their major biologic effects depend on their rapid synthesis.

Nitric oxide

NO is the main vasorelaxing factor produced by EC. In the early 1980s, Furchgott and Zawadzki demonstrated experimentally a role of EC in the obligatory vascular relaxation in response to factors like acetylcholine, thus postulating the existence of an endothelium-derived vascular relaxing factor (EDRF) [8]. In 1987, two research groups independently demonstrated that the relaxing factor was NO, an odorless gas previously known as an atmospheric pollutant [38–40].

NO arises from the conversion of L-arginine to L-citrulline in the presence of nicotinamide adenine dinucleotide phosphate (NADPH) derived electrons, a reaction catalyzed by NO synthase (NOS), which exists as three isoforms [41]. NOS III, or endothelial NOS (eNOS), is a constitutive EC enzyme that continuously produces small amounts of NO. The high-capacity inducible form (type II) and the constitutive neuronal form (type I) comprise the two other forms of NOS. Exposure of macrophages, SMC, and EC to cytokines such as interleukin (IL)-1 and TNF-α can induce type II NOS, which produces large amounts of NO during inflammatory processes [41].

The three NOS isoforms share structural similarities and have nearly identical catalytic mechanisms

Table 1.2 Vasoregulatory substances synthesized by the endothelium.

Substance	Properties	Secretion/expression	Compound chemistry	Precursor compound
NO	Vasorelaxing agent; inhibits leukocyte adhesion, exerts antiplatelet properties, inhibits SMC migration and proliferation.	Constitutive and inducible expression. Production is increased by thrombin, ADP, shear stress, cyclic strain, and cytokines	Heterodiatomic free radical	L-arginine
PGI$_2$	Antiplatelet and vasorelaxing agent	Constitutive and inducible expression at sites of vascular perturbation by proinflammatory agents	Eicosanoid	AA
EDHF	Vasorelaxing agent	Induced by acetylcholine, bradykinin, and shear stress	5,6 EET or Potassium, or Myoendothelial gap junction, or ?	AA
ACE	Catalyzes the conversion of Ang I into Ang II, which causes vasoconstriction. Also catalyzes the degradation of bradykinin	Endothelial surface	Enzyme	Ang I
ET-1	Cause vasoconstriction and proliferation of SMC	Induced by hypoxia, shear stress, and ischemia	21-amino acid peptide	Preproendothelin-1 (203-amino acids)

NO: nitric oxide; PGI$_2$: prostacyclin; EDHF: endothelium-derived hyperpolarizing factor; ACE: angiotensin-converting enzyme; Ang I and II: angiotensin I and II; ET-1: endothelin-1; SMC: smooth muscle cells; ADP: adenosine diphosphate; EET: epoxyeicosatrienoic acid; AA: arachidonic acid.

[42]. They all require a number of cofactors and prosthetic groups for their activity, including flavin adenine dinucleotide (FAD), flavin mononucleotide (FMN), heme, calmodulin (CaM), and tetrahydro-biopterin (BH$_4$). The catalytic activity of NOS isoforms requires three distinct domains. The C-terminus requires a reductase domain, a CaM-binding domain, and an oxygenase domain. The reductase domain contains the FAD and FMN moieties, and also transfers electrons from the NADPH to the oxygenase domain. The oxygenase domain catalyzes the conversion of arginine into citrulline and NO, and contains the binding sites for heme, BH$_4$, and arginine. The obligatory CaM cofactor functions as a sensor of intracellular calcium concentrations, exerting its activity only in response to elevated levels of intracellular calcium.

In EC, eNOS localizes mainly in *caveolae*, small cholesterol-rich invaginations of the plasma membrane [43] that contain the transmembrane protein caveolin and a number of signaling molecules such as G-protein-coupled receptors (including the muscarinic and the bradykinin receptors) and protein kinases [44]. eNOS binds caveolin or CaM in a mutually exclusive manner. In the resting condition, the caveolin binding suppresses eNOS activity; during activation, increased cytosolic calcium promotes a reversible dissociation of eNOS from caveolin and induces CaM binding, which augments eNOS activity [44]. Although eNOS depends primarily on calcium and CaM, recent evidence indicates the possibility of calcium-independent activation of this enzyme. The response to shear stress involves this type of eNOS activation. Signal transduction processes that lead to calcium-independent activation of eNOS involve tyrosine phosphorylation and the activation of phospholipase C-γ [43,45].

Although originally considered constitutive, current evidence suggests that different stimuli regulate eNOS at several levels. The best-known physiologic activators of endothelial NO formation include physical stimuli, such as shear stress [46] and cyclic circumferential stretch [47]. Physical exercise, likely through such mechanisms, can stimulate NO production in human vascular beds [48], and also can induce eNOS gene expression in experimental animals [49]. Moreover, endothelial NO production rises in response to hormones such as estrogens [50,51], autacoids such as bradykinin [52] and histamine [53], and platelet-derived factors such as serotonin and adenosine diphosphate (ADP), as well as products of blood coagulation such as thrombin [54]. Moreover, transforming growth factor beta (TGF-β) [55] and high glucose concentrations [56] can enhance eNOS expression, and inflammatory cytokines such as TNF-α [57] and LDL [58] can limit eNOS activity.

NO has a half-life of $\approx$3–5 s [59]; when produced by EC, it can diffuse into the underlying tissues. By permeating the SMC plasma membrane, NO interacts with the iron atom of the heme prosthetic group of guanylate cyclase, causing its activation, which leads to increased cyclic guanosine monophosphate (cGMP) formation [60]. The ensuing prevention of calcium entry into SMC produces vascular relaxation [61]. Furthermore, EC release NO into the bloodstream where, before inactivation by oxyhemoglobin, NO can remain biologically active in close proximity to the endothelial surface, thus inhibiting leukocyte adhesion [11], augmenting fibrinolysis, and inhibiting platelet adhesion and activation synergistically with PGI$_2$ [62].

The loss of endothelium-dependent NO-mediated vasodilation occurs early during endothelial dysfunction [63]. Indeed, dysregulation of NO bioavailability (production or stabilization or disposal) accompanies numerous vascular diseases, including atherosclerosis [64]. NO bioavailability decreases in patients with established coronary artery disease [65,66]. Correspondingly, pharmacologic inhibition of NO synthesis in animal models of hypercholesterolemia accelerates atherosclerosis [67]; conversely, increased availability of NO decreases formation and may cause regression of atherosclerotic lesions [68–74]. However, although results of oral L-arginine supplementation in hypercholesterolemic animals have generally shown beneficial effects, the data in humans vary [75–78]. The inactivation of NO by reactive oxygen species can contribute to the development of endothelial dysfunction. Indeed, experimental studies show that antioxidants may re-establish NO-dependent

endothelial function [79,80]. Finally, an increase in endogenous inhibitors of NO synthesis may also participate in the genesis of endothelial dysfunction. For example, levels of asymmetric dimethylarginine, which may compete with L-arginine in the synthesis of NO, increase in young individuals with hypercholesterolemia; this increase associates with endothelium-dependent vasomotor dysfunction [81].

Prostacyclin, thromboxane, and other eicosanoids

The term "eicosanoids" encompasses prostaglandins (PGs), thromboxanes (TX), leukotrienes, and hydroxyl-eicosatetraenoic acids formed from polyunsaturated 20-carbon fatty acids, including the most abundant and the most biologically prominent precursor, arachidonic acid (AA). AA, a normal component of cell membrane phospholipids, becomes available for eicosanoid synthesis only after its release from phospholipids through the action of several phospholipases, principally phospholipase A$_2$. Released AA serves as a substrate for PG H synthases-1 and -2, also known as cyclooxygenases (COX)-1 and -2; lipoxygenases (5-, 12-, or 15-lipoxygenase); or cytochrome P450 enzymes [82]. Both COX-1 and -2 catalyze the conversion of AA to PGH$_2$. While most tissues express COX-1 constitutively, COX-2 expression rises markedly only upon cell activation, such as in inflammation [82]. The direct product of COX catalysis, PGH$_2$, has a half-life of $\approx$5 min in aqueous media, causes vasoconstriction, and undergoes further enzymatic conversion into several PGs, such as PGD$_2$, PGE$_2$, PGF$_2$-α or PGI$_2$, and TX, depending on the local tissue distribution of specific PG or TX synthases. Thus, the synthesis of specific PGs varies among tissues or cell types. For example, EC primarily contain PGI synthase (PGIS), which catalyzes PGH$_2$ conversion into PGI$_2$. Prostanoids signal through a series of seven-membrane spanning G-protein-coupled receptors. Through activation of the IP receptor present on SMC and platelets, PGI$_2$ causes vasodilation and inhibits platelet aggregation. Activation of adenylyl cyclase mediates most biologic effects of PGI$_2$, with the consequent increase in intracellular levels of cyclic adenosine monophosphate (cAMP) [83]. COX-1 and PGIS constitutive actions produce PGI$_2$ in resting EC [84]. However, although IL-1β stimulation of human umbilical vein EC leads to increased accumulation of PGI$_2$, PGD$_2$ and PGE$_2$ also arise largely via COX-2 through both PGH_2 non-enzymatic transformation [85] and, particularly for PGE_2, through the additive effect of an inducible PG E synthase (PGES) activity [86]. Additionally, EC can synthesize TX, a vasoconstrictor primarily produced by platelets, as recently proven by the cloning of an endothelial TX synthase [82,87]. An interesting interaction between platelets and EC can occur in this regard. EC stimulated by thrombin can restore TX production of aspirin-treated platelets by supplying them with PGH_2 in a juxtacrine manner [84,88], one of the many known examples of eicosanoid transcellular metabolism. Other potential COX products include a variety of compounds termed isoprostanes, e.g., 8-iso-$PGF_{2\alpha}$. The isoprostanes, a family of oxygenated arachidonate products, share structural similarities with eicosanoids. Under conditions of oxidative stress, the production of isoprostanes from arachidonate requires reactive oxygen species but not COX activity [89]. Conditions that induce increased generation or impaired disposal of free radicals, however, also involve parallel COX-2 expression and the production of 8-isoprostanes, a process inhibitable by indomethacin [89]. One interpretation for endothelial COX-2-dependent production of isoprostanes involves reactive oxygen species, produced by COX-2 activity (having an oxygenase and a peroxidase activity), that lead themselves to the production of isoprostanes. Therefore, COX-2 activity may also affect vascular function by enhancing oxidative stress within the cell.

Despite extensive study, the specific roles of vascular COX-1 vs COX-2 and their contribution to the pathophysiology of atherosclerosis remain undetermined. We have demonstrated the presence of COX-1 and -2 mRNA and protein in atherosclerotic plaques, macrophages, and SMC; COX-2 resides in the endothelium of atherosclerotic vessels [90]. Overexpression of functionally coupled COX-2, PGES, and some matrix metalloproteinases (MMP) occurs simultaneously in symptomatic atherosclerotic lesions. Since MMP may participate in the digestion of the fibrous cap, the functionally coupled overexpression of COX-2 and inducible PGES may contribute to a destabilization of the atherosclerotic plaque [91]. Additionally, COX-2, MMP-9, and membrane type 1 MMP colocalize in the EC lining of *vasa vasorum* in human atherosclerotic aortas [92]. Moreover, several lines of evidence now indicate a proangiogenic role of COX-2 activity [93], a process that might further contribute to plaque destabilization [94]. Therefore, COX-2 inhibition emerged as a potential therapy to mitigate complications of atherosclerosis. Clinical trials, however, have proven controversial [95], and overall suggest a detrimental effect [96–99] on cardiovascular outcomes in recipients of COX-2 inhibitors, in common with many other non-steroidal anti-inflammatory agents. One explanation involves reduced production of COX-2-derived PGI_2 [100]. Slight but sustained increases in blood pressure also may tend to worsen cardiovascular outcomes in individuals treated with COX-2 inhibitors and other non-steroidal anti-inflammatory agents. Fuller understanding of the specific roles of endothelial COX-1 and -2 in the modulation of vascular function and in the formation, progression, and destabilization of atherosclerosis requires further study.

Endothelium-derived hyperpolarizing factor

In the early 1980s, several lines of evidence began to indicate that the release of either NO or PGI_2 did not fully explain endothelium-dependent relaxation. Indeed, pharmacologic inhibition or genetic inactivation of NOS and inhibition of PGI_2 production do not greatly affect endothelium-dependent relaxation in response to either chemical (acetylcholine, bradykinin) or mechanical (shear stress) stimulations, especially in small resistance arteries. The observation that this process involves hyperpolarization of the target vascular SMC (and of the endothelium itself), causing relaxation without increased intracellular levels of cyclic nucleotides, led to the concept of an "endothelium-derived hyperpolarizing factor" (EDHF) [101,102]. EDHF would transduce its cellular effects by either directly or indirectly opening K^+ channels on vascular SMC, or through a hyperpolarization of EC, facilitating the electrical coupling between EC and vascular SMC [103].

The chemical identity of EDHF has received considerable attention, but thus far has yielded no consensus. Tissue and species heterogeneity implies the existence of multiple such factors. Four major candidates for EDHF exist. Substantial evidence supports the hypothesis that AA metabolites may share some EDHF properties. Epoxy-eicosatrienoic acids (EET), metabolites of AA through the P450 epoxygenase pathway, exert EDHF activity in at least some vascular beds upon stimulation of endothelial receptors. EET would be either synthesized or released from stored pools in the endothelium. Once released, EET would diffuse to the vascular SMC, where they would increase the probability of opening big conductance calcium-activated potassium channels (BK_{Ca}), and hyperpolarize vascular SMC [104]. Alternatively or additionally, another AA product, the endogenous cannabinoid anandamide, may act as EDHF: anandamide activates cannabinoid receptors in both EC and vascular SMC, and can hyperpolarize SMC [105]. A third hypothesis implicates potassium ions (K^+) as EDHF: stimulated endothelial receptors activate small and intermediate conductance calcium-activated potassium channels (SK_{Ca} and IK_{Ca}) and increase the probability that they will open in EC, leading to the efflux of K^+ from EC and increased levels of extracellular K^+. Moderately increased concentrations of endothelial K^+, such as that occurring upon stimulation of EC in the rat hepatic artery, can induce hyperpolarization and relaxation of vascular SMC by activating the inward rectifying K^+ channels (K_{IR}) and the Na^+-K^+-ATPase between EC and SMC gap junctions [103], which provide a low-resistance electrical pathway between these two cell layers [106]. The number of these "heterocellular" gap junctions increases as artery diameter decreases, paralleling the predominance of EDHF relevance in microvessels. Cell activation by an agonist facilitates myoendothelial gap junctional communication. Thus, gap junctions would transmit EC stimulation and subsequent hyperpolarization to the underlying vascular SMC. If cations (or a current) move through the gap junction to hyperpolarize vascular SMC, "EDHF" does not involve a factor *per se* but rather a process of current movement between cells. Although gap junctions also would allow movement of low molecular weight water-soluble molecules such as cAMP or cGMP from the endothelium to vascular SMC, thus accounting for EDHF properties, it is more likely that no "factor" transfer participates in the dynamic regulation of gap junctional communication. Other mechanisms remain unsubstantiated or await fuller scrutiny. However, several mechanisms for EDHF likely operate simultaneously or sequentially and act additively or synergistically in a given site of the circulation. The relative proportions of each mechanism likely depend on numerous variables including the activation state of the vascular smooth muscle, the density of myoendothelial gap junctions, expression level of cytochrome P450, and the appropriate isoforms of Na^+-K^+-ATPase and/or K_{IR} channels.

Pulsatile stretch [107] or receptor-dependent calcium-elevating agents result in EDHF release [104]. Biologic effects of EDHF decrease in vascular abnormalities, including those associated with aging and hypercholesterolemia [108]. Therefore, decreased EDHF may account, at least in part, for the alterations of vascular responses that occur in atherosclerosis [109].

Endothelins

In sharp contrast with the less well-defined substances described above, ET are well-characterized and potent vasoconstrictors [110]. ET, 21-amino acid peptides closely related to the snake venom safaratoxin, arise from different tissues as three different isoforms: ET-1, -2 and -3. ET-1, first discovered in 1988, was isolated from the conditioned medium of porcine aortic EC [111]. EC can only synthesize ET-1, a 203-amino acid precursor named preproendothelin, which cleaves to big ET (39-amino acids) and then, in a reaction catalyzed by an ET-converting enzyme (ECE), further converts to the 21-amino acid active peptide [112]. ECE exists as several different isoforms, e.g., ECE-1a, -1b, and -2. EC only appear to express the ECE-1a isoform [113,114].

EC release 75% of their ET abluminally, toward SMC; the remainder enters the vessel lumen, so that the plasma of normal healthy subjects has low levels of ET-1. ET-1 exerts its biologic effects by stimulating specific G-protein-coupled receptors, termed A (ET_A) and B (ET_B) receptors. SMC express ET_A and, at lower levels, ET_B receptors. Stimulation of SMC ET receptors induces vasoconstriction by two different mechanisms: increased intracellular calcium influx and activation of phospholipase C and A_2 [115]. EC also have ET_B receptors, whose stimulation promotes the formation of NO and PGI_2, a reaction that could serve as a feedback mechanism to restore normal vascular tone. Increased production and/or activity of ET may participate in several pathologic states related to a dysfunctional endothelium, such as pulmonary and systemic hypertension, heart failure, and atherosclerosis [116,117]. Factors implicated in atherogenesis, e.g., inflammatory cytokines [118,119] and oxidized LDL [120–123], also induce ET-1 production by EC. Jones et al. observed increased expression of ET-1 in human atherosclerotic vessels at sites directly overlying atherosclerotic plaques [124]. The pathologic role of ET-1 in the development of atherosclerosis may involve not only local perturbation of blood flow but also mitogenic effects on SMC [115], stimulation of adhesion molecule expression [125], and leukocyte chemoattraction [126]. In early atherosclerosis or even in the presence of the sole risk factors, abnormal vasoconstriction arises in part from enhanced local production of ET [127].

The endothelial renin–angiotensin system

The renin–angiotensin–aldosterone system contributes to the regulation of electrolyte balance, fluid volume, and blood pressure by angiotensin II (Ang II) and, subsequently, aldosterone production. The elements of this system comprise a cascade of enzymatic reaction in which a first enzyme, renin, converts angiotensinogen to angiotensin I (Ang I), and a second enzyme termed ACE further cleaves Ang I into Ang II [128]. Ang II, a potent vasoconstrictor, increases blood pressure and stimulates aldosterone secretion, in turn promoting sodium retention. ACE arises in large part from EC [129]. In normal vessels, ACE localizes on the surface of EC, where it is easily available for the cleavage of plasma Ang I [129]. In addition to converting Ang I to Ang II, ACE degrades and inactivates bradykinin, a potent indirect vasodilator, by inducing endothelial NO, EDHF, and PGI_2.

Specific receptors termed angiotensin II receptor type 1 (with subclasses AT_{1A} and AT_{1B}) and angiotensin II receptor type 2 mediate the biologic effects of Ang II. AT_1 stimulation on SMC mediates the main physiologic effects of Ang II, vasoconstriction, and SMC proliferation [130]. However, EC contain AT_1 and, in smaller amounts, AT_2 [131]. Recent experimental evidence suggests an important role of Ang II in the development of atherosclerosis, through direct action on the endothelium. Ang II exerts proinflammatory effects on vascular endothelium by inducing the most important inflammatory genes implicated in the inception of atherosclerotic lesion, i.e., intercellular adhesion molecule (ICAM)-1 and vascular cell adhesion molecule (VCAM)-1 (see below). The stimulation of AT_1 receptors appears to mediate

this effect, since AT_1 receptor blockers prevent the inflammatory effect of angiotensin [132,133].

The endothelial control of hemostasis

The endothelium plays a key role in the control of hemostasis, exerting effects on platelets, the coagulation system, and fibrinolysis. In normal physiologic conditions, the endothelium displays antiplatelet, anticoagulant, and fibrinolytic properties, but dysfunctional EC promote a prothrombotic, antifibrinolytic state.

Control of platelet function

Normally, circulating platelets do not interact with the EC surface, due in part to the release of NO and PGI_2, and in part to catabolism of the proaggregatory mediator ADP that results from the constitutive expression of an ecto-ADPase (CD39). Endothelium-derived NO exerts a strong vasorelaxing action and also potently inhibits platelet adhesion, activation, secretion, and aggregation through a cyclic guanosine monophosphate (cGMP)-dependent mechanism [134].

Similarly, endothelial PGI_2 contributes to endothelial vasorelaxing properties even more efficiently than NO, and inhibits platelet aggregation through the activation of the IP receptor present on platelets [135]. NO also inhibits P-selectin expression on the platelet surface and, by inhibiting agonist-dependent increase in intraplatelet calcium [136], suppresses the calcium-sensitive conformational change in the heterodimeric integrin glycoprotein(GP) IIb–IIIa required for fibrinogen binding [137]. Additionally, NO appears to promote platelet disaggregation indirectly by impairing the activity of phosphoinositide 3-kinase, which normally supports conformational changes in GP IIb–IIIa, rendering its association with fibrinogen irreversible [138].

Another long-recognized antiplatelet property of normal EC involves ecto-ADPase/CD39, a membrane-associated ectonucleotidase. Released by platelets and other cells, ADP strongly activates platelets by interacting with the platelet $P2Y_{12}$ receptor [139,140]. The constitutive expression of ecto-ADPase, an adenosine triphosphate (ATP)-diphosphohydrolase, by EC allows efficient metabolism of this platelet agonist to AMP, thus maintaining platelets in their resting state [141].

Anticoagulant properties

Hemostatic clots form due to the polymerization of fibrinogen into fibrin, a conversion catalyzed by thrombin, a serine protease that cleaves fibrinogen, activates several other coagulation enzymes and cofactors and, in conjunction, activates platelets and EC [142]. Therefore, it is not surprising that several highly regulated pathways have evolved to constrain the generation and activity of thrombin [143]. The endothelium employs at least three anticoagulant strategies, i.e., heparin–antithrombin; tissue factor (TF) pathway inhibitor (TFPI); and thrombomodulin–protein C anticoagulant.

The matrix surrounding the endothelium contains cell surface heparan sulfate and related glycosaminoglycans that promote antithrombin III (AT-III) activity [144,145]. This complex inactivates thrombin and factors Xa, IXa, and XIa. The expression of heparan sulfate and proteoglycans likely responds to inflammatory conditions, as indicated by suppression during sepsis [146,147]. The endothelium also prevents thrombin formation by expressing TFPI, which binds to factor Xa within the TF/FVIIa/FXa complex [148]. TFPI and AT-III both contribute to physiologic hemostasis, and both show impairment in acquired thrombotic states [149,150].

Of these three anticoagulant systems, the thrombomodulin–protein C system has the greatest complexity. EC synthesize thrombomodulin present on the endothelial luminal surface of most vessels, in capillaries, arteries, veins, and lymphatics. Human umbilical vein EC contain 40,000–50,000 thrombomodulin molecules per cell [151]. Thrombin bound to thrombomodulin loses its procoagulant activity, and the complex instead becomes a potent activator of protein C, an anticoagulant protein synthesized by the liver [152], which circulates in plasma at a concentration of $\approx 4\,\mu g/mL$ [153]. The activation rate of protein C increases when it binds to the endothelial protein C receptor (EPCR), a specific receptor on EC [154]. Once activated (activated protein C, APC), protein C retains its binding affinity for EPCR, but appears to lose anticoagulant activity [155]. Indeed, APC reversibly binds to EPCR ($K_d \approx 30\,nM$); when APC dissociates from EPCR, it binds to protein S, a molecule synthesized both in the liver and EC [156]. This complex proteolytically inactivates factors Va and VIIIa [157]. Inflammatory cytokines such as TNF-α or IL-1β can reduce thrombomodulin expression.

Indeed, TNF-α both inhibits transcription of thrombomodulin mRNA and augments the lysosomal degradation of the mature protein [158]. Recent data showing a lower degree of expression in patients with unstable angina also suggests a role for regulation of the anticoagulant protein S in vascular disease [159].

Procoagulant properties

The pivotal step in transforming the inner vessel surface from an anticoagulant to a procoagulant surface involves the induction of TF, a 263-amino acid residue membrane-bound GP comprised of a 219-amino acid residue extracellular domain, a single transmembrane sequence, and a short cytoplasmic domain [160]. TF dramatically accelerates factor VIIa-dependent activation of factors X and IX. Therefore, it is not surprising that the unperturbed endothelium in physiologic conditions does not express TF, at least in the adult [161]. TF participates importantly in various pathologic states, including atherosclerosis. TF accumulates in experimentally injured vessels and in atherosclerotic plaques [162]. The accumulation of TF likely accounts for the high thrombogenicity of some plaques [163]. Diverse agonists including thrombin, endotoxin [164], several cytokines such as IL-1α and β [165] and TNF-α [166], shear stress [167], and oxidized lipoproteins [168] induce endothelial synthesis of TF *in vitro*. The ligation of CD40, the expression of which rises after exposure to interferon-γ, by CD40 ligand (CD154) on T-cells or activated platelets also increases TF expression [169,170]. TF mRNA and protein levels decline despite continued exposure to agonists, a mechanism that may help to limit the extent of fibrin formation. Cells in culture also shed microvesicles containing TF, which may propagate the activation of thrombosis distal to the initial site of TF exposure [171]. Patients with disseminated intravascular coagulation have elevated plasma levels of TF [172].

EC also express several receptors for fibrin and specific fibrin degradation products, including a 130-kDa GP [173], a tissue transglutaminase [174], and the integrin $\alpha_v\beta_3$ (vitronectin receptor) [175]. The endothelial expression of this receptor is important, since the binding of fibrin promotes endothelial adhesion, spreading, proliferation, migration, retraction, and leukocyte adhesion and also inhibits PGI$_2$ synthesis [107].

Control of fibrinolysis

Fibrinolysis depends primarily on the action of plasmin, an active protease formed from its precursor, plasminogen, upon stimulation by tissue-type plasminogen activator (tPA). The contribution of EC to fibrinolysis varies with their metabolic status, i.e., quiescent vs activated, their site in the vasculature, and the concentration of other hemostatically active molecules in the local plasma milieu. Although several studies with EC cultured from various tissues originally indicated that all EC can produce and secrete tPA [176], more recent studies using *in situ* hybridization and immunohistochemistry have demonstrated tPA antigen and mRNA only in a distinct subset of quiescent microvascular EC of both primates and mice [177]. Hence, contrary to assumptions based on work with cultured EC, tPA production *in vivo* likely associates only with a distinct subpopulation of EC in the microvasculature. The urokinase-type plasminogen activator (uPA) appears absent in quiescent endothelium [178]. Consistent with the hypothesized importance of uPA in cell migration and tissue remodeling, EC involved in wound repair or angiogenesis express uPA as a fibrin-specific precursor termed prourokinase [179]. However, uPA has obvious importance for vascular homeostasis, since mice genetically deficient in uPA develop thrombosis and show thrombotic tissue injury in response to lipopolysaccharide (LPS) [180].

The endothelium also can produce large amounts of plasminogen activator inhibitor (PAI)-1 [181]. Experiments in mice have identified the liver at the major source of plasma PAI-1, and shown that quiescent EC express little or no PAI-1 [182]. However, the endothelium overexpresses this inhibitor of fibrinolysis in virtually all tissues after exposure to inflammatory stimuli [182].

With regard to the endothelial regulation of fibrinolysis, it is also important to consider the dual role exhibited by thrombomodulin. Binding of thrombin to thrombomodulin accelerates its capacity to activate a protein known as thrombin-activatable fibrinolysis inhibitor (TAFI) [183]. TAFI is a procarboxypeptidase-B-like molecule that, when activated, cleaves basic carboxyterminal residues within fibrin and other proteins, resulting in the loss of plasminogen/plasmin and tPA binding sites on fibrin and thus retarded fibrinolysis [183]. In this manner, through the regulated expression of thrombomodulin, EC could decrease the rate of intravascular fibrinolysis.

Control of leukocyte traffic during inflammatory reactions (see also Chapter 2)

The development of inflammatory reactions by the vascular endothelium participates integrally in normal host defense mechanisms initiated by injury or infection. Physiologically, such reactions maintain and/or repair normal structure and function of the vessel wall and of the entire organism, defending it from external insults or foreign agents. Mice lacking the selectin family of adhesion molecules suffer recurrent infections [184]. On the other hand, the initiation of abundant inflammatory reactions can lead to severe tissue damage, possibly including the development of atherosclerosis [185].

The interaction between EC and leukocytes depends on the expression of adhesion molecules and production of inflammatory cytokines, both critical factors in initiating and sustaining inflammatory processes. Among different chemokines, IL-8 [186] and monocyte chemoattractant protein-1 (MCP-1) [187] likely play key roles in the recruitment of polymorphonuclear leukocytes, lymphocytes, and monocytes into the vessel wall. Among several other cell types, EC produce IL-8 and MCP-1 through mechanisms mediated by nuclear factor kappa (NF-κB) [187,188].

During inflammation, loosely tethered leukocytes first roll over the EC surface, then arrest and spread, and finally emigrate between EC to reach the underlying tissues. The interaction between EC and leukocytes initially involves a relatively loose adhesion of leukocytes to EC, so that leukocytes "roll" over the endothelium [189]. Firmer adhesion and transmigration of leukocytes across EC follow this process. Leukocyte rolling involves molecules belonging to the selectin family of adhesion molecules, e.g., P-, E-, and L-selectin, typically characterized by an amino-terminal Ca^{2+}-dependent lectin domain, an epidermal growth factor (EGF) domain, a series of short consensus repeats, a transmembrane domain, and a cytoplasmic tail [190,191]. While E-selectin expression occurs only on activated EC, L-selectin expresses on most leukocytes and binds to ligands constitutively expressed on high endothelial venules of lymphoid tissues; ligands induced on the endothelium at sites of inflammation; and ligands exposed on other leukocytes. P-selectin rapidly redistributes from secretory granules to the surface of platelets and EC stimulated with thrombin or histamine. In general, selectins bind to sialylated and fucosylated oligosaccharides that attach to proteins and lipids on most leukocytes and some EC. In particular, E-selectin preferentially binds to the GP E-selectin ligand (ESL)-1 [192,193]. L- and P-selectin bind preferentially to sialomucins. Involvement of individual types of selectins in the initial leukocyte rolling depends primarily on the type of stimuli. For example, immediate stimulation of leukocyte rolling induced by histamine or thrombin depends primarily on P-selectin stored in Weibel–Palade bodies [194]. EC activation can induce a rapid translocation and fusion of these organelles with plasma membranes and, therefore, the swift appearance, within minutes, of P-selectin on the EC surface. However, activated EC express P-selectin only temporarily; 30 min following the initial stimulus, surface levels of this adhesion molecule already wane [195]. In contrast to histamine or thrombin, TNF or IL-1 can stimulate delayed leukocyte rolling and adhesion to EC primarily through the induction of E-selectin. In contrast to P-selectin, EC do not store preformed E-selectin. Following stimulation with TNF or IL-1, the expression of E-selectin typically rises after ≈4 h, peaks at ≈12 h, and declines after 24 h [189]. Studies demonstrating the presence of both E- and P-selectin on the surface of EC overlying atherosclerotic plaques affirm the importance of the selectin family of adhesion molecules in the development of atherosclerosis [196]. Moreover, the absence of P-selectin delays fatty streak formation in mice predisposed to the development of atherosclerosis [197].

Firmer adhesion of leukocytes to the vascular endothelium involves adhesion molecules of the immunoglobulin superfamily, i.e., ICAM-1, -2, -3, VCAM-1, and PECAM-1 [198]. ICAM 1, 2 and -3 are closely related, and bind to the same leukocyte integrin receptors, i.e., CD11/CD18 [199]. Unstimulated, resting EC constitutively express low levels of ICAM-1, but exposure of EC to stimuli such as IL-1, TNF and interferon-γ [200] markedly

increases ICAM-1 expression. After stimulation, ICAM-1 peaks at 6 h, and its levels remain sustained for at least 72 h [201]. ICAM-1 expression depends predominantly on transcriptional regulation. The ICAM-1 promoter region contains several enhancer sequences. Although several other transcription factors such as specificity protein (SP)1; activator protein (AP)-1, retinoic acid responsive element (RARE), and CCAAT/enhancer binding protein (C/EBP) participate in the activation of the ICAM-1 gene, particularly in EC, NF-κB likely is the most important regulatory element [202].

VCAM-1 principally mediates the adhesion of monocytes, lymphocyte, eosinophils, and basophils, but not neutrophils, to the surface of the vascular endothelium [203,204]. The best-known inducers of VCAM-1 include cytokines such as TNF-α, IL-1 [205,206], modified LDL [207], and advanced glycation end products (AGEs) [208,209]. Similar to ICAM-1 and E-selectin, the transcriptional regulation of VCAM-1 also requires NF-κB and AP-1 [210]. Recent findings in genetically engineered mice that express a form of VCAM-1 with reduced function have established the causal role of VCAM-1 in early atherogenesis [211].

The final phase of leukocyte emigration through the endothelium involves PECAM-1, another member of the immunoglobulin superfamily. PECAM-1, which likely participates in the regulation of endothelial permeability and leukocyte adhesion [18], localizes preferentially in the intercellular junctions of EC, where it forms homodimers linking two EC. Additionally, the leukocyte surface contains PECAM-1. The dissociation of homotypic PECAM-1 dimers between EC to form heterotypic dimers between emigrating leukocytes and EC appears critical for leukocyte diapedesis [212], through a mechanism that apparently involves a reactive oxygen species-induced phosphorylation of this adhesion molecule [213]. However, the role of PECAM-1 in the stimulation of leukocyte adhesion and migration during atherogenesis remains uncertain, since levels of PECAM 1 expression do not occur in human atherosclerotic coronary arteries [214] or atheromata in ApoE$^{-/-}$ mice [215]. Figure 1.4 provides a summary of endothelial functions and illustrates how the loss of homeostatic balance leads to the development of the atherosclerotic plaque.

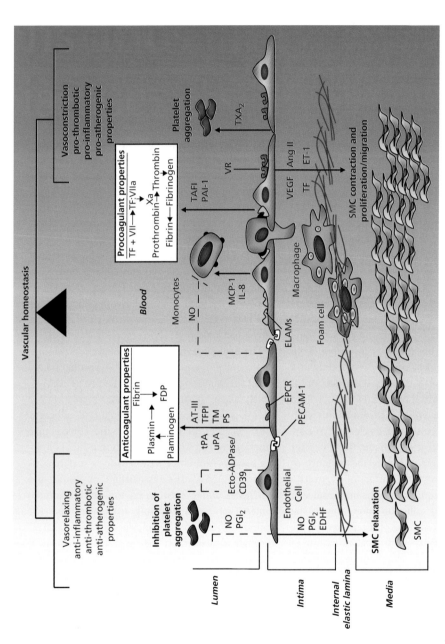

Figure 1.4 Molecular and cellular mediators of the antithrombotic and antiatherogenic properties of the endothelium. The normally functioning endothelium (left and white) produces several vasodilatory substances, e.g., prostacyclin (PGI$_2$), nitric oxide (NO), and endothelium-derived hyperpolarizing factor (EDHF), that maintain normal vascular tone, counteract platelet aggregation, exert anticoagulant properties that control fibrin production (thrombomodulin (TM), endothelial cell protein C receptor (EPCR), protein S (PS), tissue factor pathway inhibitor (TFPI)), inhibit tissue factor (TF) activity, and enhance fibrinolysis (tissue- and urokinase-type plasminogen activators (tPA, uPA)).

A dysfunctional endothelium (right and red) favors atherothrombosis, enhancing the production of pro-coagulants such as TF, anti-fibrinolytic factors such as plasminogen activator inhibitor (PAI)-1, and vasoconstrictors such as endothelin (ET)-1 and angiotensin (Ang)-II) and promoting leukocyte adhesion and migration through the production of endothelial-leukocyte adhesion molecules (ELAMs) and chemoattractants such as monocyte chemotactic protein (MCP-1) and interleukin (IL)-8, thus overall favoring inflammation, plaque formation, and growth as well as vasoconstriction and thrombosis. → induces; ─── inhibits; FDP: = fibrin-degrading products; TXA$_2$ = thromboxane A$_2$; VEGF = vascular endothelial growth factor; TAFI = thrombin-activatable fibrinolysis inhibitor; AT-III = antithrombin-III; VR: = vitronectin receptor.

Role of transcriptional factor NF-κB in endothelial dysfunction

The activation of NF-κB likely plays a key role in the development of endothelial dysfunction [216]. NF-κB comprises a family of transcription factors originally identified in B cells, expressed ubiquitously and highly phylogenetically conserved. Family members include Re1A (p65), Re1B, c-Re1, NF-κB1 (p50), NF-κB2 (p52), and their inhibitory subunits IκBα, IκBβ , and IκBε. NF-κB subunits form homo- and heterodimers, the most prominent being the p65/p50 heterodimer, and bind to the decameric consensus sequence GGG*RNNT*YCC (R = G or A, Y = C or T, N = nucleotide), thus inducing the expression of target genes. Interaction with IκB to form a heterotrimer retains NF-κB in the cytoplasm in an inactive state under basal conditions. NF-κB activates rapidly in response to a variety of stimuli that always lead to IκB degradation. Important stimuli include TNF-α, IL-1, bacterial LPS, hyperglycemia, PAF, shear stress, oxidized lipids, oxidant stress, and hypoxia/reperfusion [217]. NF-κB exhibits very rapid and transient activation, making it well suited for the expression of many immune- and "stress"-response genes that require action on demand for only a limited period of time. Independent of the type of stimuli, co-treatment with antioxidants or metal chelators can inhibit NF-κB activation. Therefore, changes in the cellular redox balance may alter NF-κB activation [210,218,219].

The promoter regions of most transcriptionally regulated genes expressed in EC in response to inflammatory mediators such as LPS, IL-1, or TNF-α contain functional NF-κB binding sites. Genes regulated by NF-κB include VCAM-1, E-selectin, IL-1, -6, -8, TF, PAI-1, COX-2, and iNOS, all strategically involved in endothelial activation and dysfunction. In addition, atherosclerotic lesions contain activated NF-κB [220,221]. Interestingly, the expression of inflammatory cytokines depends on activated NF-κB and, in turn, these cytokines can stimulate its activation. Thus, inflammatory cytokines may use NF-κB to amplify their own signals [216]. On the other hand, inhibition of basal endothelial NO production can activate NF-κB and augment the expression of NF-κB-regulated genes, i.e., genes encoding for VCAM-1 and ICAM-1 [11,222], and treating EC with NO donors decreases TNF-induced NF-κB activation and attenuates cytokine-induced expression of VCAM-1 and ICAM-1 [11].

General conclusions

We can no longer view the endothelium as a static physical barrier that simply separates blood from tissue. Healthy EC are vital for the correct maintenance of vascular homeostasis. By secretion or surface expression of a series of specific molecules, EC ensure appropriately regulated blood flow under normal conditions, and avoid intravascular activation of platelets and coagulation. In response to pathophysiologic mediators, EC properties modulate dynamically to support vessel growth or repair and guide the resolution of inflammatory or infectious processes. In most instances, this transient alteration of EC phenotype contributes to the successful restoration of vascular homeostasis. Certain disease states such as atherosclerosis, however, may involve a chronically perturbed EC behavior critical for disease progression. Increased understanding of EC biology has defined many endothelial functions at the molecular level and several mechanisms that cause acute and chronic changes in EC functions. Efforts to understand the physiologic features of the endothelium and mechanisms underlying long-term changes in endothelial properties as well as strategies to alleviate endothelial dysfunction provide a promising pathway for the treatment of diseases characterized by altered endothelial functions.

References

1 Fishman AP. Endothelium: a distributed organ of diverse capabilities. *Ann NY Acad Sci* 1982;401:1–8.
2 Toffoletto E. *Discorso su Malpighi*. Bologna: Migrizia; 1965.
3 von Rocklinghausen F. Eine method, mikroskopische hohle und solide gebilde voneinander zu unterscheiden. *Virckow Arch* 1860;19:451.
4 Majno G. Maude Abbott lecture – 1991. The capillary then and now: an overview of capillary pathology. *Mod Pathol* 1992;5:9–22.
5 Palade G. Fine structure of blood capillaries. *J Appl Physiol* 1953;24:1424–1428.
6 Gowans J. The recirculation of lymphocytes from blood to lymph in the rat. *J Physiol* 1959;146:54–69.

7 Cines DB, Pollak ES, Buck CA, et al. Endothelial cells in physiology and in the pathophysiology of vascular disorders. *Blood* 1998;91:3527–3561.

8 Furchgott RF, Zawadzki JV. The obligatory role of endothelial cells in the relaxation of arterial smooth muscle by acetylcholine. *Nature* 1980;288:373–376.

9 Gimbrone MA, Kume N, Cybulsky MI. Vascular endothelium dysfunction and the pathogenesis of atherosclerosis. In: Weber PC, Leaf A, eds. *Atherosclerosis Reviews.* New York: Reaven Press; 1993.

10 Gimbrone MA. Vascular endothelium in health and disease. In: Haber E, ed. *Molecular Cardiovascular Medicine.* New York: Scientific American Medicine; 1995:67B–70B.

11 De Caterina R, Libby P, Peng HB, et al. Nitric oxide decreases cytokine-induced endothelial activation. *J Clin Invest* 1995;96:60–68.

12 Augustin HG, Kozian DH, Johnson RC. Differentiation of endothelial cells: analysis of the constitutive and activated endothelial cell phenotypes. *Bioessays* 1994;16:901–906.

13 Dejana E, Corada M, Lampugnani MG. Endothelial cell-to-cell junctions. *Faseb J* 1995;9:910–918.

14 Risau W, Flamme I. Vasculogenesis. *Ann Rev Cell Dev Biol* 1995;11:73–91.

15 Lampugnani MG, Dejana E. Interendothelial junctions: structure, signalling and functional roles. *Curr Opin Cell Biol* 1997;9:674–682.

16 Lum H, Malik AB. Mechanisms of increased endothelial permeability. *Can J Physiol Pharmacol* 1996;74:787–800.

17 Firth J. Endothelial barriers: from hypothetical pores to membrane proteins. *J Anat* 2002;200:541–548.

18 Dejana E, Valiron O, Navarro P, et al. Intercellular junctions in the endothelium and the control of vascular permeability. *Ann NY Acad Sci* 1997;811:36–43; discussion 43–34.

19 Dejana E, Lampugnani MG, Martinez-Estrada O, et al. The molecular organization of endothelial junctions and their functional role in vascular morphogenesis and permeability. *Int J Dev Biol* 2000;44:743–748.

20 Okano M, Yoshida Y. Influence of shear stress on endothelial cell shapes and junction complexes at flow dividers of aortic bifurcations in cholesterol-fed rabbits. *Front Med Biol Eng* 1993;5:95–120.

21 Yoshida Y, Okano M, Wang S, et al. Hemodynamic-force-induced difference of interendothelial junctional complexes. *Ann NY Acad Sci* 1995;748:104–120; discussion 120–101.

22 Okano M, Yoshida Y. Junction complexes of endothelial cells in atherosclerosis-prone and atherosclerosis-resistant regions on flow dividers of brachiocephalic bifurcations in the rabbit aorta. *Biorheology* 1994;31:155–161.

23 Kumar N, Gilula N. The gap junction communication channel. *Cell* 1996;84:381–388.

24 White T, Paul D. Genetic diseases and gene knockouts reveal diverse connexin functions. *Annu Rev Physiol* 1999;61:283–310.

25 Kwak B, Mulhaupt F, Veillard N, et al. Altered pattern of vascular connexin expression in atherosclerotic plaques. *Arterioscler Thromb Vasc Biol* 2002;22:225–230.

26 Inoguchi T, Yu HY, Imamura M, et al. Altered gap junction activity in cardiovascular tissues of diabetes. *Med Electron Microsc* 2001;34:86–91.

27 Dejana E, Spagnuolo R, Bazzoni G. Interendothelial junctions and their role in the control of angiogenesis, vascular permeability and leukocyte transmigration. *Thromb Haemost* 2001;86:308–315.

28 Petzelbauer P, Halama T, Groger M. Endothelial adherens junctions. *J Investig Dermatol Symp Proc* 2000;5:10–13.

29 Blaschuk OW, Rowlands TM. Cadherins as modulators of angiogenesis and the structural integrity of blood vessels. *Cancer Metastasis Rev* 2000;19:1–5.

30 Bobryshev YV, Cherian SM, Inder SJ, et al. Neovascular expression of VE-cadherin in human atherosclerotic arteries and its relation to intimal inflammation. *Cardiovasc Res* 1999;43:1003–1017.

31 Lim MJ, Chiang ET, Hechtman HB, et al. Inflammation-induced subcellular redistribution of VE-cadherin, actin, and gamma-catenin in cultured human lung microvessel endothelial cells. *Microvasc Res* 2001;62:366–382.

32 Vuong PT, Malik AB, Nagpala PG, et al. Protein kinase C beta modulates thrombin-induced Ca^{2+} signaling and endothelial permeability increase. *J Cell Physiol* 1998;175:379–387.

33 Lum H, Podolski JL, Gurnack ME, et al. Protein phosphatase 2b inhibitor potentiates endothelial PKC activity and barrier dysfunction. *Am J Physiol Lung Cell Mol Physiol* 2001;281:L546–L555.

34 He P, Liu B, Curry FE. Effect of nitric oxide synthase inhibitors on endothelial $[Ca^{2+}]i$ and microvessel permeability. *Am J Physiol* 1997;272:H176–H185.

35 Baldwin AL, Thurston G. Mechanics of endothelial cell architecture and vascular permeability. *Crit Rev Biomed Eng* 2001;29:247–278.

36 Bove K, Neumann P, Gertzberg N, et al. Role of ECNOS-derived NO in mediating TNF-induced endothelial barrier dysfunction. *Am J Physiol Lung Cell Mol Physiol* 2001;280:L914–L922.

37 Essler M, Retzer M, Bauer M, et al. Mildly oxidized low density lipoprotein induces contraction of human endothelial cells through activation of rho/rho kinase and inhibition of myosin light chain phosphatase. *J Biol Chem* 1999;274:30361–30364.

38 Ignarro LJ, Byrns RE, Buga GM, et al. Endothelium-derived relaxing factor from pulmonary artery and vein possesses pharmacologic and chemical properties identical to those of nitric oxide radical. *Circ Res* 1987;61:866–879.

39 Palmer RM, Ferrige AG, Moncada S. Nitric oxide release accounts for the biological activity of endothelium-derived relaxing factor. *Nature* 1987;327:524–526.

40 Palmer RM, Ashton DS, Moncada S. Vascular endothelial cells synthesize nitric oxide from L-arginine. *Nature* 1988;333:664–666.

41 Stamler JS, Singel DJ, Loscalzo J. Biochemistry of nitric oxide and its redox-activated forms. *Science* 1992;258:1898–1902.

42 Marletta MA. Nitric oxide synthase: aspects concerning structure and catalysis. *Cell* 1994;78:927–930.

43 Fleming I, Busse R. Signal transduction of ENOS activation. *Cardiovasc Res* 1999;43:532–541.

44 Michel T, Feron O. Nitric oxide synthases: which, where, how, and why? *J Clin Invest* 1997;100:2146–2152.

45 Fleming I, Busse R. Molecular mechanisms involved in the regulation of the endothelial nitric oxide synthase. *Am J Physiol Regul Integr Comp Physiol* 2003;284:R1–R12.

46 Boo YC, Hwang J, Sykes M, et al. Shear stress stimulates phosphorylation of ENOS at ser(635) by a protein kinase A-dependent mechanism. *Am J Physiol Heart Circ Physiol* 2002;283:H1819–H1828.

47 Ziegler T, Silacci P, Harrison VJ, et al. Nitric oxide synthase expression in endothelial cells exposed to mechanical forces. *Hypertension* 1998;32:351–355.

48 Hambrecht R, Adams V, Erbs S, et al. Regular physical activity improves endothelial function in patients with coronary artery disease by increasing phosphorylation of endothelial nitric oxide synthase. *Circulation* 2003;16:16.

49 Tanabe T, Maeda S, Miyauchi T, et al. Exercise training improves ageing-induced decrease in ENOS expression of the aorta. *Acta Physiol Scand* 2003;178:3–10.

50 Chambliss KL, Shaul PW. Estrogen modulation of endothelial nitric oxide synthase. *Endocr Rev* 2002;23:665–686.

51 Prorock AJ, Hafezi-Moghadam A, Laubach VE, et al. Vascular protection by estrogen in ischemia–reperfusion injury requires endothelial nitric oxide synthase. *Am J Physiol Heart Circ Physiol* 2003;284:H133–H140.

52 Bae SW, Kim HS, Cha YN, et al. Rapid increase in endothelial nitric oxide production by bradykinin is mediated by protein kinase A signaling pathway. *Biochem Biophys Res Commun* 2003;306:981–987.

53 Li H, Burkhardt C, Heinrich UR, et al. Histamine upregulates gene expression of endothelial nitric oxide synthase in human vascular endothelial cells. *Circulation* 2003;107:2348–2354.

54 Arnal JF, Dinh-Xuan AT, Pueyo M, et al. Endothelium-derived nitric oxide and vascular physiology and pathology. *Cell Mol Life Sci* 1999;55:1078–1087.

55 Inoue N, Venema RC, Sayegh HS, et al. Molecular regulation of the bovine endothelial cell nitric oxide synthase by transforming growth factor-beta 1. *Arterioscler Thromb Vasc Biol* 1995;15:1255–1261.

56 Cosentino F, Hishikawa K, Katusic ZS, et al. High glucose increases nitric oxide synthase expression and superoxide anion generation in human aortic endothelial cells. *Circulation* 1997;96:25–28.

57 Yoshizumi M, Perrella MA, Burnett Jr JC, et al. Tumor necrosis factor downregulates an endothelial nitric oxide synthase mRNA by shortening its half-life. *Circ Res* 1993;73:205–209.

58 Mukherjee S, Coaxum SD, Maleque M, et al. Effects of oxidized low density lipoprotein on nitric oxide synthetase and protein kinase C activities in bovine endothelial cells. *Cell Mol Biol (Noisy-le-grand)* 2001;47:1051–1058.

59 Moncada S, Palmer RM, Higgs EA. Nitric oxide: physiology, pathophysiology, and pharmacology. *Pharmacol Rev* 1991;43:109–142.

60 Arnold WP, Mittal CK, Katsuki S, et al. Nitric oxide activates guanylate cyclase and increases guanosine 3':5'-cyclic monophosphate levels in various tissue preparations. *Proc Natl Acad Sci USA* 1977;74:3203–3207.

61 Loscalzo J, Welch G. Nitric oxide and its role in the cardiovascular system. *Prog Cardiovasc Dis* 1995;38:87–104.

62 Gryglewski RJ. Interactions between endothelial mediators. *Pharmacol Toxicol* 1995;77:1–9.

63 Bonetti PO, Lerman LO, Lerman A. Endothelial dysfunction: a marker of atherosclerotic risk. *Arterioscler Thromb Vasc Biol* 2003;23:168–175.

64 Behrendt D, Ganz P. Endothelial function. From vascular biology to clinical applications. *Am J Cardiol* 2002;90:40L–48L.

65 Cox DA, Vita JA, Treasure CB, et al. Atherosclerosis impairs flow-mediated dilation of coronary arteries in humans. *Circulation* 1989;80:458–465.

66 Vita JA, Treasure CB, Ganz P, et al. Control of shear stress in the epicardial coronary arteries of humans: impairment by atherosclerosis. *J Am Coll Cardiol* 1989;14:1193–1199.

67 Cayatte AJ, Palacino JJ, Horten K, et al. Chronic inhibition of nitric oxide production accelerates neointima formation and impairs endothelial function in hypercholesterolemic rabbits. *Arterioscler Thromb* 1994;14:753–759.

68 Bult H, De Meyer GR, Herman AG. Influence of chronic treatment with a nitric oxide donor on fatty streak development and reactivity of the rabbit aorta. *Br J Pharmacol* 1995;114:1371–1382.

69 De Meyer GR, Bult H, Ustunes L, et al. Effect of nitric oxide donors on neointima formation and vascular reactivity in the collared carotid artery of rabbits. *J Cardiovasc Pharmacol* 1995;26:272–279.

70 Creager MA, Gallagher SJ, Girerd XJ, et al. L-arginine improves endothelium-dependent vasodilation in hypercholesterolemic humans. *J Clin Invest* 1992;90:1248–1253.

71 Sato J, Mohacsi T, Noel A, et al. *In vivo* gene transfer of endothelial nitric oxide synthase to carotid arteries from hypercholesterolemic rabbits enhances endothelium-dependent relaxations. *Stroke* 2000;31:968–975.

72 Boger RH, Bode-Boger SM, Brandes RP, et al. Dietary L-arginine reduces the progression of atherosclerosis in

cholesterol-fed rabbits: comparison with lovastatin. *Circulation* 1997;96:1282–1290.

73 Phivthong-ngam L, Bode-Boger SM, Boger RH, et al. Dietary L-arginine normalizes endothelin-induced vascular contractions in cholesterol-fed rabbits. *J Cardiovasc Pharmacol* 1998;32:300–307.

74 Boger RH, Bode-Boger SM, Phivthong-ngam L, et al. Dietary L-arginine and alpha-tocopherol reduce vascular oxidative stress and preserve endothelial function in hypercholesterolemic rabbits via different mechanisms. *Atherosclerosis* 1998;141:31–43.

75 Preli RB, Klein KP, Herrington DM. Vascular effects of dietary L-arginine supplementation. *Atherosclerosis* 2002;162:1–15.

76 Lekakis JP, Papathanassiou S, Papaioannou TG, et al. Oral L-arginine improves endothelial dysfunction in patients with essential hypertension. *Int J Cardiol* 2002;86:317–323.

77 de Nigris F, Lerman LO, Ignarro SW, et al. Beneficial effects of antioxidants and L-arginine on oxidation-sensitive gene expression and endothelial NO synthase activity at sites of disturbed shear stress. *Proc Natl Acad Sci USA* 2003;100:1420–1425.

78 Piatti P, Fragasso G, Monti LD, et al. Acute intravenous L-arginine infusion decreases endothelin-1 levels and improves endothelial function in patients with angina pectoris and normal coronary arteriograms: correlation with asymmetric dimethylarginine levels. *Circulation* 2003;107:429–436.

79 Keaney Jr JF, Gaziano JM, Xu A, et al. Dietary antioxidants preserve endothelium-dependent vessel relaxation in cholesterol-fed rabbits. *Proc Natl Acad Sci USA* 1993;90:11880–11884.

80 Keaney Jr JF, Xu A, Cunningham D, et al. Dietary probucol preserves endothelial function in cholesterol-fed rabbits by limiting vascular oxidative stress and superoxide generation. *J Clin Invest* 1995;95:2520–2529.

81 Boger RH, Bode-Boger SM, Szuba A, et al. Asymmetric dimethylarginine (ADMA): a novel risk factor for endothelial dysfunction: its role in hypercholesterolemia. *Circulation* 1998;98:1842–1847.

82 Maclouf J, Folco G, Patrono C. Eicosanoids and iso-eicosanoids: constitutive, inducible and transcellular biosynthesis in vascular disease. *Thromb Haemost* 1998;79:691–705.

83 Moncada S, Vane JR. Prostacyclin and its clinical applications. *Ann Clin Res* 1984;16:241–252.

84 Camacho M, Vila L. Transcellular formation of thromboxane a(2) in mixed incubations of endothelial cells and aspirin-treated platelets strongly depends on the prostaglandin i-synthase activity. *Thromb Res* 2000;99:155–164.

85 Camacho M, Lopez-Belmonte J, Vila L. Rate of vasoconstrictor prostanoids released by endothelial cells depends on cyclooxygenase-2 expression and prostaglandin I synthase activity. *Circ Res* 1998;83:353–365.

86 Uracz W, Uracz D, Olszanecki R, et al. Interleukin 1beta induces functional prostaglandin e synthase in cultured human umbilical vein endothelial cells. *J Physiol Pharmacol* 2002;53:643–654.

87 Tazawa R, Green ED, Ohashi K, et al. Characterization of the complete genomic structure of human thromboxane synthase gene and functional analysis of its promoter. *Arch Biochem Biophys* 1996;334:349–356.

88 Karim S, Habib A, Levy-Toledano S, et al. Cyclooxygenase-1 and -2 of endothelial cells utilize exogenous or endogenous arachidonic acid for transcellular production of thromboxane. *J Biol Chem* 1996;271:12042–12048.

89 Watkins MT, Patton GM, Soler HM, et al. Synthesis of 8-epi-prostaglandin f2alpha by human endothelial cells: role of prostaglandin h2 synthase. *Biochem J* 1999;344:747–754.

90 Schönbeck U, Sukhova G, Graber P, et al. Augmented expression of cyclooxygenase-2 in human atherosclerotic lesions. *Am J Pathol* 1999;155:1281–1291.

91 Cipollone F, Prontera C, Pini B, et al. Overexpression of functionally coupled cyclooxygenase-2 and prostaglandin e synthase in symptomatic atherosclerotic plaque as a basis of prostaglandin e_2-dependent plaque instability. *Circulation* 2001;104:921–927.

92 Hong BK, Kwon HM, Lee BK, et al. Coexpression of cyclooxygenase-2 and matrix metalloproteinases in human aortic atherosclerotic lesions. *Yonsei Med J* 2000;41:82–88.

93 Leahy K, Koki A, Masferrer J. Role of cyclooxygenase in angiogenesis. *Curr Med Chem* 2000;7:1163–1170.

94 Kumamoto M, Nakashima Y, Sueishi k. Intimal neovascularization in human atherosclerosis. Its origin and pathophysiological significance. *Human Pathol* 1995;20.

95 Massy ZA, Swan SK. Cyclooxygenase-2 and atherosclerosis: friend or foe? *Nephrol Dial Transplant* 2001;16:2286–2289.

96 Fitzgerald GA. Coxibs and cardiovascular disease. *N Engl J Med* 2004;351:1709–1711.

97 Topol EJ. Failing the public health – Rofecoxib, Merck, and the FDA. *N Engl J Med* 2004;351:1707–1709.

98 Furberg CD, Psaty BM, FitzGerald GA. Parecoxib, valdecoxib, and cardiovascular risk. *Circulation* 2005;111:249.

99 Okie S. Raising the safety bar – the FDA's coxib meeting. *N Engl J Med* 2005;352:1283–1285.

100 Egan KM, Lawson JA, Fries S, et al. Cox-2-derived prostacyclin confers atheroprotection on female mice. *Science* 2004;306:1954–1957.

101 Triggle C, Dong H, Waldron G, et al. Endothelium-derived hyperpolarizing factor(s). Species and tissue heterogenity. *Clin Exp Pharmacol Physiol* 1999;26:176–179.

102 Ding H, McGuire J, Triggle C. The other endothelium-derived relaxating factor. A review of recent findings concerning the nature and the cellular actions of endothelium-derived hyperpolarizing factor (EDHF). *Biomed Res* 2000;11:119–129.

103 Triggle CR, Ding H. Endothelium-derived hyperpolarizing factor: is there a novel chemical mediator? *Clin Exp Pharmacol Physiol* 2002;29:153–160.

104 Campbell WB, Gebremedhin D, Pratt PF, et al. Identification of epoxyeicosatrienoic acids as endothelium-derived hyperpolarizing factors. *Circ Res* 1996;78:415–423.

105 Randall MD, Alexander SPH, Bennett T. An cndogenous cannabinoid as an endothelium-derived vasorelaxant. *Biochem Biophys Res Commun* 1996;229:114–120.

106 Chaytor AT, Evans WH, Griffith TM. Central role of heterocellular gap junctional communication in endothelium-dependent relaxations of rabbit arteries. *J Physiol* 1998;508.

107 Popp R, Fleming I, Busse R. Pulsatile stretch in coronary arteries elicits release of endothelium-derived hyperpolarizing factor: a modulator of arterial compliance. *Circ Res* 1998;82:696–703.

108 Urakami-Harasawa L, Shimokawa H, Nakashima M, et al. Importance of endothelium-derived hyperpolarizing factor in human arteries. *J Clin Invest* 1997;100:2793–2799.

109 Feletou M, Vanhoutte PM. The alternative: EDHF. *J Mol Cell Cardiol* 1999;31:15–22.

110 Yanagisawa M, Kurihara H, Kimura S, et al. A novel peptide vasoconstrictor, endothelin, is produced by vascular endothelium and modulates smooth muscle Ca^{2+} channels. *J Hypertens Suppl* 1988;6:S188–S191.

111 Yanagisawa M, Inoue A, Ishikawa T, et al. Primary structure, synthesis, and biological activity of rat endothelin, an endothelium-derived vasoconstrictor peptide. *Proc Natl Acad Sci USA* 1988;85:6964–6967.

112 Xu D, Emoto N, Giaid A, et al. ECE-1: a membrane-bound metalloprotease that catalyzes the proteolytic activation of big endothelin-1. *Cell* 1994;78:473–485.

113 Corder R, Barker S. The expression of endothelin-1 and endothelin-converting enzyme-1 (ECE-1) are independently regulated in bovine aortic endothelial cells. *J Cardiovasc Pharmacol* 1999;33:671–677.

114 Muller L, Valdenaire O, Barret A, et al. Expression of the endothelin-converting enzyme-1 isoforms in endothelial cells. *J Cardiovasc Pharmacol* 2000;36:S15–S18.

115 Schiffrin EL, Touyz RM. Vascular biology of endothelin. *J Cardiovasc Pharmacol* 1998;32:S2–S13.

116 Lerman A, Edwards BS, Hallett JW, et al. Circulating and tissue endothelin immunoreactivity in advanced atherosclerosis. *N Engl J Med* 1991;325:997–1001.

117 Lerman A, Kubo SH, Tschumperlin LK, et al. Plasma endothelin concentrations in humans with end-stage heart failure and after heart transplantation. *J Am Coll Cardiol* 1992;20:849–853.

118 Corder R, Carrier M, Khan N, et al. Cytokine regulation of endothelin-1 release from bovine aortic endothelial cells. *J Cardiovasc Pharmacol* 1995;26:S56–S58.

119 Herman WH, Holcomb JM, Hricik DE, et al. Interleukin-1 beta induces endothelin-1 gene by multiple mechanisms. *Transplant Proc* 1999;31:1412–1413.

120 Boulanger CM, Tanner FC, Bea ML, et al. Oxidized low density lipoproteins induce mRNA expression and release of endothelin from human and porcine endothelium. *Circ Res* 1992;70:1191–1197.

121 Horio T, Kohno M, Yasunari K, et al. Stimulation of endothelin-1 release by low density and very low density lipoproteins in cultured human endothelial cells. *Atherosclerosis* 1993;101:185–190.

122 Achmad TH, Winterscheidt A, Lindemann C, et al. Oxidized low density lipoprotein acts on endothelial cells in culture to enhance endothelin secretion and monocyte migration. *Methods Find Exp Clin Pharmacol* 1997;19:153–159.

123 Unoki H, Fan J, Watanabe T. Low-density lipoproteins modulate endothelial cells to secrete endothelin-1 in a polarized pattern: a study using a culture model system simulating arterial intima. *Cell Tissue Res* 1999;295:89–99.

124 Jones GT, van Rij AM, Solomon C, et al. Endothelin-1 is increased overlying atherosclerotic plaques in human arteries. *Atherosclerosis* 1996;124:25–35.

125 Ishizuka T, Takamizawa-Matsumoto M, Suzuki K, et al. Endothelin-1 enhances vascular cell adhesion molecule-1 expression in tumor necrosis factor alpha-stimulated vascular endothelial cells. *Eur J Pharmacol* 1999;369:237–245.

126 Hofman FM, Chen P, Jeyaseelan R, et al. Endothelin-1 induces production of the neutrophil chemotactic factor interleukin-8 by human brain-derived endothelial cells. *Blood* 1998;92:3064–3072.

127 Lerman A, Holmes Jr DR, Bell MR, et al. Endothelin in coronary endothelial dysfunction and early atherosclerosis in humans. *Circulation* 1995;92:2426–2431.

128 Unger T. The role of the renin–angiotensin system in the development of cardiovascular disease. *Am J Cardiol* 2002;89:3A–9A; discussion 10A.

129 Igic R, Behnia R. Properties and distribution of angiotensin I converting enzyme. *Curr Pharm Des* 2003;9:697–706.

130 Stoll M, Meffert S, Stroth U, et al. Growth or anti-growth: angiotensin and the endothelium. *J Hypertens* 1995;13:1529–1534.

131 Pueyo ME, Michel JB. Angiotensin II receptors in endothelial cells. *Gen Pharmacol* 1997;29:691–696.

132 Pastore L, Tessitore A, Martinotti S, et al. Angiotensin II stimulates intercellular adhesion molecule-1 (ICAM-1)

expression by human vascular endothelial cells and increases soluble ICAM-1 release *in vivo. Circulation* 1999;100:1646–1652.

133 Pueyo ME, Gonzalez W, Nicoletti A, et al. Angiotensin II stimulates endothelial vascular cell adhesion molecule-1 via nuclear factor-kappa b activation induced by intracellular oxidative stress. *Arterioscler Thromb Vasc Biol* 2000;20:645–651.

134 Cannon R. Role of nitric oxide in cardiovascular disease: focus on endothelium. *Clin Chem* 1998;44:1808–1819.

135 Gryglewski RJ, Chlopicki S, Swies J, et al. Prostacyclin, nitric oxide, and atherosclerosis. *Ann NY Acad Sci* 1995;748:194–206; discussion 206–197.

136 Mendelsohn ME, O'Neill S, George D, et al. Inhibition of fibrinogen binding to human platelets by *s*-nitroso-*n*-acetylcysteine. *J Biol Chem* 1990;265:19028–19034.

137 Michelson AD, Benoit SE, Furman MI, et al. Effects of nitric oxide/EDRF on platelet surface glycoproteins. *Am J Physiol* 1996;270:H1640–H1648.

138 Pigazzi A, Heydrick S, Folli F, et al. Nitric oxide inhibits thrombin receptor-activating peptide-induced phosphoinositide 3-kinase activity in human platelets. *J Biol Chem* 1999;274:14368–14375.

139 Hollopeter G, Jantzen HM, Vincent D, et al. Identification of the platelet ADP receptor targeted by antithrombotic drugs. *Nature* 2001;409:202–207.

140 Gachet C. ADP receptors of platelets and their inhibition. *Thromb Haemost* 2001;86:222–232.

141 Marcus A, Broekman M, Drosopoulos J, et al. Metabolic control of excessive extracellular nucleotide accumulation by CD39/ecto-nucleotidase-1: implications for ischemic vascular diseases. *JPET* 2003;305:9–16.

142 Mann KG. Thrombosis: theoretical considerations. *Am J Clin Nutr* 1997;65:1657S–1664S.

143 Rosenberg RD, Rosenberg JS. Natural anticoagulant mechanisms. *J Clin Invest* 1984;74:1–6.

144 Marcum JA, Rosenberg RD. Anticoagulantly active heparin-like molecules from vascular tissue. *Biochemistry* 1984;23:1730–1737.

145 Marcum JA, McKenney JB, Rosenberg RD. Acceleration of thrombin–antithrombin complex formation in rat hindquarters via heparinlike molecules bound to the endothelium. *J Clin Invest* 1984;74:341–350.

146 Heyderman RS, Klein NJ, Shennan GI, et al. Reduction of the anticoagulant activity of glycosaminoglycans on the surface of the vascular endothelium by endotoxin and neutrophils: evaluation by an amidolytic assay. *Thromb Res* 1992;67:677–685.

147 Klein NJ, Shennan GI, Heyderman RS, et al. Alteration in glycosaminoglycan metabolism and surface charge on human umbilical vein endothelial cells induced by cytokines, endotoxin and neutrophils. *J Cell Sci* 1992;102:821–832.

148 Broze Jr GJ. Tissue factor pathway inhibitor. *Thromb Haemost* 1995;74:90–93.

149 Jesty J, Lorenz A, Rodriguez J, et al. Initiation of the tissue factor pathway of coagulation in the presence of heparin: control by antithrombin III and tissue factor pathway inhibitor. *Blood* 1996;87:2301–2307.

150 Bombeli T, Karsan A, Tait JF, et al. Apoptotic vascular endothelial cells become procoagulant. *Blood* 1997;89:2429–2442.

151 Maruyama I, Majerus PW. The turnover of thrombin–thrombomodulin complex in cultured human umbilical vein endothelial cells and a549 lung cancer cells. Endocytosis and degradation of thrombin. *J Biol Chem* 1985;260:15432–15438.

152 Bombeli T, Mueller M, Haeberli A. Anticoagulant properties of the vascular endothelium. *Thromb Haemost* 1997;77:408–423.

153 Esmon CT. Coagulation and inflammation. *J Endotoxin Res* 2003;9:192–198.

154 Stearns-Kurosawa DJ, Kurosawa S, Mollica JS, et al. The endothelial cell protein C receptor augments protein C activation by the thrombin–thrombomodulin complex. *Proc Natl Acad Sci USA* 1996;93:10212–10216.

155 Liaw PC, Neuenschwander PF, Smirnov MD, et al. Mechanisms by which soluble endothelial cell protein C receptor modulates protein C and activated protein C function. *J Biol Chem* 2000;275:5447–5452.

156 Lu D, Kalafatis M, Mann KG, et al. Comparison of activated protein C/protein S-mediated inactivation of human factor VIII and factor V. *Blood* 1996; 87: 4708–4717.

157 Esmon CT. Protein C, protein S and thrombomodulin. In: Robert W, Colman M, Hirsh J, et al., eds. *Hemostasis and Thrombosis: Basic Principles and Clinical Practice.* Philadelphia: Lippincott Williams & Wilkins; 2001:335–353.

158 Grey ST, Csizmadia V, Hancock WW. Differential effect of tumor necrosis factor-alpha on thrombomodulin gene expression by human monocytoid (THP-1) cell versus endothelial cells. *Int J Hematol* 1998;67:53–62.

159 Randi AM, Biguzzi E, Falciani F, et al. Identification of differentially expressed genes in coronary atherosclerotic plaques from patients with stable or unstable angina by cDNA array analysis. *J Thromb Haemost* 2003;1:829–835.

160 Morrissey JH, Fakhrai H, Edgington TS. Molecular cloning of the cDNA for tissue factor, the cellular receptor for the initiation of the coagulation protease cascade. *Cell* 1987;50:129–135.

161 Drake TA, Morrissey JH, Edgington TS. Selective cellular expression of tissue factor in human tissues. Implications for disorders of hemostasis and thrombosis. *Am J Pathol* 1989;134:1087–1097.

162 Marmur JD, Thiruvikraman SV, Fyfe BS, et al. Identification of active tissue factor in human coronary atheroma. *Circulation* 1996;94:1226–1232.

163 Taubman MB, Fallon JT, Schecter AD, et al. Tissue factor in the pathogenesis of atherosclerosis. *Thromb Haemost* 1997;78:200–204.

164 Colucci M, Balconi G, Lorenzet R, et al. Cultured human endothelial cells generate tissue factor in response to endotoxin. *J Clin Invest* 1983;71:1893–1896.

165 Bevilacqua MP, Pober JS, Majeau GR, et al. Interleukin 1 (IL-1) induces biosynthesis and cell surface expression of procoagulant activity in human vascular endothelial cells. *J Exp Med* 1984;160:618–623.

166 Mulder AB, Hegge-Paping KS, Magielse CP, et al. Tumor necrosis factor alpha-induced endothelial tissue factor is located on the cell surface rather than in the subendothelial matrix. *Blood* 1994;84:1559–1566.

167 Lin MC, Almus-Jacobs F, Chen HH, et al. Shear stress induction of the tissue factor gene. *J Clin Invest* 1997;99:737–744.

168 Drake TA, Hannani K, Fei HH, et al. Minimally oxidized low-density lipoprotein induces tissue factor expression in cultured human endothelial cells. *Am J Pathol* 1991;138:601–607.

169 Slupsky JR, Kalbas M, Willuweit A, et al. Activated platelets induce tissue factor expression on human umbilical vein endothelial cells by ligation of CD40. *Thromb Haemost* 1998;80:1008–1014.

170 Miller DL, Yaron R, Yellin MJ. CD40l–CD40 interactions regulate endothelial cell surface tissue factor and thrombomodulin expression. *J Leukoc Biol* 1998;63:373–379.

171 Bona R, Lee E, Rickles F. Tissue factor apoprotein: intracellular transport and expression in shed membrane vesicles. *Thromb Res* 1987;48:487–500.

172 Shimura M, Wada H, Wakita Y, et al. Plasma tissue factor and tissue factor pathway inhibitor levels in patients with disseminated intravascular coagulation. *Am J Hematol* 1996;52:165–170.

173 Erban JK, Wagner DD. A 130-kDa protein on endothelial cells binds to amino acids 15–42 of the b beta chain of fibrinogen. *J Biol Chem* 1992;267:2451–2458.

174 Greenberg CS, Birckbichler PJ, Rice RH. Transglutaminases: multifunctional cross-linking enzymes that stabilize tissues. *Faseb J* 1991;5:3071–3077.

175 Okada Y, Copeland BR, Hamann GF, et al. Integrin alphavbeta3 is expressed in selected microvessels after focal cerebral ischemia. *Am J Pathol* 1996;149:37–44.

176 Hirsh J, Salzman E, Marder V, et al. Overview of the thrombotic process and its therapy. In: Colman R, Hirsh J, Marder V, et al., eds. *Hemostasis and Thrombosis, Basic Principles and Clinical Practice.* Philadelphia: Lippincott Williams & Wilkins; 1994:1151–1161.

177 Levin EG, Santell L, Osborn KG. The expression of endothelial tissue plasminogen activator *in vivo*: a function defined by vessel size and anatomic location. *J Cell Sci* 1997;110:139–148.

178 Wojta J, Hoover RL, Daniel TO. Vascular origin determines plasminogen activator expression in human endothelial cells. Renal endothelial cells produce large amounts of single chain urokinase type plasminogen activator. *J Biol Chem* 1989;264:2846–2852.

179 Bacharach E, Itin A, Keshet E. *In vivo* patterns of expression of urokinase and its inhibitor PAI-1 suggest a concerted role in regulating physiological angiogenesis. *Proc Natl Acad Sci USA* 1992;89:10686–10690.

180 Yamamoto K, Loskutoff DJ. Fibrin deposition in tissues from endotoxin-treated mice correlates with decreases in the expression of urokinase-type but not tissue-type plasminogen activator. *J Clin Invest* 1996;97:2440–2451.

181 Levin EG, Santell L. Association of a plasminogen activator inhibitor (PAI-1) with the growth substratum and membrane of human endothelial cells. *J Cell Biol* 1987;105:2543–2549.

182 Sawdey MS, Loskutoff DJ. Regulation of murine type 1 plasminogen activator inhibitor gene expression *in vivo*. Tissue specificity and induction by lipopolysaccharide, tumor necrosis factor-alpha, and transforming growth factor-beta. *J Clin Invest* 1991;88:1346–1353.

183 Bajzar L, Morser J, Nesheim M. TAFI, or plasma procarboxypeptidase b, couples the coagulation and fibrinolytic cascades through the thrombin–thrombomodulin complex. *J Biol Chem* 1996;271:16603–16608.

184 Frenette PS, Mayadas TN, Rayburn H, et al. Susceptibility to infection and altered hematopoiesis in mice deficient in both P- and E-selectins. *Cell* 1996;84:563–574.

185 Ross R. Atherosclerosis – an inflammatory disease. *N Engl J Med* 1999;340:115–126.

186 Lukacs NW, Strieter RM, Elner V, et al. Production of chemokines, interleukin-8 and monocyte chemoattractant protein-1, during monocyte: endothelial cell interactions. *Blood* 1995;86:2767–2773.

187 Martin T, Cardarelli PM, Parry GC, et al. Cytokine induction of monocyte chemoattractant protein-1 gene expression in human endothelial cells depends on the cooperative action of NF-kappa b and AP-1. *Eur J Immunol* 1997;27:1091–1097.

188 Shono T, Ono M, Izumi H, et al. Involvement of the transcription factor NF-kappa b in tubular morphogenesis of human microvascular endothelial cells by oxidative stress. *Mol Cell Biol* 1996;16:4231–4239.

189 McIntyre TM, Modur V, Prescott SM, et al. Molecular mechanisms of early inflammation. *Thromb Haemost* 1997;78:302–305.

190 McEver RP, Moore KL, Cummings RD. Leukocyte traf-
     ficking mediated by selectin–carbohydrate interactions.
     J Biol Chem 1995;270:11025–11028.

191 Gonzalez-Amaro R, Sanchez-Madrid F. Cell adhesion
     molecules: selectins and integrins. *Crit Rev Immunol*
     1999;19:389–429.

192 Steegmaier M, Borges E, Berger J, et al. The E-selectin-
     ligand ESL-1 is located in the golgi as well as on micro-
     villi on the cell surface. *J Cell Sci* 1997;110:687–694.

193 Wild MK, Huang MC, Schulze-Horsel U, et al. Affinity,
     kinetics, and thermodynamics of E-selectin binding to E-
     selectin ligand-1. *J Biol Chem* 2001;276:31602–31612.

194 Yao L, Pan J, Setiadi H, et al. Interleukin 4 or oncostatin
     m induces a prolonged increase in P-selectin mRNA
     and protein in human endothelial cells. *J Exp Med*
     1996;184:81–92.

195 Subramaniam M, Koedam JA, Wagner DD. Divergent
     fates of P- and E-selectins after their expression on the
     plasma membrane. *Mol Biol Cell* 1993;4:791–801.

196 Wood KM, Cadogan MD, Ramshaw AL, et al. The dis-
     tribution of adhesion molecules in human atheroscle-
     rosis. *Histopathology* 1993;22:437–444.

197 Johnson RC, Chapman SM, Dong ZM, et al. Absence of
     P-selectin delays fatty streak formation in mice. *J Clin
     Invest* 1997;99:1037–1043.

198 Springer TA. Traffic signals for lymphocyte recircula-
     tion and leukocyte emigration: the multistep paradigm.
     Cell 1994;76:301–314.

199 Binnerts ME, van Kooyk Y, Simmons DL, et al. Distinct
     binding of t lymphocytes to ICAM-1, -2 or -3 upon acti-
     vation of LFA-1. *Eur J Immunol* 1994;24:2155–2160.

200 Dustin ML, Rothlein R, Bhan AK, et al. Induction by IL
     1 and interferon-gamma: tissue distribution, biochem-
     istry, and function of a natural adherence molecule
     (ICAM-1). *J Immunol* 1986;137:245–254.

201 Scholz D, Devaux B, Hirche A, et al. Expression of adhe-
     sion molecules is specific and time-dependent in
     cytokine-stimulated endothelial cells in culture. *Cell
     Tissue Res* 1996;284:415–423.

202 Stade BG, Messer G, Riethmuller G, et al. Structural
     characteristics of the 5′ region of the human ICAM-1
     gene. *Immunobiology* 1990;182:79–87.

203 Schleimer RP, Sterbinsky SA, Kaiser J, et al. IL-4 induces
     adherence of human eosinophils and basophils but not
     neutrophils to endothelium. Association with expres-
     sion of VCAM-1. *J Immunol* 1992;148:1086–1092.

204 Libby P, Galis ZS. Cytokines regulate genes involved in
     atherogenesis. *Ann NY Acad Sci* 1995;748:158–168; dis-
     cussion 168–170.

205 Osborn L, Hession C, Tizard R, et al. Direct expression
     cloning of vascular cell adhesion molecule 1, a
     cytokine-induced endothelial protein that binds to
     lymphocytes. *Cell* 1989;59:1203–1211.

206 Marui N, Offermann MK, Swerlick R, et al. Vascular cell
     adhesion molecule-1 (VCAM-1) gene transcription
     and expression are regulated through an antioxidant-
     sensitive mechanism in human vascular endothelial
     cells. *J Clin Invest* 1993;92:1866–1874.

207 Lin JH, Zhu Y, Liao HL, et al. Induction of vascular cell
     adhesion molecule-1 by low-density lipoprotein.
     Atherosclerosis 1996;127:185–194.

208 Basta G, Lazzerini G, Massaro M, et al. Advanced glycation
     end products activate endothelium through signal-trans-
     duction receptor rage: a mechanism for amplification of
     inflammatory responses. *Circulation* 2002;105:816–822.

209 Basta G, Schmidt AM, De Caterina R. Advanced glyca-
     tion end products and vascular inflammation: implica-
     tions for accelerated atherosclerosis in diabetes.
     Cardiovasc Res 2004;63:582–592.

210 Collins T, Read MA, Neish AS, et al. Transcriptional reg-
     ulation of endothelial cell adhesion molecules: NF-
     kappa b and cytokine-inducible enhancers. *Faseb J*
     1995;9:899–909.

211 Cybulsky MI, Iiyama K, Li H, et al. A major role for
     VCAM-1, but not ICAM-1, in early atherosclerosis. *J
     Clin Invest* 2001;107:1255–1262.

212 Newman PJ. The biology of PECAM-1. *J Clin Invest*
     1997;99:3–8.

213 Rattan V, Sultana C, Shen Y, et al. Oxidant stress-
     induced transendothelial migration of monocytes is
     linked to phosphorylation of PECAM-1. *Am J Physiol*
     1997;273:E453–E461.

214 Davies MJ, Gordon JL, Gearing AJ, et al. The expression
     of the adhesion molecules ICAM-1, VCAM-1, PECAM,
     and E-selectin in human atherosclerosis. *J Pathol*
     1993;171:223–229.

215 Nakashima Y, Raines EW, Plump AS, et al. Upregulation
     of VCAM-1 and ICAM-1 at atherosclerosis-prone sites
     on the endothelium in the ApoE-deficient mouse.
     Arterioscler Thromb Vasc Biol 1998;18:842–851.

216 De Martin R, Hoeth M, Hofer-Warbinek R, et al. The
     transcription factor NF-kappa b and the regulation of
     vascular cell function. *Arterioscler Thromb Vasc Biol*
     2000;20:E83–E88.

217 Pahl HL. Activators and target genes of REL/NF-kappa
     b transcription factors. *Oncogene* 1999;18:6853–6866.

218 Baeuerle PA. The inducible transcription activator NF-
     kappa b: regulation by distinct protein subunits.
     Biochim Biophys Acta 1991;1072:63–80.

219 Schreck R, Albermann K, Baeuerle PA. Nuclear factor
     kappa b: an oxidative stress-responsive transcription
     factor of eukaryotic cells (a review). *Free Radic Res
     Commun* 1992;17:221–237.

220 Brand K, Page S, Rogler G, et al. Activated transcription
     factor nuclear factor-kappa b is present in the athero-
     sclerotic lesion. *J Clin Invest* 1996;97:1715–1722.

221 Bourcier T, Sukhova G, Libby P. The nuclear factor kappa-b signaling pathway participates in dysregulation of vascular smooth muscle cells *in vitro* and in human atherosclerosis. *J Biol Chem* 1997;272:15817–15824.

222 Khan BV, Harrison DG, Olbrych MT, et al. Nitric oxide regulates vascular cell adhesion molecule 1 gene expression and redox-sensitive transcriptional events in human vascular endothelial cells. *Proc Natl Acad Sci USA* 1996;93:9114–9119.

223 Singer C. A short history of anatomy and physiology from Greeks to Harvey. New York: Dover Publications; 1957.

224 Galen C. *Whether Blood Is Naturally Contained in the Arteries.* Princenton University Press; 1984.

225 Harvey W. *Exercitatio anatomica de motu cordis et sanguinis in animalibus.* Springfield; 1928.

226 Leeuwenhoek A. Letter to royal society no. 110. In: Palm L, ed. *Collected letters of antoni van leeuwenhoek.* Lisse: Swetz & Zeitlinger; 1983.

227 Starling E. On the absorption of fluids from the connective tissue space. *J Physiol* 1896;19:312–326.

228 Pappenheimer J. Passage of molecules through capillary walls. *Physiol Rew* 1953;33:387–399.

229 Moncada S, Gryglewski R, Bunting S, et al. An enzyme isolated from arteries transforms prostaglandin endoperoxides to an unstable substance that inhibits platelet aggregation. *Nature* 1976;263:663–665.

CHAPTER 2

Endothelial activation and the initiation of atherosclerosis

Raffaele De Caterina, MD, PhD, *Antonella Zampolli,* DBiol, PhD, *Guido Lazzerini,* BSc, *& Peter Libby,* MD

Medical scientists once hypothesized that athero-sclerosis begins as a "response to injury" caused by damage to the intima during endothelial cell (EC) detachment. Our current concept of atherogenesis focuses instead on the role of inflammation in an otherwise morphologically intact endothelium. Sound experimental and clinical evidence linking hypercholesterolemia and other risk factors for atherosclerosis suggests a central role for inflam-matory mechanisms that occur within the broader concept of endothelial dysfunctions [1–3]. Indeed, inflammatory mechanisms that induce endothelial dysfunction can promote lesion inception, devel-opment, and complications. Therefore, we now con-sider atherosclerosis an inflammatory disease [4,5].

Early phases of atherosclerosis: the "fatty streak"

Atherosclerotic lesions originate mainly at bifurca-tion sites, branching points, and convex areas of bending arteries – critical areas where low or oscillat-ing shear stress [6] likely favors passive transport of arterial blood components inside the vascular wall. A complex of functional phenotypic alterations ren-ders the endothelium adhesive to circulating leuko-cytes, more permeable to solutes, and capable of enhanced synthesis of mitogenic, chemoattractive, and inflammatory mediators. This concerted tran-scriptional activation of genes that recruit leuko-cytes into the intima, i.e., "endothelial activation," [7] participates importantly in the initiation, pro-gression, and clinical emergence of atherosclerotic vascular disease.

Although complex lesions contain different mor-phological aspects that reflect the various stages of plaque evolution and possibly a different natural his-tory [8], the arterial fatty streak represents the earliest stage of plaque development. Autopsy sometimes detects fatty streaks in the fetus [9], and also reveals their presence in the coronary arteries of 50% of young subjects 10–14 years old [10]. Characterized by areas of intimal thickening derived from circu-lating monocytes and sustained by the intimal accumulation of lipid-laden macrophages (foam cells), fatty streaks contain varying numbers of T-lymphocytes [11,12] (Figures 2.1–2.3). Many consider these lesions reversible. Fatty streaks from animal models, particularly moderately hyper-cholesterolemic primates [13,14], foreshadow the more advanced lesions that later appear in the same critical areas of the arterial vasculature. Thus, the initial phases of atherosclerosis begin with fatty streak pathogenesis.

Molecular mechanisms of endothelial activation and leukocyte binding

Recruitment of monocytes into the intima occurs early in the formation of the atherosclerotic plaque. In general, leukocyte extravasation initiates any inflammatory process. While leukocytes do not adhere to a normal endothelium, they do adhere to an activated endothelium. In any type of inflamma-tion, molecules expressed on the surface of activated EC mediate leukocyte adhesion and transmigration in the intima (Figure 2.4). Simultaneously, an array of pro-inflammatory mediators coordinates leuko-cyte homing; ultimately, both EC and leukocyte

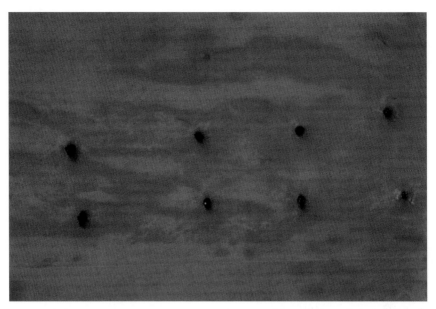

Figure 2.1 Fatty streaks from a human aorta, longitudinally cut, mounted en face, and stained in red with Oil Red-O for lipids, of a young male dying of accidental causes. Such lesions occur commonly in the young, and many think they are fully reversible. However, they localize in the same sites of the arterial tree where "raised" lesions later develop. Note the preferential locations of fatty streaks around the orifices of intercostal arteries, where hemodynamic forces likely contribute to their pathogenesis. (From Davies MJ, *Colour Atlas of Cardiovascular Pathology*. Oxford, Harvey Miller Publishers-Oxford University Press, 1986, with permission of the Publisher).

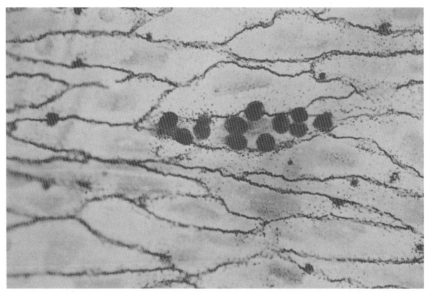

Figure 2.2 Adhesion of monocytes to vascular endothelium in early atherogenesis in the rat model. The endothelial monolayer in the inner surface of a rat aorta stained *en face* with silver nitrate delineates EC borders in this low-power scanning electron micrograph. Monocytes adhere in clusters to an EC morphologically indistinguishable from neighboring cells, thus configuring, by definition, a situation of endothelial "dysfunction". (Reprinted from Ref. [72] by permission from the American Society for Investigative Pathology).

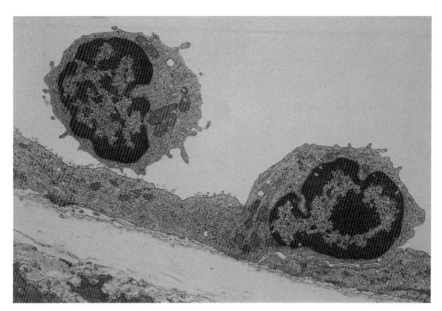

Figure 2.3 Transmission electron micrograph of the endothelial surface of the aorta in a hypercholesterolemic rat model. One monocyte (left) approaches the endothelial surface, and another passes into the sub-endothelial intima through junctions between adjacent EC. Monocytes are clearly identified by the characteristic "kidney-shaped" nuclei. (Reprinted from Ref. [72] by permission from the American Society for Investigative Pathology).

activation provide traffic signals for such homing [15]. The molecules involved in such signaling events are mainly endothelial leukocyte adhesion molecules and chemoattractants.

Endothelial leukocyte adhesion molecules involved specifically in atherogenesis belong to the selectin and integrin families and also to a sub-group of the immunoglobulin superfamily [16] (Table 2.1). By binding to sialyl Lewis^x (SLe^x) or closely related carbohydrate structures as their ligands, P- and E-selectin mediate transient labile contact, or "rolling," of leukocytes with the endothelium. P-selectin, which localizes in EC overlying human atheroma [17], participates in early atherogenesis. Indeed, atheroma formation decreases in hyperlipidemic atherosclerosis-prone mice lacking P-selectin [18,19]. However, vascular cell adhesion molecule-1 (VCAM-1), a member of the immunoglobulin superfamily, plays a more prominent role, mediating steady leukocyte adhesion to the endothelium by binding to the cognate integrin ligand very late antigen (VLA)-4, which expresses specifically on the surface of circulating monocytes and T-lymphocytes [20]. In rabbit and mouse models of cholesterol-induced atherosclerosis, EC selectively express VCAM-1 at sites prone to lesion development [21,22]. Crossbreeding VCAM-1 hypomorphic mice expressing VCAM-1 with one IgG domain genetically deleted, with atherosclerosis-prone LDLR$^{-/-}$ mice yields offspring characterized by reduced lesion formation [23]. Interestingly, such reduction does not occur with intercellular adhesion molecule-1 (ICAM-1), another inflammatory adhesion molecule [23].

Pro-inflammatory cytokines such as interleukin (IL)-1, tumor-necrosis factor (TNF)-α, and CD40 ligand (CD40L) induce the expression of VCAM-1, ICAM-1, E-selectin, and soluble endothelial products including monocyte chemoattractant protein-1 (MCP-1), macrophage-colony stimulating factor (M-CSF), IL-6, and IL-8 (see below). Components of oxidized lipoproteins such as oxidized phospholipids and short-chain aldehydes [24,25] as well as in some experiments advanced glycation endproducts (AGE) [26,27] also induce VCAM-1 expression.

Nuclear factor-κB activation: a common denominator in vascular disease

Nuclear factor-kappa B (NF-κB), a transcription factor that participates in the expression of most molecules implicated in endothelial activation discussed thus far (Figure 2.5), provides a common link that

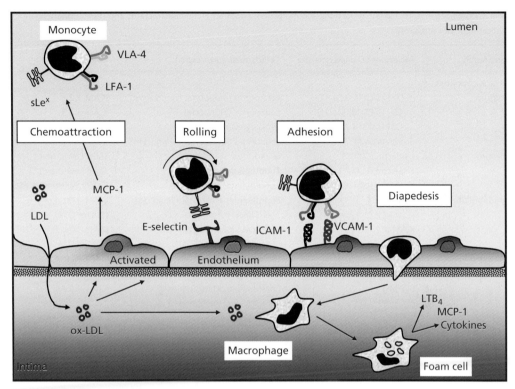

Figure 2.4 The different phases of monocyte adhesion to the endothelium together with molecular ligands presumably implicated in the process. The first phase, denoted as "rolling," involves a slowing-down of monocytes when activated EC expressing E-selectin tether flowing monocytes via labile binding of E-selectin to carbohydrate ligands (sialyl-Lexis^x) already constitutively expressed on the monocyte surface. By considerably decreasing monocyte speed, rolling allows monocytes to "sense" the atmosphere of specific chemoattractants, i.e., the chemokine monocyte chemoattractant protein-1 (MCP-1). Through inside-out signaling, intracellular signal transduction in the monocyte following MCP-1 stimulation allows a conformational change of integrin-type receptors (leukocyte function associated antigen-1 (LFA-1), Mac-1, and VLA4) that recognize immunoglobulin ligands expressed *de novo* on the surface of activated EC, i.e., intercellular adhesion molecule-1 (ICAM-1) and vascular cell adhesion molecule (VCAM)-1, leading to labile and then firm attachment of monocytes on the endothelial surface ("arrest" and "spreading") and their subsequent "diapedesis". Diapedesis occurs through other types of intermolecular interactions that likely involve platelet-EC adhesion molecule-1 (PECAM-1) on the endothelial surface. Although susceptible to further refinement and evolution, this conceptual framework, largely adapted from similar models developed for neutrophil and lymphocyte adhesion, aids our understanding of the role of different adhesion molecules and soluble cytokines in monocyte adhesion, and also allows us to interpret the selective recruitment of monocytes in early atherogenesis. See also Table 2.1 and text for abbreviations and further details on the molecules involved.

can explain the coordinate expression of various endothelial genes involved in endothelial activation. Moreover, its signaling pathway activates in areas of disturbed blood flow and in response to cytokines, i.e., IL-1 and TNF-α, and other inflammatory stimuli such as bacterial lipopolysaccharide (LPS) and AGE [28]. All such stimuli induce oxidative stress by increasing production of reactive oxygen species (ROS). Because activated NF-κB occurs in atherosclerotic lesions but not in normal vessels [29], this factor may play a central role in endothelial activation

and atherogenesis. Since the targeted deletion of genes encoding some NF-κB components are lethal embryonically, direct evidence for its direct causal role remains undetermined.

Molecular mechanisms of chemoattraction and intimal monocyte–macrophage activation

After adhering to the vascular endothelium, leukocytes enter the arterial wall by diapedesis through the space between adjacent EC, a process coordinated

Table 2.1 Selected endothelial leukocyte adhesion molecules, endothelial chemoattractants and their cognate ligands implicated in atherosclerosis.

Gene family	Molecules/CD nomenclature	Cellular/tissue expression	Cognate ligand
Surface associated			
Integrins	β_2 CD11a/CD18 (LFA-1)	Leukocytes (monocyte, lymphocyte)	ICAM-1,2,3
	CD11b/CD18 (Mac-1)	Leukocytes (monocyte)	ICAM-1,2,3
	CD11c/CD18	Leukocytes (monocyte)	
	β_1 $\alpha_4\beta_1$ (VLA-4)	Leukocytes (monocyte, lymphocyte)	VCAM-1
Selectins	L-selectin (CD62L)	Leukocytes	Sialyl Lewis[x] and [a]
	E-selectin (ELAM-1, CD62E)	Endothelium	Sialyl Lewis[x] and [a]
	P-selectin (CD62P, PADGEM)	Endothelium, platelets	Sialyl Lewis[x] and [a], PSGL
Immunoglobulins	ICAM-1	Endothelium and certain leukocyte cell lines	LFA-1, Mac-1, CD11c/CD18
	ICAM-2	Endothelium, platelets	LFA-1, Mac-1, CD11c/CD18
	ICAM-3	Leukocytes	LFA-1, Mac-1, CD11c/CD18
	VCAM-1	Endothelium, smooth muscle	$\alpha_4\beta_1$ (VLA-4)
	PECAM-1 (CD31)	Endothelium, platelets, leukocytes	
Mucin-like	PSGL-1	Leukocytes	Sialyl Lewis[x] and [a]
Secreted			
Cytokine	Interleukin-1	Monocytes, smooth muscle	IL-1 receptor
	Tumor-necrosis factor	Monocytes, smooth muscle	TNF-receptor
	MCP-1	Endothelium, smooth muscle	MCP-1 receptor
	M-CSF	Endothelium, smooth muscle	M-CSF receptor
Lipid	PAF	Endothelium, leukocytes	PAF receptor

ELAM-1: endothelial leukocyte adhesion molecule-1; PECAM-1: platelet-EC adhesion molecule-1; LFA-1: leukocyte function associated antigen-1; IL-1:interleukin-1; TNF: tumor-necrosis factor; MCP-1: monocyte chemoattractant protein-1; M-CSF: macrophage-colony stimulating factor; PAF: platelet activating factor; PSGL: P-selectin glycoprotein ligand.

during atherogenesis by chemoattractive chemokines. MCP-1 plays a major role. Mice lacking MCP-1 or its receptor, C–C chemokine receptor-2 (CCR-2), develop less atherosclerosis and show reduced accumulation of mononuclear phagocytes in the arterial intima [30,31]. Synthesized by the vascular wall in response to interferon-γ and produced in turn by the same T-cells, chemokines including interferon-inducible protein-10 (IP-10), monokine induced by interferon-γ (MIG), and interferon-inducible T-cell alpha chemoattractant (I-TAC) likely orchestrate T-cell migration in the intima [32]. Additionally, recent studies in mice with targeted deletion of the 5-lipoxygenase (5-LO) gene suggest non-cell specific chemoattraction by the 5-LO product leukotrienes (LT), especially LTB$_4$, in atherogenesis [33]. Once accumulated in the intima, mononuclear leukocytes transform into active macrophages through a process supported by the cytokine M-CSF, a mitogen that activates monocytes

and induces their differentiation. Produced by EC and smooth muscle cells, M-CSF localizes in human and experimental atheroma [34].

Macrophages can internalize oxidized lipids, thus leading to the formation of lipid peroxides that facilitate the accumulation of cholesterol esters [35]. Several specialized "scavenger" receptors unrelated to the classical low-density lipoprotein (LDL) receptor whose expression is elicited in part by M-CSF, mediate lipid internalization [36]. Scavenger receptors preferentially bind the protein moiety of LDL and possibly of very-LDL (VLDL), modified variously by oxidation, acetylation, and glycation during atherogenesis. Such receptors include the scavenger receptor A family [37], CD36 [38], CD68/macrosialin [39], Scavenger receptor Class B, member 1 (SCARB1) [40], and the newly cloned receptor for OxLDL (LOX-1, first found on EC) [41] and Scavenger Receptor for Phosphatidylserine and Oxidized Lipoprotein (SR-PSOX) [42].

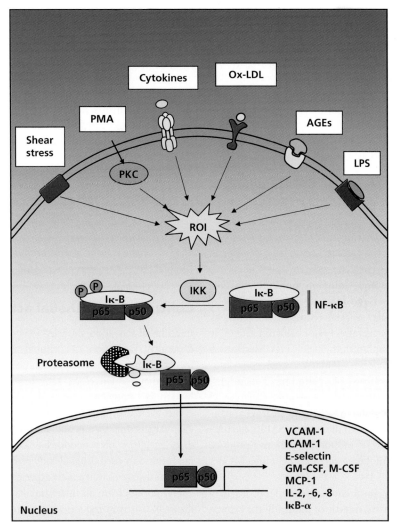

Figure 2.5 The NF-κB system of transcription factors comprises a series of heterodimeric molecules (monomers including Rel-A/p65, p50, p52, Rel-B, c-Rel) normally sequestered in the cytoplasm and bound to an inhibitor (I-κB). Upon the influence of inflammatory cytokines and likely other stimuli able to activate EC, the generation of intracellular ROS (mostly H$_2$O$_2$) leads to the binding of I-κB to ubiquitin, and the proteolytic degradation of I-κB. Heterodimers freed from the inhibitor can migrate into the nucleus, where they bind specific recognition (consen- sus) sequences in the promoter region of a variety of genes of endothelial activation, resulting in increased transcription of the respective genes. Partial overlap, or redundancy, of cytokine properties, e.g., the similarity of endothelial activation induced by IL-1 and TNF, results from likely activation by various stimuli, i.e., different cytokines. The fact that multiple genes, e.g., E-selectin, VCAM-1, and ICAM-1, animate when even a single cytokine activates the system epitomizes "pleiotropy," another property of inflammatory cytokines.

Thus, macrophages become "foam cells," the typical component of the fatty streak, by accumulating lipid droplets.

The subsequent evolution of the fatty streak likely depends on continuing inflammation. Focal chemoattraction of increased levels of monocytes and lymphocytes sustains continued lipid deposition and thickening of the vessel wall, ultimately resulting in focal macrophage apoptosis, matrix accumulation, and plaque growth.

Triggers of lesion development

The retention of lipoproteins, especially LDL and modified LDL, in the arterial intima triggers increased expression of adhesion molecules and pro-inflammatory cytokines at lesion-prone sites [43]. Proteoglycans that interact preferentially with apolipoprotein B (apoB)-containing atherogenic lipoproteins also participate importantly in this process [44]. In the sub-endothelial space, lipoproteins undergo several modifications including self-aggregation [45], complex formation with proteoglycans [46], immune complex formation [47] and degradation by hydrolytic enzymes [48,49], and oxidative modifications that enhance their uptake by macrophages *in vitro*. Oxidized LDL have undergone by far the most extensive study [50–52]. Oxidized lipoproteins, specifically LDL, contain distinctive oxidized phospholipids and biologically active determinants; some react with specific antibodies [53], and thus have been detected in the atheroma [54]. Such oxidative lipoproteins can induce expression of adhesion molecules, chemokines, and other pro-inflammatory cytokines by various vascular cellular components and by monocytes. Specifically, lysophosphatidyl choline (LPC) and lysophosphatic acid (LPA) derivatives [25,55], the valeryl-, glutaryl-, and epoxy-isoprostane derivatives of palmitoyl arachidonyl phosphatidyl choline (PAPC), stearoyl arachidonyl phosphatidyl choline (SAPC), and stearoyl arachidonyl phosphatidyl ethanolamine (SAPE) all stimulate EC binding of monocytes [56] and produce monocyte chemotactic factors, including MCP-1 and IL-8 [57].

Additionally, local shear stress alterations may promote or repress, directly or indirectly, the expression of adhesion molecules [58]. Physiological levels of laminar shear stress modulate the expression of pathophysiologically relevant genes including platelet-derived growth factors (PDGF)-A and PDGF-B, transforming growth factor-β (TGF β), fibrinolytic factors such as tPA, and adhesion molecules such as ICAM-1 and VCAM-1. Many of these genes share a common shear stress response element (SSRE) as well as binding sites for NF-κB [59]. Steady laminar shear stress but not turbulent shear stress differentially regulates genes relevant to atherogenesis, increasing the expression of inducible cyclooxygenase-2 (COX-2), manganese-dependent superoxide dismutase (Mn-SOD), and the endothelial isoform of nitric oxide synthase (eNOS). Notably, the products of such genes exert

potent anti-adhesive, anti-inflammatory, and anti-oxidant effects [60].

Although LDL levels contribute importantly to atherogenesis, lipid lowering does not eliminate acute coronary events. Under conditions of increased atherosclerotic risk, other triggers may act through similar mechanisms, independent of the lipid profile. Such triggers include AGE, which accelerate in diabetic hyperglycemia and in end-stage renal disease; lipoprotein(a), a modified LDL particle associated with atherosclerotic lesions; high levels of homocysteine achieved in homocystinuria or in cases of enzymatic defects (either genetic or acquired) of the homocysteine biosynthetic pathway; oxidative stress; and infective agents such as *Herpes* viruses or *Chlamydia pneumoniae* (see Chapters 5–11).

Control of endothelial activation

Endothelial activation, modeled *in vitro* by cytokine-dependent activation of cultured EC, results in increased expression of adhesion molecules and soluble mediators. Therefore, activated EC provide a model for studying early molecular intracellular events elicited by atherogenic stimuli, and also provide targets for therapeutic interventions. Several drug categories affect endothelial activation, including commonly used drugs already proven effective in vascular disease as well as new experimental agents.

NO donors form an interesting category of such drugs. NO actively reduces the transcription of pro-inflammatory, pro-atherogenic genes by decreasing the expression of adhesion molecules and thus reducing leukocyte adhesion to arteries [61]. Exogenously administered through different donors, NO reduces mononuclear leukocyte adhesion to human EC challenged *in vitro* with inflammatory cytokines, i.e., IL-1 or TNF-α, by counteracting VCAM-1 expression [62]. Such inhibition occurs transcriptionally by interfering with the NF-κB signaling pathway through a cyclic guanosin-monophosphate (GMP)-independent mechanism. NO also inhibits NF-κB by inducing its endogenous inhibitor, IκBα [63]. Thus, tonic synthesis of NO, i.e., induced by shear stress, may contribute to the physiological anti-adhesive state of the normal endothelium. On the other hand, endothelial dysfunction, characterized by impaired

NO production, also involves augmented expression of endothelial adhesion molecules and monocyte chemoattractants. Therefore, therapeutic interventions aimed at counteracting endothelial activation and atherogenesis potentially may restore availability of NO.

Statins improve the bioavailability of NO in at least two ways. Blocking geranylgeranylation of the small guanosin-triphosphate (GTP)-binding Ras-like protein Rho [64] post-transcriptionally augments eNOS. Furthermore, statins rapidly activate the serine/threonine kinase Akt, leading in turn to phosphorylation, increased activity of eNOS, and enhanced NO production [65]. Such action suggests that statins influence all stages of atherosclerosis. Drugs that interfere with the renin-angiotensin system also repress endothelial activation, likely through effects mediated by NF-κB [66], and may elucidate cardiovascular benefits not explained fully by reduced blood pressure in trials involving such drugs [67]. Administration of n-3 (omega-3) polyunsaturated fatty acids (PUFA) may provide a useful therapeutic strategy as well. The n-3 PUFA associate epidemiologically with cardiovascular protection, and likely act at various levels of atherosclerosis and its clinical consequences. By reducing VCAM-1 expression elicited *in vitro* by cytokines such as IL-1, n-3 PUFA may act directly on the vessel wall [68,69]. Oleic acid displays qualitatively similar anti-inflammatory and anti-adhesive properties [70,71]. The examples discussed above highlight possible preventive interventions in vascular disease that might interfere with molecular mechanisms during early atherogenesis.

References

1 The Scandinavian Simvastatin Survival Study Group. Randomised trial of cholesterol lowering in 4444 patients with coronary heart disease: the Scandinavian Simvastatin Survival Study (4S). *Lancet* 1994;344:1383–1389.

2 Cholesterol and Recurrent Events (CARE) Trial Investigators. The effect of pravastatin on coronary events after myocardial infarction in patients with average cholesterol levels. *N Engl J Med* 1996;335:1001–1009.

3 Expert Panel on Detection, Evaluation, and Treatment of High Blood Cholesterol in Adults. Executive Summary of the Third Report of the National Cholesterol Education Program (NCEP) Expert Panel on Detection, Evaluation,

and Treatment of High Blood Cholesterol in Adults (Adult Treatment Panel III). *J Am Med Assoc* 2001; 285:2486–2497.

4 Ross R. Atherosclerosis – an inflammatory disease. *N Engl J Med* 1999;340:115–126.

5 Libby P, Ridker P, Maseri A. Inflammation and atherosclerosis. *Circulation* 2002;105:1135–1143.

6 Glagov S, Zarins C, Giddens D, et al. Hemodynamics and atherosclerosis. Insights and perspectives gained from studies of human arteries. *Arch Pathol Lab Med* 1988; 112:1018–1031.

7 Gimbrone MA, Kume N, Cybulsky MI. Vascular endothelial dysfunction and the pathogenesis of atherosclerosis. In: Weber P, Leaf A, eds. *Atherosclerosis Reviews*. New York: Raven Press; 1993.

8 Stary HC, Chandler AB, Dinsmore RE. A definition of advanced types of atherosclerotic lesions and a histological classification of atherosclerosis: a report from the Committee on Vascular Lesions of the Council on Atherosclerosis, American Heart Association. *Circulation* 1995;92:1355–1374.

9 Napoli C, D'Armiento F, Mancini F, et al. Fatty streak formation occurs in human fetal aortas and is greatly enhanced by maternal hypercholesterolemia. *J Clin Invest* 1997;100:2680–2690.

10 Stary HC. Macrophage, macrophage-foam cell, and eccentric intimal thickening in the coronary arteries of young children. *Atherosclerosis* 1987;64:91–108.

11 Gerrity R. The role of monocyte in atherogenesis. *Am J Pathol* 1981;103:181–200.

12 Stary H, Chandler A, Glagov S. A definition of initial, fatty streak, and intermediate lesions of atherosclerosis: a report from the Committee on Vascular Lesions of the Council on Atherosclerosis, American Heart Association. *Circulation* 1994;89:2462–2478.

13 Faggiotto A, Ross R, Harker L. Studies of hypercholesterolemia in the nonhuman primate. I. Changes that lead to fatty streak formation. *Arteriosclerosis* 1984;4:323–340.

14 Faggiotto A, Ross R. Studies of hypercholesterolemia in the nonhuman primate. II. Fatty streak conversion to fibrous plaque. *Arteriosclerosis* 1984;4:341–356.

15 Springer TA. Traffic signals for lymphocyte recirculation and leukocyte emigration: the multistep paradigm. *Cell* 1994;76:301–314.

16 Carlos TM, Harlan JM. Leukocyte-endothelial adhesion molecules. *Blood* 1994;84:2068–2101.

17 Vora DK, Fang ZT, Liva SM, et al. Induction of P-selectin by oxidized lipoproteins. Separate effects on synthesis and surface expression. *Circ Res* 1997;80:810–818.

18 Johnson RC, Chapman SM, Dong ZM, et al. Absence of P-selectin delays fatty streak formation in mice. *J Clin Invest* 1997;99:1037–1043.

19 Dong Z, Chapman S, Brown A, et al. The combined role of P- and E-selectins in atherosclerosis. *J Clin Invest* 1998;102.

20 Cybulsky MI, Gimbrone MA. Endothelial expression of a mononuclear leukocyte adhesion molecule during atherogenesis. *Science* 1991;251:788–791.

21 Li H, Cybulsky MI, Gimbrone MA, et al. An atherogenic diet rapidly induces VCAM-1, a cytokine regulatable mononuclear leukocyte adhesion molecule, in rabbit endothelium. *Arterioscler Thromb* 1993;13:197–204.

22 Iiyama K, Hajra L, Iiyama M, et al. Patterns of vascular cell adhesion molecule-1 and intercellular adhesion molecule-1 expression in rabbit and mouse atherosclerotic lesions and at sites predisposed to lesion formation. *Circ Res* 1999;85:199–207.

23 Cybulsky MI, Iiyama K, Li H, et al. Major role for VCAM-1 but not ICAM-1, in early atherosclerosis. *J Clin Invest* 2001;107:1255–1262.

24 Berliner J, Territo M, Sevanian A, et al. Minimally modified low density lipoprotein stimulates monocyte endothelial interactions. *J Clin Invest* 1990;85:1260–1266.

25 Kume N, Cybulsky MI, Gimbrone MA. Lysophosphatidylcholine, a component of atherogenic lipoproteins, induces mononuclear leukocyte adhesion molecules in cultured human and rabbit arterial endothelial cells. *J Clin Invest* 1992;90:1138–1144.

26 Schmidt AM, Hori O, Chen JX, et al. Advanced glycation endproducts interacting with their endothelial receptor induce expression of vascular cell adhesion molecule-1 (VCAM-1) in cultured human endothelial cells and in mice. A potential mechanism for the accelerated vasculopathy of diabetes. *J Clin Invest* 1995;96:1395–1403.

27 Basta G, Lazzerini G, Massaro M, et al. Advanced glycation end products activate endothelium through signal-transduction receptor RAGE: a mechanism for amplification of inflammatory responses. *Circulation* 2002; 105:816–822.

28 Collins T. Biology of disease: endothelial nuclear factor-κB and the initiation of the atherosclerotic lesion. *Lab Invest* 1993;88:499–508.

29 Brand K, Page S, Rogler G, et al. Activated transcription factor nuclear factor-kappa B is present in the atherosclerotic lesion. *J Clin Invest* 1996; 97:1715–1722.

30 Boring L, Gosling J, Cleary M, et al. Decreased lesion formation in CCR2-/-mice reveals a role for chemokines in the initiation of atherosclerosis. *Nature* 1998; 394:894–897.

31 Gu L, Okada Y, Clinton S, et al. Absence of monocyte chemoattractant protein-1 reduces atherosclerosis in low-density lipoprotein-deficient mice. *Mol Cel* 1998;2:275–281.

32 Mach F, Sauty A, Iarossi A, et al. Differential expression of three T lymphocyte-activating CXC chemokines by human atheroma associated cells. *J Clin Invest* 1999;104:1041–1050.

33 Mehrabian M, Allayee H, Wong J, et al. Identification of 5-lipoxygenase as a major gene contributing to atherosclerosis susceptibility in mice. *Circ Res* 2002;91:120–126.

34 Clinton SK, Underwood R, Sherman ML, et al. Macrophage-colony stimulating factor gene expression in vascular cells and in experimental and human atherosclerosis. *Am J Path* 1992;140:301–316.

35 Ross R. The pathogenesis of atherosclerosis: a perspective for the 1990s. *Nature* 1993;362:801–809.

36 Qiao JH, Tripathi J, Mishia NK, et al. Role of machrophage colony-stimulating factor in atherosclerosis: studies of osteopetrotic mice. *Am J Pathol* 1997;150: 1687–1699.

37 Krieger M, Acton S, Ashkenas J, et al. Molecular flypaper, host defense, and atherosclerosis. Structure, binding properties, and functions of macrophage scavenger receptors. *J Biol Chem* 1993; 268:4569–4572.

38 Endemann G, Stanton L, Madden K, et al. CD36 is a receptor for oxidized low density lipoprotein. *J Biol Chem* 1993;268:11811–11816.

39 Ramprasad MP, Terpstra V, Kondratenko N, et al. Cell surface expression of mouse macrosialin and human CD68 and their role as macrophage receptors for oxidized low density lipoprotein. *Proc Natl Acad Sci USA* 1996;93:14833–14838.

40 Acton S, Rigotti A, Landschulz KT, et al. Identification of scavenger receptor SR-BI as a high density lipoprotein receptor. *Science* 1996;271: 518–520.

41 Sawamura T, Kume N, Aoyama T, et al. An endothelial receptor for oxidized low-density lipoprotein. *Nature* 1997;386:73–77.

42 Minami M, Kume N, Shimaoka T, et al. Expression of SR-PSOX, a novel cell-surface scavenger receptor for phosphatidylserine and oxidized LDL in human atherosclerotic lesions. *Atheroscl Thromb Vasc Biol* 2000; 2001:1796–1800.

43 Williams KJ, Tabas I. The response-to-retention theory of early atherogenesis. *Arterioscler Thromb Vasc Biol* 1995;15:551.

44 Skalen K, Gustafsson M, Rydberg EK, et al. Subendothelial retention of atherogenic lipoproteins in early atherosclerosis. *Nature* 2002;417:750–754.

45 Khoo JC, Miller E, McLoughlin P, et al. Enhanced macrophage uptake of low density lipoprotein after self-aggregation. *Arteriosclerosis* 1988;8:348–358.

46 Hurt E, Camejo G. Effect of arterial proteoglycans on the interaction of LDL with human monocyte-derived macrophages. *Atherosclerosis* 1987;67:115–126.

47 Klimov AN, Denisenko AD, Popov AV, et al. Lipoprotein-antibody immune complexes: their catabolism and role in foam cell formation. *Atherosclerosis* 1985;58:1–15.

48 Heinecke J, Suits A, Aviram M, et al. Phagocytosis of lipase-aggregated low density lipoprotein promotes macrophage foam cell formation: sequential morphological and biochemical events. *Arterioscler Thromb* 1991; 11:1643–1651.

49 Bhakdi S, Dorweiler B, Kirchmann R, et al. On the pathogenesis of atherosclerosis: enzymatic transformation of human low density lipoprotein to an atherogenic moiety. *J Exp Med* 1995;182:1959–1971.

50 Parthasarathy S, Rankin SM. Role of oxidized low density lipoprotein in atherogenesis. *Prog Lipid Res* 1992;31.

51 Steinberg D. Oxidative modification of LDL and atherogenesis. *Circulation* 1997;95:1062–1071.

52 Kita T, Kume N, Minami M, et al. Role of oxidized LDL in atherosclerosis. *Ann NY Acad Sci* 2001;947:199–205.

53 Friedman P, Horkko S, Steinberg D, et al. Correlation of antiphospholipid antibody recognition with the structure of synthetic oxidized phospholipids: importance of Schiff base formation and Aldol condensation. *J Biol Chem* 2001;14:14.

54 Witzum JL, Berliner J. Oxidized phospholipids and isoprostanes in atherosclerosis. *Curr Opin Lipidol* 1998; 9:441–448.

55 Rizza C, Leitinger N, Yue J, et al. Lysophosphatidic acid as a regulator of endothelial/leukocyte interaction. *Lab Invest* 1999;79:1227–1235.

56 Leitinger N, Tyner TR, Oslund L, et al. Structurally similar oxidized phospholipids differentially regulate endothelial binding of monocytes and neutrophils. *Proc Natl Acad Sci USA* 1999;96:12010–12015.

57 Subbanagounder G, Wong JW, Lee H, et al. Epoxyisoprostane and epoxycyclopentenone phospholipids regulate monocyte chemotactic protein-1 and interleukin-8 synthesis. Formation of these oxidized phospholipids in response to interleukin-1 beta. *J Biol Chem* 2001;277:7271–7281.

58 Gimbrone MA, Topper JN, Nagel T, et al. Endothelial dysfunction, hemodynamic forces, and atherogenesis. *Ann NY Acad Sci* 2000; 902: 230–239.

59 Gimbrone MA, Nagel T, Topper JN. Biomechanical activation: an emerging paradigm in endothelial adhesion biology. *J Clin Invest* 1997;99.

60 Topper JN, Cai J, Falb D, et al. Identification of vascular endothelial genes differentially responsive to fluid mechanical stimuli: cyclooxygenase-2, manganese superoxide dismutase, and endothelial cell nitric oxide synthase are selectively up-regulated by steady laminar shear stress. *Proc Natl Acad Sci USA* 1996; 93: 10417–10422.

61 Lefer AM, Ma XL. Decreased basal nitric oxide release in hypercholesterolemia increases neutrophil adherence to rabbit coronary artery endothelium. *Arterioscler Thromb* 1993;13:771–776.

62 De Caterina R, Libby P, Peng H-B, et al. Nitric oxide decreases cytokine-induced endothelial activation. *J Clin Invest* 1995;96:60–68.

63 Peng H-B, Libby P, Liao JK. Induction and stabilization of I kappa B alpha by nitric oxide mediates inhibition of NF-kappa B. *J Biol Chem* 1995;270:14214–14219.

64 Laufs U, Liao JK. Targeting Rho in cardiovascular disease. *Circ Res* 2000;87:526–528.

65 Kureishi Y, Luo Z, Shiojima I, et al. The HMG-CoA reductase inhibitor simvastatin activates the protein kinase Akt and promotes angiogenesis in normocholesterolemic animals. *Nat Med* 2000;6:1004–1010.

66 De Caterina R, Manes C. Inflammation in early atherogenesis: impact of ACE-inhibition. *Eur Heart J Suppl* 2003;5(Suppl A):A15–A24.

67 Heart Outcomes Prevention Evaluation (HOPE) Study Group. Heart Outcomes Prevention Evaluation (HOPE): main results. In: American Heart Association 72nd *Scientific Sessions – Special Session IV – Clinical Trial Results – November 10 1999*. Atlanta, Georgia; 1999.

68 De Caterina R, Cybulsky MI, Clinton SK, et al. Omega-3 fatty acids and endothelial leukocyte adhesion molecules. *Prostagl Leukot Ess Fatty Acid* 1995;52:192–195.

69 Massaro M, Carluccio MA, Bonfrate C, et al. The double bond in unsaturated fatty acids is the necessary and sufficient requirement for the inhibition of expression of endothelial leukocyte adhesion molecules through interference with nuclear factor-kappa B activation. *Lipids* 1999;34:S213–S214.

70 Carluccio MA, Massaro M, Bonfrate C, et al. Oleic acid inhibits endothelial activation: a direct vascular antiatherogenic mechanism of a nutritional component in the mediterranean diet. *Arterioscler Thromb Vasc Biol* 1999;19:220–228.

71 Massaro M, Carluccio MA, Paolicchi A, et al. Mechanisms for reduction of endothelial activation by oleate: inhibition of nuclear factor-kappa B through antioxidant effects. *Prostagl Leukot Ess Fatty Acid* 2002 ;67:175–181.

72 Joris I, Zand T, Nunnari JJ, et al. Studies on the pathogenesis of atherosclerosis. I. Adhesion and emigration of mononuclear cells in the aorta of hypercholesterolemic rats. *Am J Pathol* 1983; 113: 341–358.

CHAPTER 3

Mechanisms of plaque progression and complications

Raffaele De Caterina, MD, PhD, *Antonella Zampolli*, DBiol, PhD, *Serena Del Turco*, DBiol, PhD, & *Peter Libby*, MD

General morphology of the atheroma

Several different variables and developmental stages influence the transformation of the fatty streak into a more complex lesion and ultimately into an athero-sclerotic plaque, a process that results in a large variety of plaque morphologies. The histological classification and nomenclature proposed by the American Heart Association's Committee of Vascular Lesion Evaluation of the Council on Atherosclerosis implies a linear chronology of plaque progression not quite ascertained (Table 3.1) [1]. Indeed, coronary patients tend to have more than one type of lesion, and transition among the different stages does not always appear linear. In addition, plaque growth often seems discontinuous, and phases of sudden progression may alternate with long periods of stability or minimal growth [2,3]. Generally, the morphology of atherosclerotic lesions comprises three main categories: fibroatheromatous, fibrous, and complicated plaques.

Fibroatheromatous plaques

Although the fatty streak (see Chapter 2) may regress, a persistent inflammatory milieu, i.e., continuous recruitment of inflammatory cells and lipid deposition, eventually results in the accumulation of extracellular lipids within the lesion. Foam cells – derived mostly from monocyte–macrophages attracted from the circulating blood, but also from

Table 3.1 American Heart Association (AHA) classification of atherosclerotic lesions (from Refs [1,14]).

	AHA nomenclature	*Corresponding terms*	
Type I	Initial lesion		
Type IIa	Progression-prone type II lesion	Fatty dot, fatty streak	Early lesions
Type IIb	Progression-resistant type II lesion		
Type III	Intermediate lesion (preatheroma)		
Type IV	Atheroma	Atheromatous plaque, fibrolipid	
Type Va	Fibroatheroma/type V lesion	plaque, fibrous plaque, plaque	
Type Vb	Calcific lesion (type VII lesion)	Calcified plaque	Advanced lesions,
Type Vc	Fibrotic lesions (type VIII lesion)	Fibrous plaque	raised lesions
Type VI	Lesion with surface defect and/or thrombotic deposit	Complicated lesion, complicated plaque	

Lumen

Lumen

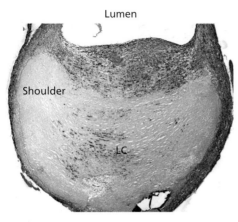

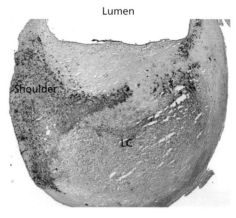

SMC × 20

MΦ × 20

Figure 3.1 An example of an atherosclerotic plaque with a large lipid core (LC). The section on the left is immunostained (in red) with an antibody against smooth muscle cells (SMC), while the serial section on the right shows staining for macrophages (MΦ) in red. Notice the complementarity of the areas stained with SMC co-localizing, with the fibrous cap, i.e., the layers of collagen separating the lipid core (LC) from the lumen, and the areas stained with macrophages, co-localizing with the LC and the shoulder region of the plaque. The most intense staining for macrophages is in the shoulder area, while a weaker staining is present in the LC, probably in relation to the lipid gruel. Original magnification ×20. (Courtesy of Dr. Galina Sukhova, Brigham and Women's Hospital, Boston, MA).

smooth muscle cells (SMC) replicating in the intima of the developing plaque – may undergo programmed cell death, or apoptosis, releasing stored lipids and creating a self-sustained cycle of events that determines the formation of the so-called *lipid* or *necrotic core* [4,5] (Figure 3.1). The lipid core contains extracellular lipids that derive from foam cell apoptosis and intimal infiltration of circulating low-density lipoproteins (LDL). Extracellular lipids, i.e., cholesterol, cholesteryl esters, and cholesterol crystals as well as other molecules secreted by resident cells such as tissue factor (TF) derived from macrophages, confer thrombogenicity to the lipid core [6]. The collagen-rich *fibrous cap* arises from the secretory activity of SMC and separates the lipid core from the circulating blood. SMC secrete a matrix rich in collagen, elastin, and proteoglycans in a regulated fashion that determines the amount of matrix deposited and the morphology of the cap. SMC reside in a type I collagen-rich matrix in the fibrous cap; the thickness of the fibrous cap likely determines plaque stability. Foam cells and T-lymphocytes that sustain inflammatory processes inside the plaque localize near the fibrous cap. Interestingly, many layers of fibrous tissue may contain more than one lipid core, thus forming a multi-layered fibroatheromatous plaque. Calcium deposits are found scattered in either the

lipid core of the lesion or SMC organelles [7]. The fibroatheromatous plaque may evolve into a fibrous or complicated plaque.

Fibrous plaques

Although current understanding suggests that fibrous plaques evolve from fibroatheromatous plaques, the relationship between them remains unclear (Figure 3.2). Indeed fibrous plaques, which represent the majority of plaques observed at autopsy, contain little or no lipid core [8]. Some fibrous caps overlie large accumulations of intimal calcium, with minimal or absent lipid necrotic core. It remains unclear whether such lesions derive from fibrous lesions or represent the evolution of disrupted plaques after healing and calcification [9].

Complicated plaques

Complicated plaques contain superimposed thrombi, either occluding or non-occluding. Such plaques can undergo *plaque rupture*, or *fissuring*, i.e., documented physical discontinuity of the cap, which connects the lipid core to the lumen [10] (Figure 3.3). Autopsy studies show that 70–80% of coronary thrombi result from plaque rupture. Thrombus propagation occurs mainly upstream from the site of rupture [11,12].

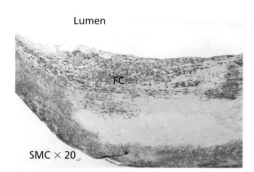

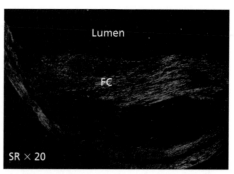

Figure 3.2 Serial sections of a prevalently fibrous plaque, immunostained in red with an antibody against smooth muscle cells (SMC) |(left panel), or stained with Sirius Red (SR) for type I–III interstitial collagen fibers and photographed under polarized light (right panel). FC denotes the fibrous cap, which is particularly thick in this case. Notice the abundance of SMC and interstitial collagen in the FC. Original magnification ×20. (Courtesy of Dr. Galina Sukhova, Brigham and Women's Hospital, Boston, MA).

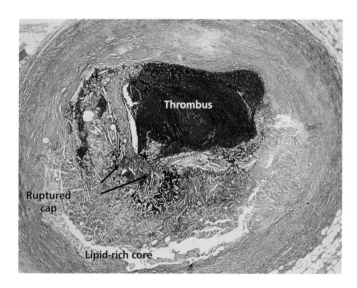

Figure 3.3 A ruptured plaque. The image shows the fissuring of fibrous cap in a plaque causing a tight stenosis. Fissuring (arrows) allows the sudden contact of the circulating blood with the highly thrombogenic content of the lipid core. Trichromic staining. Original magnification ×20. (Courtesy of Dr. Erling Falk, Skejby Hospital, Aarhus, Denmark).

Thrombosis also occurs in the absence of frank plaque rupture, sometimes with disruption of the endothelial lining (Figure 3.4) and usually associated with fibrous plaques or less frequently with fibroatheromatous plaques that contain a major fibrous component. Such *plaque erosions* occur more frequently in young individuals, especially women, and also in patients with hypertriglyceridemia and diabetes. Erosion may participate in the development of approximately 20–40% of coronary thrombi [13]. A minor, undefined fraction of plaque complications result from erosions near calcified nodules [14].

Intraplaque hemorrhage, a complication often observed in advanced coronary atherosclerotic lesions, usually associates with ruptured plaques and occurs more frequently in fibroatheromas with cores in late-stage necrosis or with thin caps. The extent of intraplaque hemorrhage correlates with increased risk of plaque instability [15].

Molecular mechanisms of lesion progression

Accumulating macrophage-derived foam cells characteristic of the fatty streak foreshadow its evolution toward a more advanced atherosclerotic lesion that results from ongoing lipid deposition, SMC accumulations that migrate from the media and replicate in the intima, and their elaboration of

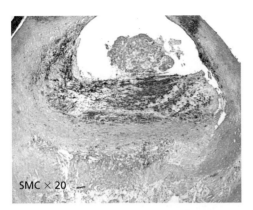
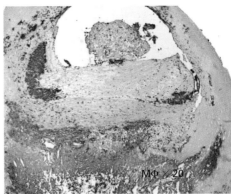

Figure 3.4 Plaque erosion. Two serial sections from the same plaque show thrombosis in the vessel lumen in the absence of a clear fissuring. The section on the left is immunostained with an antibody against smooth muscle cells (SMC), while the section on the right with an antibody against macrophages (MΦ). Note the thick fibrous cap, rich in collagen and SMC, and poor in macrophages in the area of erosion with superimposed thrombosis. The diagnosis of erosion is only possible by excluding plaque fissuring in serial sections of the same plaque. Original magnification ×20. (Courtesy of Dr. Galina Sukhova, Brigham and Women's Hospital, Boston, MA).

extracellular matrix. Inflammatory mechanisms likely participate in all such processes. Endothelial activation presumably persists due to the expression of adhesion molecules in the evolving lesion, particularly in the microvasculature, where they favor leukocyte recruitment [16,17]. Such expression of adhesion molecules also occurs on SMC, mediating cell–cell and cell–matrix interaction.

Other changes in endothelial function also contribute to lesion progression. Normally functioning endothelial cells (EC) synthesize anti-thrombotic mediators such as prostacyclin and nitric oxide (NO), express on their surface heparin-like glycosaminoglycans and thrombomodulin, and contribute to the fibrinolytic balance by producing plasminogen activators (see Chapter 1). The loss of normal endothelial function on the endothelium overlying an evolving plaque may interfere with such mechanisms, eventually resulting in platelet adhesion and mural microthrombosis [18].

Moreover, inflammatory phenomena within the plaque likely play a prominent role in plaque progression. The expression of adhesion molecules exemplifies the smouldering inflammation that accompanies lesion growth.

Inflammatory mechanisms in plaque progression

Inflammatory mechanisms involved in atherosclerosis in general and lesion progression in particular typify chronic inflammatory response, wherein macrophages and T-lymphocytes, the major cellular participants, synthesize an array of mediators responsible for the fibro-proliferative mechanisms observed at this stage.

One such mediator, platelet-derived growth factor (PDGF), promotes SMC chemoattraction, proliferation, and synthesis of extracellular matrix [19]. PDGF is a homodimer or heterodimer deriving from the combination of two polypeptide moieties, termed A and B chains. Many cell types in the fatty streak can express PDGF, and EC produce both isoforms. Vascular SMC, at least *in vitro*, express only the A chain; macrophages express PDGF and a variety of other growth factors such as heparin-binding epidermal growth factor (HB-EGF), fibroblast growth factor (FGF), and insulin-like growth factors (IGF) [20]. Inflammatory cytokines regulate growth factor expression. For example, interleukin (IL)-1 increases the production of PDGF-A chain by human vascular SMC and also augments basic FGF expression by human SMC, inducing both SMC and fibroblast proliferation [21,22].

Transforming growth factor (TGF)-β, a potent inducer of collagenolysis, also promotes SMC proliferation. The T-lymphocyte-derived cytokine interferon (IFN)-γ and heparin-like glycosaminoglycans inhibit both SMC proliferation and matrix secretion. As discussed earlier, SMC proliferation and matrix deposition likely influence plaque stability,

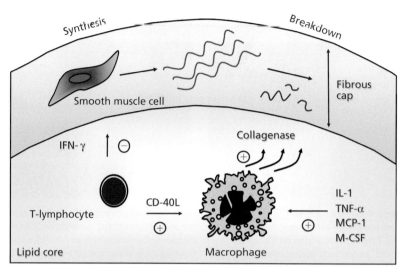

Figure 3.5 Matrix metabolism and the integrity of the plaque fibrous cap. Pathways of synthesis and degradation of the extracellular matrix components within the plaque, influencing plaque stability, are shown together with mediators and cellular sources. (Adapted from Ref. [48]) See text for additional details. IFN-γ: interferon-γ MCP-1: monocyte chemoattractant protein-1; M-CSF: macrophage-colony stimulating factor.

which depends upon the balance between proliferative and anti-proliferative stimuli on the one hand and secretory/anti-secretory stimuli on the other (Figure 3.5).

A similar situation likely occurs during calcium deposition. Action on vascular wall cells by TGF family members may promote mineralization of the atheroma by producing a molecule termed bone morphogenetic protein [23]. On the other hand, animal studies have shown that macrophages within the atheroma probably act like osteoclasts, the cells responsible for bone reabsorption [24]. Impaired balance between calcification and reabsorption can determine the evolution of extended calcifications.

T-lymphocytes may contribute to plaque growth by not only synthesizing soluble cytokines but also by expressing CD40 ligand (CD40L, CD154), a cell surface protein and immunomodulatory cytokine homologous to tumor necrosis factor (TNF), the role of which in atherosclerosis development remains unclear. CD40 ligation occurs in the presence of activated CD4$^+$ T-cells and elicits *in vitro* the expression of a wide array of inflammatory mediators [25] including TF, collagenases, and matrix metalloproteinase (MMP)-11, all critical to plaque thrombogenicity and instability [26,27] as well as vascular endothelial growth factor (VEGF) [28,29] and cyclooxygenase-2 (COX-2) [30], which potentially contribute to plaque neovascularization (see below). In atherosclerosis-susceptible mice, antibody blockade of CD40L reduces lesion development and inhibits the growth of pre-existing atheromas [31,32]. However, bone marrow transplantation experiments suggest that the progression of atherosclerosis does not require leukocyte-derived CD40L [33]. Studies on human plaque specimens demonstrated that CD40 and CD40L expression localizes mainly in the intima, notably in the endothelium that lines the arterial lumen, in microvessel EC [28,34] and in platelets [34]. Recent results from the Dallas Heart Study did not positively associate sCD40L with atherosclerotic risk factors or subclinical atherosclerosis, suggesting that any role for sCD40L as a predictor of events likely occurs in the context of atherothrombosis-related clinical conditions [35].

Overall, cytokines and growth factors can control lesion progression by recruiting inflammatory cells and directing the expression of growth-regulatory genes, which in turn regulate intimal cell proliferation, collagen deposition, and lesion mineralization.

Mechanisms of plaque complications

Most acute manifestations of atherosclerosis, i.e., unstable angina, acute myocardial infarction, and

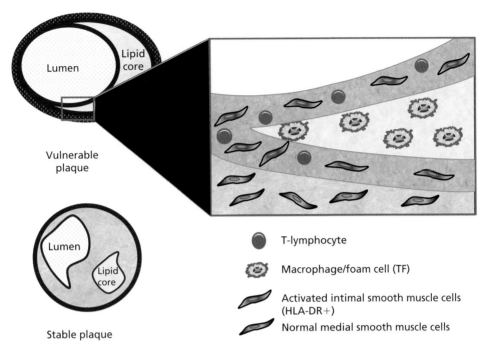

T-lymphocyte

Macrophage/foam cell (TF)

Activated intimal smooth muscle cells
(HLA-DR+)

Normal medial smooth muscle cells

Figure 3.6 Characteristics of the stable vs the unstable (vulnerable) plaque. This diagram shows the two extremes of plaque stability. The upper panel depicts a prototypic unstable plaque with minimal lumen reduction, and therefore poorly appreciated at angiography. This plaque usually has a large lipid core and a thin fibrous cap, particularly prone to rupture in the shoulder region (magnified in the right hand panel) where inflammatory cells (macrophages) producing matrix-degrading enzymes accumulate. The lower panel depicts a prototypic stable plaque, usually with a thick fibrous cap and minimal or absent lipid core. (Adapted from Libby P, *Nature Medicine*, 1995.) See text for additional details.

stroke, causally implicate thrombosis. In 1966, Constantinides promoted plaque rupture as the immediate precipitating cause of coronary thrombosis [36]. Davies and coworkers [37–40] and Falk and coworkers [12,41–43] subsequently established the role of plaque rupture and ensuing thrombosis in myocardial infarction, unstable angina, and sudden ischemic death. What makes one plaque more likely to rupture? Some typical features of rupture-prone, or vulnerable, plaques include structural, cellular, and functional characteristics (Figure 3.6).

Determinants of plaque vulnerability

Lipid core

Independently of size, thick-capped collagen-rich plaques appear more stable, while thin-capped lipid-rich plaques are more likely to rupture [44]. A rupture-prone, or "vulnerable," plaque contains up to 40% lipid [45]. This observation may explain in part the reduction of coronary events that follows lipid-lowering therapy with statins.

Fibrous cap

The fibrous cap consists of collagen, elastin, and proteoglycans, all components of the extracellular matrix derived mostly from SMC. Interstitial collagen accounts for most of the cap's tensile strength [46]. Accordingly, caps from ruptured plaques are usually thinner than intact plaques and also contain fewer matrix components and SMC [47]. Cap thickness likely results from the balance between the rate of biosynthesis and the rate of degradation of such components, most importantly collagen [48,49]. A large eccentric lipid core presumably increases vulnerability by distributing maximal circumferential stress on the "shoulder" of the cap, i.e., the region where the cap connects to the vessel wall [50]. Approximately 60% of all plaque ruptures occur in this region [51].

Degree of stenosis and remodeling

The degree of lumen stenosis in an artery correlates only very loosely with the probability of thrombosis.

Indeed, most acute myocardial infarctions result from atheromas that cause <50% stenosis of the arterial lumen [52,53], which outnumber tight stenoses. Lumen diameter depends on plaque size and "compensatory" enlargement, i.e., large plaques that expand outwardly toward the vessel wall (outward or positive remodeling) and hence do not affect lumen caliber. Studies using intravascular ultrasound show that outward arterial expansion resulting from positive remodeling occurs more commonly at sites of culprit lesions in patients with unstable angina, while inward or negative remodeling occurs more commonly in patients with stable angina [54]. Therefore, positive remodeling may increase the likelihood of plaque rupture, since wall tension relates directly to vessel radius (the Laplace relationship). Indeed, circumferential stress, which should favor cap disruption, increases in the presence of a larger lumen [50].

Plaque inflammation

Ruptured plaques are characterized by increased levels of inflammatory cells, mainly macrophage/foam cells and T-lymphocytes, in the lipid core, fibrous cap, and the adventitia underlying the plaque, in conjunction with neomicrovessels [48]. Inflammatory cytokines, either soluble or cell-surface bound (such as CD40L), mediate inflammatory processes that take place in the atheroma; they also play a major role in the regulation of matrix deposition and degradation (see below). Inflammation predisposes plaques to rupture by thinning the fibrous cap.

Other inflammatory mechanisms influence also plaque stability. In humans, overexpression of the inflammatory enzyme COX-2 associates with plaque complications [55]. Macrophage-derived angiogenic factors such as VEGF promote plaque neovascularization, thereby providing new access routes for inflammatory cells in the plaque [56]. Macrophages also furnish most of the TF, which initiates the extrinsic pathway of the coagulation cascade.

Neovascularization and intraplaque hemorrhage

Frequently observed in relation with the presence of an atherosclerotic lesion [57], neoangiogenesis potentially contributes to the growth and development of neointimal thickening [58]. Immunohistochemical studies demonstrate that intimal capillaries originate in the adventitial network near the plaque [59]. Such capillaries may promote plaque growth by providing a route for infiltrating inflammatory cells and the deposition of plasma constituents [60]. Moulton et al. observed retarded lesion progression concomitant with markedly decreased macrophage accumulation and inflammation in ApoE$^{-/-}$ mice with already developed atherosclerotic lesions and treated with angiostatin, an inhibitor of plaque neovascularization [61].

Further, neoangiogenesis associates directly with plaque instability as a source of intraplaque hemorrhage [29,62,63]. A recent study examining multiple coronary lesions from patients who died suddenly of coronary events suggests that intraplaque hemorrhage predominates in disrupted coronary plaques and also correlates with a larger necrotic lipid core and increased plaque vulnerability. Thus, hemorrhage may provide a potent atherogenic stimulus that likely increases the risk of plaque destabilization [15].

Lesion complications: pathobiology of the fibrous cap

Among the various matrix components of the fibrous cap, collagen has great importance due to its abundance and its contribution to the plaque's structural integrity and tensile resistance to shear stress. Plaque collagen, mainly types I and III, derives from protocollagen precursors synthesized in the intima by SMC. As discussed previously, cytokines importantly determine collagen "homeostasis." TGF-β and PDGF originate in macrophages and localize in the atherosclerotic plaque, where they induce SMC proliferation and collagen synthesis. At the same time, SMC respond to T-lymphocyte-derived IFN-γ by decreasing matrix deposition [48]. Factors that impair the balance between the rate of synthesis and the rate of degradation of matrix components in general and collagen in particular can determine fibrous cap vulnerability. T-lymphocytes have particular relevance in this context. Activated T-lymphocytes co-localize with macrophages at sites of plaque disruption or erosion in human atherosclerotic plaques, and SMC and leukocytes in these regions express the histocompatibility antigen HLA-DR, an index of IFN-γ activation [64,65]. Accordingly, T-cells correlate inversely with collagen type-I expression in atherosclerotic lesions as both immunoreactive protein and mRNA [66].

Table 3.2 Members of the MMP family expressed in vascular tissues (adapted from Ref. [69]).

Group/members	MMP#	Substrate
Collagenases		
Interstitial collagenase	1	Collagen types I, II, III, VII, X, gelatin, proteoglycans
Neutrophil collagenase	8	Collagen types I, II, III, proteoglycans
Collagenase-3	13	Collagen types I, II, III
Gelatinases		
Gelatinase-A	2	Collagen types IV, V, VII, X, gelatin
Gelatinase-B	9	Collagen types IV, V, VII, X, gelatin
Stromelysins		
Stromelysin-1	3	Collagen types III, IV, V, IX, laminin, fibronectin, elastin, gelatin, proteoglycans
Stromelysin-2	10	Collagen types III, IV, V, IX, laminin, fibronectin, elastin, gelatin, proteoglycans
Stromelysin-3	11	Gelatin, fibronectin, proteoglycans
Matrilysin	7	Gelatin, fibronectin, laminin, collagen type IV, proteoglycan core protein
Membrane-type (MT) MMPs		
MT1-MMP	14	Fibronectin, laminin, collagen type I, II, IV
MT2-MMP	15	Fibronectin, laminin, collagen type I, II, IV
MT3-MMP	16	Gelatin, collagen types III, IV, fibronectin
MT4-MMP	17	Gelatin, collagen type III, IV
Others		
Metallo-elastase	12	Elastin

Combined with IL-1 and TNFα, IFN-γ can lead to SMC apoptosis [67]. Indeed, markers of cell death occur on cells localizing at plaque shoulders, and very few SMC localize at sites of ruptures. Such observations suggest that cytokine-induced cell death may contribute to plaque instability by depriving the lesion of SMC [68].

The expression of matrix-degrading metalloproteinases (MMP) likely participates critically in matrix degradation. Classified according to substrate specificity as collagenases, gelatinases, stromelysins, and membrane-type MMP, members of the MMP family can degrade all components of the extracellular matrix [69] (Table 3.2). Inflammatory cytokines, growth factors, and oncogene products tightly regulate the very low constitutive expression of MMP at the transcriptional level. Moreover, MMP are generally expressed as inactive zymogens that require further autolytic, proteolytic, or oxidative cleavage to achieve the appropriate active conformation. Tissue inhibitors of metalloproteinases (TIMP), a family of endogenous inhibitors synthesized mainly by SMC, also control MMP activity in normal conditions. An imbalance in the MMP–TIMP ratio may contribute to plaque instability [70]. Indeed,

some studies have demonstrated that elevated levels of various MMP in human atherosclerotic plaques correspond with macrophage-rich areas [71–76]. Co-culturing macrophages with human atherosclerotic plaques induces MMP-dependent collagen breakdown [77]. Although macrophages express most MMP in atherosclerotic lesions, SMC and EC also participate in such expression in response to a variety of stimuli including oxidized lipids [78], thrombin [79], *Chlamydia pneumoniae* heat shock proteins [80], and hemodynamic stress [81]. Notably, specific inflammatory signals such as IL-1, TNF-α, and T-cell interaction involving CD40L (CD154) can induce MMP [82]. In addition to specific matrix-degrading activities, other effects of macrophage-derived MMP may participate in plaque vulnerability. Some MMP have indirect proliferative effects on vascular cells [83,84]. MMP-11, characterized by weak matrix-degrading activity, specifically degrades serine-protease inhibitors (serpins). Because serpins inhibit proteases such as cathepsins, plasmin, and leukocyte elastase, MMP-11 may enhance indirectly the activity of proteolytic enzymes potentially involved in matrix degradation [74].

Mechanisms involving cell death and MMP activation may participate importantly in plaque erosion. Virmani et al. determined that erosion associates with bland inflammation [14], and others have reported a major involvement of macrophages and T-lymphocytes [65]. EC detachment occurs commonly, possibly due to apoptosis triggered by cooperating inflammatory cytokines [85]. MMP with substrate specificity for matrix components of the basal lamina, i.e., non-fibrillar collagen, may loosen the connections between EC and the basement membrane, and thus promote endothelial desquamation.

Plaques with a thin and weakened fibrous cap seem to rupture without an obvious trigger or a particular precipitating event. Putative triggers of plaque rupture include physical exercise, emotional stress, acute infections, and consumption of illicit drugs (causing increased cardiac output and hemodynamic forces, and/or vasoconstriction).

EC apoptosis and endothelial regeneration

Widely documented in atherosclerosis, apoptosis particularly associates with areas of inflammation in the developing plaque, usually in relation with macrophages and SMC [86]. However, apoptosis also occurs in the endothelial lining [87]. EC apoptosis may contribute to atherothrombosis by exposing a thrombogenic surface secondary to endothelial denudation, and increasing the thrombogenicity of the blood environment by shedding TF microparticles. Endothelial senescence and denudation with platelet deposition both occur in advanced plaques [88,89], and both correlate with areas of diminished or disturbed flow, a condition typically found downstream of stenosis. A recent study examining non-ruptured carotid plaques observed preferential EC apoptosis in the downstream portion of the plaque with respect to blood flow [90]. This link between low shear stress and endothelial apoptosis possibly may provide a mechanism to explain plaque erosion [91]. Apoptotic cells increase the exposure of anionic phospholipids, particularly phosphatidylserine, in the outer layer of cell membrane [92], and TF activity increases in association with such phospholipid species [93]. Indeed, cultured human EC, which normally offer an anticoagulant and non-platelet-adhesive surface, become

procoagulant after increased exposure of phosphatidylserine in the outer layer of the cell membrane, and adhesive for non-activated platelets after the induction of apoptosis [94,95]. Therefore, re-endothelialization strategies provide promising therapeutic targets, especially in light of recent exciting observations on endothelial progenitor cells (EPC), derived from hematopoietic stem cells, and their relation to cardiovascular disease [96]. Positive for CD34 and CD133 and observed in the blood of adult humans, bone marrow-derived EPC, or angioblasts, contribute to neovascularization, both as angiogenesis, i.e., new vessel formation from pre-existing EC, and vasculogenesis, i.e., *in situ* formation of vessels through cell clusters and blood islands, the same process active in the embryo [97,98]. Increased neovascularization by EPC or CD34-positive cells improves cardiac function [99,100]. Further, levels of circulating EPC correlate inversely with risk factors for coronary artery disease [101,102] and the combined Framingham risk factor score, and also predict vascular vasoreactivity [103]. Therefore, EPC that normally circulate in the peripheral blood may mobilize actively in pathological conditions such as acute myocardial ischemia, and thus contribute to endothelial repair or neovascularization [104]. Impaired EC mobilization could affect vascular disease progression. Notably, statins improve EPC mobilization through a NO-dependent mechanism [105–107]. Moreover, *in vivo* studies have demonstrated that EPC participate in the re-endothelialization of a damaged artery and that statins accelerate healing in such models [108,109]. Estrogens that, like statins, increase NO bioavailability may achieve a similar effect [110].

Not all plaque disruptions result in acute coronary syndromes

In the majority of cases, ruptured or eroded plaque with superimposed thrombosis underlie acute coronary syndromes [111]. The clinical presentation of acute coronary syndromes depends on the location, severity, and duration of myocardial ischemia. A non-occlusive or transiently occlusive thrombus (mostly formed by platelets: white thrombus) usually associates with unstable angina, pain at rest, and non-ST elevation myocardial infarction. On the other hand, an occlusive thrombus causes ST elevation myocardial infarction [112], which responds best to fibrinolytic drugs due to a large propagation component caused by upstream (mostly) and downstream activation of coagulation (red thrombus). The organization and healing of a mural thrombus at the site of plaque disruption may determine rapid plaque growth and rapid progression from severe stenosis to occlusion, often with the underlying aspect of a multi-layered plaque [113].

However, while plaque fissuring (or sometimes erosion) certainly correlates with acute coronary syndromes, autopsy studies have shown that coronary artery rupture may not generate clinical manifestations, which are rather the exception than the rule [114]. Indeed, patients who succumb to noncoronary events frequently have fissured plaques in their coronary arteries [115].

Explanations for the occlusive/ non-occlusive nature of coronary thrombosis

Local rheological conditions likely determine whether contact between the thrombogenic lipid core and the blood results in an occlusive or a mural thrombus. Flow patterns may explain why highly severe stenoses more likely associate with an occlusive thrombus [12,116]. After plaque rupture, the intensity of the thrombogenic stimulus may modulate the risk of subsequent thrombosis, correlating with the amount and composition of the lipid core and its TF content. Thus, the degree of lipid core thrombogenicity might explain the variable frequency of occlusive thrombosis following plaque rupture [117,118]. The activity of the hemostatic system, i.e., platelet function, coagulation activation, and the status of fibrinolysis, likely influence subsequent acute events. Indeed, the levels of fibrinogen [119], coagulation factor VII, and factor VIII-von Willebrand factor [120] may predict the risk of acute myocardial infarction and death in selected populations. The beneficial effect of anti-platelet drugs, heparin-like anticoagulants, and oral anti-platelet agents suggests a crucial role for the hemostatic system in arterial thrombosis and acute coronary syndromes. Therefore, the rare but catastrophic occlusive coronary thrombosis likely requires the interplay of a wide range of hemodynamic and hemostatic factors. While such an event likely provokes an ST elevation acute myocardial infarction, mural, or intermittent thrombosis more likely causes a non-ST segment elevation infarction or unstable angina [112].

Even in the presence of an acute occlusive thrombosis due to plaque rupture and intimal hemorrhage, variables including the presence and extent of collateral circulation, previous exposure to ischemia, and the presence and extent of ischemic preconditioning modulate the risk of developing an acute coronary syndrome. Despite the frequency of plaque complications, an acute coronary syndrome occurs relatively rarely, and actually may result from the alignment of a constellation of events of which plaque rupture or erosion likely comprise necessary but insufficient elements. Some systemic factors contribute, e.g., inflammation or a tendency to thrombosis or impaired fibrinolysis, and may explain multiple ruptures in different sites of the same artery or different arteries in the same patient. Therefore, recent attention shifted from the concept of the "vulnerable plaque" to that of the "vulnerable patient" [121,122].

Finally, serial angiography [2] has documented rapid, discontinuous lesion progression that can occur without clinical manifestation. Pathological examination reveals mural thrombus with histological features of a multi-layered lesion [41] (Figure 3.7) within a plaque. These observations explain how healing of disrupted plaque may lead to atheroma progression.

The relationship between acute coronary syndromes and coronary anatomy as assessed from angiography – searching for the vulnerable plaque or the vulnerable patient?

When plaque growth in the coronary arteries reduces lumen diameter even to a very large extent, myocardial blood flow at rest remains constant due to the compensatory dilation of resistance arterioles located distally to the stenosis (coronary reserve) [123]. However, when myocardial oxygen requirements increase, e.g., with the increased heart rate accompanying physical exercise, further compensatory dilation becomes impossible beyond a certain threshold (exhaustion of coronary reserve). The balance between oxygen requirement and availability determines the occurrence of myocardial ischemia. This hemodynamic mechanism of ischemia, caused by increased myocardial oxygen requirements in the presence of an exhausted coronary reserve, largely

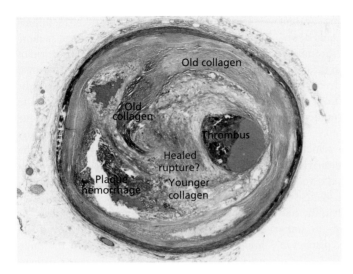

Figure 3.7 Healing plaque rupture with layered thrombus. Cross-sectioned coronary artery illustrating plaque rupture with multi-layered thrombus superimposed. Three layers are readily seen, with the oldest part of the thrombus incorporated into the fibrous cap (healing rupture) and the most recent part located centrally and consisting predominantly of platelets (acute thrombus). Trichromic staining. Original magnification ×20. (By courtesy of Dr. Erling Falk, Skejby Hospital, Aarhus, Denmark).

determines effort stable angina, where symptoms correlate with the degree of angiographically determined lumen stenosis in a main coronary artery. However, the degree of lumen stenosis in acute coronary syndromes, as assessed by angiography even shortly before the acute event, does not correlate with the occurrence of symptoms at rest. The outward growth, or "positive remodeling," of many plaques renders them difficult to detect by angiography, which assesses the lumen and not the vessel wall. Therefore, most acute plaque complications occur at sites of angiographically mild stenoses, which outnumber severe stenoses [52], or can even arise in angiographically "normal" regions of vessels. In many cases, the abrupt vessel closure does not permit adaptation to ischemia, e.g., the growth of collaterals or the occurrence of preconditioning that otherwise may limit myocardial necrosis in the depending myocardial territory. Therefore, we currently recognize that angiography does not predict accurately acute manifestations of coronary artery disease. Alternative approaches to identifying rupture-prone, i.e., "vulnerable," plaques and examining plaque characteristics other than lumen impingement include morphological techniques such as intravascular ultrasound [124], optical coherence tomography [125] and magnetic resonance imaging [126], or functional techniques such as thermography [127] or elastography [128]. However, instability is largely a multi-focal process [129,130]. Systemic elevation of markers such as C-reactive protein [131–133], IL-6 [134], myeloperoxidase [135], or glutathione peroxidase [136], which predict acute coronary events in various populations, likely reflect not single "vulnerable" lesions but rather a generalized and diffuse vascular inflammatory process characteristic of coronary and extra-coronary arterial beds. Therefore, current attention focuses more intently on the unstable patient than the unstable plaque [121,122]. The current clinical practice of targeting single lesions with percutaneous coronary interventions presents evident limitations to this regard. Recent appreciation of the systemic nature of acute coronary syndromes likely will introduce new diagnostic criteria for determining the risk of acute events [121,122,137].

Recent lessons and future directions

Many practical consequences emerge from the improved understanding of the pathogenetic mechanisms that lead from fatty streaks to vascular events. Clearly, knowledge of obligatory or ancillary steps in these processes will allow the selection of molecular targets to devise preventive strategies. Screening for new drugs will include *in vitro* models that allow quick evaluation of the role played by specific molecules. However, such knowledge already permits fuller understanding of major drug categories such as statins, omega-3 fatty acids, and angiotensin converting enzyme (ACE) inhibitors.

Statins decrease vascular events, such as stroke, not linked clearly to serum cholesterol, possibly

Table 3.3 A list of new molecular targets and new agents (in parentheses) of potential use in| vascular disease based on knowledge on the pathogenesis of lesion development and complications.

Lesion inception
  Expression of endothelial-leukocyte adhesion molecules (e.g., VCAM-1)
  Chemokines (e.g., MCP-1)
  Other cytokines and growth factors (e.g., M-CSF)
  Cytokine receptors
  Fatty acids and fatty acid analogues
  Inhibitors of cytokine signal transduction (e.g., tyrosine kinases, MAP kinases, antioxidants)
  Transcription factors (e.g., NF-κB, Egr-1)
  LDL oxidation (new antioxidants)
  Novel NO donors and stimulators of NO synthesis
Lesion progression
  All of the above plus
  New inhibitors of cholesterol synthesis
  Farnesyl transferase and Geranyl transferase
  Cell cycle regulators
  Cytostatic agents, rapamycin
  CD40–CD40 ligand interactions
Plaque fissuring
  MMP (MMP inhibitors)
  PPAR-α and -γ agonists
  CD40–CD40 ligand interactions
  Inhibitors of plaque neovascularization
Thrombosis
  Platelet adhesion and aggregation (new anti-platelet agents, such as antagonists of $\alpha_v\beta_3$)
  Thrombin (new direct thrombin inhibitors)
  New inhibitors of factor VII-TF interaction (e.g., TFPI)
  New fibrinolytic agents

Myocardial consequences of ischemia
  Collateral vessels, neovascularization (VEGF, FGF)
  Phenotypic transformation of cardiac cells (e.g., acquisition of a contractile phenotype from fibroblasts)
  Stem cells, progenitor cells

VCAM-1: Vascular cell adhesion molecule-1; MCP-1: monocyte chemoattractant protein-1, M-CSF: macrophage-colony stimulating factor; MAP: mitogen-activated protein; NF-κB: nuclear factor-κB; Egr-1: early growth response protein 1, PPAR: peroxisome proliferator activated receptors; TFPI: tissue factor pathway inhibitor; VEGF: vascular endothelial growth factor; FGF: fibroblast growth factor.

highlighting cholesterol-independent (so-called "pleiotropic") effects of this class of drugs [138,139]. Lipid lowering certainly modifies plaque composition by decreasing intraplaque lipids and stabilizing the plaque. However, other effects of statins may relate more closely to "stabilizing" the vulnerable plaque. For example, statin reduction of intracellular oxidative stress [139] may interfere with many pro-inflammatory positive-feedback loops activated by reactive oxygen species, including the expression of adhesion molecules and MMP

activation [140]. By stabilizing endothelial NO synthase (eNOS) messenger RNA [141] and increasing eNOS phosphorylation, in turn augmenting eNOS activity [142], statins improve coronary vasomotion and endothelium-dependent relaxation. In addition to – and possibly independent of – cholesterol reduction, such effects of statins may participate in protection against ischemic stroke (see also Chapters 17 and 21).

Peroxisome proliferator-activated receptor (PPAR) agonists including fibrates and thiazolidinediones

[143] belong to another class of drugs with "new" and potentially pleiotropic effects on atherosclerosis and plaque stability. As regulators of lipid and lipoprotein metabolism, PPAR agonists such as fibrates control plasma levels of cholesterol and triglycerides, directly affecting the main risk factors for cardiovascular disease. Additionally, recent studies suggest that PPAR agonists also affect various cellular and molecular mechanisms of atherosclerosis development and progression, possibly by promoting cholesterol efflux from macrophages, thus reducing foam cell formation [144,145]. Furthermore, such mechanisms might blunt inflammation by inhibiting nuclear factor-κB (NF-κB) activation [146] that affects in turn the synthesis of pivotal mediators (vascular cell adhesion molecule-1 (VCAM-1) [147], monocyte chemoattractant protein-1 (MCP-1) [148], and various cytokines [149]) as well as T-lymphocyte activation [150,151]. Additionally, PPAR may affect plaque stability by inhibiting the expression of MMP-9 [152] and TF [153,154] and the proliferation of vascular SMC [155]. Animal studies suggest that PPAR agonists inhibit atherosclerosis and stabilize plaque [156–159]. Data from angiographic intervention trials [160–162] and some but not all clinical trials [163,164] support the clinical relevance of such effects (see also Chapter 24).

Omega-3 fatty acids associate epidemiologically with protection from atherosclerosis [165,166]. Their general "anti-inflammatory" effects [167–169], likely achieved by inhibiting NF-κB [170], may explain their inhibition of early atherogenesis, e.g., the reduction in fatty streaks in young individuals [165], as well as plaque stabilization, demonstrated histologically in subjects who consume high levels of these nutrients [171] (see also Chapter 20). In addition to reducing blood pressure, ACE inhibitors may inhibit intracellular reactive oxygen species and transcription factor NF-κB [172,173] (see also Chapter 23).

Concurrently, new approaches aiming to inhibit or modulate crucial steps in the development or complication of atherosclerosis already show promise *in vitro* or in animals. All such strategies are unconventional in the sense that they seek targets other than plasma lipids (Table 3.3). Thus, molecular understanding of the evolution of atherosclerosis should aid the design of new therapeutic approaches.

References

1 Stary HC, Chandler AB, Dinsmore RE, et al. A definition of advanced types of atherosclerotic lesions and a histological classification of atherosclerosis. A report from the Committee on Vascular Lesions of the Council on Arteriosclerosis, American Heart Association. *Arterioscler Thromb Vasc Biol* 1995; 15:1512–1531.

2 Bruschke AV, Kramer JR, Bal ET, et al. The dynamics of progression of coronary atherosclerosis studied in 168 medically treated patients who underwent coronary arteriography three times. *Am Heart J* 1989;117:296–305.

3 Yokoya K, Takatsu H, Suzuki T, et al. Process of progression of coronary artery lesions from mild or moderate stenosis to moderate or severe stenosis: a study based on four serial coronary arteriograms per year. *Cicru* 1999;1000:903–909.

4 Ball RY, Stowers EC, Burton JH, et al. Evidence that the death of macrophages contributes to the lipid core of atheroma. *Atherosclerosis* 1995;114:45–54.

5 Björkerud S, Björkerud B. Apoptosis is abundant in human atherosclerotic lesion, especially in inflammatory cells (macrophages and T cells) and may contribute to the accumulation of gruel and plaque instability. *Am J Pathol* 1996;149:367.

6 Badimon JJ, Lettino M, Toschi V, et al. Local inhibition of tissue factor reduces the thrombogenicity of disrupted human atherosclerotic plaques: effect of tissue factor pathway inhibitor on plaque thrombogenicity under flow conditions. *Circulation* 1999;99:1780–1787.

7 Stary HC. Natural history of calcium deposits in atherosclerosis progression and regression. *Z Kardiol* 2000; 89:II28.

8 Roberts W. Coronary atherosclerosis: is the process focal or diffused among patient with symptomatic or fatal myocardial ischemia? *Am J Cardiol* 1998;82:41T–44T.

9 Kragel AH, Reddy SG, Wittes JT, et al. Morphometric analysis of the composition of atherosclerotic plaques in the four major epicardial coronary arteries in acute myocardial infarction and in sudden coronary death. *Circulation* 1989;80:1747–1756.

10 Leary T. Coronary spasm as a possible factor in producing sudden death. *Am Heart J* 1934;10:328–337.

11 Levin DC, Fallon JT. Significance of the angiographic morphology of localized coronary stenosis: histopathological correlations. *Circulation* 1982;66:316–320.

12 Falk E. Plaque rupture with severe pre-existing stenosis precipitating coronary thrombosis. Characteristics of coronary atherosclerotic plaques underlying fatal occlusive thrombi. *Br Heart J* 1983;50:127–134.

13 Farb A, Burke AP, Tang AL, et al. Coronary plaque erosion without rupture into a lipid core. A frequent cause of coronary thrombosis in sudden coronary death. *Circulation* 1996;93: 1354–1363.

14 Virmani R, Kolodgie FD, Burke AP, et al. Lessons from sudden coronary death: a comprehensive morphological classification scheme for atherosclerotic lesions. *Atheroscl Thromb Vasc Biol* 2000;20:1262–1275.

15 Kolodgie FD, Gold HK, Burke AP, et al. Intraplaque hemorrhage and progression of coronary atheroma. *N Engl J Med* 2003;349:2316–2325.

16 Davies MJ, Gordon JL, Gearing AJ, et al. The expression of the adhesion molecules ICAM-1, VCAM-1, PECAM, and E-selectin in human atherosclerosis. *J Pathol* 1993;171:223–229.

17 O'Brien KD, Allen MD, McDonald TO, et al. Vascular cell adhesion molecule-1 is expressed in human coronary atherosclerotic plaques. Implications for the mode of progression of advanced coronary atherosclerosis. *J Clin Invest* 1993;92:945–951.

18 Ross R. Atherosclerosis – an inflammatory disease. *N Engl J Med* 1999;340:115–126.

19 Ferns GA, Raines EW, Sprugel KH, et al. Inhibition of neointimal smooth muscle accumulation after angioplasty by an antibody to PDGF. *Science* 1991; 253: 1129–1132.

20 Libby P. Changing concepts of atherogenesis. *J Int Med* 2000;247:349.

21 Raines EW, Dower SK, Ross R. Interleukin-1 mitogenic activity for fibroblasts and smooth muscle cells is due to PDGF-AA. *Science* 1989;243:393–396.

22 Gay CG, Winkles JA. Interleukin 1 regulates heparin-binding growth factor 2 gene expression in vascular smooth muscle cells. *Proc Natl Acad Sci USA* 1991;88:296–300.

23 Bostrom K, Watson KE, Horn S, et al. Bone morphogenetic protein expression in human atherosclerotic lesion. *J Clin Invest* 1993;91:1800–1809.

24 Rajavashisth T, Quiao J, Tripathi S, et al. Heterozygous osteopetrotic (op) mutation reduces atherosclerosis in LDL receptor-deficient mice. *J Clin Invest* 1998;101: 2072–2110.

25 Schonbeck U, Libby P. CD40 signaling and plaque instability. *Circ Res* 2001;89:1092–1103.

26 Schonbeck U, Mach F, Sukhova GK, et al. Regulation of matrix metalloproteinase expression in human vascular smooth muscle cells by T lymphocytes: a role for CD40 signaling in plaque rupture? *Circ Res* 1997;81:448–454.

27 Schonbeck U, Mach F, Sukhova GK, et al. CD40 ligation induces tissue factor expression in human vascular smooth muscle cells. *Am J Pathol* 2000;156:7–14.

28 Mach F, Schonbeck U, Sukhova G, et al. Functional CD40 ligand is expressed on human vascular endothelial cells, smooth muscle cells, and macrophages: implications for CD40–CD40 ligand signaling in atherosclerosis. *PNAS* 1997;94:1931–1936.

29 de Boer OJ, van der Wal AC, Teeling P, et al. Leucocyte recruitment in rupture prone regions of lipid-rich plaques: a prominent role for neovascularization? *Cardiovasc Res* 1999;41:443–449.

30 Schonbeck U, Sukhova GK, Graber P, et al. Augmented expression of cyclooxygenase-2 in human atherosclerotic lesions. *Am J Pathol* 1999;155:1281–1291.

31 Mach F, Schonbeck U, Sukhova GK, et al. Reduction of atherosclerosis in mice by inhibition of CD40 signalling. *Nature* 1998;394:200–203.

32 Schonbeck U, Sukhova GK, Shimizu K, et al. Inhibition of CD40 signaling limits evolution of established atherosclerosis in mice. *Proc Natl Acad Sci USA* 2000;97:7458–7463.

33 Bavendiek U, Zirlik A, LaClair S, et al. Atherogenesis in mice does not require CD40 ligand from bone marrow-derived cells. *Arterioscler Thromb Vasc Biol* 2005;25: 1244–1249.

34 Büchner K, Henn V, Gräfe M, et al. CD40 ligand is selectively expressed on CD4+ T cells and platelets: implications for CD40–CD40L signalling in atherosclerosis. *J Pathol* 2003;201:288–295.

35 de Lemos JA, Zirlik A, Schonbeck U, et al. Associations between soluble CD40 ligand, atherosclerosis risk factors, and subclinical atherosclerosis: results from the Dallas Heart Study. *Arterioscler Thromb Vasc Biol* 2005; 25:2192–2196.

36 Constantinides P. Plaque fissures in human coronary thrombosis. *J Atheroscler Res* 1966;6:1–17.

37 Davies MJ, Woolf N, Robertson W. Pathology of acute myocardial infarction with particular reference to occlusive coronary thrombi. *Br Hear J* 1976;38:659–664.

38 Davies MJ, Fulton WF, Robertson WB. The relation of coronary thrombosis to ischaemic myocardial necrosis. *J Pathol* 1979;127:99–110.

39 Davies MJ, Thomas T. The pathological basis and microanatomy of occlusive thrombus formation in human coronary arteries. *Philos Trans R Soc Lond B Biol Sci* 1981;294:225–229.

40 Davies MJ, Thomas T. Thrombosis and acute coronary-artery lesions in sudden cardiac ischemic death. *N Engl J Med* 1984;310:1137–1140.

41 Falk E. Unstable angina with fatal outcome: dynamic coronary thrombosis leading to infarction and/or sudden death. Autopsy evidence of recurrent mural thrombosis with peripheral embolization culminating in total vascular occlusion. *Circulation* 1985;71:699–708.

42 Falk E. Morphologic features of unstable atherothrombotic plaques underlying acute coronary syndromes. *Am J Cardiol* 1989;63:114E–120E.

43 Falk E, Shah PK, Fuster V. Coronary plaque disruption. *Circulation* 1995;92:657–671.

44 Falk E. Why do plaques rupture? *Circulation* 1992;86: III30–III42.

45 Felton CV, Crook D, Davies MJ, et al. Relation of plaque lipid composition and morphology to the stability of

human aortic plaques. *Arterioscler Thromb Vasc Biol* 1997;17:1337–1345.

46 Lee RT, Libby P. The unstable atheroma. *Atheroscl Thromb Vasc Biol* 1997;17:1859–1867.

47 Burleigh MC, Briggs AD, Lendon CL, et al. Collagen types I and III, collagen content, GAGs and mechanical strength of human atherosclerotic plaque caps: span-wise variations. *Atherosclerosis* 1992;96:71–81.

48 Libby P. Molecular basis of the acute coronary syndromes. *Circulation* 1995;91:2844–2850.

49 Shah PK. Plaque disruption and thrombosis: potential role of inflammation and infection. *Cardiol Rev* 2000; 8:31–39.

50 Loree HM, Kamm RD, Stringfellow RG, et al. Effects of fibrous cap thickness on peak circumferential stress in model atherosclerotic vessels. *Circ Res* 1992;71: 850–858.

51 Cheng GC, Loree HM, Kamm RD, et al. Distribution of circumferential stress in ruptured and stable atherosclerotic lesions. A structural analysis with histopathological correlation. *Circulation* 1993;87:1179–1187.

52 Ambrose JA, Tannenbaum MA, Alexopoulos D, et al. Angiographic progression of coronary artery disease and the development of myocardial infarction. *J Am Coll Cardiol* 1988;12:56–62.

53 Smith Jr S. Risk-reduction therapy: the challenge to change. *Circulation* 1996;93:2205–2211.

54 Schoenhagen P, Ziada KM, Kapadia SR, et al. Extent and direction of arterial remodeling in stable versus unstable coronary syndromes: an intravascular ultrasound study. *Circulation* 2000;101:598–603.

55 Cipollone F, Prontera C, Pini B, et al. Overexpression of functionally coupled cyclooxygenase-2 and prostaglandin E synthase in symptomatic atherosclerotic plaque as a basis of prostaglandin E_2-dependent plaque instability. *Circulation* 2001;104:921–927.

56 Ramos MA, Kuzuya M, Esaki T, et al. Induction of macrophage VEGF in response to oxidized LDL and VEGF accumulation in human atherosclerotic lesions. *Atheroscl Thromb Vasc Biol* 1988;18:1188–1196.

57 Barger AC, Beekes RM, Lecompte PM. Vasa vasorum and neovascularization of human coronary arteries: a possible role in the pathophysiology of atherosclerosis. *N Engl J Med* 1984;310:175–177.

58 Celletti F, Waugh J, Amabile P, et al. Inhibition of vascular endothelial growth factor-mediated neointima progression with angiostatin or paclitaxel. *J Vasc Interv Radiol* 2002;13:703–707.

59 Zhang Y, Cliff WJ, Shoefl G, et al. Immunohistochemical study of intimal microvessels in coronary atherosclerosis. *Am J Pathol* 1993;143:164–172.

60 Moulton KS, Heller E, Konerding MA, et al. Angiogenesis inhibitors endostatin od TNP-470 reduce intimal neovascularization and plaque growth in apolipoprotein E-deficient mice. *Circulation* 1999;99: 1726–1732.

61 Moulton K, Vakili K, Zurakovski D, et al. Inhibition of plaque neovascularization reduces macrophage accumulation and progression of advanced atherosclerosis. *Proc Natl Acad Sci USA* 2003;1000: 4736–4741.

62 Barger A, Beeuwkes R. Rupture of coronary vasa vasorum as a trigger of acute myocardial infarction. *Am J Cardiol* 1990;66:41G–43G.

63 McCarthy MJ, Loftus IM, Thompson MM, et al. Angiogenesis and the atherosclerotic carotid plaque: an association between symptomatology and plaque morphology. *J Vasc Surg* 1999;30:261–268.

64 Hansson GK, Jonasson L, Lojsthed B, et al. Localization of T lymphocytes and macrophages in fibrous and complicated human atherosclerotic plaques. *Atherosclerosis* 988;72:135–141.

65 van der Wal AC, Becker AE, van der Loos CM, et al. Site of intimal rupture or erosion of thrombosed coronary atherosclerotic plaques is characterized by an inflammatory process irrespective of the dominant plaque morphology. *Circulation* 1994;89:36–44.

66 Rekhter M, Zhang K, Narayanan AS, et al. Type I collagen gene expression in human atherosclerosis. Localization to specific plaque regions. *Am J Pathol* 1993;143: 1634–1648.

67 Geng Y, Muszynski M, Hansson G, et al. Apoptosis of vascular smooth muscle cells induced by *in vitro* stimulation with interferon-gamma, tumor necrosis factor-alpha, and interleukin-1 beta. *Arterioscler Thromb Vasc Biol* 1996;16:19–27.

68 Geng Y-J, Libby P. Progression of atheroma: a struggle between death and procreation. *Arterioscler Thromb Vasc Biol* 2002;22:1370–1380.

69 Nagase H, Woessner Jr JF. Matrix metalloproteinases. *J Biol Chem* 1999;274:21491–21494.

70 George SJ. Therapeutic potential of matrix metalloproteinase inhibitors in atherosclerosis. *Exp Opin Invest Drug* 2000;9:993–1007.

71 Galis ZS, Sukkova GK, Lark MW, et al. Increased expression of matrix metalloproteinases and matrix degrading activity in vulnerable regions in human atherosclerotic plaque. *J Clin Invest* 1994;94:2493–2503.

72 Galis Z, Sukhova G, Kranzhofer R, et al. Macrophage foam cells from experimental atheroma constitutively produce matrix-degrading metalloproteinases. *Proc Natl Acad Sci USA* 1995;92:402–406.

73 Halpert I, Sires UI, Roby JD, et al. Matrilysin is expressed in lipid-laden macrophages at sites of potential rupture in atherosclerotic lesions and localizes to areas of versica deposition, a proteoglycan substrate for the enzyme. *Proc Natl Acad Sci USA* 1996;93:9748–9753.

74 Schonbeck U, Mach F, Sukhova G, et al. Expression of stromelysin-3 in atherosclerotic lesions: regulation via

CD40–CD40 ligand signalling *in vitro* and *in vivo*. *J Exp Med* 1999;189:843–853.

75 Sukhova G, Schonbeck U, Rabkin E, et al. Evidence for increased collageolysis by interstitial collagenases-1 and -3 in vulnerable human atheromatous plaques. *Circulation* 1999;99:2503–2509.

76 Rajavashisth T, Xu X, Jovinge S, et al. Membrane type 1 matrix metalloproteinase expression in human atherosclerotic plaques-evidence for activation by proinflammatory mediators. *Circulation* 1999;99:3103–3109.

77 Shah P, Falk E, Badimon J, et al. Human monocyte-derived macrophages induce collagen breakdown in fibrous caps of atherosclerotic plaques: potential role of matrix-degrading metalloproteinases and implications for plaque rupture. *Circulation* 1995;92: 1565–1569.

78 Xu XP, Meisel SR, Ong JM, et al. Oxidized low-density lipoprotein regulates matrix metalloproteinase-9 and its tissue inhibitor in human monocyte-derived macrophages. *Circulation* 1999;99:993–998.

79 Galis Z, Kranzhofer R, Fenton JW, et al. Thrombin promotes activation of matrix metalloproteinase-2 produced by cultured vascular smooth muscle cells. *Arterioscler Thromb Vasc Biol* 1997;17:483–489.

80 Kol A, Sukhova G, Lichtman AH, et al. Chlamydial heat shock protein 60 localizes in human atheroma and regulates macrophage tumor necrosis factor-alpha and matrix metalloproteinase expression. *Circulation* 1998; 28:300–307.

81 Lee R, Schoen F, Loree H, et al. Circumferential stress and matrix metalloproteinase 1 in human coronary atherosclerosis. Implications for plaque rupture. *Arterioscler Thromb Vasc Biol* 1996;16:1070–1073.

82 Mach F, Schonbeck U, Bonnefroy J, et al. Activation of monocyte/macrophage functions related to acute atheroma complication by ligation of CD40: induction of collagenase, stromelysin, and tissue factor. *Circulation* 1997;96:396–399.

83 Chandler S, Cossins J, Lury J, et al. Macrophage metalloelastase degrade matrix and myeli protein and processes a tumor necrosis factor-a fusion protein. *Biochem Biophys Res Commun* 1996;228:421–429.

84 Fowlkes JL, Enghild JJ, Suzuki K, et al. Matrix metalloproteinases degrade insulin-like growth factor-binding protein-3 in dermal fibroblast cultures. *J Biol Chem* 1994;269:25742–25746.

85 Slowik MR, Min W, Ardito T, et al. Evidence that tumor necrosis factor triggers apoptosis in human endothelial cells by interleukin-1-converting enzyme-like protease-dependent and -independent pathways. *Lab Invest* 1997; 77:257–267.

86 Kockx MM. Apoptosis in the atherosclerotic plaque: quantitative and qualitative aspects. *Atheroscl Thromb Vasc Biol* 1998;18:1519–1522.

87 Mallat Z, Tedgui A. Apoptosis in the vasculature: mechanisms and functional importance. *Br J Pharmacol* 2000; 130:947–962.

88 Constantinides P, Harkey M. Electron microscopic exploration of human endothelium in step-serial sections of early and advanced atherosclerotic lesions. *Ann NY Acad Sci* 1990;598:113–124.

89 Burrig KF. The endothelium of advanced arteriosclerotic plaques in humans. *Arterioscler Thromb* 1991;11: 1678–1689.

90 Tricot O, Mallat Z, Heymes C, et al. Relation between endothelial cell apoptosis and blood flow direction in human atherosclerotic plaques. *Circulation* 2000;101: 2450–2453.

91 Mallat Z, Tedgui A. Current perspective on the role of apoptosis in atherothrombotic disease. *Circ Res* 2001; 88:998–1003.

92 Fadok VA, Savil JS, Haslett C, et al. Different populations of macrophages use either the vitronectin receptor or the phosphatidylserine receptor to recognize and remove apoptotic cells. *J Immunol* 1992;149:4029–4035.

93 Bach R, Rifkin DB. Expression of tissue factor procoagulant activity: regulation by cytosolic calcium. *PNAS* 1990;87:6995–6999.

94 Bombeli T, Karsan A, Tait JF, et al. Apoptotic vascular endothelial cells become procoagulant. *Blood* 1997; 89:2429–2442.

95 Bombeli T, Schwartz BR, Harlan JM. Endothelial cells undergoing apoptosis become proadhesive for nonactivated platelets. *Blood* 1999;93:3831–3838.

96 Takahashi T, Kalka C, Masuda H, et al. Ischemia- and cytokine-induced mobilization of bone marrow-derived endothelial progenitor cells for neovascularization. *Nat Med* 1999;5:434–438.

97 Asahara T, Murohara T, Sullivan A, et al. Isolation of putative progenitor endothelial cells for angiogenesis. *Science* 1997;275:964–997.

98 Shi Q, Rafi S, Wu MH, et al. Evidence for circulating bone marrow-derived endothelial cells. *Blood* 1998;92: 362–367.

99 Kawamoto A, Gwon HG, Iwaguro H, et al. Therapeutic potential of *ex vivo* expanded endothelial progenitor cells for myocardial ischemia. *Circulation* 2001;103: 634–637.

100 Kocher AA, Schuster MD, Szablocs MJ, et al. Neovascularization of ischemic myocardium by human bone marrow-derived angioblasts prevents cardiomyocyte apoptosis, reduces remodeling and improves cardiac function. *Nat Med* 2001;7:430–436.

101 Vasa M, Fichtlscherer S, Aicher A, et al. Number and migratory activity of circulating endothelial progenitor cells inversely correlate with risk factors for coronary artery disease. *Circ Res* 2001;89:E1–E7.

102 Tepper OM, Galiano RD, Capla JM, et al. Human endothelial progenitor cells from type II diabetics exhibit impaired proliferation, adhesion, and incorporation into vascular structures. *Circulation* 2002;106: 2781–2786.

103 Hill JM, Zalos G, Halcox JP, et al. Circulating endothelial progenitor cells, vascular function, and cardiovascular risk. *N Engl J Med* 2003;348:581–582.

104 Shintani S, Murohara T, Ikeda H, et al. Mobilization of endothelial progenitor cells in patients with acute myocardial infarction. *Circulation* 2001;103:2776–2779.

105 Dimmeler S, Aicher A, Vasa M, et al. HMG-CoA reductase inhibitors (statins) increase endothelial progenitor cells via the PI 3-kinase/ Akt pathway. *J Clin Invest* 2001;108:391–397.

106 Llevadot J, Murasawa S, Kureishi Y, et al. HMG-CoA reductase inhibitor mobilizes bone marrow-derived endothelial progenitor cells. *J Clin Invest* 2001;108: 399–405.

107 Aicher A, Heeschen C, Mildner-Rihm C, et al. Essential role of endothelial nitric oxide synthase for mobilization of stem and progenitor cells. *Nat Med* 2003;9: 1370–1376.

108 Walter DH, Rittig K, Bahlmann FH, et al. Statin therapy accelerates reendothelialization: a novel effect involving mobilization and incorporation of bone marrow-derived endothelial progenitor cells. *Circulation* 2002;105:3017–3024.

109 Werner N, Priller J, Laufs U, et al. Bone marrow-derived progenitor cells modulate vascular reendothelialization and neointimal formation: effect of 3-hydroxy-3-methylglutaryl coenzyme a reductase inhibition. *Atheroscl Thromb Vasc Biol* 2002;22:1567–1572.

110 Strehlow K, Werner N, Berweiler J, et al. Estrogen increases bone marrow-derived endothelial progenitor cell production and diminishes neointima formation. *Circulation* 2003;107:3059–3065.

111 Davies MJ. The pathophysiology of acute coronary syndromes. *Heart* 2000;83:361–366.

112 Falk E, Fernandez-Ortiz A. Role of thrombosis in atherosclerosis and its complications. *Am J Cardiol* 1995; 75:3B–11B.

113 Burke AP, Kolodgie FD, Farb A, et al. Healed plaque ruptures and sudden coronary death: evidence that subclinical rupture has a role in plaque progression. *Circulation* 2001;103: 934–940.

114 Mann J, Davies MJ. Mechanisms of progression in native coronary artery disease: role of healed plaque disruption. *Heart* 1999;82:265–268.

115 Arbustini E, Grasso M, Diegoli M, et al. Coronary thrombosis in non-cardiac death. *Coron Artery Dis* 1993;4:751–759.

116 El Fawal MA, Berg GA, Wheatley DJ, et al. Sudden coronary death in Glasgow: nature and frequency of acute coronary lesions. *Br Heart J* 1987;57:329–335.

117 Fernandez-Ortiz A, Badimon JJ, Falk E, et al. Characterization of the relative thrombogenicity of atherosclerotic plaque contents: implications for consequences of plaque rupture. *J Am Coll Cardiol* 1994;23: 1562–1569.

118 Toschi V, Gallo R, Lettino M, et al. Tissue factor modulates the thrombogenicity of human atherosclerotic plaques. *Circulation* 1997;95.

119 Danesh J, Collins R, Appelby P, et al. Association of fibrinogen, C-reactive protein, albumin, or leukocyte count with coronary heart disease: meta-analyses of prospective studies. *J Am Med Assoc* 1998;279:1477–1482.

120 Saito I, Folsom A, Brancati F, et al. Nontraditional risk factors for coronary heart disease incidence among persons with diabetes: the Atherosclerosis Risk in Communities (ARIC) Study. *Ann Intern Med* 2000; 133:81–91.

121 Naghavi M, Libby P, Falk E, et al. From vulnerable plaque to vulnerable patient: a call for new definitions and risk assessment strategies: Part I. *Circulation* 2003;108:1664–1672.

122 Naghavi M, Libby P, Falk E, et al. From vulnerable plaque to vulnerable patient: a call for new definitions and risk assessment strategies: Part II. *Circulation* 2003; 108:1772–1778.

123 Gould KL. *Coronary Artery Stenosis*. New York: Elsevier; 1991.

124 Schwartz L, Bui S. The role of intravascular ultrasound in the diagnosis and treatment of patients with coronary artery disease. *Compr Ther* 2003;29:54–65.

125 Jang IK, Bouma BE, Kang DH, et al. Visualization of coronary atherosclerotic plaques in patients using optical coherence tomography: comparison with intravascular ultrasound. *J Am Coll Cardiol* 2002;39: 604–609.

126 Fayad ZA, Choudhury RP, Fuster V. Magnetic resonance imaging of coronary atherosclerosis. *Curr Atheroscler Rep* 2003;5:411–417.

127 Stefanadis C, Toutouzas K, Vaina S, et al. Thermography of the cardiovascular system. *J Interv Cardiol* 2002; 15:461–466.

128 Schaar JA, De Korte CL, Mastik F, et al. Characterizing vulnerable plaque features with intravascular elastography. *Circulation* 2003;108:2636–2641.

129 Rioufol G, Finet G, Ginon I, et al. Multiple atherosclerotic plaque rupture in acute coronary syndrome: a three-vessel intravascular ultrasound study. *Circulation* 2002;106:804–808.

130 Buffon A, Biasucci LM, Liuzzo G, et al. Widespread coronary inflammation in unstable angina. *N Engl J Med* 2002;347:5–12.

131 Ridker PM, Haughie P. Prospective studies of C-reactive protein as a risk factor for cardiovascular disease. *J Investig Med* 1998;46:391–395.

132 Ridker PM, Bassuk SS, Toth PP. C-reactive protein and risk of cardiovascular disease: evidence and clinical application. *Curr Atheroscler Rep* 2003;5:341–349.

133 Ridker PM. High-sensitivity C-reactive protein and cardiovascular risk: rationale for screening and primary prevention. *Am J Cardiol* 2003;92:17K–22K.

134 Biasucci LM, Vitelli A, Liuzzo G, et al. Elevated levels of interleukin-6 in unstable angina. *Circulation* 1996;94:874–877.

135 Brennan ML, Penn MS, Van Lente F, et al. Prognostic value of myeloperoxidase in patients with chest pain. *N Engl J Med* 2003;349:1595–1604.

136 Blankenberg S, Rupprecht HJ, Bickel C, et al. Glutathione peroxidase 1 activity and cardiovascular events in patients with coronary artery disease. *N Engl J Med* 2003;349:1605–1613.

137 Schoenhagen P, Tuzcu M, Ellis S. Plaque vulnerability, plaque rupture and acute coronary syndromes. (Multi)-Focal manifestations of a systemic disease process. *Circulation* 2002;106:760–762.

138 Takemoto M, Liao JK. Pleiotropic effects of 3-hydroxy-3-methylglutaryl coenzyme A reductase inhibitors. *Atheroscl Thromb Vasc Biol* 2001;21:1712–1719.

139 Di Napoli P, Taccardi AA, Oliver M, et al. Statins and stroke: evidence for cholesterol-independent effects. *Eur Heart J* 2002;23:1908–1921.

140 Aikawa M, Rabkin E, Okada Y, et al. Lipid lowering by diet reduces matrix metalloproteinases activity and increases collagen content of rabbit atheroma. A potent mechanism of lesion stabilization. *Circulation* 1998;97:2433–2444.

141 Laufs U, La Fata V, Plutzky J, et al. Upregulation of endothelial nitric oxide synthase by HMG CoA reductase inhibitors. *Circulation* 1998;97:1129–1135.

142 Kureishi Y, Luo Z, Shiojima I, et al. The HMG-CoA reductase inhibitor simvastatin activates the protein kinase Akt and promotes angiogenesis in normocholesterolemic animals. *Nat Med* 2000;6:1004–1011.

143 Barbier O, Pineda Torra I, Duguay Y, et al. Pleiotropic actions of peroxisome proliferator-activated receptors in lipid metabolism and atherosclerosis. *Atheroscl Thromb Vasc Biol* 2002;22:717.

144 Moore KJ, Rosen ED, Fitzgerald ML, et al. The role of PPAR-gamma in macrophage differentiation and cholesterol uptake. *Nat Med* 2001;7:41–47.

145 Chawla A, Barak Y, Nagy L, et al. PPAR-gamma dependent and independent effects on macrophage-gene expression in lipid metabolism and inflammation. *Nat Med* 2001;7:48–52.

146 Delerive P, De Bosscher K, Besnard S, et al. Peroxisome proliferator-activated receptor alpha negatively regulates the vascular inflammatory gene response by negative cross-talk with transcription factors NF-kappaB and AP-1. *J Biol Chem* 1999;274: 32048–32054.

147 Marx N, Sukhova G, Collins T, et al. PPAR alpha activators inhibit cytokine-induced vascular cell adhesion molecule-1 expression in human endothelial cells. *Circulation* 1999;99:3125–3131.

148 Murao K, Imachi H, Momoi A, et al. Thiazolidinedione inhibits the production of monocyte chemoattractant protein-1 in cytokine-treated human vascular endothelial cells. *FEBS Lett* 1999;454:27–30.

149 Ricote M, Huang JT, Welch JS, et al. The peroxisome proliferator-activated receptor (PPARgamma) as a regulator of monocyte/macrophage function. *J Leukoc Biol* 1999;66:733–739.

150 Jones DC, Ding X, Daynes RA. Nuclear receptor PPARalpha is expressed in resting murine lymphocytes: the PPARalpha in T and B lymphocytes is both transactivation and transrepression competent. *J Biol Chem* 2002;277:6838–6845.

151 Wang P, Anderson PO, Chen S, et al. Inhibition of the transcription factors AP-1 and NF-kappaB in CD4 T cells by peroxisome proliferator-activated receptor gamma ligands. *Int Immunopharmacol* 2001;1:803–812.

152 Marx N, Sukhova G, Murphy C, et al. Macrophages in human atheroma contain PPARgamma: differentiation-dependent peroxisomal proliferator-activated receptor gamma (PPARgamma) expression and reduction of MMP-9 activity through PPARgamma activation in mononuclear phagocytes *in vitro*. *Am J Pathol* 1998;153:17–23.

153 Neve B, Corseaux D, Chinetti G, et al. PPARalpha agonists inhibit tissue factor expression in human monocytes and macrophages. *Circulation* 2001;103:207–212.

154 Marx N, Mackman N, Schonbeck U, et al. PPARalpha activators inhibit tissue factor expression and activity in human monocytes. *Circulation* 2001;103:213–219.

155 Goetze S, Kintscher U, Kim S, et al. Peroxisome proliferator-activated receptor-gamma ligands inhibit nuclear but not cytosolic extracellular signal-regulated kinase/mitogen-activated protein kinase-regulated steps in vascular smooth muscle cell migration. *J Cardiovasc Pharmacol* 2001;38:909–921.

156 Pasceri V, Wu HD, Willerson JT, et al. Modulation of vascular inflammation *in vitro* and *in vivo* by peroxisome proliferator-activated receptor-gamma activators. *Circulation* 2000;101:235–238.

157 Li AC, Brown KK, Silvestre MJ, et al. Peroxisome proliferator-activated receptor gamma ligands inhibit development of atherosclerosis in LDL receptor-deficient mice. *J Clin Invest* 2000;106:523–531.

158 Collins AR, Meehan WP, Kintscher U, et al. Troglitazone inhibits formation of early atherosclerotic lesions in diabetic and nondiabetic low density lipoprotein receptor-deficient mice. *Arterioscler Thromb Vasc Biol* 2001;21:365–371.

159 Duez H, Chao YS, Hernandez M, et al. Reduction of atherosclerosis by the peroxisome proliferator-activated receptor alpha agonist fenofibrate in mice. *J Biol Chem* 2002;277:48051–48057.

160 Frick M, Syvanne M, Nieminen M, et al. Prevention of the angiographic progression of coronary and vein-graft atherosclerosis by gemfibrozil after coronary bypass surgery in men with low levels of HDL cholesterol: Lipid Coronary Angiography Trial (LOCAT) Study Group. *Circulation* 1997;96:2137–2143.

161 Ericcson CG, Hamsten A, Nilsson J, et al. Angiographic assessment of effects of bezafibrate on progression of coronary artery disease in young male postinfarction patients. *Lancet* 1996;347:849–853.

162 Diabetes Atherosclerosis Intervention Study Group. DAIS: effect of fenofibrate on progression of coronary-artery disease in type 2 diabetes: the Diabetes Atherosclerosis Intervention Study, a randomised study. *Lancet* 2001;357:905–910.

163 Frick MH, Elo O, Haapa K, et al. Helsinki Heart Study primary-prevention trial with gemfibrozil in middle-aged men with dyslipidemia: safety of treatment, changes in risk factors, and incidence of coronary heart disease. *N Engl J Med* 1987;317:1237–1245.

164 Rubins HB, Robins SJ, Collins D, et al. Gemfibrozil for the secondary prevention of coronary heart disease in men with low levels of high-density lipoprotein cholesterol: Veterans Affairs High-Density Lipoprotein Cholesterol Intervention Trial Study Group. *N Engl J Med* 1999;341:410–418.

165 Newman WP, Middaugh JP, Propst MT, et al. Atherosclerosis in Alaska natives and non-natives. *Lancet* 1993;341:1056–1057.

166 De Caterina R, Zampolli A. n-3 fatty acids: antiatherosclerotic effects. *Lipids* 2001;36(Suppl):S69–S78.

167 De Caterina R, Cybulsky MI, Clinton SK, et al. The omega-3 fatty acid docosahexaenoate reduces cytokine-induced expression of proatherogenic and proinflammatory proteins in human endothelial cells. *Arterioscler Thromb* 1994;14:1829–1836.

168 De Caterina R, Cybulsky MA, Clinton SK, et al. Omega-3 fatty acids and endothelial leukocyte adhesion molecules. *Prostagl Leukot Ess Fatty Acid* 1995;52:191–195.

169 De Caterina R, Libby P. Control of endothelial leukocyte adhesion molecules by fatty acids. *Lipids* 1996; 31(Suppl):S57–S63.

170 De Caterina R, Liao JK, Libby P. Fatty acid modulation of endothelial activation. *Am J Clin Nutr* 2000;71: 213S–223S.

171 Thies F, Garry JM, Yaqoob P, et al. Association of n-3 polyunsaturated fatty acids with stability of atherosclerotic plaques: a randomised controlled trial. *Lancet* 2003;361:477–485.

172 De Caterina R, Manes C. Inflammation in early atherogenesis: impact of ACE inhibition. *Eur Heart J Suppl* 2003; 5(Suppl A):A15–A24.

173 Yusuf S, Sleight P, Pogue J, et al. Effects of an angiotensin-converting-enzyme inhibitor, ramipril, on cardiovascular events in high-risk patients. The Heart Outcomes Prevention Evaluation Study Investigators. *N Engl J Med* 2000;342:145–153.

CHAPTER 4

Angiogenesis in cardiovascular disease

Karen S. Moulton, MD

Introduction

Angiogenesis is a complex biologic response enacted by endothelial cells. Several cardiovascular pathologies, including atherosclerosis, myocardial infarction, and cardiac growth and hypertrophy are accompanied by angiogenesis, which imparts physiologic functions for injured and ischemic tissues, but has pathologic effects when it is sustained, as in chronic inflammation. Understanding functional consequences of angiogenesis in various cardiovascular conditions could elucidate disease mechanisms or new treatments. Analysis of endothelial cell responses to mechanical forces, soluble growth factors and inhibitors, extracellular matrix (ECM) molecules, inflammation and coagulation factors during the specialized process of angiogenesis can further enhance our knowledge of endothelial and vascular cell biology.

Cell mechanisms of angiogenesis can also operate in non-angiogenic cardiovascular conditions that are related to the more broadly defined concept of vascular remodeling. Similar to steps required for the formation of new blood vessels, vascular remodeling involves proliferation, apoptosis, and migration of vascular wall cells, as well as turnover of the ECM [1]. Adaptive vascular remodeling occurs in systemic and pulmonary hypertension, restenosis after angioplasty or stenting, closure of the ductus arteriosus, arterial remodeling of vein bypass grafts and shunts, and compensatory dilation of atherosclerotic vessels due to hemodynamic flow disturbances in the proximity of atherosclerotic plaques.

Vasculogenesis, angiogenesis, and arteriogenesis

The formation of new blood vessels is a fundamental process involved in the development of the embryo, reproduction, inflammation, and wound repair [2]. Blood vessels and the circulation are absent in the earliest stages of development, when the embryo receives its nutrition by diffusion; however, a functional vascular network is essential for survival and subsequent development of the embryo. Blood vessel formation in the embryo arises by two primary mechanisms: vasculogenesis and angiogenesis [3]. The prevalence of both developmental processes varies temporally and spatially in different regions of the embryo. For instance, the dorsal aorta forms by vasculogenesis, and the cerebral vasculature develops predominantly by mechanisms of angiogenesis [4].

Vasculogenesis

Vasculogenesis involves the migration and expansion of endothelial cell precursor angioblasts into sites of blood vessel formation in the embryo and yolk sac, *in situ* differentiation of angioblasts into endothelial cells, and the assembly of endothelial cells into a primary vascular plexus that connects with endocardial tubes and the extra embryonic vasculature [5,6]. Vasculogenesis and angioblast differentiation are dependent on vascular endothelial growth factor (VEGF), VEGF receptor-2 (VEGFR-2) and VEGF receptor-1 (VEGFR-1), and neuropilin-1 [7–11]. Commitment of hemangioblasts to the angioblast fate is not fully understood, but involves

VEGF and its receptors, products of the Notch gene family, and various transcription factors including Ets-1, members of the GATA family and their cofactors Friend of Gata (FOG) [12–14]. The fate of vascular cells to become arteries is regulated by Notch signaling, the bHLH factor Gridlock, ephrin B2, and neuropilin [10,15]. Venous identity is promoted by the orphan receptor COUP-TFII [16]. Interestingly, arterial and venous patterns in the embryo are determined by molecular events prior to the start of the circulation; however, this molecular determination of vascular patterns in development does not diminish the importance of hemodynamic factors on vascular patterning in the adult. Knowledge of arterial- and venous-specific signaling could reveal molecular changes in venous bypass grafts exposed to arterial blood flow, arterial–venous fistulas, vascular malformations, and reopened arteries after percutaneous interventions.

Angiogenesis

During late stages of fetal growth until adulthood, new blood vessels originate predominantly by mechanisms of angiogenesis. The primary vascular plexus formed by vasculogenesis is subsequently expanded and remodeled into a mature vascular network by diverse mechanisms of angiogenesis. Angiogenesis mechanisms include: (i) sprouting, wherein new vessels branch from the sides or ends of pre-existing blood vessels; (ii) bridging or intussusception, wherein connections between endothelial cells develop across the lumen to subdivide blood vessels along its length into smaller parallel vessels; and (iii) intercalation, which incorporates additional endothelial cells to increase the length and caliber of blood vessels in the growing fetus [3].

During the maturation phase of angiogenesis, vascular networks become extensively remodeled to create mature three-dimensional vascular networks comprised of appropriate arterial and venous patterns with a more optimal circulation. Vascular pruning involves the regression of some newly formed vessels, which become filled in with matrix, and the simultaneous fortification of adjacent blood vessels. Often vascular regression and growth both occur in close proximity, raising skepticism that vascular patterns could arise simply by modulating soluble angiogenic growth factors that saturate angiogenic microenvironments.

Current knowledge of angiogenesis has been advanced by the discovery of molecular factors critical for vascular development and maturation in mice, including Tie2 receptors and their angiopoietin ligands, VE-cadherin, activin receptor-like kinase-1, platelet-derived growth factor (PDGF), transforming growth factor beta (TGF-β), and hypoxia-inducing factor-1 alpha (HIF-1α) among others [17–20]. The formation of normal vascular patterns requires vascular cells to integrate and exhibit differential responses to diverse molecular and environmental factors such as hypoxia. Vascular maturation requires recruitment of pericytes that stabilize early endothelial sprouts and promote vascular maturation by elaborating paracrine factors and secreting ECM molecules to form the vascular basement membrane [21]. ECM molecules and hemodynamic forces mechanically control endothelial cell behavior during angiogenesis [22].

Important signals for vascular patterning also arise outside the vasculature. For example, molecules expressed by nerves have reciprocal effects on vascular cells and progenitors, which account for the parallel organization of nerves and blood vessels in the embryo and adult [23]. Coronary artery development requires the expression of the transcription factor FOG-2 by the myocardium, which directs the migration and differentiation of endothelial cells and smooth muscle cells into the epicardial layer of the heart [14]. Hematopoietic cells of the lymphocyte and myeloid lineages (megakaryocytes, monocytes, granulocytes, mast cells) express angiogenic factors and proteases that modulate both developmental and postnatal angiogenesis [24–27].

Vascular development in the embryo must also be coordinated with organogenesis, because the vascular architecture of many organs, such as the lung, the liver, the kidney, and the endocrine glands, is closely integrated with the physiology of that organ. Blood vessels induce development of the pancreas in some species [28]. Angiogenesis and organogenesis are sometimes coordinated by organ-specific factors, as indicated by the discovery of an endocrine-gland-specific endothelial cell growth factor and its receptor that have little activities on endothelial cells derived from other organs [29]. Other organ-specific factors may still be identified to link the formation of vascular anatomy with different types of organogenesis.

Postnatal mechanisms of blood vessel formation

Postnatal vasculogenesis

The discovery of endothelial precursor cells has suggested additional mechanisms for postnatal blood vessel formation. Endothelial cell colonies seeded on impermeable endovascular grafts in dogs after bone marrow transplants were found to be derived from donor bone marrow cells [30]. Other studies similarly identified small numbers of endothelial precursor cells that circulate in the adult and are mobilized from the bone marrow by VEGF,

granulocyte–monocyte colony-stimulating factor (GM-CSF), insulin-like growth factor-1(IGF-1), and by the activation of VEGFR-1 by placental growth factor (PlGF) [31,32]. Likewise, some inhibitors of angiogenesis impair the release of endothelial precursors from the bone marrow [33,34].

Recent careful studies have shown that "true" endothelial precursor cells intercalate into the endothelium of vascular structures and differentiate into mature endothelial cells as depicted in Figure 4.1. Many bone-marrow-derived precursor cells express hematopoietic markers and recruit to

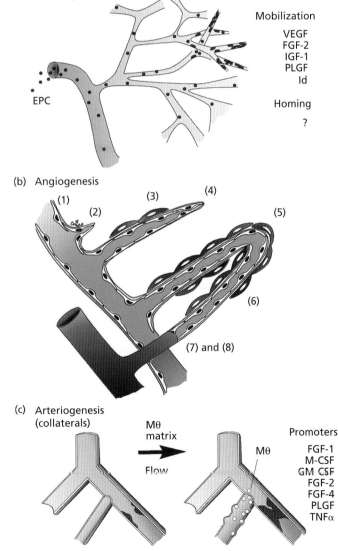

Figure 4.1 Mechanisms of postnatal angiogenesis and or arteriogenesis. (a) Vasculogenesis occurs in the adult via mobilization of endothelial precursor cells from the bone marrow niche. Vascular progenitors home to sites of angiogenesis where they differentiate, migrate, and incorporate into newly formed vessels or repair areas of injured endothelium. Hematopoietic progenitors are recruited to perivascular locations around developing new blood vessels. Growth factors and chemokines promote the release of these cells, but the homing mechanisms are not fully understood. (b) Angiogenesis sprouting is diagramed showing eight stages as outline in the text: (1) vasodilation of the parent vessel, (2) degradation of basement membrane, (3) endothelial cell migration and proliferation, (4) lumen formation, (5) capillary loop formation, (6) synthesis of new basement membrane, (7) stabilization and maturation of sprouts,and (8) Regulation of endothelial cell survival. (c) Arteriogenesis involves the expansion or formation of new larger-caliber conduit vessels that supply blood to capillary beds. Macrophages (Mθ) and flow can significantly enhance collateral growth. Several angiogenic factors promote both angiogenesis (capillary formation) and collateral development. The listed factors provide additional signals that are necessary to complete the arteriogenesis program. (Illustration by Silvia Sonn).

perivascular locations near new blood vessels where they exert paracrine effects on angiogenesis [35,36]. Only small numbers of precursor-derived endothelial cells are found in sites of angiogenesis, which originally raised questions about their functional significance. Later studies showed that endothelial cell precursors could compensate for genetically suppressed angiogenesis mechanisms in Id-deficient mice, which could not grow tumors until wild-type bone marrow stem cells or endothelial precursor cells were transplanted [13,37].

Despite their low numbers, newly arrived progenitors provide critical paracrine and recruiting functions for local endothelial cells [38]. New cell-based strategies delivering stem cells or endothelial cell precursor cells have shown positive results in preclinical models of collateral formation and re-endothelialization of injured arteries or thrombosed blood vessels. Several animal and clinical studies of transplant recipients now indicate that vascular smooth muscle cells in the neointima of atherosclerotic and transplant-associated arteriosclerotic lesions can arise from circulating smooth muscle progenitors, not just from medial wall cells [39,40].

Postnatal angiogenesis

Mechanisms of postnatal vessel formation in physiologic and pathologic disease models most commonly involve sprouting and adhere to the following general series of morphologic and biochemical events (Figure 4.1):

1 *Vasodilation of the parent vessel*: Vasodilation is mediated by the production of nitric oxide. The permeability of angiogenic vessels is enhanced by VEGF and its downstream signaling targets, as well as by VE-cadherin, which all promote the extravasation of plasma proteins to form a provisional matrix for cell migration.

2 *Remodeling of basement membrane*: Endothelial cells in the parent vessel alter their attachments to basement membrane and pericytes. Changes in flow and mechanical forces transmitted through the endothelium activates proteases that remodel the vascular basement membrane causing it to thin and change its composition [41,42]. Matrix remodeling has several consequences for regulating angiogenesis: mechanical forces converge on thinned regions of the basement membrane to facilitate sprouting. Remodeled ECM alters endothelial cell responsiveness to

growth factors and releases growth factors or inhibitors sequestered in the matrix to potentiate or limit angiogenesis [43,44].

3 *Endothelial cell migration and proliferation*: Endothelial cell proliferation and migration both contribute to the increasing length of developing vessels, but migrating endothelial cells form the tip of the capillary sprout [45]. Most angiogenesis factors, including members of the VEGF and fibroblast growth factor (FGF) families, modulate both proliferation and migration of endothelial cells. Complexes of activated metalloproteases and $\alpha_v\beta_3$ integrins on endothelial cells coordinate migration with the exposure of matrix molecules to facilitate adhesion [46].

4 *Lumen formation*: As the endothelial cells align in the developing capillary, they attach to each other and to the ECM in a manner that creates a lumen. The lumen develops proximally in the developing sprout as a continuation of the lumen from the parent vessel. Lumen formation can also occur by vacuolization within the endothelial cell. Lumen formation requires the production of fibronectin and laminin matrix, and depends on adhesion molecules and cell surface glycoproteins [47–49].

5 *Loop formation*: Parallel capillaries fuse and coalesce along their length or at their tips to form a loop capable of handling blood flow. Blood flow causes further vascular remodeling. Blood cells such as platelets carry several endothelial factors that facilitate the maturation of the newly perfused vessel [26].

6 *Maturation of the basement membrane*: The new capillary continues to remodel the basement membrane by enhancing its content in collagen type IV, collagen XV, and collagen XVIII [50].

7 *Stabilization/incorporation of pericytes*: Maturation of the new vessel requires the recruitment of pericytes, which have long protruding cytoplasmic processes that run lengthwise and around the capillary wall [21]. Pericytes help synthesize basement membranes, regulate blood flow and permeability, and produce paracrine signals, including VEGF, PDGF, TGF-β, and angiopoietin-1 (Ang1) [51]. Several studies have shown that pericytes stabilize the newly formed blood vessel and inhibit vascular regression after angiogenic factors subside [52].

8 *Endothelial cell survival/apoptosis*: Endothelial cells of quiescent blood vessels survive with little cell turnover. The regulation of endothelial cell survival and apoptosis in angiogenic vessels is a natural mechanism for vascular pruning to create vascular patterns. Endothelial cell apoptosis is enhanced by disruption of cell attachments to the matrix or to other endothelial cells (VE-cadherin), the withdrawal of growth factors VEGF and Ang1, and by changes in nitric oxide and hemodynamic shear forces [19,53,54]. Some angiogenesis inhibitors, including thrombospondin-1 (TSP-1), endostatin and antagonists of $\alpha_v\beta_3$ and VEGF, induce endothelial cell apoptosis [55–57].

Arteriogenesis

Arteriogenesis is the formation of larger-caliber blood vessels with a more complex structure, consisting of an endothelium plus incorporated smooth muscle cells and ECM that form the media, elastin fibers, and the adventitia. Angiogenesis and arteriogenesis programs share common endothelial cell regulators; however, the molecular mechanisms and spatial cues to generate or remodel large-caliber conduit blood vessels most likely differ from those necessary to create simple capillaries, which are comprised of an endothelium, basement membrane, and fewer mural cells. Angiogenesis is usually induced by hypoxia, but arteriogenesis develops proximal to local tissue hypoxia. Pressure gradients across the collateral network and regional shear forces on endothelial cells may initiate cellular and ECM remodeling events [58]. Endothelial activation on remodeling collaterals and monocyte adhesion are critical factors.

Monocytes release growth factors and proteases that attenuate and remodel the internal elastic lamina and the medial layers. Smooth muscle cells proliferate and are incorporated into the widened media. Often the expanded internal elastic lamina has a helical orientation in remodeled collaterals, which accounts for their tortuosity [59]. High cardiac flow states associated with chronic anemia and arterio-venous fistulas stimulate the development of tortuous epicardial coronary collaterals.

Molecular distinctions of arteriogenesis from angiogenesis programs are emerging. PlGF and monocyte chemotactic protein-1 (MCP-1) promote arteriogenesis due to their added effects on inflammatory cells that cooperate with endothelial cells in collateral formation [60–63]. Agents that recruit smooth muscle cells to form the muscular and matrix components of the blood vessel wall, such as basic FGF, PDGF-B, and TGF-β, may have added effects compared to factors with primary effects on endothelial cells. The transcription factor MEF2C is necessary for the differentiation of smooth muscle cells that incorporate into larger-caliber blood vessels. Fibrillin-1 and elastin are required to form stable arteries [64].

Basic questions in arteriogenesis remain under debate: Do collateral blood vessels form *de novo* or do they arise by expanding existing arterioles? What signals are derived from the downstream ischemic vascular bed and sensed by the proximal conduit vessels? What contributions do vascular and hematopoietic progenitor cells make in angiogenesis and arteriogenesis? Future advances in our molecular understanding in the mechanisms of angiogenesis and arteriogenesis are essential to design more effective treatments, particularly in patients with cardiovascular risk factors and endothelial cell dysfunction.

Physiologic and pathologic postnatal angiogenesis

In the adult, endothelial cell turnover is relatively quiescent, with only 0.01% of cells in the cell division cycle at any given time [65]. Angiogenesis is stimulated for discrete periods during physiologic angiogenesis involved in ovulation, postnatal growth and tissue regeneration, menstrual changes of the endometrium, and wound healing [66]. In contrast, pathologic angiogenesis is abnormally sustained in tumors, diabetic retinopathy, ischemic tissues, and chronic inflammatory conditions, such as rheumatoid arthritis and atherosclerosis [2,67]. Many cellular events and regulatory molecules are shared by both categories of angiogenesis; however, inflammation is a distinguishing feature that accompanies postnatal pathologic angiogenesis. Immune cells including macrophages, mast cells, and T cells modulate various steps of angiogenesis by elaborating several angiogenic growth factors, releasing matrix-associated proteases able to remodel vascular basement membranes and facilitate endothelial cell invasion, and producing chemokines that recruit precursor cells from the bone marrow [24,68,69]. Differences between physiologic and pathologic angiogenesis could explain why molecules such as PlGF, endothelial nitric oxide synthase (eNOS), chemokines and cyclooxygenase-2, which modulate immune cells, have minimal effects on embryonic angiogenesis, yet significant effects on disease-associated angiogenesis [63,70,71].

Differences between physiologic and pathologic angiogenesis can be exploited for selective treatments. Tumor vessels express unique molecules and have exposed intercellular gaps that may be exploited for drug delivery and targeting to specific vascular addresses [72,73]. Molecular distinctions of other types of pathologic angiogenesis could identify unique pathways that could be selectively regulated without interference of physiologic angiogenesis. For example, angiogenesis associated with chronic inflammation may be more responsive to agents that target chemokines, tumor necrosis factor alpha (TNF-α), or other factors regulated by immune cells.

One caveat to consider is that many diseases are associated with angiogenesis, but not all angiogenesis-related diseases depend on angiogenesis for pathologic progression [74]. The distinction between "angiogenic" and "angiogenic-dependent" diseases is determined empirically, based on collective results from genetic and pharmacologic interventions that independently manipulate neovascularization and alter the disease course. As an example, wound healing is an angiogenic process; however, it is only modestly inhibited by a variety of angiogenesis inhibitors that significantly inhibit angiogenesis in tumors, atherosclerosis, or arthritis models [53,63,75].

Assays of angiogenesis

Advances in the understanding of angiogenesis were facilitated by culture techniques for the isolation and growth of endothelial cells [76,77]. *In vitro* angiogenesis assays enabled the discovery of molecules that regulate proliferation, migration, tube formation, and endothelial cell survival or apoptotic pathways involved in angiogenesis [78]. Aorta explants produce more complex endothelial cell sprouts in a matrix and facilitate the comparisons of endothelial cell outgrowth from aortas of genetically modified mice [79,80]. *In vitro* assays help to determine mechanisms of angiogenesis regulators; however, no single assay is sufficient proof of their activity *in vivo*. Disruption of tube formation

in tube morphogenesis assays is sometimes misinterpreted as evidence for negative regulators of angiogenesis. Scatter factor (hepatocyte growth factor) was so named because it increased endothelial cell motility and disrupted endothelial cell tubes, yet functions as a pro-angiogenesis regulator *in vivo* [81,82]. Results of tube morphogenesis are sometimes misinterpreted as endothelial cell differentiation, even though fully differentiated primary endothelial cells derived from large veins or arteries are sometimes used to evaluate microvascular tube formation [83,84].

Although *in vitro* assays are useful to examine specific endothelial cell responses relevant to angiogenesis, angiogenesis-related molecules require functional validation *in vivo*. Culture systems have higher oxygen and different growth factors and serum conditions compared with the angiogenesis microenvironment *in vivo*. Endothelial cell regulators may be metabolized differently *in vivo*, require additional cofactors, or have secondary effects on other cell types. Perhaps most importantly, matrix turnover and mechanical factors are not well represented *in vitro*. The initiation of blood flow in early endothelial cell sprouts trigger further vascular remodeling and synthesis of the vascular basement membrane [85].

The corneal micropocket and Matrigel® (tumor-derived extract of basement membranes) or sponge implant assays are common *in vivo* assays that measure neovascularization induced by growth factors released from implants or matrix [86]. The corneal micropocket model has advantages because the entire area of newly formed vessels in the avascular cornea is easily measured *in situ*, monitored temporally, and its arterial, venous, and lymphatic connections can be identified [86,87]. Both methods are useful to evaluate mechanisms of postnatal angiogenesis in mice with genetic mutations. Advances with specialized video microscopy chambers and multiphoton intravital microscopy allow real-time analysis of cellular and molecular events during angiogenesis *in vivo* [88,89].

Angiogenic growth factors

The importance of angiogenesis in normal development and various pathologic conditions prompted investigators to identify angiogenesis regulators.

Table 4.1 Endogenous angiogenic factors.

Factor	Molecular weight	Endothelial mitogen	Year reported
Basic fibroblast growth factor [91]	18,000	Yes	1984
Acidic fibroblast growth factor [92]	16,400	Yes	1984
Angiogenin	14,100	No	1985
Transforming growth factorTGF alpha	5,500	Yes	1986
Transforming growth factorTGF beta	25,000	No	1986
Tumor necrosis factor alpha	17,000	No	1987
Vascular endothelial growth factor [195]	45,000	Yes	1983
Platelet-derived endothelial growth factor	45,000	Yes	1989
Granulocyte–monocyte stimulating factor	17,000	Yes	1991
Placental growth factor	25,000	Weak	1991
Interleukin-8	40,000	Yes	1992
Hepatocyte growth factor	92,000	Yes	1993
Angiopoietin-1 [122]	40,000	Weak	1996

Table 4.1 lists a number of identified naturally occurring factors that promote angiogenesis [90]. Selected angiogenesis stimulators and inhibitors with expression relevant to the cardiovascular system are discussed below.

Fibroblast growth factors

FGF constitute a large family of related polypeptides that are potent endothelial cell mitogens, yet also stimulate smooth muscle cells and other cell types. Basic FGF (FGF-2) was the first isolated angiogenesis factor, followed quickly by acidic FGF (FGF-1) [91,92]. FGF-1 and FGF-2 do not contain secretion signals, suggesting that cell injury is one mechanism for their release [93]. Affinity of FGF-2 for heparan sulfate glycosaminoglycans on the cell surface facilitates FGF ligand binding to its native receptors and provides reservoirs of factors in ECM, which are released during wounding or by inflammatory cells [94].

The roles of FGF-1 and FGF-2 have been evaluated in vascular diseases. The adventitial delivery of FGF-2 augmented neointimal smooth muscle cell proliferation and neovascularization after balloon injury of the carotid artery [95]. Direct gene transfer of FGF-1 in endothelial cells of porcine arteries promoted intimal hyperplasia and stimulated intimal neovascularization [96]. Human atherosclerotic tissues express increased FGF-1 compared with normal vessels, which may promote plaque neovascularization and restenosis [97]. The administration of FGF-1 or FGF-2 enhanced myocardial and peripheral limb collateral vessels [98–100]. FGF members have advantages for arteriogenesis programs due to their added effects on smooth muscle cells that are recruited into larger-caliber collaterals, and to the induction of reduced permeability compared to VEGF [101,102].

VEGF and its receptors

VEGF, also known as vascular permeability factor, is a potent cytokine regulating multiple functions in the vascular endothelium [103]. The VEGF family of growth factors includes the prototype member VEGF-A, and other members VEGF-B, VEGF-C, VEGF-D, and VEGF-E, which differ by their tissue distributions and affinities for various VEGF receptors. Similar to FGF, VEGF stimulates endothelial cell proliferation and migration and has high heparin-binding affinity. As its alternative name implies, VEGF increases the permeability of capillaries and promotes the development of a fenestrated endothelium [104]. Permeability properties of VEGF facilitate physiologic and pathologic angiogenesis by extravasating plasma proteins that form a provisional matrix favoring cell migration [105].

VEGF and its receptors are required for blood vessel growth during development. Interruption of only one VEGF gene allele is embryonic lethal, which indicates that VEGF expression is tightly regulated during development [8,106]. VEGF binds to tyrosine kinase receptors VEGF receptor-1 (VEGFR-1), also known as Flt-1 (*fms*-like tyrosine kinase-1), and VEGF receptor-2 (VEGFR-2), also known as

Kdr (kinase insert domain containing receptor) or Flk-1 (fetal liver kinase). VEGFR-2 is expressed early in the developing endothelium of the yolk sac and later in angioblasts and all endothelial cells [9]. Null mutations of VEGFR-2 blocked the formation of blood islands, hematopoiesis, vasculogenesis, and endothelial cell differentiation [7,12].

VEGFR-1 is similarly expressed during early vascular development and postnatal angiogenesis; however, VEGFR-1 is also expressed on inflammatory cells such as monocytes and macrophages, which coordinates inflammation and pathologic angiogenesis associated with atherosclerosis and arthritis [63,107,108]. Deletion of VEGFR-1 allowed endothelial cell differentiation, but endothelial cells assembled into abnormal vascular channels [109]. VEGFR-1 also binds PlGF.

Postnatal VEGF functions have been evaluated with conditional knockout mice and pharmacologic inhibitors. The loss of VEGF impairs ovarian angiogenesis and ovulation, bone vascularization, postnatal growth, and retinal neovascularization [52,110,111]. In the vascular system, VEGF has protective effects that ameliorate cerebral and tissue ischemia, yet its accumulation in advanced atherosclerotic lesions may promote the pathologic recruitment of monocytes and neovascularization [63,112]. VEGF agents have been tested in several clinical trials for therapeutic angiogenesis; however, clinical results were less optimal compared to preclinical studies [113].

VEGF-A has several splice variants, of which $VEGF_{121}$, $VEGF_{165}$, and $VEGF_{189}$ are the most common isoforms. All splice variants stimulate endothelial cell proliferation by binding VEGFR-1 and VEGFR-2, but they have different affinities for heparan sulfate proteoglycans that influence their biologic functions [114]. The most soluble $VEGF_{121}$ isoform shows little binding to ECM and neuropilin, a co-receptor for VEGF; whereas the longer isoforms $VEGF_{165}$, $VEGF_{189}$, and $VEGF_{206}$ are primarily associated with matrix and bind neuropilin receptors, which may coordinate neural axon and vascular patterning [115]. Interestingly, VEGF activation of neuropilin on T cells is necessary for primary immune responses, thereby providing another molecular link between angiogenesis and chronic inflammation [116].

The differences in matrix affinities and receptor binding suggest that VEGF splice variants have differential functions in physiologic and pathologic angiogenesis [117]. Mouse strains that express single VEGF isoforms have shown that matrix-associated VEGF isoforms are required to direct coronary artery development and normal vessel patterning in the eye [118]. In other tissues, soluble forms of VEGF are needed to guide and attract the invasion of vessels into avascular tissues, such as joints and retina [114,119]. Thus, a complement of different VEGF-A isoforms may be required to harness VEGF for therapeutic purposes.

Tie2 receptors and angiopoietins

The endothelial cell Tie1 and Tie2 receptors are important for vascular development [120]. Tie1-deficient embryos have abnormal vascular integrity and develop edema and hemorrhage. The physiologic ligands for Tie1 receptors are not yet identified, but Tie1 signaling might be regulated by some angiopoietin ligands [121]. Tie2-deficient embryos have abnormal angiogenesis and immature vascular networks. Angiopoietins comprise a family of ligands that bind Tie2 receptors and have effects on multiple steps of the angiogenic remodeling process, particularly for the interactions between endothelial cells themselves and with pericytes and the basement membrane [122,123]. The most abundant angiopoietin members are Ang1 and Ang2, which function as agonist and relative antagonist, respectively. Ang1 inhibits vascular permeability, but has little mitogenic activity on endothelial cells [124]. In combination with VEGF, Ang1 enhances angiogenesis and collateral vessel formation without the induction of excessive permeability and the recruitment of inflammatory cells compared to VEGF alone [125,126].

Neural and vascular system regulators

Neuropilin and semaphorin

Nerves and blood vessels resemble each other in their ability to form branching networks and are organized in parallel patterns, suggesting possible molecular interactions. Neuropilins, NRP1 and NRP2, were first identified as receptors for semaphorins and mediators of neuronal guidance. NRP1 was subsequently identified as another receptor for VEGF on endothelial cells that regulated angiogenesis. NRP1 is expressed preferentially on arterial endothelial cells and binds Semaphorin 3A, whereas NRP2 is expressed preferentially on venous and lymphatic vessels, and binds Semaphorin 3F. Mutational studies and the use of soluble NRP receptors have revealed essential roles in vascular and cardiac development and in postnatal angiogenesis. Semaphorin 3A binds endothelial cells and inhibits angiogenesis, in part due to direct competition for VEGF binding to NRP1 [127].

EphrinB2 and EphB4 receptors

Ephrins and their Eph receptors are a large family of ligands and tyrosine kinase receptors involved in many developmental processes including the nervous system and angiogenesis. EphrinB2, a transmembrane ligand for EphB4 receptor, is expressed by arterial, but not venous endothelial cells [10]. Conversely, the EphB4 receptor is expressed on veins. EphrinB2-deficient mice developed abnormal capillary networks in the brain and yolk sac and abnormal myocardial trabeculation. A similar phenotype of embryos lacking the EphB4 receptor indicated that normal capillary patterns require reciprocal signaling by the receptor and transmembrane ligand pair [11]. Smooth muscle cells acquire the ephrinB2 transmembrane ligand as they incorporate into arterial structures, suggesting a role in arteriogenesis [128].

EphrinB2 provides a molecular mechanism for the parallel development of nerves and blood vessels [23,129]. The extracellular domains of ephrinB2 provide guidance cues for nerves, but internal signals generated by this receptor on endothelial cells are required for normal vascular patterning [130]. The biologic effects of these arterial and venous receptors during postnatal angiogenesis may elucidate pathologic mechanisms for vein grafts implanted into arterial circuits and arterio-venous malformations.

Other neuronal guidance factors with reciprocal effects in vascular development include Slit ligands and their Robo receptors and Netrin ligands. Robo-4 is selectively expressed on endothelial cells and contributes to developmental and tumor angiogenesis [131]. Strategies for angiogenesis often focus on the quantitative effects of various molecules; however, providing guidance cues may be equally important to direct normal vascular patterns.

Matrix remodeling proteases

Proteases of the matrix metalloprotease (MMP), heparanase, plasminogen activator, and cathepsin families regulate angiogenesis by a variety of mechanisms [42,132–134]. Proteases facilitate endothelial cell migration and tissue invasion. By binding to integrins on the endothelial cell surface, MMPs are postured to coordinate cell adhesion, migration, and matrix remodeling during sprouting [46]. Infiltrations of hematopoietic cells such as monocytes, mast cells, T or B cells release proteases that temporally correlate with the angiogenic switch in different tumors [27,135]. The above mechanisms support a positive role for various protease activities during angiogenesis; however, their angiogenesis-related functions are more complex because proteolytically released fragments derived from ECM components exert negative effects on angiogenesis [44,136].

MMP activity correlates with inflammatory cells in atherosclerotic lesions and may promote plaque rupture that triggers heart attacks or strokes [137]. Despite the clear association of MMP with pathologic vascular remodeling and aneurysm formation, treatment strategies that target various proteases are challenged by their redundant activities and diverse protein substrates with broad biologic effects.

Clinical assays that detect MMP activities in the urine and the blood of patients with vascular inflammation, aneurysms, vasculitis, and malignancy show promise in providing sensitive biomarkers for predicting clinical risk or assessing treatments [138]. Molecular probes activated by various MMPs can sense or directly image MMP activity *in vivo* [139].

Chemokines and other angiogenic molecules

Several factors, including leptin, chemokines, hepatocyte growth factor, and interleukins, induce angiogenesis when given exogenously, but have minimal roles in vascular development. Different chemokines act either as inhibitors or stimulators of angiogenesis [140]. Stromal cell-derived factor-1 binds to the chemokine receptor CXCR-4, which in turn mobilizes endothelial cell precursors [32,141].

Inhibitors of angiogenesis

Control of angiogenesis also involves negative regulators, some of which are listed in Table 4.2 [90]. Most endothelial cells in the body are maintained in a quiescent state and are stabilized presumably by mural cells and basement membranes. The abundant growth factors with angiogenic potential in the blood and ECM that bathe the endothelium led to the conceptual hypothesis that these growth factors must be antagonized by endogenous inhibitors in order to maintain endothelial cell quiescence [142]. Soon after the discovery of FGF-2 and VEGF, *in vitro* and *in vivo* angiogenesis screens were established to identify molecules that inhibit endothelial cell proliferation and migration.

Interferon alpha

Interferon alpha inhibits angiogenesis in the cornea assay and inhibits both endothelial cell proliferation and migration in culture [143]. Currently, interferon alpha is administered at low doses to inhibit the growth of life-threatening hemangiomas and certain tumors [144]. Interferon alpha acts as an indirect inhibitor of angiogenesis, due in part to its inhibition of FGF-2 release.

Thrombospondin-1

TSP-1 is a component of ECM that acts as a negative regulator of angiogenesis. The anti-angiogenesis function of TSP-1 was discovered in a model of tumor progression, wherein inactivation of the tumor suppressor gene p53 resulted in loss of TSP-1 and increased tumor angiogenesis by the parent tumor cells [145]. Subsequently, TSP-1 was purified and shown to inhibit endothelial cell migration and neovascularization in the cornea assay. Progesterone-dependent expression of TSP-1 during the menstrual cycle modulates regression of endometrial vessels [146]. TSP-1-induced endothelial cell apoptosis is mediated by the CD36 receptor, which also functions as a scavenger receptor important for the clearance of apoptotic bodies and lipids in atherosclerosis [57,147]. Inhibition of endothelial cell migration by TSP-1 also depends on β1 integrins [148]. Maturation of capillaries in developing lungs and pancreas are restored by TSP-1 peptides that activate latent secreted forms of transforming growth factor beta1 (TGF-β1) [149]. Clinical trials of anti-angiogenic TSP-1-derived peptides are being evaluated in cancer patients [150].

TSP-1 agents have been studied in a limited number of models of cardiovascular disease. Atherosclerotic tissues express TSP-1, but a pathogenic role has not yet been shown [151]. In the rat carotid balloon injury model, neutralizing antibodies to TSP-1 enhanced re-endothelialization and inhibited smooth muscle cell proliferation [152]. Interestingly, missense polymorphism variants of TSP-1 and TSP-4 were associated with an increased odds ratio for premature coronary artery disease [153]. Since TSPs are large multidomain proteins with diverse effects on leukocytes and platelets, it is not yet conclusive that the increased cardiovascular risk is related to loss of TSP anti-angiogenesis functions.

Tissue inhibitors of metalloproteases

The activities of metalloproteases are tightly regulated during angiogenesis at many levels, including activation by proteolytic processing of pro-enzymes and inhibition by forming complexes with a specific inhibitor, which itself can be a product of a protease [154]. Tissue inhibitors of metalloproteases (TIMPs) are stoichiometrically balanced relative to their respective metalloprotease partners and therefore function as angiogenesis inhibitors *in vivo* [155]. Additionally, TIMP-2 contains a non-enzymatic domain that binds endothelial cells via integrins and inhibits proliferation and migration [156,157]. Mice with genetic alterations in TIMPs or various MMP family members have demonstrated diverse effects of these molecules in the cardiovascular system [158].

Cryptic regulators of angiogenesis

Several cryptic angiogenesis regulators are released by proteolysis of parent molecules. TSP-1 and platelet factor-4 parent molecules inhibit angiogenesis, yet can be modified to truncated forms with more potent activity [43,159]. Plasminogen, fibronectin, and prolactin have no initial effect, but their proteolytically released-peptides inhibit angiogenesis [160–162]. Angiostatin, generated from plasminogen by elastases and metalloprotease-2, binds

Table 4.2 Endogenous negative regulators of endothelial cell proliferation.

Factor	Inhibits proliferation	Inhibits chemotaxis	Parent molecule	Year
Platelet factor-4 [159]	Yes	Yes	–	1995
TSP-1 [145]	Yes	Yes	–	1989
TIMP-1	No	Yes	–	1991
TIMP-2 [155]	Yes	Yes	–	1990
Prolactin (16-kDa fragment) [162]	Yes	Yes	Prolactin	1993
Angiostatin [160]	Yes	Yes	Plasminogen	1994
Endostatin [44]	Yes	–	Collagen XVIII	1997
Tumstatin [165]	Yes	Yes	Collagen IV	2002
Restin	Yes	Yes	Collagen XV	2000
Endorepellin [166]	Yes	Yes	Perlecan	2003

angiomotin receptors on endothelial cells and inhibits endothelial cell migration and proliferation [136,163]. Several molecules with inhibitory effects on endothelial cells are released from vascular basement membrane components including collagen XVIII, collagen XV, collagen IV, and perlecan (Table 4.2) [44,164–166]. Common features of endostatin, restin, tumstatin, and endorepellin include their affinity for heparan sulfates and derivation from the C-terminal non-collagenous domains of their parent molecules, which are oriented toward the endothelial interface. Heparan sulfate affinity is necessary for anti-angiogenesis functions, presumably by facilitating interactions on the endothelial cell surface [167]. Although high-affinity signaling receptors for these different inhibitory proteins have not been widely recognized, these proteins interact with different integrins to mediate their effects on angiogenesis [168–170]. Thus, the endogenous interactions of these matrix molecules with endothelial cells likely modulate adhesion and migration capacities of endothelial cells during the sprouting and maturation phases of angiogenesis.

Lymphangiogenesis

Mechanisms of lymphangiogenesis have been elucidated by the identification of lymphatic-specific endothelial markers and growth factors. Whereas Notch family members and COUP-TFIII promote arterial and venous specification, respectively, the homeobox gene Prox-1 induces lymphatic commitment [171]. The VEGF receptor-3 (VEGFR-3) is expressed on lymphatic endothelium in the embryo and adult, but it may have a broader role on vascular development. VEGFR-3-deficient mice undergo vasculogenesis and angiogenesis, but have defective lumens in large vessels, which results in pericardial effusion, cardiovascular failure, and lethality prior to the onset of lymphatic development [172]. A dominant inactivating VEGFR-3 mutation results in lymphedema, abnormal lymphatics, and mimics Milroy's disease in patients with hereditary congenital lymphedema syndromes linked to VEGFR-3 mutations [173,174]. VEGFR-3 is activated by VEGF-C and VEGF-D to induce lymphangiogenesis; however, upregulated expression of VEGF-C also induces angiogenesis, mediated by binding to other VEGF receptors [175–177]. Loss of NRP2 in veins and lymphatic vessels interferes with small lymphatics, but has no obvious effect on larger collecting lymphatics [178].

Some factors have dual roles in both angiogenesis and lymphangiogenesis; but selective regulation of either process may be beneficial to a variety of inflammatory, vascular, edematous, and malignant diseases. VEGF-C treatments induce angiogenesis and lymphangiogenesis, which may ameliorate lymphedema syndromes [174,176]. VEGF-C mutants have been designed that specifically activate VEGFR-3 and induce lymphangiogenesis without angiogenesis [179]. Circulating endothelial cell precursors express VEGFR-3 and sometimes incorporates into lymphatic channels, which raises questions about their therapeutic potential and from what point of entry these cells leave the blood to enter the lymphatic circulation [180].

Pulmonary vascular remodeling

Pulmonary hypertension is a complex condition associated with vascular remodeling in the pulmonary circulation, either as a primary intrinsic defect or as a secondary response to hemodynamic changes associated with cardiac defects, pulmonary embolus, or hypoxic conditions. Genetic studies in families prone to develop pulmonary hypertension have identified susceptibility genes in the TGF receptor and growth factor families. Pathologic changes in pulmonary vessels include endothelial cell and smooth muscle cell proliferation, endothelial cell activation, enhanced growth factors and protease activation [181,182]. Plexiform lesions in some types of pulmonary hypertension consist of clonal endothelial cell populations, resulting from local clonal expansion. Intimal hyperplasia in pulmonary arteries can also develop neovascularization similar to atherosclerotic lesions of systemic arteries. Characterization of the responses of endothelial cells and smooth muscle cells during pathologic angiogenesis may provide further understanding as to potential mediators of pulmonary vascular diseases.

Angiogenesis in cardiac growth and hypertrophy

During late fetal and early postnatal periods of development, rapid growth of cardiac myocytes is accompanied by a proportional growth of capillaries and enlargement of large-caliber coronary vessels [183]. Body growth exposes the ventricle to increased stretch and pressure loads, which induce hypertrophy and hyperplasia of cardiac myocytes. During this rapid phase of cardiac growth, myocardial capillary density increases by sprouting and intussusception mechanisms and capillary diameters decrease, which maximizes oxygen transport efficiency, as the relative area of endothelium to vessel volume is increased [184]. The number of main coronary arteries remains fixed after birth, but large vessels increase their length and diameter [185]. Outward caliber growth of blood vessels requires endothelial cell intercalation, basement membranes remodeling, and proliferation of mural cells and adventitial vasa vasorum to perfuse the outer vessel wall [186].

Cardiac growth decreases rapidly with maturity, but cardiomyocyte hypertrophy and hyperplasia can be stimulated by hormonal, hemodynamic, and pathologic circumstances in the adult. Hearts at older ages are often exposed to hypertension, increased vascular resistance, or valvular abnormalities that alter pressure or volume loads. Alterations in myocardial mass and dimensions are accompanied by concomitant changes in coronary vessels and capillaries, which can be either compensatory or pathologic. Typically, capillary growth is inadequate to meet the demands of hypertrophied myocytes, thereby contributing to myocardial dysfunction [187].

During adult cardiac hypertrophy, angiogenesis is observed at the capillary level. Larger coronary vessels do not increase significantly, but coronary arterioles enlarge and branch. Myocardial vascular growth can be assessed by a variety of methods. Capillary density is measured as a ratio of capillary to myofibril area in heart tissue fixed at the same systolic or diastolic period. Incorporation of bromodeoxyuridine indicates endothelial cell proliferation or repair [185]. The functional capacity of the coronary circulation is determined from the maximal blood flow after vasodilation relative to resting blood flow. Nuclear medicine, magnetic resonance or positron emission technologies, and vascular targeted microbubbles are newer methods to quantify changes in collateral circulation or tissue perfusion [188].

Angiogenesis and cardiac mass regulation

Studies suggest a paracrine relationship for VEGF that coordinates changes in the endothelial and myocardial compartments. Ischemic cardiomyopathy resulted from inadequate coronary artery development in genetically altered mice expressing only soluble VEGF$_{120}$ [118]. Ablation of VEGF expression by cardiac myocytes induced a dilated cardiomyopathy with reduced capillary density, ventricular dysfunction, and the induction of hypoxia-responsive genes involved in energy metabolism. These two examples of impaired myocardial angiogenesis during postnatal cardiac growth indicate that normal cardiac function and dimensions require coordinated changes in the vasculature [189]. Endothelial-directed interventions could hypothetically modulate cardiac mass and restrict hypertrophy; however, the therapeutic window may be narrow to maintain adequate myocardial perfusion and avoid ischemic cardiomyopathy and dilation. The vascular remodeling that accompanies most forms of pathologic cardiac hypertrophy is already inadequate to meet the demands of increased myocyte mass and pressure or volume loads. Thus, pathologic cardiac hypertrophy may be an angiogenic disease with practical constraints for attempts to suppress cardiac remodeling by direct control of myocardial angiogenesis, unless better clinical methods exist to assess myocardial perfusion demands.

Factors influencing myocardial angiogenesis

Cardiac growth and the cardiac vasculature are influenced by hormonal and certain physiologic conditions. Elevated or reduced thyroxin levels increase myocardial size and capillary density without inducing significant endothelial cell proliferation, suggesting that endothelial cells elongate or increase in size [190]. Mechanical forces exerted by contraction and blood flow influence vessel development. Forces are transmitted from the apical endothelial cell surface, across the actin cytoskeleton, to the vascular basement membrane and adjacent cardiomyocytes and back again. Molecular mechanisms activated by mechanical stimuli involve integrins and their signaling pathways, cell–cell junction molecules, structural molecules in the cytoskeleton, activation of flow-sensitive ion channels, and regulation of cell–matrix interactions [22,191]. Shear stress and stretch activation of endothelial cells alter patterns of gene expression, cell shape and release of prostacyclins, nitric oxide and other vasoactive molecules [1,192]. Chronic vasodilators have been employed to increase coronary blood flow and increase capillary density in the myocardium.

Hypoxia in tissues is a potent inducer of angiogenesis. Hypoxia or hypoglycemia increase HIF-1α, that regulates several genes involved in angiogenesis and erythropoiesis to restore homeostasis in tissues deprived of oxygen or nutrients [193]. Increased expression of HIF-1α in transgenic mice induced blood vessels with increased calibers and more smooth muscle cells compared to capillaries induced by VEGF alone [194]. HIF-1α regulation of cell cycle and metabolic pathways enhance immune and endothelial cell survival while invading hypoxic microenvironments during angiogenesis [195,196].

The effects of hypoxia on coronary vessels and the heart *in vivo* are more complex, because chronic hypoxia in patients induces other physiologic adaptations. For example, chronic hypoxia induces pulmonary hypertension, right ventricular hypertrophy, and alterations in capillaries and arterioles due to the altered pressure load rather than reduced oxygen delivery in the right ventricle. Hypoxia induces microscopic foci of myocardial necrosis associated with inflammation and angiogenesis. Patients with chronic megaloblastic and iron deficiency anemia have increased cardiac output and develop more coronary anastomoses and collaterals [197].

Angiogenesis after myocardial infarction

Abrupt closure of the coronary vessels results in myocardial infarction and a subsequent release of angiogenic growth factors including FGF-2 and VEGF. Serial angiograms performed on patients receiving thrombolytic agents allowed temporal observations of coronary collaterals, which can either grow or regress after an acute myocardial infarction. A significant fraction of patients with acute infarcts have pre-existing collaterals, which correlate with preserved left ventricular function [198]. In patients with persistent coronary occlusions, the incidence of collaterals increased from 33% at baseline to 90% after the event. In contrast, the incidence of collaterals, assessed by contrast filling on angiogram, decreased from 38% to 7% in those patients with sustained reperfusion [199]. Thus, collaterals develop and new myocardial capillaries proliferate and invade the periphery of the infarct zone within 14 days after a myocardial infarction.

Therapeutic regulation of collaterals

Growing new blood vessels is a desired clinical intervention. Established collaterals reduce the extent of transmural infarction and left ventricular aneurysm incidence following myocardial infarction by providing basal perfusion and possibly by enabling the recruitment of progenitors involved in tissue repair

[198]. Collateral formation is a normal physiologic response, yet it is usually inadequate and too late to compensate for the loss of native major blood vessels.

Therapeutic angiogenesis methods attempt to augment the native collateral response to spare limbs from amputation, improve wound healing, and preserve ventricular function. Perfusion capillaries are already closely spaced in most organs and normal tissues; therefore, the expansion of capillary networks by angiogenesis yields at most 2–3-fold increases in blood flow. In contrast, collaterals, which are conduit vessels, have the capacity to increase blood flow 10–30-fold. Human coronary collaterals consist of dilated epicardial vessels and intramyocardial collateral vessels, ranging in diameters from 20 to 200 μm, which develop in association with microscopic foci of myocardial necrosis and monocyte infiltrates [59]. Postnatal vasculogenesis driven by vascular precursor cells may contribute to either process, but the extent of its contribution is currently not known.

Initial trials of therapeutic collateral used single growth factors that primarily target endothelial cell proliferation and migration. Treatment rationales were empiric, and little selection criterion for agents seemed necessary because a wide variety of agents including VEGF and FGF family members were beneficial. An inherent assumption of these treatments was that applied factors would initiate or amplify an endogenous physiologic program. Clinical results on patients with vascular disease and cardiovascular risk factors were less impressive compared to preclinical studies, which typically employed younger animal subjects without co-morbid diseases. The discrepancies suggest the physiologic program is not intact in many clinical subjects or that additional factors are needed. Challenges for translation of these new concepts remain, because arteriogenesis programs are complex, poorly understood, and likely involve an orchestrated cascade of events involving multiple genes.

Renewed efforts to optimize clinical responses follow four general strategies. The first addresses the need to target accessory cells that are necessary for arteriogenesis programs beyond just endothelial cells. Shortcomings of single agents may be compensated by a rational combination of agents, particular agents that activate monocytes and macrophages. Macrophage colony-stimulating factor (MCSF),

GM-CSF, PlGF, MCP-1 and TNF-α enhance arteriogenesis [24,63]. A randomized double-blind placebo-controlled clinical trial showed that the short-term administrations of GM-CSF improved coronary collateral blood flow index [200]. PDGF and FGF molecules have dual effects on smooth muscle cells and endothelial cells to facilitate the growth of larger-caliber vessels [201].

A second general strategy casts a wider net to activate broad gene programs in order to compensate for deficient factors, both known and unknown. Gene therapy with the transcription factor HIF-1α stimulates larger vascular structures with more mural cells and stabilized permeability [194]. Cell-based therapies of vascular precursor cells, infused systemically or delivered locally, are presumed to release diverse paracrine factors that may recruit and guide other vascular cells involved in angiogenesis or arteriogenesis [202]. Challenges remain for progenitor cell therapies because the heterogeneity of these cell populations are undefined, age-related changes alter their repair and inflammatory actions, and local injections do not necessarily restrict cell trafficking or mimic native maturation signals induced by transendothelial migration [203]. Another theoretical concern is the risk of inducing pathologic angiogenesis in dormant and subclinical malignancies, retinal diseases, and vulnerable atherosclerotic lesions, which necessitate close screening and monitoring of subjects.

A third strategy seeks to enhance efficacy by targeting treatments and improving the pharmacokinetics of agents for sufficient duration. Longer-acting gene therapy systems are needed to sustain treatments over 4 weeks, because initial collaterals continue to remodel over several months and symptom relief may be delayed [204]. Clinical tools map ischemic regions for local delivery of angiogenesis factors [205]; however, factors may still redistribute systemically, as shown by changes in blood pressure [113]. Gains in molecular targeting can take advantage of endothelial heterogeneity to deliver treatments to specific vascular beds for more selective control [73]. Although local agents can boost regional responses, systemic mobilization of endothelial precursors could still be required if vasculogenesis indeed plays an important role in angiogenesis in the adult [206].

The fourth approach to augment collateral responses of patients is to correct clinical conditions or compensate for suboptimal steps impaired by hypercholesterolemia, hypertension, endothelial cell dysfunction, diabetes, and advanced age [207–210]. Some of these clinical conditions correlate with reduced growth factors, which can be supplemented. Impaired responses measured at one time point might actually be delayed responses, which would require longer treatment periods [211]. Defects in post-receptor signaling mechanisms attenuate angiogenesis and collateral responses. More research is required to identify the molecular basis of receptor signaling defects to determine whether they can be restored. Monocytes isolated from diabetic patients have reduced VEGF–VEGFR-1 activation and migration responses [212]. Endothelial cell dysfunction and reduced eNOS activity associated with hypercholesterolemia were not fully restored by increased VEGF exposure [70,207]. Finally, genetic variability in clinical populations could account for differences in individual responses to angiogenic therapy [213]. Screens to identify predictors of collateral response might allow the use of tailored regimens for individual patients.

The initial benefits of some placebo-controlled clinic trials, including the TRAFFIC trial for peripheral vascular disease and GM-CSF induction of coronary perfusion, provide a basis for continued progress [200,201]. Clinical trials with myocardial injection of CD34+ progenitors are emerging [214]. Our knowledge about the potential benefits and consequences of pro- and anti-angiogenesis strategies in different clinical settings is still limited, but destined to increase rapidly with clinical experience. For example, GM-CSF improved coronary conductance in chronic ischemia, but it increased in-stent restenosis when used to augment collaterals in acute myocardial infarction [215]. Clinical trials will see further advances with the use of biomarkers and improved methods to objectively measure new vessel formation and perfusion.

A final caveat emphasizes the palliative nature of angiogenic treatments, which are necessitated by the ravages of atherosclerosis and other vascular diseases. Collateral treatments have similar goals as percutaneous interventions and arterial bypass surgeries that improve functional capacity and relieve symptoms; however, benefits on cardiovascular mortality might be modest or manifested only in subsets of patients [216]. Collaterals are unlikely to compensate for proximal left main coronary artery stenosis, where a large myocardial territory is at risk and where bridging collaterals have more difficulty in growing from the thick-walled aorta beyond the left main obstruction. Significant clinical and survival endpoints are gained by current and future advances in primary and secondary preventive treatments for the underlying disease, which would obviate the need to develop collaterals in the first place.

Angiogenesis in atherosclerotic plaques and chronic vascular inflammation

Normal vessels have a microvasculature known as vasa vasorum that is confined to the adventitial and outer medial layers, yet proliferates and extends into the intima in association with atherosclerosis and other types of large-vessel vasculitis including giant cell arteritis, transplant-associated vasculitis, and thromboembolic occlusions in arteries and vein (Figure 4.2) [217–219]. Extensive neovascularization in atherosclerotic plaques was vividly demonstrated by images of coronary arteries after perfusion casting with polymers [67]. Anatomically, plaque capillaries arise more frequently from the native adventitial vasa vasorum, which are supplied by vessels that originate at branch points of coronary arteries and run lengthwise along arteries. Micro-computed tomography techniques image the three-dimensional anatomy of vasa vasorum, which connect with venous and arteriolar support vessels, yet rarely anastomose with the artery lumen [220,221].

Clinical significance

The clinical importance of plaque microvessels is suggested by studies showing their higher prevalence in cellular and inflammatory lesions that have a higher incidence of plaque rupture [222]. Plaque neovascularization is often observed in shoulder regions near the fibrous cap and along the base of plaques adjacent to macrophage, T cell, and mast cell infiltrates [223]. Invading capillaries in these vulnerable regions may mechanically weaken atheromas and increase susceptibility to plaque rupture and late ischemic complications of atherosclerosis [224]. Plaque capillaries are fragile and prone to cause intraplaque hemorrhage, similar to new

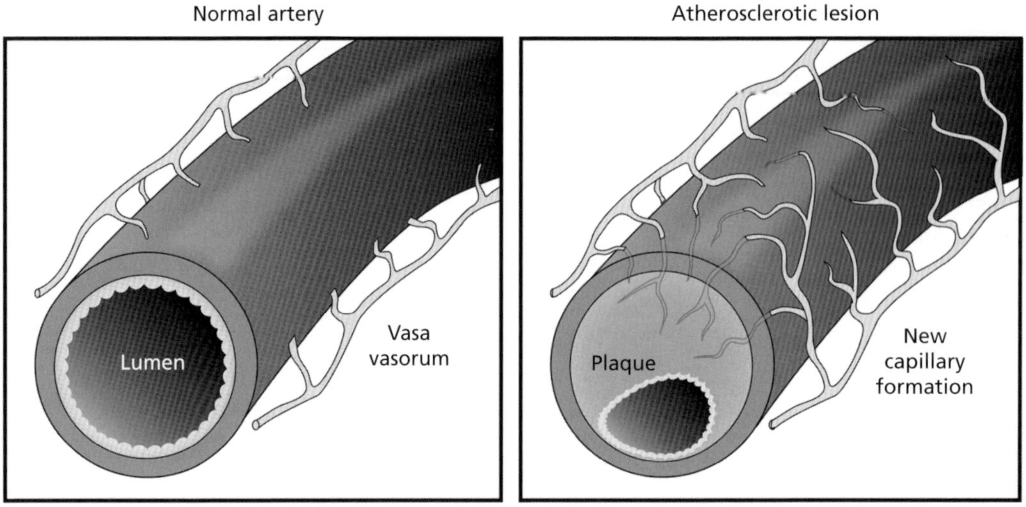

Normal artery   Atherosclerotic lesion

Figure 4.2 Diagram of vasa vasorum in normal and diseased arteries. Vasa vasorum in normal arteries have a well-defined architecture of first- and second-order small-caliber end vessels that supply blood to the outer adventitial and medial layers. In major blood vessel affected by atherosclerosis, vasa vasorum networks become more extensive, disorganized and extend inward to the intimal layer of atheromas where they bleed, deposit proatherogenic molecules, and recruit additional leukocytes. The extent of neovascularization in atheromas correlates with plaque growth and immune cell contents. (Illustration by Steven Moskowitz).

vessels formed in proliferative diabetic retinopathy [225]. Intraplaque hemorrhage and deposition of cholesterol-rich erythrocytes from angiogenic plaque capillaries may provide a mechanism for plaque progression and instability [226,227]. Finally, the availability of positive and negative regulators of neovascularization may yield new treatments directed at angiogenesis-related complications of atherosclerosis and vasculitis, which would complement our current preventive regimens directed at hypercholesterolemia, hypertension, and inflammation.

Functions of plaque angiogenesis

Plaque neovascularization contributes to atherosclerosis and vascular diseases by performing several functions. First, multiple evidence indicates that vasa vasorum provide perfusion to the thickened vessel wall. Atherectomy specimens from primary atherosclerotic lesions show a correlation between proliferating endothelial cells in plaque capillaries and the proliferation of other cells in growing plaques [228]. Vasa vasorum are observed in arteries of humans and large species when the wall thickness exceeds approximately $300\,\mu m$ [186,229]. Interruption of vasa vasorum results in medial necrosis [230]. Diffusible blood tracers localize near plaque

capillaries [231]. Vasodilators and vasoconstrictors regulate blood flow in the outer vessel wall supplied by plaque capillaries and vasa vasorum [232].

Second, plaque neovascularization provides conduits for immune cell exchange in the plaque. Consistent with this function, plaque neovascularization spatially and quantitatively correlates with immune cell infiltrates [80,233]. Neovascular expression of E-selectin, vascular cell adhesion molecule-1 (VCAM-1), intercellular adhesion molecule-1 (ICAM-1) or other adhesion molecules facilitate leukocyte exchange into deep regions of advanced atheromas in addition to the overlying macrovascular endothelium [234]. Alternatively, the proximity of plaque capillaries and inflammatory cells in atheromas may occur because these cells release angiogenic factors necessary for their formation. Regardless of the initiating event, once neovascularization is established in a chronic inflammatory process, a positive feedback loop may operate, whereby immune cells stimulate neovascularization that promotes further leukocyte recruitment. Macrophages are present in early lesions before the ingrowth of vasa vasorum [21]. Thus, the "chicken or egg question" may be less clinically relevant than the question whether either or both immune- and endothelial-cell-directed treatments are needed to terminate this feedback loop [63,80].

A third hypothesized function of plaque angiogenesis is to directly and indirectly promotes plaque rupture [67,222]. Direct mechanisms of plaque rupture mediated by plaque neovascularization include intraplaque bleeding and the activation of proteases by invading endothelial cells [132]. Intraplaque hemorrhage traps blood cells and other proatherogenic molecules and induces acute inflammation, which could abruptly trigger a period of plaque instability [226,227]. Indirect mechanisms of rupture enhanced by plaque neovascularization include its capacity to recruit immune cells and deposit proatherogenic substances into regions more prone to erode or rupture. Vulnerable plaque morphologies require additional characterization of their neovascular composition; however, plaque neovascularization is more frequent in culprit and diabetic atheromas [235,236].

Regulation of plaque neovascularization is a promising strategy to ameliorate atherosclerosis morbidity and mortality, but these strategies require experimental verification in both basic and clinical investigations. 3-hydroxy-3-methyl glutaryl coenzyme A (HMG-CoA) reductase inhibitors and antagonists of the angiotensin pathway have recognized antiangiogenic effects; however, these properties alone may not account for their plaque-stabilizing mechanisms observed in their widespread clinical use [237,238]. Furthermore, various inhibitors of angiogenesis have diverse mechanisms of action and variable effects on non-endothelial cells; therefore, the effects of angiogenesis inhibitors on atherosclerosis are not likely to be similar.

Plaque angiogenesis is a control point in advanced vascular disease

A functional correlation of plaque growth and plaque neovascularization was initially demonstrated by the stage-dependent inhibition of advanced atherosclerosis by various angiogenesis inhibitors administered to atherosclerosis-prone mice [239]. Conversely, two separate stimulators of angiogenesis promoted plaque growth [240,241]. Perivascular delivery of growth factors and antagonists of these growth factors indicated a close correlation between intimal hyperplasia and the extent of vasa vasorum, but stimulation of adventitial angiogenesis alone

would not initiate intimal proliferation [242]. Although the mechanisms whereby these diverse positive and negative endothelial cell regulators alter plaque growth are not yet determined, together these results support the hypothesis that plaque neovascularization promotes the progression of atherosclerosis.

The correlation between intimal neovascularization and plaque growth does not necessarily mean that plaque size is the sole determinant for the distribution and abundance of neovascularization, or that plaques grow or regress only due to changes in perfusion and intimal hypoxia. Primary human and murine atheromas have variable matrix, lipid, and cellular composition. Plaques with intimal thickness greater than 250 µm are more likely to contain intimal capillaries; however, some advanced fibrous lesions contain no intimal neovascularization [228,231]. Neovascular densities are more highly correlated with immune cells, rather than plaque thickness [80]. Increased plaque thickness resulting in intimal hypoxia may be one prerequisite for the intimal extension of vasa vasorum, but it would not exclude a possible contribution from inflammatory mediators.

If plaque capillaries promote leukocyte exchange or sustain growth beyond critical dimensions, then atheromas that acquire neovascularization would grow at different rates compared to atheromas that lack it. The arterial endothelium is the primary interface with blood in non-vascularized early atheromas, which have a high surface area-to-plaque volume ratio. When plaques thicken and expand outward in the vessel wall, the ratio of macrovascular endothelial area to the atheroma volume diminishes (Figure 4.3). The plaque microvasculature may therefore surpass the area of exchange provided by the arterial endothelium over plaques, which may in part explain the relative insensitivity of early atheromas to angiogenesis inhibitors that effectively inhibited advanced atheromas [239]. Recent studies with other animal and arterial injury models confirm the late-stage dependence of plaque growth and intimal hyperplasia on neovascularization [242].

The plaque microvascular network may have additional significance because of recent data showing that smooth muscle and endothelial cell precursors may be derived from the circulation [40]. The number of these precursor cells may not contribute

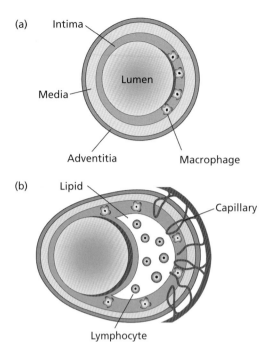

(a)

Intima

Lumen

Media

Adventitia

Macrophage

(b)

Lipid

Capillary

Lymphocyte

Figure 4.3 Macrovascular endothelium is the major interface with blood in early atherosclerotic lesions and fatty streaks. Ratios of macrovascular endothelial surface area-to-plaque volume are highest during early stages of atherosclerosis. In advanced atheromas, the plaque microvasculature acts as an additional endothelial interface between blood and plaque tissues besides the overlying arterial endothelium. Atheroma growth at advanced stages of atherosclerosis is accompanied by outward remodeling of the artery. Microvascular endothelial surface areas ultimately surpass the relative area of exchange provided by the macrovascular endothelium. The functional contributions of plaque neovascularization increase in advanced atheromas, which correspond to later stages of atherosclerosis when clinical symptoms of the disease are manifested.

a significant "local mass" of cells compared to mature immune and vascular wall cells; however, the paracrine effects of these progenitor populations may dictate critical commands to influence resident cell behaviors and recruit more bone-marrow-derived cells.

Physiologic and pathologic effects of vascular progenitors

The effect of bone-marrow-derived cells on vascular repair and disease is an active field of investigation likely to change our understanding of disease

mechanisms [243]. As discussed earlier, several studies illustrated the ability of progenitor cells to promote vascular repair, endothelialization of denuded large arteries and angiogenesis responses, either by true vasculogenesis or paracrine mechanisms [35,202]. Bone marrow progenitors are identified by expression of cell lineage and stem cell antigens; however, this freeze-frame selection captures a cell population with diverse potentials. Furthermore, bone marrow populations from young and old subjects have different therapeutic effects on angiogenesis and vascular repair [244]. Homing of bone-marrow-derived cells induces distinctly different repair or proinflammatory effects in aortas of atherosclerosis-prone mice [203]. Young animal-derived progenitors result in reduced proinflammatory effects, whereas older animals have fewer progenitors but they have a higher tendency to induce inflammatory responses. These results support the hypothesis that atherosclerosis results from failed vascular repair mechanisms exhausted by risk factors, such as advanced age, hypercholesterolemia, and diabetes. Patterns of gene expression in aortas of chimeric mice receiving bone marrow from young or old mice showed broad differences, indicating that aged bone marrow cells are qualitatively different, and the homing of these cells in aortas results in enhanced expression of proinflammatory genes [245]. The molecular basis of age-dependent changes remain unknown; however, this data may be clinically relevant to the choice of progenitor cell donors for patients receiving cell-based angiogenesis treatments.

Regulation of plaque angiogenesis

Despite the intriguing clinical and functional significance of intimal neovascularization in atherosclerotic plaques, the mechanisms regulating intimal angiogenesis are not fully known [246]. Several angiogenic factors including VEGF, FGF family members, chemokines, PlGF, and PDGF are abundantly expressed in human atherosclerotic lesions [97,112,247]. Macrophages in atherosclerotic lesions also express interleukin-8, TGF-β, and other cytokines, which can further augment the production of some angiogenic factors by other vascular wall cells. VEGF abundance increases during the progression of atherosclerosis [112], but VEGF receptor-2 antagonists did not inhibit plaque neovascularization when provided for a short period [63]. Compensation by other angiogenic factors could in principle alter the efficacy of VEGF antagonists on plaque neovascularization and atherosclerosis.

The abundance of angiogenic factors in early atheromas prior to the onset of plaque angiogenesis suggests that angiogenic stimulators may be necessary but not sufficient to initiate angiogenesis. The complex regulation of plaque angiogenesis also includes microenvironment factors, such as local hypoxia or oxidative stress, ECM turnover, and the presence of endogenous factors that antagonize the proliferation of vasa vasorum. TSP-1 and collagen XVIII, the parent molecule of endostatin, are abundant in the vessel wall, which impede the inward growth of vasa vasorum across the media into atheromas [248]. Collagen XVIII in the artery becomes depleted in advanced atheromas. Mice lacking collagen XVIII develop increased atherosclerosis and a 4-fold higher incidence of intimal neovascularization in atheromas at high predilection sites [249]. Other protective effects of collagen XVIII and endostatin in vascular basement membranes maintain normal barrier function of small and large blood vessels and interfere with the retention of lipoproteins in subendothelial matrix [250, 251]. Thus, loss of collagen XVIII is both a consequence and a pathologic mechanism for the progression of atherosclerosis.

In principle, the results for collagen XVIII may be true for other artery wall components with anti-angiogenesis and barrier functions, including perlecan and collagen IV, that could impede the intimal extension of vasa vasorum in atherosclerosis and other types of vasculitis [165,166]. Complete ablation of vasa vasorum, both in the intima and adventitia, may be less ideal than just stopping intimal invasion across the media, where fragile capillaries are closer to the atheroma surface and exposed to greater mechanical strain. Neovascular bleeding and leukocyte recruitment in superficial intimal areas of atheromas could have a higher chance of inducing an uncontained rupture and the consequent thrombotic occlusion of an artery. If this is true, then replacement of protective components that are depleted in diseased arteries could be a novel treatment strategy for many vascular diseases.

Angiogenesis in restenosis

Both positive and negative angiogenesis regulators have been employed to modify restenosis, with conflicting results depending on the agent, dose, and delivery route. Retrospective analyses of results provide some clarifying insights. Loss of macrovascular endothelium on the instrumented large vessel is the primary injury after balloon dilation or stent deployment, which exposes underlying vascular cells to abundant growth factors, platelets, and immune cells, and allows the deposition of fibrinogen and fibrin, which all promote intimal hyperplasia [252]. Second, the physical dilation of the outer vessel layers mechanically stimulates the proliferation of adventitial vasa vasorum, which also favors intimal hyperplasia [253]. The primary loss of arterial endothelium is uniform; however, the extent of adventitial injury to vasa vasorum may not be uniform, depending on the animal species and the methods of arterial injury (wire, dilation, etc). Positive or negative regulators have been delivered to the injured artery by different routes: systemically, locally along the artery surface (adenovirus and plasmid gene therapy, catheter delivery), or in the adventitia (sustained-released vehicles). Considerations of these "front door" and "back door" differences in injury and treatment routes provide insights for disparate results in various studies. For example, the systemic delivery of VEGF promoted plaque neovascularization and intimal hyperplasia [101], whereas local VEGF on the denuded artery surface enhanced repair of arterial endothelium and limited intimal hyperplasia [254]. Arterial surface delivery of an endothelial cell inhibitor inhibited the arterial re-endothelialization and increased intimal hyperplasia, whereas adventitial delivery inhibited adventitial angiogenesis and intimal hyperplasia [255,256]. Future combined selective strategies might be employed to deliver inhibitors to the adventitia, while promoting growth factor restoration of a functional endothelium on the main artery [152].

Putting it all together: making arteries grow and blocking plaque angiogenesis

The potential use of both endothelial cell growth factors and inhibitors for patients with cardiovascular diseases raises a number of important and clinically relevant questions. This discussion does not seek to vilify or vindicate any single strategy. Rather, the clinical setting will dictate which strategy is indicated – either to palliate severe vascular occlusion or to prevent disease progression and acute complications. Second, the general effects of inhibitors and stimulators with diverse mechanisms and differences in cell targets should not be generalized to all agents with either positive or negative effects. For example, "anti-VEGF" is not equivalent to "anti-angiogenesis." Basal levels of VEGF may be beneficial to endothelial cells, while higher doses can be pathologic [117]. Conversely, it could be argued that physiologic levels of inhibitors in the vascular basement membrane may maintain endothelial quiescence, but excessive doses applied at times when angiogenesis is desired might reduce endothelial cell survival.

Reviews of positive and negative endothelial cell regulators reveal inherent trade-offs in the functions of these molecules during arterial repair, ischemia-associated angiogenesis, and atherosclerosis [257]. The capacity of exogenous growth factors to promote plaque angiogenesis and atherosclerosis is recognized, but the level of this risk may be acceptable or managed. Atheromas already have a significant reservoir of local angiogenic growth factors; therefore, low levels of systemic growth factors that do not induce vascular permeability may have limited effects on plaque growth over a restricted treatment period. Risks of promoting vascular occlusion may be acceptable in patients with defined vascular anatomy. On the other hand, if mobilized progenitor cells from the bone marrow contribute to atherosclerosis and are needed to create collaterals, then systemically released cells could travel to either location, producing either deleterious or beneficial effects. Even locally injected progenitors may not stay put. More knowledge about homing mechanisms and local effects of progenitor cells are needed to modify this risk.

The more dangerous risks of promoting plaque angiogenesis, instability, and acute ischemic syndromes cannot be currently estimated without new clinical tools to monitor plaque neovascularization or follow biomarkers that predict plaque hemorrhage. More optimal collateral treatments will minimize undesired regulation of pathologic angiogenesis in other tissues by the rationale choice of agents

(arteriogenic vs angiogenesis, organ-specific angiogenesis factors) and delivery mechanisms (adventitial, local sustained-release, molecularly targeted agents to specific vascular beds).

Converse questions also arise concerning the clinical use of angiogenesis inhibitors. Will angiogenesis inhibitors block collateral development? The clinical setting often dictates this potential outcome. The angiogenesis inhibitors TSP and platelet factor-4 impair collateral formation when given at the time of vascular occlusion, but were not effective if treatments were delayed [258]. Once formed and stabilized by incorporated smooth muscle cells, perfused collateral vessels often remain patent in ischemic tissue, even after growth factor levels subside [52]. Current clinical uses of angiogenesis inhibitors for cancer, macular degeneration, and arthritis require chronic treatments. Given the high prevalence of cardiovascular disease, these agents are likely to have concurrent cardiovascular effects in patients, either beneficial or deleterious, depending on the type and severity of co-morbid clinical conditions and the molecules targeted by different agents. Some patients receiving non-selective VEGF antagonists develop mild systemic and pulmonary hypertension, presumably due to downstream effects of VEGF on NOS activity. Even though the mild hypertensive response is readily controlled by anti-hypertension medications, it is possible that the downstream effects of VEGF antagonists contribute to the intended anti-angiogenic effect by improving vascular pruning and drug delivery into the tumor interior [259].

A second question arises whether angiogenesis inhibitors will induce necrosis in plaques, which would destabilize atheromas. The ultimate answer to this question requires clinical results with various agents; however, this question implies two assumptions, which are flawed: (i) the metabolic demands of intimal cells in growing plaques are sufficiently satisfied by plaque neovascularization and (ii) the innermost layer of atheromas is not perfused by the artery. The distribution of neovascularization is not uniform in plaques, and the expression of HIF-1α in atheromas suggests that ischemia persists even when neovascularization is present [238]. Hemodynamic flow in plaque capillaries is poorly understood and is most likely very inefficient. Plaques causing flow-limiting stenosis reduce afferent perfusion pressure to vasa vasorum, which are supplied by downstream vessels. High transmural pressures in arteries compared to vasa vasorum suggest that plaque perfusion is greatest during diastole. The well-defined architecture of first- and second-order vasa vasorum in normal vessels may optimize perfusion of high-pressure arteries, whereas the disorganized and poorly pruned vasa vasorum in atherosclerotic arteries create geometric resistance that impairs microcirculation. Ultimately, atheroma changes resulting from angiogenesis inhibition may depend on the rate of vascular regression and the microcirculatory effects of vascular pruning [259].

Future applications

The study of tumor and developmental angiogenesis has improved our understanding of angiogenesis mechanisms and identified important growth factors, inhibitors, and ECM molecules that regulate this process postnatally. This information has provided new insights into cardiovascular diseases that involve vascular remodeling, angiogenesis, and arteriogenesis, which will hopefully result in new therapeutic options. It is commonly assumed that major life-threatening illnesses such as cancer and atherosclerosis will demand the most potent and rapidly acting therapies; however, chronic sustained control may only need maintenance therapy. Just as chemotherapy drugs are combined in effective regimens that balance untoward side effects and cardiovascular drugs are combined to control different risk factors, more selective angiogenesis and anti-angiogenesis strategies will evolve based on clinical experience. Future development of more selective and targeted angiogenesis agents will facilitate the rationale use of combined therapies to inhibit different phases of pathologic blood vessel growth and enhance defective pathways in physiologic collaterals.

References

1 Gibbons GH, Dzau VJ. The emerging concept of vascular remodeling. *N Engl J Med* 1994;330:1431–1438.

2 Folkman J. Angiogenesis in cancer, vascular, rheumatoid and other disease. *Nat Med* 1995;1:27–31.

3 Carmeliet P. Mechanisms of angiogenesis and arteriogenesis. *Nat Med* 2000;6:389–395.

4 Drexler H, Schnurch H, Breier G, et al. Regulation of embryonic blood vessel formation. In: Maragoudakis M, Gullino P, Lelkes P, eds. *Angiogenesis in Health and Disease*. New York: Plenum Press; 1992:17–26.

5 Carmeliet P. Angiogenesis in life, disease and medicine. *Nature* 2005;438:932–936.

6 Coultas L, Chawengsaksophak K, Rossant J. Endothelial cells and VEGF in vascular development. *Nature* 2005; 438:937–945.

7 Shalaby F, Rossant J, Yamaguchi TP, et al. Failure of blood-island formation and vasculogenesis in Flk-1-deficient mice. *Nature* 1995;376:62–66.

8 Carmeliet P, Ferreira V, Breier G, et al. Abnormal blood vessel development and lethality in embryos lacking a single VEGF allele. *Nature* 1996;380:435–439.

9 Millauer B, Wizigmann-Voos S, Schnurch H, et al. High affinity VEGF binding and developmental expression suggest Flk-1 as a major regulator of vasculogenesis and angiogenesis. *Cell* 1993;72:835–846.

10 Wang HU, Chen ZF, Anderson DJ. Molecular distinction and angiogenic interaction between embryonic arteries and veins revealed by ephrin-B2 and its receptor Eph-B4. *Cell* 1998;93:741–753.

11 Gerety SS, Wang HU, Chen ZF, et al. Symmetrical mutant phenotypes of the receptor EphB4 and its specific transmembrane ligand ephrin-B2 in cardiovascular development. *Mol Cell* 1999;4:403–414.

12 Shalaby F, Ho J, Stanford WL, et al. A requirement for Flk1 in primitive and definitive hematopoiesis and vasculogenesis. *Cell* 1997;89:981–990.

13 Lyden D, Young AZ, Zagzag D, et al. Id1 and Id3 are required for neurogenesis, angiogenesis and vascularization of tumour xenografts. *Nature* 1999;401: 670–677.

14 Tevosian SG, Deconinck AE, Tanaka M, et al. FOG-2, a cofactor for GATA transcription factors, is essential for heart morphogenesis and development of coronary vessels from epicardium. *Cell* 2000;101:729–739.

15 Zhong TP, Rosenberg M, Mohideen MA, et al. Gridlock, an HLH gene required for assembly of the aorta in zebrafish. *Science* 2000;287:1820–1824.

16 You LR, Lin FJ, Lee CT, et al. Suppression of Notch signalling by the COUP-TFII transcription factor regulates vein identity. *Nature* 2005;435: 98–104.

17 Suri C, Jones PF, Patan S, et al. Requisite role of angiopoietin-1, a ligand for the TIE2 receptor, during embryonic angiogenesis. *Cell* 1996;87: 1171–1180.

18 Urness LD, Sorensen LK, Li DY. Arteriovenous malformations in mice lacking activin receptor-like kinase-1 *Nat Genet* 2000;26:328–331.

19 Carmeliet P, Lampugnani MG, Moons L, et al. Targeted deficiency or cytosolic truncation of the VE-cadherin gene in mice impairs VEGF-mediated endothelial survival and angiogenesis. *Cell* 1999;98:147–157.

20 Ryan HE, Lo J, Johnson RS. HIF-1 alpha is required for solid tumor formation and embryonic vascularization. *Embo J* 1998;17:3005–3015.

21 Hirschi KK, D'Amore PA. Pericytes in the microvasculature. *Cardiovasc Res* 1996;32:687–698.

22 Ingber DE. Mechanical signaling and the cellular response to extracellular matrix in angiogenesis and cardiovascular physiology. *Circ Res* 2002;91:877–887.

23 Mukouyama YS, Shin D, Britsch S, et al. Sensory nerves determine the pattern of arterial differentiation and blood vessel branching in the skin. *Cell* 2002;109:693–705.

24 Arras M, Ito WD, Scholz D, et al. Monocyte activation in angiogenesis and collateral growth in the rabbit hindlimb. *J Clin Invest* 1998;101:40–50.

25 Reinders ME, Sho M, Izawa A, et al. Proinflammatory functions of vascular endothelial growth factor in alloimmunity. *J Clin Invest* 2003;112:1655–1665.

26 Mohle R, Green D, Moore MA, et al. Constitutive production and thrombin-induced release of vascular endothelial growth factor by human megakaryocytes and platelets. *Proc Natl Acad Sci USA* 1997;94:663–668.

27 Coussens LM, Raymond WW, Bergers G, et al. Inflammatory mast cells up-regulate angiogenesis during squamous epithelial carcinogenesis. *Gene Dev* 1999;13: 1382–1397.

28 Lammert E, Cleaver O, Melton D. Induction of pancreatic differentiation by signals from blood vessels. *Science* 2001;294:564–567.

29 LeCouter J, Kowalski J, Foster J, et al. Identification of an angiogenic mitogen selective for endocrine gland endothelium. *Nature* 2001;412:877–884.

30 Shi Q, Rafii S, Wu MH, et al. Evidence for circulating bone marrow-derived endothelial cells. *Blood* 1998;92: 362–367.

31 Asahara T, Murohara T, Sullivan A, et al. Isolation of putative progenitor endothelial cells for angiogenesis. *Science* 1997;275:964–967.

32 Peichev M, Naiyer AJ, Pereira D, et al. Expression of VEGFR-2 and AC133 by circulating human CD34(+) cells identifies a population of functional endothelial precursors. *Blood* 2000;95:952–958.

33 Beaudry P, Force J, Naumov GN, et al. Differential effects of vascular endothelial growth factor receptor-2 inhibitor ZD6474 on circulating endothelial progenitors and mature circulating endothelial cells: implications for use as a surrogate marker of antiangiogenic activity. *Clin Cancer Res* 2005;11:3514–3522.

34 Schuch G, Heymach JV, Nomi M, et al. Endostatin inhibits the vascular endothelial growth factor-induced mobilization of endothelial progenitor cells. *Cancer Res* 2003;63:8345–8350.

35 O'Neill TJt, Wamhoff BR, Owens GK, et al. Mobilization of bone marrow-derived cells enhances the angiogenic response to hypoxia without transdifferentiation into endothelial cells. *Circ Res* 2005;97:1027–1035.

36 Duda DG, Cohen KS, Kozin SV, et al. Evidence for bone marrow-derived endothelial cells incorporation into perfused blood vessels in tumors. *Blood* 2006;107: 2774–2776.

37 Lyden D, Hattori K, Dias S, et al. Impaired recruitment of bone-marrow-derived endothelial and hematopoietic precursor cells blocks tumor angiogenesis and growth. *Nat Med* 2001;7:1194–1201.

38 Asahara T, Masuda H, Takahashi T, et al. Bone marrow origin of endothelial progenitor cells responsible for postnatal vasculogenesis in physiological and pathological neovascularization. *Circ Res* 1999;85:221–228.

39 Quaini F, Urbanek K, Beltrami AP, et al. Chimerism of the transplanted heart. *N Engl J Med* 2002;346:5–15.

40 Sata M, Saiura A, Kunisato A, et al. Hematopoietic stem cells differentiate into vascular cells that participate in the pathogenesis of atherosclerosis. *Nat Med* 2002;8: 403–409.

41 Liotta LA, Steeg PS, Stetler-Stevenson WG. Cancer metastasis and angiogenesis: an imbalance of positive and negative regulation. *Cell* 1991;64:327–336.

42 Gross JL, Moscatelli D, Rifkin DB. Increased capillary endothelial cell protease activity in response to angiogenic stimuli *in vitro*. *Proc Natl Acad Sci USA* 1983; 80:2623–2627.

43 Tolsma SS, Volpert OV, Good DJ, et al. Peptides derived from two separate domains of the matrix protein thrombospondin-1 have anti-angiogenic activity. *J Cell Biol* 1993;122:497–511.

44 O'Reilly MS, Boehm T, Shing Y, et al. Endostatin: an endogenous inhibitor of angiogenesis and tumor growth. *Cell* 1997;88:277–285.

45 Ausprunk DH, Folkman J. Migration and proliferation of endothelial cells in preformed and newly formed blood vessels during tumor angiogenesis. *Microvasc Res* 1977;14:53–65.

46 Brooks PC, Stromblad S, Sanders LC, et al. Localization of matrix metalloproteinase MMP-2 to the surface of invasive cells by interaction with integrin alpha v beta 3. *Cell* 1996;85:683–693.

47 Leavesley DI, Schwartz MA, Rosenfeld M, et al. Integrin beta 1- and beta 3-mediated endothelial cell migration is triggered through distinct signaling mechanisms. *J Cell Biol* 1993;121:163–170.

48 Nguyen M, Strubel NA, Bischoff J. A role for sialyl Lewis-X/A glycoconjugates in capillary morphogenesis. *Nature* 1993;365:267–269.

49 Grant DS, Tashiro K, Segui-Real B, et al. Two different laminin domains mediate the differentiation of human endothelial cells into capillary-like structures *in vitro*. *Cell* 1989;58:933–943.

50 Ausprunk DH, Dethlefsen S, Higgins E. Distribution of fibronectin, laminin and type IV collagen during development of blood vessels in the chick chorioallantoic membrane. In: Feinberg R, Sherer G, Auerbach R, eds. *The Development of the Vascular System.* Basel: Karger; 1991:93–108.

51 Leveen P, Pekny M, Gebre-Medhin S, et al. Mice deficient for PDGF B show renal, cardiovascular, and hematological abnormalities. *Gene Dev* 1994;8:1875–1887.

52 Benjamin LE, Hemo I, Keshet E. A plasticity window for blood vessel remodelling is defined by pericyte coverage of the preformed endothelial network and is regulated by PDGF-B and VEGF. *Development* 1998;125: 1591–1598.

53 Hood JD, Bednarski M, Frausto R, et al. Tumor regression by targeted gene delivery to the neovasculature. *Science* 2002;296:2404–2407.

54 Friedlander M, Brooks PC, Shaffer RW, et al. Definition of two angiogenic pathways by distinct alpha v integrins. *Science* 1995;270:1500–1502.

55 Brooks PC, Montgomery AM, Rosenfeld M, et al. Integrin alpha v beta 3 antagonists promote tumor regression by inducing apoptosis of angiogenic blood vessels. *Cell* 1994;79:1157–1164.

56 Holmgren L, O'Reilly MS, Folkman J. Dormancy of micrometastases: balanced proliferation and apoptosis in the presence of angiogenesis suppression. *Nat Med* 1995; 1:149–153.

57 Jimenez B, Volpert OV, Crawford SE, et al. Signals leading to apoptosis-dependent inhibition of neovascularization by thrombospondin-1. *Nat Med* 2000;6: 41–48.

58 Kass RW, Kotler MN, Yazdanfar S. Stimulation of coronary collateral growth: current developments in angiogenesis and future clinical applications. *Am Heart J* 1992;123:486–496.

59 Schaper W. Control of coronary angiogenesis. *Eur Heart J* 1995;16:66–68.

60 Heil M, Ziegelhoeffer T, Wagner S, et al. Collateral artery growth (arteriogenesis) after experimental arterial occlusion is impaired in mice lacking CC-chemokine receptor-2. *Circ Res* 2004;94:671–677.

61 Ito WD, Arras M, Winkler B, et al. Monocyte chemotactic protein-1 increases collateral and peripheral conductance after femoral artery occlusion. *Circ Res* 1997;80: 829–837.

62 Buschmann IR, Hoefer IE, van Royen N, et al. GM-CSF: a strong arteriogenic factor acting by amplification of monocyte function. *Atherosclerosis* 2001;159:343–356.

63 Luttun A, Tjwa M, Moons L, et al. Revascularization of ischemic tissues by PlGF treatment, and inhibition of tumor angiogenesis, arthritis and atherosclerosis by anti-Flt1. *Nat Med* 2002;8:831–840.

64 Li DY, Brooke B, Davis EC, et al. Elastin is an essential determinant of arterial morphogenesis. *Nature* 1998;393: 276–280.

65 Engerman RL, Pfaffenbach D, Davis MD. Cell turnover of capillaries. *Lab Invest* 1967;17:738–743.

66 Reynolds LP, Killilea SD, Redmer DA. Angiogenesis in the female reproductive system. *Faseb J* 1992;6:886–892.

67 Barger AC, Beeuwkes III R, Lainey LL, et al. Hypothesis: vasa vasorum and neovascularization of human coronary arteries. A possible role in the pathophysiology of atherosclerosis. *N Engl J Med* 1984;310:175–177.

68 Polverini PJ, Cotran RS, Gimbrone Jr MA, et al. Activated macrophages induce vascular proliferation. *Nature* 1977;269:804–806.

69 Heissig B, Hattori K, Dias S, et al. Recruitment of stem and progenitor cells from the bone marrow niche requires MMP-9 release of kit-ligand *Cell* 2002;109:625–637.

70 Murohara T, Asahara T, Silver M, et al. Nitric oxide synthase modulates angiogenesis in response to tissue ischemia. *J Clin Invest* 1998;101:2567–2578.

71 Jones MK, Wang H, Peskar BM, et al. Inhibition of angiogenesis by nonsteroidal anti-inflammatory drugs: insight into mechanisms and implications for cancer growth and ulcer healing. *Nat Med* 1999;5:1418–1423.

72 St Croix B, Rago C, Velculescu V, et al. Genes expressed in human tumor endothelium. *Science* 2000;289:1197–1202.

73 Arap W, Kolonin MG, Trepel M, et al. Steps toward mapping the human vasculature by phage display. *Nat Med* 2002;8:121–127.

74 Folkman J. Angiogenesis. In: Braunwald E, Fauci AS, Kasper DL, Hauser SL, Longo DL, Jameson JL, eds. *Harrison's Textbook of Internal Medicine*, 15th edn. New York: McGraw-Hill; 2001:517–530.

75 Clark RA, Tonnesen MG, Gailit J, et al. Transient functional expression of alphaVbeta 3 on vascular cells during wound repair. *Am J Pathol* 1996;148:1407–1421.

76 Jaffe EA, Nachman RL, Becker CG, et al. Culture of human endothelial cells derived from umbilical veins: identification by morphologic and immunologic criteria. *J Clin Invest* 1972;52:2745–2756.

77 Folkman J, Haudenschild C, Zetter BR. Long-term culture of capillary endothelial cells. *Proc Natl Acad Sci USA* 1979;76:5217–5221.

78 Auerbach W, Auerbach R. *In vivo* assays of angiogenesis. In: Maragoudakis M, Gullino P, Lelkes P, eds. *Angiogenesis, Molecular Biology, Clinical Aspects.* New York: Plenum Press; 1994:283–290.

79 Nicosia RF, Ottinetti A. Growth of microvessels in serum-free matrix culture of rat aorta. A quantitative assay of angiogenesis *in vitro*. *Lab Invest* 1990;63: 115–122.

80 Moulton KS, Vakili K, Zurakowski D, et al. Inhibition of plaque neovascularization reduces macrophage

accumulation and progression of advanced atherosclerosis. *Proc Natl Acad Sci USA* 2003;100:4736–4741.

81 Van Belle E, Witzenbichler B, Chen D, et al. Potentiated angiogenic effect of scatter factor/hepatocyte growth factor via induction of vascular endothelial growth factor: the case for paracrine amplification of angiogenesis. *Circulation* 1998;97:381–390.

82 Kumar R, Yoneda J, Bucana CD, et al. Regulation of distinct steps of angiogenesis by different angiogenic molecules. *Int J Oncol* 1998;12:749–757.

83 Rikitake Y, Hirata K, Kawashima S, et al. Involvement of endothelial nitric oxide in sphingosine-1-phosphate-induced angiogenesis. *Arterioscler Thromb Vasc Biol* 2002;22:108–114.

84 Miura S, Fujino M, Matsuo Y, et al. High density lipoprotein-induced angiogenesis requires the activation of Ras/MAP kinase in human coronary artery endothelial cells. *Arterioscler Thromb Vasc Biol* 2003;23:802–808.

85 Baluk P, Lee CG, Link H, et al. Regulated angiogenesis and vascular regression in mice overexpressing vascular endothelial growth factor in airways. *Am J Pathol* 2004; 165:1071–1085.

86 Kenyon BM, Browne F, D'Amato RJ. Effects of thalidomide and related metabolites in a mouse corneal model of neovascularization. *Exp Eye Res* 1997;64:971–978.

87 Chang LK, Garcia-Cardena G, Farnebo F, et al. Dose-dependent response of FGF-2 for lymphangiogenesis. *Proc Natl Acad Sci USA* 2004;101:11658–11663.

88 Leunig M, Yuan F, Menger M, et al. Angiogenesis, microvascular architecture, microhemodynamics, and interstitial fluid pressure during early growth of human adenocarcinoma LS174T in SCID mice. *Cancer Res* 1992; 52:6553–6560.

89 Sipkins DA, Wei X, Wu JW, et al. *In vivo* imaging of specialized bone marrow endothelial microdomains for tumour engraftment. *Nature* 2005;435:969–973.

90 Folkman J. Seminars in Medicine of the Beth Israel Hospital, Boston. Clinical applications of research on angiogenesis. *N Engl J Med* 1995;333:1757–1763.

91 Shing Y, Folkman J, Sullivan R, et al. Heparin affinity: purification of a tumor-derived capillary endothelial cell growth factor. *Science* 1984;223:1296–1299.

92 Thomas KA, Rios-Candelore M, Fitzpatrick S. Purification and characterization of acidic fibroblast growth factor from bovine brain. *Proc Natl Acad Sci USA* 1984;81: 357–361.

93 Vlodavsky I, Folkman J, Sullivan R, et al. Endothelial cell-derived basic fibroblast growth factor: synthesis and deposition into subendothelial extracellular matrix. *Proc Natl Acad Sci USA* 1987;84:2292–2296.

94 Maciag T, Mehlman T, Friesel R, et al. Heparin binds endothelial cell growth factor, the principal endothelial cell mitogen in bovine brain. *Science* 1984;225:932–935.

95 Edelman ER, Nugent MA, Smith LT, et al. Basic fibroblast growth factor enhances the coupling of intimal hyperplasia and proliferation of vasa vasorum in injured rat arteries. *J Clin Invest* 1992;89:465–473.

96 Nabel EG, Yang ZY, Plautz G, et al. Recombinant fibroblast growth factor-1 promotes intimal hyperplasia and angiogenesis in arteries *in vivo*. *Nature* 1993;362:844–846.

97 Brogi E, Winkles JA, Underwood R, et al. Distinct patterns of expression of fibroblast growth factors and their receptors in human atheroma and nonatherosclerotic arteries. Association of acidic FGF with plaque microvessels and macrophages. *J Clin Invest* 1993;92: 2408–2418.

98 Baffour R, Berman J, Garb JL, et al. Enhanced angiogenesis and growth of collaterals by *in vivo* administration of recombinant basic fibroblast growth factor in a rabbit model of acute lower limb ischemia: dose–response effect of basic fibroblast growth factor. *J Vasc Surg* 1992; 16:181–191.

99 Pu LQ, Sniderman AD, Brassard R, et al. Enhanced revascularization of the ischemic limb by angiogenic therapy. *Circulation* 1993;88:208–215.

100 Yanagisawa-Miwa A, Uchida Y, Nakamura F, et al. Salvage of infarcted myocardium by angiogenic action of basic fibroblast growth factor. *Science* 1992;257: 1401–1403.

101 Lazarous DF, Shou M, Scheinowitz M, et al. Comparative effects of basic fibroblast growth factor and vascular endothelial growth factor on coronary collateral development and the arterial response to injury. *Circulation* 1996;94:1074–1082.

102 Simons M, Annex BH, Laham RJ, et al. Pharmacological treatment of coronary artery disease with recombinant fibroblast growth factor-2: double-blind, randomized, controlled clinical trial. *Circulation* 2002;105: 788–793.

103 Ferrara N, Houck KA, Jakeman LB, et al. The vascular endothelial growth factor family of polypeptides. *J Cell Biochem* 1991;47:211–218.

104 Roberts WG, Palade GE. Increased microvascular permeability and endothelial fenestration induced by vascular endothelial growth factor. *J Cell Sci* 1995;108 (Pt 6):2369–2379.

105 Dvorak HF, Brown LF, Detmar M, et al. Vascular permeability factor/vascular endothelial growth factor, microvascular hyperpermeability, and angiogenesis. *Am J Pathol* 1995;146:1029–1039.

106 Ferrara N, Carver-Moore K, Chen H, et al. Heterozygous embryonic lethality induced by targeted inactivation of the VEGF gene. *Nature* 1996;380:439–442.

107 Peters KG, De Vries C, Williams LT. Vascular endothelial growth factor receptor expression during embryogenesis and tissue repair suggests a role in endothelial

differentiation and blood vessel growth. *Proc Natl Acad Sci USA* 1993;90:8915–8919.

108 Barleon B, Sozzani S, Zhou D, et al. Migration of human monocytes in response to vascular endothelial growth factor (VEGF) is mediated via the VEGF receptor flt-1. *Blood* 1996;87:3336–3343.

109 Fong GH, Zhang L, Bryce DM, et al. Increased hemangioblast commitment, not vascular disorganization, is the primary defect in flt-1 knock-out mice. *Development* 1999;126:3015–3025.

110 Ferrara N, Chen H, Davis-Smyth T, et al. Vascular endothelial growth factor is essential for corpus luteum angiogenesis. *Nat Med* 1998;4:336–340.

111 Gerber HP, Vu TH, Ryan AM, et al. VEGF couples hypertrophic cartilage remodeling, ossification and angiogenesis during endochondral bone formation. *Nat Med* 1999;5:623–628.

112 Inoue M, Itoh H, Ueda M, et al. Vascular endothelial growth factor (VEGF) expression in human coronary atherosclerotic lesions: possible pathophysiological significance of VEGF in progression of atherosclerosis. *Circulation* 1998;98:2108–2116.

113 Henry TD, Annex BH, McKendall GR, et al. The VIVA trial: vascular endothelial growth factor in ischemia for vascular angiogenesis. *Circulation* 2003;107:1359–1365.

114 Ng YS, Rohan R, Sunday ME, et al. Differential expression of VEGF isoforms in mouse during development and in the adult. *Dev Dynam* 2001;220:112–121.

115 Soker S, Takashima S, Miao HQ, et al. Neuropilin-1 is expressed by endothelial and tumor cells as an isoform-specific receptor for vascular endothelial growth factor. *Cell* 1998;92:735–745.

116 Tordjman R, Lepelletier Y, Lemarchandel V, et al. A neuronal receptor, neuropilin-1, is essential for the initiation of the primary immune response. *Nat Immunol* 2002;3: 477–482.

117 Ishida S, Usui T, Yamashiro K, et al. VEGF164-mediated inflammation is required for pathological, but not physiological, ischemia-induced retinal neovascularization. *J Exp Med* 2003;198:483–489.

118 Carmeliet P, Ng YS, Nuyens D, et al. Impaired myocardial angiogenesis and ischemic cardiomyopathy in mice lacking the vascular endothelial growth factor isoforms VEGF164 and VEGF188. *Nat Med* 1999;5:495–502.

119 Maes C, Stockmans I, Moermans K, et al. Soluble VEGF isoforms are essential for establishing epiphyseal vascularization and regulating chondrocyte development and survival. *J Clin Invest* 2004;113:188–199.

120 Sato TN, Tozawa Y, Deutsch U, et al. Distinct roles of the receptor tyrosine kinases Tie-1 and Tie-2 in blood vessel formation. *Nature* 1995;376:70–74.

121 Saharinen P, Kerkela K, Ekman N, et al. Multiple angiopoietin recombinant proteins activate the Tie1 receptor tyrosine kinase and promote its interaction with Tie2. *J Cell Biol* 2005;169:239–243.

122 Davis S, Aldrich TH, Jones PF, et al. Isolation of angiopoietin-1, a ligand for the TIE2 receptor, by secretion-trap expression cloning. *Cell* 1996;87: 1161–1169.

123 Maisonpierre PC, Suri C, Jones PF, et al. Angiopoietin-2, a natural antagonist for Tie2 that disrupts *in vivo* angiogenesis. *Science* 1997;277:55–60.

124 Thurston G, Rudge JS, Ioffe E, et al. Angiopoietin-1 protects the adult vasculature against plasma leakage. *Nat Med* 2000;6:460–463.

125 Shyu KG, Manor O, Magner M, et al. Direct intramuscular injection of plasmid DNA encoding angiopoietin-1 but not angiopoietin-2 augments revascularization in the rabbit ischemic hindlimb. *Circulation* 1998;98:2081–2087.

126 Thurston G, Suri C, Smith K, et al. Leakage-resistant blood vessels in mice transgenically overexpressing angiopoietin-1. *Science* 1999;286:2511–2514.

127 Bielenberg DR, Hida Y, Shimizu A, et al. Semaphorin 3F, a chemorepulsant for endothelial cells, induces a poorly vascularized, encapsulated, nonmetastatic tumor phenotype. *J Clin Invest* 2004;114:1260–1271.

128 Shin D, Garcia-Cardena G, Hayashi S, et al. Expression of ephrinB2 identifies a stable genetic difference between arterial and venous vascular smooth muscle as well as endothelial cells, and marks subsets of microvessels at sites of adult neovascularization. *Dev Biol* 2001;230: 139–150.

129 Wang HU, Anderson DJ. Eph family transmembrane ligands can mediate repulsive guidance of trunk neural crest migration and motor axon outgrowth. *Neuron* 1997;18:383–396.

130 Adams RH, Diella F, Hennig S, et al. The cytoplasmic domain of the ligand ephrinB2 is required for vascular morphogenesis but not cranial neural crest migration. *Cell* 2001;104:57–69.

131 Park KW, Morrison CM, Sorensen LK, et al. Robo4 is a vascular-specific receptor that inhibits endothelial migration. *Dev Biol* 2003;261:251–267.

132 Galis ZS, Sukhova GK, Lark MW, et al. Increased expression of matrix metalloproteinases and matrix degrading activity in vulnerable regions of human atherosclerotic plaques. *J Clin Invest* 1994;94:2493–2503.

133 Hiraoka N, Allen E, Apel I, et al. Matrix metalloproteinases regulate neovascularization by acting as pericellular fibrinolysins. *Cell* 1998;95:365–377.

134 Shi GP, Sukhova GK, Kuzuya M, et al. Deficiency of the cysteine protease cathepsin S impairs microvessel growth. *Circ Res* 2003;92:493–500.

135 Bergers G, Brekken R, McMahon G, et al. Matrix metalloproteinase-9 triggers the angiogenic switch during carcinogenesis. *Nat Cell Biol* 2000;2:737–744.

136 O'Reilly MS, Wiederschain D, Stetler-Stevenson WG, et al. Regulation of angiostatin production by matrix metalloproteinase-2 in a model of concomitant resistance. *J Biol Chem* 1999;274:29568–29571.

137 Aikawa M, Rabkin E, Okada Y, et al. Lipid lowering by diet reduces matrix metalloproteinase activity and increases collagen content of rabbit atheroma. A potential mechanism of lesion stabilization. *Circulation* 1998;97: 2433–2444.

138 Fernandez CA, Yan L, Louis G, et al. The matrix metalloproteinase-9/neutrophil gelatinase-associated lipocalin complex plays a role in breast tumor growth and is present in the urine of breast cancer patients. *Clin Cancer Res* 2005;11:5390–5395.

139 Bremer C, Tung CH, Weissleder R. *In vivo* molecular target assessment of matrix metalloproteinase inhibition. *Nat Med* 2001;7:743–748.

140 Strieter RM, Polverini PJ, Kunkel SL, et al. The functional role of the ELR motif in CXC chemokine-mediated angiogenesis. *J Biol Chem* 1995;270: 27348–27357.

141 Naiyer AJ, Jo DY, Ahn J, et al. Stromal derived factor-1-induced chemokinesis of cord blood CD34(+) cells (long-term culture-initiating cells) through endothelial cells is mediated by E-selectin. *Blood* 1999;94:4011–4019.

142 Hanahan D, Folkman J. Patterns and emerging mechanisms of the angiogenic switch during tumorigenesis. *Cell* 1996;86:353–364.

143 Brouty-Boye D, Zetter BR. Inhibition of cell motility by interferon. *Science* 1980;208:516–518.

144 Ezekowitz RA, Mulliken JB, Folkman J. Interferon alfa-2a therapy for life-threatening hemangiomas of infancy. *N Engl J Med* 1992;326:1456–1463.

145 Rastinejad F, Polverini PJ, Bouck NP. Regulation of the activity of a new inhibitor of angiogenesis by a cancer suppressor gene. *Cell* 1989;56:345–355.

146 Iruela-Arispe ML, Porter P, Bornstein P, et al. Thrombospondin-1, an inhibitor of angiogenesis, is regulated by progesterone in the human endometrium. *J Clin Invest* 1996;97:403–412.

147 Febbraio M, Hajjar DP, Silverstein RL. CD36: a class B scavenger receptor involved in angiogenesis, atherosclerosis, inflammation, and lipid metabolism. *J Clin Invest* 2001;108:785–791.

148 Short SM, Derrien A, Narsimhan RP, et al. Inhibition of endothelial cell migration by thrombospondin-1 type-1 repeats is mediated by beta1 integrins. *J Cell Biol* 2005;168:643–653.

149 Crawford SE, Stellmach V, Murphy-Ullrich JE, et al. Thrombospondin-1 is a major activator of TGF-beta1 *in vivo*. *Cell* 1998;93:1159–1170.

150 Hoekstra R, de Vos FY, Eskens FA, et al. Phase I safety, pharmacokinetic, and pharmacodynamic study of the thrombospondin-1-mimetic angiogenesis inhibitor ABT-510 in patients with advanced cancer. *J Clin Oncol* 2005;23:5188–5197.

151 Roth JJ, Gahtan V, Brown JL, et al. Thrombospondin-1 is elevated with both intimal hyperplasia and hypercholesterolemia. *J Surg Res* 1998;74:11–16.

152 Chen D, Asahara T, Krasinski K, et al. Antibody blockade of thrombospondin accelerates reendothelialization and reduces neointima formation in balloon-injured rat carotid artery. *Circulation* 1999;100:849–854.

153 Topol EJ, McCarthy J, Gabriel S, et al. Single nucleotide polymorphisms in multiple novel thrombospondin genes may be associated with familial premature myocardial infarction. *Circulation* 2001;104:2641–2644.

154 Kleiner Jr DE, Tuuttila A, Tryggvason K, et al. Stability analysis of latent and active 72-kDa type IV collagenase: the role of tissue inhibitor of metalloproteinases-2 (TIMP-2). *Biochemistry* 1993;32:1583–1592.

155 Moses MA, Sudhalter J, Langer R. Identification of an inhibitor of neovascularization from cartilage. *Science* 1990;248:1408–1410.

156 Fernandez CA, Butterfield C, Jackson G, et al. Structural and functional uncoupling of the enzymatic and angiogenic inhibitory activities of tissue inhibitor of metalloproteinase-2 (TIMP-2): loop 6 is a novel angiogenesis inhibitor. *J Biol Chem* 2003;278:40989–40995.

157 Seo DW, Li H, Guedez L, et al. TIMP-2 mediated inhibition of angiogenesis: an MMP-independent mechanism. *Cell* 2003;114:171–180.

158 Lemaitre V, Soloway PD, D'Armiento J. Increased medial degradation with pseudo-aneurysm formation in apolipoprotein E-knockout mice deficient in tissue inhibitor of metalloproteinases-1. *Circulation* 2003;107: 333–338.

159 Gupta SK, Hassel T, Singh JP. A potent inhibitor of endothelial cell proliferation is generated by proteolytic cleavage of the chemokine platelet factor 4. *Proc Natl Acad Sci USA* 1995;92:7799–7803.

160 O'Reilly MS, Holmgren L, Shing Y, et al. Angiostatin: a novel angiogenesis inhibitor that mediates the suppression of metastases by a Lewis lung carcinoma. *Cell* 1994;79:315–328.

161 Homandberg GA, Williams JE, Grant D, et al. Heparin-binding fragments of fibronectin are potent inhibitors of endothelial cell growth. *Am J Pathol* 1985;120:327–332.

162 Clapp C, Martial JA, Guzman RC, et al. The 16-kilodalton N-terminal fragment of human prolactin is a potent inhibitor of angiogenesis. *Endocrinology* 1993;133:1292–1299.

163 Bratt A, Birot O, Sinha I, et al. Angiomotin regulates endothelial cell–cell junctions and cell motility. *J Biol Chem* 2005;280:34859–34869.

164 Sasaki T, Fukai N, Mann K, et al. Structure, function and tissue forms of the C-terminal globular domain of

collagen XVIII containing the angiogenesis inhibitor endostatin. *EMBO J* 1998;17:4249–4256.

165 Maeshima Y, Sudhakar A, Lively JC, et al. Tumstatin, an endothelial cell-specific inhibitor of protein synthesis. *Science* 2002;295:140–143.

166 Mongiat M, Sweeney SM, San Antonio JD, et al. Endorepellin, a novel inhibitor of angiogenesis derived from the C terminus of perlecan. *J Biol Chem* 2003;278: 4238–4249.

167 Iozzo RV. Basement membrane proteoglycans: from cellar to ceiling. *Nat Rev Mol Cell Biol* 2005;6:646–656.

168 Rehn M, Veikkola T, Kukk-Valdre E, et al. Interaction of endostatin with integrins implicated in angiogenesis. *Proc Natl Acad Sci USA* 2001;98:1024–1029.

169 Sudhakar A, Sugimoto H, Yang C, et al. Human tumstatin and human endostatin exhibit distinct antiangiogenic activities mediated by alpha v beta 3 and alpha 5 beta 1 integrins. *Proc Natl Acad Sci USA* 2003;100: 4766–4771.

170 Bix G, Fu J, Gonzalez EM, et al. Endorepellin causes endothelial cell disassembly of actin cytoskeleton and focal adhesions through alpha2beta1 integrin. *J Cell Biol* 2004;166:97–109.

171 Wigle JT, Oliver G. Prox1 function is required for the development of the murine lymphatic system. *Cell* 1999;98:769–778.

172 Dumont DJ, Jussila L, Taipale J, et al. Cardiovascular failure in mouse embryos deficient in VEGF receptor-3. *Science* 1998;282:946–949.

173 Irrthum A, Karkkainen MJ, Devriendt K, et al. Congenital hereditary lymphedema caused by a mutation that inactivates VEGFR3 tyrosine kinase. *Am J Human Genet* 2000;67:295–301.

174 Karkkainen MJ, Saaristo A, Jussila L, et al. A model for gene therapy of human hereditary lymphedema. *Proc Natl Acad Sci USA* 2001;98:12677–12682.

175 Jeltsch M, Kaipainen A, Joukov V, et al. Hyperplasia of lymphatic vessels in VEGF-C transgenic mice. *Science* 1997;276:1423–1425.

176 Cao Y, Linden P, Farnebo J, et al. Vascular endothelial growth factor C induces angiogenesis *in vivo*. *Proc Natl Acad Sci USA* 1998;95:14389–14394.

177 Saaristo A, Veikkola T, Enholm B, et al. Adenoviral VEGF-C overexpression induces blood vessel enlargement, tortuosity, and leakiness but no sprouting angiogenesis in the skin or mucous membranes. *FASEB J* 2002;16:1041–1049.

178 Yuan L, Moyon D, Pardanaud L, et al. Abnormal lymphatic vessel development in neuropilin 2 mutant mice. *Development* 2002;129:4797–4806.

179 Saaristo A, Veikkola T, Tammela T, et al. Lymphangiogenic gene therapy with minimal blood vascular side effects. *J Exp Med* 2002;196:719–730.

180 Salven P, Mustjoki S, Alitalo R, et al. VEGFR-3 and CD133 identify a population of CD34+lymphatic/vascular endothelial precursor cells. *Blood* 2003;101:168–172.

181 Cowan KN, Jones PL, Rabinovitch M. Elastase and matrix metalloproteinase inhibitors induce regression, and tenascin-C antisense prevents progression, of vascular disease. *J Clin Invest* 2000;105:21–34.

182 Rosenberg HC, Rabinovitch M. Endothelial injury and vascular reactivity in monocrotaline pulmonary hypertension. *Am J Physiol* 1988;255:H1484–H1491.

183 Rakusan K, Cicutti N, Flanagan MF. Changes in the microvascular network during cardiac growth, development, and aging. *Cell Mol Biol Res* 1994;40:117–122.

184 van Groningen JP, Wenink AC, Testers LH. Myocardial capillaries: increase in number by splitting of existing vessels. *Anat Embryol (Berlin)* 1991;184:65–70.

185 Hudlicka O, Brown MD. Postnatal growth of the heart and its blood vessels. *J Vasc Res* 1996;33:266–287.

186 Wolinsky H, Glagov S. A lamellar unit of aortic medial structure and function in mammals. *Circ Res* 1967;20: 99–111.

187 Tomanek RJ, Torry RJ. Growth of the coronary vasculature in hypertrophy: mechanisms and model dependence. *Cell Mol Biol Res* 1994;40:129–136.

188 Leong-Poi H, Christiansen J, Klibanov AL, et al. Noninvasive assessment of angiogenesis by ultrasound and microbubbles targeted to alpha(v)-integrins. *Circulation* 2003;107:455–460.

189 Giordano FJ, Gerber HP, Williams SP, et al. A cardiac myocyte vascular endothelial growth factor paracrine pathway is required to maintain cardiac function. *Proc Natl Acad Sci USA* 2001;98:5780–5785.

190 Heron MI, Rakusan K. Geometry of coronary capillaries in hyperthyroid and hypothyroid rat heart. *Am J Physiol* 1994;267:H1024–H1031.

191 Cooke JP, Rossitch Jr E, Andon NA, et al. Flow activates an endothelial potassium channel to release an endogenous nitrovasodilator. *J Clin Invest* 1991;88:1663–1671.

192 Topper JN, Cai J, Falb D, et al. Identification of vascular endothelial genes differentially responsive to fluid mechanical stimuli: cyclooxygenase-2, manganese superoxide dismutase, and endothelial cell nitric oxide synthase are selectively up-regulated by steady laminar shear stress. *Proc Natl Acad Sci USA* 1996;93: 10417–10422.

193 Carmeliet P, Dor Y, Herbert JM, et al. Role of HIF-1 alpha in hypoxia-mediated apoptosis, cell proliferation and tumour angiogenesis. *Nature* 1998;394:485–490.

194 Elson DA, Thurston G, Huang LE, et al. Induction of hypervascularity without leakage or inflammation in transgenic mice overexpressing hypoxia-inducible factor-1alpha. *Gene Dev* 2001;15:2520–2532.

195 Tang N, Wang L, Esko J, et al. Loss of HIF-1alpha in endothelial cells disrupts a hypoxia-driven VEGF

autocrine loop necessary for tumorigenesis. *Cancer Cell* 2004;6:485–495.

196 Cramer T, Yamanishi Y, Clausen BE, et al. HIF-1alpha is essential for myeloid cell-mediated inflammation. *Cell* 2003;112:645–657.

197 Pepler W, Meyer B. Interarterial coronary anastomoses and coronary artery pattern: a comparative study of South African Bantu and European hearts. *Circulation* 1960;22:14–24.

198 Rentrop KP, Thornton JC, Feit F, et al. Determinants and protective potential of coronary arterial collaterals as assessed by an angioplasty model. *Am J Cardiol* 1988;61:677–684.

199 Rentrop KP, Feit F, Sherman W, et al. Serial angiographic assessment of coronary artery obstruction and collateral flow in acute myocardial infarction. Report from the second Mount Sinai-New York University Reperfusion Trial. *Circulation* 1989;80:1166–1175.

200 Seiler C, Pohl T, Wustmann K, et al. Promotion of collateral growth by granulocyte–macrophage colony-stimulating factor in patients with coronary artery disease: a randomized, double-blind, placebo-controlled study. *Circulation* 2001;104:2012–2017.

201 Lederman RJ, Mendelsohn FO, Anderson RD, TRAFFIC Investigators. Therapeutic angiogenesis with recombinant fibroblast growth factor-2 for intermittent claudication (the TRAFFIC study): a randomised trial. *Lancet* 2002;359:2053–2058.

202 Kinnaird T, Stabile E, Burnett MS, et al. Marrow-derived stromal cells express genes encoding a broad spectrum of arteriogenic cytokines and promote *in vitro* and *in vivo* arteriogenesis through paracrine mechanisms. *Circ Res* 2004;94:678–685.

203 Rauscher FM, Goldschmidt-Clermont PJ, Davis BH, et al. Aging, progenitor cell exhaustion, and atherosclerosis. *Circulation* 2003;108:457–463.

204 Dor Y, Djonov V, Abramovitch R, et al. Conditional switching of VEGF provides new insights into adult neovascularization and pro-angiogenic therapy. *Embo J* 2002;21:1939–1947.

205 Garcia L, Baim DS, Post M, et al. Therapeutic angiogenesis using endocardial approach to administration: techniques and results. *Curr Intervent Cardiol Rep* 1999; 1:222–227.

206 Kalka C, Masuda H, Takahashi T, et al. Vascular endothelial growth factor(165) gene transfer augments circulating endothelial progenitor cells in human subjects. *Circ Res* 2000;86:1198–1202.

207 Couffinhal T, Silver M, Kearney M, et al. Impaired collateral vessel development associated with reduced expression of vascular endothelial growth factor in ApoE− / −mice. *Circulation* 1999;99:3188–3198.

208 Rivard A, Fabre JE, Silver M, et al. Age-dependent impairment of angiogenesis. *Circulation* 1999;99:111–120.

209 Rivard A, Silver M, Chen D, et al. Rescue of diabetes-related impairment of angiogenesis by intramuscular gene therapy with adeno-VEGF. *Am J Pathol* 1999;154: 355–363.

210 Van Belle E, Rivard A, Chen D, et al. Hypercholesterolemia attenuates angiogenesis but does not preclude augmentation by angiogenic cytokines. *Circulation* 1997;96:2667–2674.

211 Tirziu D, Moodie KL, Zhuang ZW, et al. Delayed arteriogenesis in hypercholesterolemic mice. *Circulation* 2005;112:2501–2509.

212 Waltenberger J, Lange J, Kranz A. Vascular endothelial growth factor-A-induced chemotaxis of monocytes is attenuated in patients with diabetes mellitus: a potential predictor for the individual capacity to develop collaterals. *Circulation* 2000;102:185–190.

213 Schultz A, Lavie L, Hochberg I, et al. Interindividual heterogeneity in the hypoxic regulation of VEGF: significance for the development of the coronary artery collateral circulation. *Circulation* 1999;100:547–552.

214 Ii M, Nishimura H, Iwakura A, et al. Endothelial progenitor cells are rapidly recruited to myocardium and mediate protective effect of ischemic preconditioning via "imported" nitric oxide synthase activity. *Circulation* 2005;111:1114–1120.

215 Kang HJ, Kim HS, Zhang SY, et al. Effects of intracoronary infusion of peripheral blood stem-cells mobilised with granulocyte-colony stimulating factor on left ventricular systolic function and restenosis after coronary stenting in myocardial infarction: the MAGIC cell randomised clinical trial. *Lancet* 2004;363:751–756.

216 The BARI Study Investigators. Comparison of coronary bypass surgery with angioplasty in patients with multivessel disease. The Bypass Angioplasty Revascularization Investigation (BARI) Investigators. *N Engl J Med* 1996; 335:217–225.

217 Koester W. Endarteritis and arteritis. *Berl Klin Wochenschr* 1876;13:454–455.

218 Kaiser M, Younge B, Bjornsson J, et al. Formation of new vasa vasorum in vasculitis. Production of angiogenic cytokines by multinucleated giant cells. *Am J Pathol* 1999;155:765–774.

219 Tanaka H, Sukhova GK, Libby P. Interaction of the allogeneic state and hypercholesterolemia in arterial lesion formation in experimental cardiac allografts. *Arterioscler Thromb* 1994;14:734–745.

220 Gossl M, Malyar NM, Rosol M, et al. Impact of coronary vasa vasorum functional structure on coronary vessel wall perfusion distribution. *Am J Physiol Heart Circ Physiol* 2003;285:H2019–H2026.

221 Kwon HM, Sangiorgi G, Ritman EL, et al. Enhanced coronary vasa vasorum neovascularization in experimental hypercholesterolemia. *J Clin Invest* 1998;101: 1551–1556.

222 Paterson JC. Capillary rupture with intimal hemorrhage as a causative factor in coronary thrombosis. *Arch Pathol* 1938;25:474–487.

223 Kumamoto M, Nakashima Y, Sueishi K. Intimal neovascularization in human coronary atherosclerosis: its origin and pathophysiological significance. *Hum Pathol* 1995;26:450–456.

224 Libby P. Molecular bases of the acute coronary syndromes. *Circulation* 1995;91:2844–2850.

225 Joussen AM, Poulaki V, Le ML, et al. A central role for inflammation in the pathogenesis of diabetic retinopathy. *Faseb J* 2004;18:1450–1452.

226 Kolodgie FD, Gold HK, Burke AP, et al. Intraplaque hemorrhage and progression of coronary atheroma. *N Engl J Med* 2003;349:2316–2325.

227 Virmani R, Kolodgie FD, Burke AP, et al. Atherosclerotic plaque progression and vulnerability to rupture: angiogenesis as a source of intraplaque hemorrhage. *Arterioscler Thromb Vasc Biol* 2005;25:2054–2061.

228 O'Brien ER, Garvin MR, Dev R, et al. Angiogenesis in human coronary atherosclerotic plaques. *Am J Pathol* 1994;145:883–894.

229 Geiringer E. Intimal vascularization and atherosclerosis. *J Pathol Bacteriol.* 1951;63:210–211.

230 Werber AH, Armstrong ML, Heistad DD. Diffusional support of the thoracic aorta in atherosclerotic monkeys. *Atherosclerosis* 1987;68:123–130.

231 Zhang Y, Cliff WJ, Schoefl GI, et al. Immunohistochemical study of intimal microvessels in coronary atherosclerosis. *Am J Pathol* 1993;143:164–172.

232 Williams JK, Armstrong ML, Heistad DD. Vasa vasorum in atherosclerotic coronary arteries: responses to vasoactive stimuli and regression of atherosclerosis. *Circ Res* 1988;62:515–523.

233 Davies MJ, Richardson PD, Woolf N, et al. Risk of thrombosis in human atherosclerotic plaques: role of extracellular lipid, macrophage, and smooth muscle cell content. *Br Heart J* 1993;69:377–381.

234 O'Brien KD, McDonald TO, Chait A, et al. Neovascular expression of E-selectin, intercellular adhesion molecule-1, and vascular cell adhesion molecule-1 in human atherosclerosis and their relation to intimal leukocyte content. *Circulation* 1996;93:672–682.

235 Moreno PR, Purushothaman KR, Fuster V, et al. Plaque neovascularization is increased in ruptured atherosclerotic lesions of human aorta: implications for plaque vulnerability. *Circulation* 2004;110: 2032–2038.

236 Burke AP, Farb A, Malcom GT, et al. Coronary risk factors and plaque morphology in men with coronary disease who died suddenly. *N Engl J Med* 1997;336:1276–1282.

237 Park HJ, Kong D, Iruela-Arispe L, et al. 3-hydroxy-3-methylglutaryl coenzyme A reductase inhibitors interfere with angiogenesis by inhibiting the geranylgeranylation of RhoA. *Circ Res* 2002;91:143–150.

238 Wilson SH, Herrmann J, Lerman LO, et al. Simvastatin preserves the structure of coronary adventitial vasa vasorum in experimental hypercholesterolemia independent of lipid lowering. *Circulation* 2002;105: 415–418.

239 Moulton KS, Heller E, Konerding MA, et al. Angiogenesis inhibitors endostatin or TNP-470 reduce intimal neovascularization and plaque growth in apolipoprotein E-deficient mice. *Circulation* 1999;99: 1726–1732.

240 Heeschen C, Jang JJ, Weis M, et al. Nicotine stimulates angiogenesis and promotes tumor growth and atherosclerosis. *Nat Med* 2001;7:833–839.

241 Celletti FL, Waugh JM, Amabile PG, et al. Vascular endothelial growth factor enhances atherosclerotic plaque progression. *Nat Med* 2001;7:425–429.

242 Khurana R, Zhuang Z, Bhardwaj S, et al. Angiogenesis-dependent and independent phases of intimal hyperplasia. *Circulation* 2004;110:2436–2443.

243 Goldschmidt-Clermont PJ, Creager MA, Lorsordo DW, et al. Atherosclerosis 2005: recent discoveries and novel hypotheses. *Circulation* 2005;112:3348–3353.

244 Scheubel RJ, Zorn H, Silber RE, et al. Age-dependent depression in circulating endothelial progenitor cells in patients undergoing coronary artery bypass grafting. *J Am Coll Cardiol* 2003;42:2073–2080.

245 Karra R, Vemullapalli S, Dong C, et al. Molecular evidence for arterial repair in atherosclerosis. *Proc Natl Acad Sci USA* 2005;102:16789–16794.

246 Moulton KS. Plaque angiogenesis: its functions and regulation. *Cold Spring Harb Symp Quant Biol* 2003; LXVIII:471–482.

247 Couffinhal T, Kearney M, Witzenbichler B, et al. Vascular endothelial growth factor/vascular permeability factor (VEGF/VPF) in normal and atherosclerotic human arteries. *Am J Pathol* 1997;150:1673–1685.

248 Miosge N, Sasaki T, Timpl R. Angiogenesis inhibitor endostatin is a distinct component of elastic fibers in vessel walls. *FASEB J* 1999;13:1743–1750.

249 Moulton KS, Olsen BR, Sonn S, et al. Loss of collagen XVIII enhances neovascularization and vascular permeability in atherosclerosis. *Circulation* 2004;110: 1330–1336.

250 Zeng X, Chen J, Miller YI, et al. Endostatin binds biglycan and LDL and interferes with LDL retention to the subendothelial matrix during atherosclerosis. *J Lipid Res* 2005;46:1849–1859.

251 Pillarisetti S. Lipoprotein modulation of subendothelial heparan sulfate proteoglycans (perlecan) and atherogenicity. *Trend Cardiovasc Med* 2000;10:60–65.

252 Clowes AW, Collazzo RE, Karnovsky MJ. A morphologic and permeability study of luminal smooth muscle cells after arterial injury in the rat. *Lab Invest* 1978;39: 141–150.

253 Pels K, Labinaz M, Hoffert C, et al. Adventitial angiogenesis early after coronary angioplasty: correlation with arterial remodeling. *Arterioscler Thromb Vasc Biol* 1999;19:229–238.

254 Hiltunen MO, Laitinen M, Turunen MP, et al. Intravascular adenovirus-mediated VEGF-C gene transfer reduces neointima formation in balloon-denuded rabbit aorta. *Circulation* 2000;102:2262–2268.

255 Hutter R, Sauter BV, Reis ED, et al. Decreased reendothelialization and increased neointima formation with endostatin overexpression in a mouse model of arterial injury. *Circulation.* 2003;107:1658–1663.

256 Celletti FL, Waugh JM, Amabile PG, et al. Inhibition of vascular endothelial growth factor-mediated neointima progression with angiostatin or paclitaxel. *J Vasc Intervent Radiol* 2002;13:703–707.

257 Epstein SE, Stabile E, Kinnaird T, et al. Janus phenomenon: the interrelated tradeoffs inherent in therapies designed to enhance collateral formation and those designed to inhibit atherogenesis. *Circulation* 2004;109: 2826–2831.

258 Couffinhal T, Silver M, Zheng LP, et al. Mouse model of angiogenesis. *Am J Pathol* 1998;152:1667–1679.

259 Tong RT, Boucher Y, Kozin SV, et al. Vascular normalization by vascular endothelial growth factor receptor 2 blockade induces a pressure gradient across the vasculature and improves drug penetration in tumors. *Cancer Res* 2004;64:3731–3736.

105 Choudhury RP, Rong JX, Trogan E, et al. High-density lipoproteins retard the progression of atherosclerosis and favorably remodel lesions without suppressing indices of inflammation or oxidation. *Arterioscler Thromb Vasc Biol* 2004;24:1904–1909.

106 Stannard AK, Khan S, Graham A, et al. Inability of plasma high-density lipoproteins to inhibit cell adhesion molecule expression in human coronary artery endothelial cells. *Atherosclerosis* 2001;154:31–38.

CHAPTER 7

Advanced glycation endproducts and the accelerated atherosclerosis in diabetes

Giuseppina Basta, DBiol, *Ann Marie Schmidt,* MD, *& Raffaele De Caterina,* MD, PhD

Introduction

Both type 1 and type 2 diabetes are powerful and independent risk factors for coronary artery disease, stroke, and peripheral arterial disease [1,2].

Accelerated arterio- and atherosclerosis, as well as microvascular disease, are the major vascular complications of diabetes mellitus, constituting the main cause of morbidity and mortality in this common metabolic disorder. Atherosclerosis accounts for virtually 80% of all deaths among North American diabetic patients compared with one-third of all deaths in the general population. Thus, prevention and treatment of chronic vascular disease is a central therapeutic problem in diabetes.

The primary causal factor leading to the pathophysiological alterations in the diabetic vasculature is chronic exposure to high levels of blood glucose [3,4]. Data from the Diabetes Control and Complications Trial (DCCT), comprising two multicenter, randomized, prospective controlled clinical studies [3,5] definitely established a causal relationship between chronic hyperglycemia and diabetic microvascular disease long inferred from a variety of animal and clinical studies [6]. The update in 2003 from the DCCT and the Epidemiology of Diabetes Interventions and Complications Research Group indicated that subjects treated early by intensive glycemic control displayed smaller carotid intima–media thickness than those treated with standard therapies [7]. Several other reports also support a relationship between chronic hyperglycemia and

diabetic macrovascular disease in type 2 diabetic patients [8–10]. Thus, prolonged exposure to hyperglycemia is the primary factor for the development of diabetes-specific vascular disease, although the relationship between deranged glucose metabolism and arterial disease is complicated by many other factors that often coexist in diabetes, including hypertension, dyslipidemia, and genetic determinants of tissue response to injury [11].

Currently, three major mechanisms may explain the link between hyperglycemia and vascular complications, including: the increased intracellular oxidative stress induced by hyperglycemia itself, resulting in protein kinase C (particularly the beta isoform) activation and subsequent activation and nuclear translocation of the transcription factor nuclear factor (NF)-κB, leading to enhanced intracellular reactions [12]; increased activity of the sorbitol–aldose reductase pathway [13]; and formation of advanced glycation endproducts (AGE) [14,15]. Although multiple studies support the direct adverse effects of glucose itself in modulating cellular properties [16,17], the most important mechanism involved in the complex series of reaction associated with accelerated atherosclerosis in diabetes is the increase in non-enzymatic glycation of proteins and lipids, with the irreversible formation and deposition of reactive AGE. Indeed, recent studies by Brownlee's group suggest that elevated levels of glucose trigger these processes and indirectly cause increased intracellular generation of superoxide anion and other reactive oxygen species

Table 7.1 Non-receptor-mediated effects of AGE on atherogenesis.

Extracellular matrix
Collagen cross-linking and high resistance to collagenases
Enhanced synthesis of extracellular matrix components
  with consequent narrowing of the vessel lumen
Decreased polymer self-assembly of laminin
Impairment of matrix-bound heparan sulfate
  proteoglycans
Glycated sub-endothelial matrix quenching of NO
Trapping of LDL and IgG in the sub-endothelium

Lipoprotein modifications
Reduced LDL recognition by cellular LDL receptor
Enhanced glycated LDL uptake by macrophage scavenger
  receptor
Increased LDL susceptibility to oxidative modifications

Alterations of coagulation and fibrinolysis
Reduced biological activity of AT-III
Reduced fibrin susceptibility to degradation
Increased platelet aggregation
Reduced platelet membrane fluidity

AGE: advanced glycation endproducts; NO: nitric oxide; LDL: low density lipoproteins; IgG: immunoglobulin G; AT III: antithrombin III.

Table 7.2 Receptor-mediated effects of AGE on atherogenesis.

Mononuclear phagocytes
Induction of PDGF, IGF-1, and pro-inflammatory cytokines
  such as IL-1β and TNF-α
Chemotaxis by soluble AGE ligands
Apoptaxis by immobilized AGE
Increased macrophage uptake of AGE-LDL

Smooth muscle cells
Increased proliferative activity
Increased production of fibronectin
Increased susceptibility to oxidative modifications

Endothelial cells
Increased permeability
Decreased expression of t-PA and increased expression
  of PAI-I
Increased intracellular oxidative stress
Increased procoagulant activity
Induction of endothelin-1 and increased vasoconstriction
Increased expression of adhesion molecules

AGE: advanced glycation endproducts; PDGF: platelet derived growth factor; IGF-1: insulin-like growth factor-1; IL-1; interleukin-1; TNF: tumour necrosis factor; LDL: low density lipoproteins; tPA: tissue plasminogen activator; PAI-1: plasminogen activator inhibitor type-1.

collagen and altered function of heparan sulfate proteoglycans [81]. *In vitro*, AGE formation on intact glomerular basement membrane increases membrane permeability [82].

AGE-induced abnormalities in the function of extracellular matrix alter the structure and function of intact vessels. Thus, AGE decrease elasticity in large vessels of diabetic rats, even after the abolishment of vascular tone, and increase fluid filtration across the carotid artery [83]. Furthermore, glycation may modulate the function of molecules such as basic fibroblast growth factor (b-FGF). b-FGF mitogenic activity decreases markedly after post-translational modification of b-FGF induced by elevated intracellular glucose concentrations [84]. Such loss of functional properties due to AGE is important for vascular homeostasis.

Effect of AGE on lipids

When amine-containing lipids such as phosphatidylethanolamine and phosphatidylserine are incubated with glucose, a similar time- and concentration-dependent series of slow chemical reactions is observed as it occurs with proteins [85]. Quite interestingly, this formation of AGE associates

with fatty acid oxidation, which occurs at a parallel rate. In contrast, lipids lacking free amines, such as phosphatidylcholine, cannot react with glucose or form oxidation products. Glycation occurs on both the apoprotein B [86] and phospholipid [85] components of LDL, leading to functional alterations in LDL clearance and increased susceptibility to oxidative modifications. In fact, diabetic LDL samples revealed significantly elevated levels of both apoB- and lipid-linked AGE, which correlated with levels of oxidized LDL [85,87]. Intermediates such as glyoxales, glycolaldehydes, hydroxyaldehydes, or other carbonyl group-containing compounds may form during oxidation of carbohydrates and polyunsaturated fatty acids [88,89]. These common intermediates (see above) can in turn react with free amino groups of proteins, such as LDL apoB, to form AGE products, including imidazolone, CML, CEL, GOLD, MOLD, and others [59,62–64,90]. Glycation of LDL apoB occurs mainly on positively charged lysine residues within the putative LDL receptor binding domain, which are essential for the specific recognition of LDL by the LDL receptor [87]. Increased LDL glycation correlates with glucose levels, and AGE–ApoB binding results in a significant impairment of LDL receptor-mediated uptake, decreasing the *in vivo* clearance of LDL compared with native LDL [91]. Several studies have shown impaired degradation of glycated LDL in cultured human fibroblast, which possess the LDL receptor, compared with normal LDL; such impairment is proportional to the extent of glycation [91]. In contrast to fibroblasts, human monocyte-derived macrophages recognize glycated LDL more frequently than native LDL [92]. The uptake of glycated LDL by these cells, however, is not mediated by the LDL pathways, but rather by a high-capacity, low-affinity receptor pathway [92]. Thus, glycated LDL are poorly recognized by the specific LDL receptor and preferentially recognized by a non-specific ("scavenger") receptor present on human macrophages. Because LDL glycation enhances its uptake by human aortic intimal cells [93] and monocyte-derived macrophages [92], with the resulting stimulation of foam cell formation, the recognition of glycated LDL by the scavenger receptor pathway may promote intracellular accumulation of cholesteryl esters and, consequently, atherosclerosis.

Effects of AGE on hemostasis: alteration of platelet function

In diabetes, an increase in *ex vivo* platelet response to aggregating agents has been described [94]. This can also be demonstrated by the increased circulating levels of some *in vivo* markers of platelet activation, such as β-thromboglobulin [94] and platelet factor-4 [95]. Therefore, non-enzymatic glycation of platelet membrane proteins, found in diabetic subjects, may cause the platelet hypersensitivity to aggregating stimuli [96,97]. Additionally, other studies have shown that increased glycation of platelet membranes reduces platelet membrane fluidity, but this apparently does not correlate with platelet sensitivity to aggregating agents [97,98].

Effects of AGE on hemostasis: alterations of soluble proteins involved in coagulation and fibrinolysis

Several abnormalities in hemostatic mechanisms occur in diabetes, with an obvious tendency to thrombosis [99]. Such abnormalities involve all stages of hemostasis, including platelet function, fibrin formation, fibrinolysis, and endothelial hemostatic functions. The hypothesis that hyperglycemia may constitute a key factor of diabetic hypercoagulability and can induce changes promoting thrombosis is suggestive, and supported by several experimental pieces of evidence. Non-enzymatic glycation reduces the susceptibility of fibrin to degradation by specific enzymes such as plasmin [77]. A direct correlation between hyperglycemia and the increase of fibrinopeptide A (a marker of thrombin activation) occurs in patients with diabetes [100,101]. Finally, antithrombin III (formerly antithrombin III, AT-III), the likely most important physiological inhibitor of coagulation, shows diminished biological activity in patients with diabetes, probably directly due to glucose, which renders the molecule less active by occupying the lysine residue that allows the binding of AT-III to heparin, its natural cofactor [102]. Free radicals produced during glycation processes might also induce rapid inactivation of AT-III. Indeed, oxidative stress can reduce AT-III activity [103]. Moreover, hyperglycemia decreases the concentration and biological activity of protein C, another important physiologic inhibitor of coagulation [104].

Receptor-mediated effects of AGE in atherogenesis

Cellular uptake of AGE

Cell surface AGE receptors mediate endocytosis and degradation of AGE-modified molecules, serving an important function in AGE catabolism and turnover. The search for removal mechanisms of AGE has led to the discovery of several cellular receptors binding these irreversibly modified macromolecules. A macrophage AGE receptor distinct from the mannose/fucose receptors involved in glycoprotein uptake and from previously described macrophage scavenger receptors recognizes *in vivo*-isolated and *in vitro*-synthesized AGE [105,106]. Two new proteins, of 60 and 90 kDa, of apparently unique amino acid sequence, were later isolated from the rat liver [107], and subsequently an additional AGE-binding protein, termed *lactoferrin-like 80-kDa protein*, was identified [108]. Later, *galectin-3*, a 32-kDa macrophage protein, was identified as an AGE-binding protein [109].

The role of these binding proteins (there-fore not necessarily "receptors") for AGE in AGE-mediated cellular activation remains undetermined.

Subsequent studies led to the identification, cloning, and analysis of RAGE, a multi-ligand member of the immunoglobulin superfamily and a receptor for AGE [15,25,110]. Current opinion increasingly views RAGE as an intracellular signal-transducing peptide rather than a simple receptor involved in AGE endocytosis and turnover [111,112].

Structure of RAGE protein

RAGE is an approximately 45-kDa protein originally isolated from bovine lung endothelium on the basis of its ability to bind AGE ligands [113]. Subsequent molecular cloning revealed that RAGE is a newly identified member of the immunoglobulin super-family of cell-surface molecules [114]. The entire mature receptor consists of 403 amino acids in man, rat, and mouse. The extracellular region of RAGE consists of one V-type (variable) immunoglobu-lin domain, followed by two C-type (constant) immunoglobulin domains stabilized by internal disulfide bridges between cysteine residues. The V-type domain includes two putative N-linked gly-cation sites. In addition to the extracellular domain, RAGE displays a single putative transmembrane-spanning region and a short, highly charged cyto-solic tail.

RAGE tissue expression, ligands, and activation

RAGE is highly conserved across species and expressed in a wide variety of tissues [114]. Immunohistochemical methods including *in situ* hybridization and Northern analysis, have shown that RAGE antigen and mRNA localize at least in the endothelium, vascular SMC, macrophages, neu-ral tissue, and glomerular visceral epithelial cells, or podocytes [26,115]. Enzyme-linked immunosor-bent assay (ELISA) of various tissue extracts demonstrates that RAGE is most abundant in the heart, lung, and skeletal muscle. The presence of RAGE in multiple tissues suggests a potential rele-vance of ligand–RAGE interactions for the modula-tion of vascular properties, as well as of neural, renal, and cardiac functions, all prominently affected in diabetes and aging. Indeed, RAGE

expression increases at sites of diverse diseases including atherosclerosis, Alzheimer's disease, and amyotrophic lateral sclerosis [15,116,117]. In this context, other ligands for the receptor may be involved in homeostatic function as well as in pro-inflammatory events. For example, RAGE binds to amphoterin, a developmentally expressed neurite outgrowth-promoting protein that intriguingly increases in tumors, where its interaction with RAGE facilitates tumor cell migration and invasion [27,28]. Further, S100A12, a polypeptide of the S100/calgranulin family of pro-inflammatory cyto-kines also termed *extracellular newly identified RAGE binding protein* (EN-RAGE), interacts with RAGE in a dose-dependent and saturable manner, resulting in the activation of cellular targets and competition with another member of the S100/cal-granulin family, S100B, also capable of binding to RAGE [118]. Thus, RAGE is a receptor not only for AGE, but also for S100/calgranulins, molecules found in any inflammatory lesion, including the blood vessel wall of individuals with diabetes [119–121]. The overlapping presence of high levels of AGE, S100/calgranulins, and RAGE, together with dyslipidemia, might conspire to cause the rapid atherosclerosis observed in diabetes. Simi-larly, RAGE interacts with β-sheet fibrils composed of different subunits/monomers, including amyloid A, amyloid-β peptide, prion peptide, and amylin [71,122]. The binding by RAGE of seemingly diverse ligands deserves further research.

Another feature of RAGE is an unusual co-expression with its ligands in tissues. At sites where AGE and S100/calgranulins accumulate in the vas-cular lesions, RAGE expression increases in vessel wall cells, including the endothelium, vascular SMC, and invading macrophages [65,121,123]. This overlapping distribution of the receptor and its ligands may lead to prolonged cellular activa-tion, resulting in further increased expression of the receptor. Contrary to other receptors, such as the LDL receptor, which are downregulated by increased levels of their ligand, the RAGE–ligand interaction would thus lead to a positive feedback activation, which further increases receptor expres-sion. Currently, the only means to substantially downregulate RAGE expression involve interrupt-ing the cycle of ligand engagement of the receptor via soluble RAGE or blocking antibodies.

Signal-transduction pathways activated by RAGE–ligand interaction

The most important pathologic consequence of RAGE engagement with its ligands appears to be cellular activation, leading to the induction of oxidative stress and a broad spectrum of signaling mechanisms. Even if AGE were nothing more than accidental ligands for RAGE, interaction of RAGE with other ligands such as amphoterin or amyloid peptide likely induces similar consequences. In the vasculature, the principal pathological consequence of AGE interaction with RAGE is the induction of oxidative stress, leading to NF-κB activation and the induction of the endothelial expression of various cell adhesion molecules, including vascular cell adhesion molecule-1 (VCAM-1), intercellular adhesion molecule-1

(ICAM-1), and E-selectin [30,65,123]. The interaction of AGE with endothelial surface RAGE leads first to increased intracellular ROS [124,125], the generation of which seems linked, at least in part, to the activation of the reduced nicotinamide adenine dinucleotide (phosphate)-oxidase (NAD(P)H-oxidase) system [126]. Our studies have shown that mitochondrial sources of ROS are also evoked secondary to AGE–RAGE interaction [127]. ROS in turn would activate the redox-sensitive transcription factor NF-κB, a pleiotropic regulator of many "response-to-injury" genes. Antibodies directed against either RAGE or AGE themselves can block this signal-transduction cascade [126] (Figure 7.4).

NF-κB induced in response to oxidative stress leads to transcriptional activation of many genes

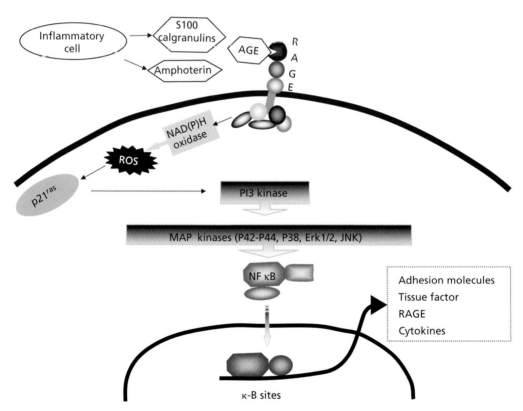

Figure 7.4 Signal-transduction pathways activated by RAGE–ligand interaction. Activation of RAGE by AGEs, amphoterin and S100/calgranulins induces the increased generation of oxygen radicals by a NAD(P)H oxidase. Free radicals then activate a Ras-MAP kinase pathway eventually leading to the activation and nuclear translocation of NF-κB. The RAGE promoter itself is controlled by NF-κB, and upregulation of the receptor provides an increasing number of binding sites for RAGE-ligands, perpetuating the cellular inflammatory response. Abbreviations: AGE: advanced glycation endproducts; NAD(P)H-oxidase: reduced nicotinamide adenine dinucleotide (phosphate)-oxidase; PI3 kinase: phosphatidyl inositol-3 kinase; MAP kinases: mitogen-activated protein kinases; Erk: extracellular regulated kinase, JNK: c-Jun N-terminal kinase; RAGE: receptor for AGE.

highly relevant for inflammation, immunity, and atherosclerosis, including tumor necrosis factors (TNF-α and -β), interleukins IL-1, -6, and -8, interferon-γ (IFN-γ), vascular cell adhesion molecule-1 (VCAM-1), intercellular adhesion molecule-1 (ICAM-1), and E-selectin [128]. Importantly, the tethering of AGE to the cell surface is not enough to generate ROS and cellular activation, since the RAGE carboxy-terminal cytosolic tail, containing known signaling phosphorylation sites, kinase domains, and other activation sites, is critical for RAGE-dependent cellular activation. Indeed, a truncated form of RAGE, lacking only the cytosolic tail and expressed in cells, retains binding to various ligands identical to wild-type RAGE, but does not mediate the induction of cellular activation [118].

Triggering of inflammatory effector mechanisms (generation of cytokines and chemokines, and expression of cell adhesion molecules) mediated by the AGE–RAGE interaction involves multiple intracellular signal-transduction pathways, including *p21ras*, MAP kinases, PI3 kinase, *cdc42/rac*, Jak/STAT, NAD(P)H oxidase, and others [31,33–36,126]. Each of these pathways is closely linked with AGE binding to RAGE, because blockade of the receptor with either anti-RAGE IgG or excess soluble (s)RAGE prevents their activation.

The presence of RAGE in all cells relevant to atherosclerosis, including EC, monocyte-derived macrophages, lymphocytes, and SMC, suggests the relevance of RAGE engagement in these processes.

Interaction of AGE with macrophages and T cells

The macrophages AGE receptor system is closely linked to AGE turnover, and may represent a mechanism that responds to the increased levels of AGE that accompany aging and the degradation of senescent proteins [129]. The interaction of AGE with macrophages induces a phenotype of activated macrophages, manifested by the induction of platelet-derived growth factor (PDGF), insulin-like growth factor 1 (IGF-1), and pro-inflammatory cytokines such as IL-1β and TNF-α [130–132]. In macrophages, AGE–RAGE interaction prompts cell migration (chemotaxis) mediated by the interaction of soluble RAGE ligands (AGE prepared *in vitro* or isolated from diabetic subjects,

AGE-β2-microglobulin or CML-adducts) with RAGE. In contrast to the effect of soluble AGE, immobilized AGE, such as those found in basement membranes, retard macrophages migration, a process known as "apoptaxis." Anti-RAGE IgG or sRAGE block both chemotactic and apoptactic responses [133,134].

More recently, EN-RAGE has been utilized as a stimulus to induce chemotaxis. The induced migration of macrophages has here been shown to be concentration- and RAGE-dependent. Similarly, the engagement of RAGE by EN-RAGE in cultured Bv2 cells (murine macrophages) induced production of IL-1β and TNF-α, in an NF-κB-dependent fashion [118]. On the other hand, when macrophages reach a site of immobilized AGE in the tissue, their migration slows down, allowing them to bind to the AGE-modified surface and to become activated. This could provide a mechanism for attracting and retaining macrophages at sites of AGE deposition in tissues, potentially contributing to the development of tissue lesions after AGE-induced macrophages migration.

An inducible system for RAGE expression also occurs in T cells [135]. The exposure to AGE of T cells pre-stimulated with phytohemagglutinin increases the synthesis and release of IFN-γ, which represents the main activating factor for macrophages and enhances diverse effects of other cytokines, such as TNF, on EC [135,136]. Since activated T cells are present in atherosclerotic lesions [137,138], combined AGE-activated T cells and macrophages may contribute to vascular damage in a hyperglycemic setting.

Interaction of AGE with vascular SMC

In the presence of AGE, cultured SMC increase their proliferative activity and fibronectin production [48,139]. The precise mechanism of this response remains unclear. *In vivo*, cytokines or growth factors induced by AGE in the MP likely mediate the effects promoting SMC growth indirectly, at least in part. Transforming growth factor-β (TGF-β) might act as an intermediate factor in AGE-induced fibronectin production by SMC [139]. These studies suggest that stimulation of SMC by AGE may contribute to the proliferative lesions commonly observed in several tissues in diabetes.

Interactions of AGE with vascular endothelium: alterations of vascular permeability and hemostatic and adhesive properties

Due to its unique position and numerous properties, the vascular endothelium is particularly important in the regulation of permeability, the maintenance of blood fluidity, the regulation of vascular growth and tone, and metabolism of hormones and vasoactive mediators. Endothelium is exposed to AGE localized on circulating proteins or cells (e.g., diabetic red blood cells) as well as those present in the underlying sub-endothelial matrix. Receptors for AGE have been found on the EC surface, and they mediate both the uptake and transcytosis of AGE as well as internal signal transduction. AGE–RAGE interaction causes perturbation of two important homeostatic properties of the endothelium: barrier function and anti-hemostatic properties.

The alteration of barrier function has been demonstrated by showing increased permeability of EC incubated with AGE, with increased transit of macromolecules through the endothelial monolayer. Alterations of the physical integrity of the endothelium is accompanied by increased permeability, as shown by the destruction of organized actin structures and alterations of cellular morphology [140,141].

AGE also determine alterations of endothelial anti-hemostatic functions *in vitro*, as shown by a reduction of thrombomodulin and the concomitant induction of tissue factor expression [142,143]. Tissue factor induction and the reduced thrombomodulin activity change the dynamic endothelial properties with regard to hemostasis from those of an anti-coagulant to those of a procoagulant surface.

In addition, cytokine (IL-1β and TNF-α), induced by the interaction of AGE with macrophages, can indirectly alter the function of EC with specific receptors for these mediators [142,143]. Such cytokines downregulate endothelial expression of tissue plasminogen activator (t-PA) and induce the transcription of its main inhibitor (type 1 plasminogen activator inhibitor, PAI-1) [144,145], causing an imbalance between these two factors that results in a reduction of endothelial fibrinolytic properties.

Binding of AGE to endothelial RAGE also results in depletion of cellular anti-oxidant defense mechanisms (e.g., glutathione and vitamin C) [32] and the generation of ROS [124] (Figure 7.2). Increased cellular oxidative stress activates NF-κB and thus promotes the expression of NF-κB-regulated genes including procoagulant tissue factor and VCAM-1 [65,140,143]. VCAM-1 expression may prime the diabetic vasculature toward enhanced interaction with circulating monocytes [146,147]. The incubation of EC with EN-RAGE or S100B causes VCAM-1 induction, in a RAGE-dependent manner, as confirmed by the inhibitory effect of anti-RAGE IgG or sRAGE [118]. It has recently been reported that AGE preparations carefully assessed to be endotoxin free would be incapable of inducing VCAM-1 or TNF-α secretion regardless of RAGE binding affinity, AGE concentration, or incubation time [148]. In contrast, the reported RAGE ligand S100b was confirmed to induce VCAM-1 expression on EC and TNF-α secretion [148]. While the validity of the former observation contrasts with a host of previous literature on this subject, the possibility that S100b acts also independent of RAGE is an interesting observation requiring attention and confirmation.

Alterations of endothelium-dependent vasodilation

AGE linked to the vascular matrix can interfere chemically with the bioavailability of nitric oxide (NO), an important regulator of vascular tone inducing SMC relaxation [149,150]. An altered endothelium-dependent vasodilation characterizes many pathological settings, including diabetes [151], aging [152], atherosclerosis [153], and some forms of hypertension [154]. AGE-modified proteins added to NO *in vitro* block NO activity in a concentration-dependent manner. Studies on animal models with experimentally induced diabetes demonstrate that an alteration of endothelium-dependent dilation occurs quickly, within 2 months, from diabetes induction [149]. Presumably, the inactivation of NO occurs through a direct reaction of the NO radical with other free radicals formed during advanced glycation reactions. In parallel, AGE induce the expression of the potent vasoconstrictor endothelin-1 and shift endothelial function toward vasoconstriction [155]. Animal models *in vivo* have provided further evidence confirming the involvement of AGE in the modulation of vascular tone in diabetes. Indeed, healthy euglycemic rats and rabbits treated with AGE show an appreciable decrease of their vasodilatory reserve [142].

AGE and RAGE in experimental animals

The first evidence of the direct pathogenetic role of AGE – independent of hyperglycemia and other possible contributory factors occurring in diabetes – has been obtained in animal models, namely healthy euglycemic rats treated with AGE. Such treatment spurs tissue deposition of AGE, accompanied by various changes in vascular function, including alterations of permeability, sub-endothelial sequestration of monocytes, and decreased sensitivity to vasodilatory agents [142,156]. Non-diabetic rabbits undergoing prolonged treatment with "physiological" amounts of AGE also manifest AGE deposition in aortic tissue and the expression of adhesion molecules such as VCAM-1 and ICAM-1 [157]. AGE administered by infusion to mice *in vivo* also induce new antigenic determinants, such as malondialdehyde in the vessel wall, markers of increased oxidative stress [23,30,124].

Peculiarly, pathological lesions characterized by AGE accumulation associate closely with increased cellular expression of RAGE and the overlapping presence of AGE epitopes. In diabetic vessels, abundant AGE lie in close proximity to cells that express high levels of RAGE [69]. Thus, rather than decreasing RAGE expression, AGE may contribute to enhanced expression of the receptor, resulting in a smoldering cellular activation in diabetic tissues. To dissect the contribution of RAGE–ligand interaction in the pathogenesis of diabetic vasculopathy, Wautier and colleagues first tested an acute animal model of diabetes-associated hyperpermeability by administering the decoy protein soluble (s)RAGE or antibodies to RAGE, able to block the access of ligands to RAGE [141]. After 9–11 weeks, rats rendered diabetic with streptozotocin showed increased vascular permeability in multiple organs, especially the intestine, skin, and kidney. RAGE blockade with either sRAGE or mono-specific antibodies normalized tissue permeability. Because increased permeability in human subjects with diabetes associates with increased morbidity and mortality from cardiovascular complications, such diabetes-associated hyperpermeability, taken here as a "surrogate" marker for diabetic vasculopathy, is likely an "intermediate" endpoint of vascular disease [157,158].

Murine models of atherosclerosis have significantly advanced our understanding of the development of accelerated diabetic macrovascular disease. Since mice inherently resist the development of atherosclerosis, in part due to their high plasma levels of high-density lipoproteins (HDL), researchers have used strains genetically susceptible to atherosclerosis. In apolipoprotein (apo)E-deficient mice, which develop spontaneous atherosclerosis on a normal chow diet, induction of diabetes with streptozotocin was associated with an approximately 5-fold increase in mean atherosclerotic lesion area at the aortic sinus after 6 weeks of diabetes compared with euglycemic apoE null mice of the same age [38]. In addition, diabetic animals displayed increased numbers of complex lesions (fibrous caps, extensive monocyte, and SMC infiltration, etc.) compared with euglycemic control mice. Diabetes-associated atherosclerotic lesions in this model featured increased AGE deposition and enhanced RAGE expression. Administration of sRAGE in diabetic apoE-null animals suppressed accelerated diabetic atherosclerosis. Here, lesions appeared arrested at the stage of fatty streak, and the number of complex atherosclerotic lesions was strikingly reduced. In parallel, plasma levels of free AGE, the vascular expression of VCAM-1 and tissue factor, and the nuclear translocation of NF-κB all decreased in sRAGE-treated mice compared with vehicle-treated littermates. The effects of RAGE blockade, interrupting the cycle of sustained cellular activation, were independent of changes in other risk factors such as blood glucose, insulin, or lipoprotein levels. Interestingly, euglycemic animals receiving sRAGE also demonstrated a trend toward diminished atherosclerosis compared to vehicle-treated animals [38]. Recent studies in diabetic apoE-null mice further support these observations. Among male apoE-null mice rendered diabetic with streptozotocin or treated with citrate buffer at the age of 6 weeks, certain mice were sacrificed or treated with once daily murine sRAGE or albumin at age 14 weeks and all mice were sacrificed at age 20 weeks. Compared with diabetic mice at the age of 14 weeks, albumin-treated animals showed increased atherosclerotic lesion area and features of plaque complexity. In diabetic mice treated with sRAGE from the age of 14–20 weeks, lesion area and complexity were significantly reduced, and were not statistically different from diabetic mice at the age of 14 weeks. In these experiments, euglycemic mice treated with sRAGE also displayed a statistically significant decrease in atherosclerosis. Taken together, these findings strongly suggest that AGE formation, which certainly forms even in the euglycemic environment exposed to oxidant stress, or plasma levels of other ligands, such as EN-RAGE, may participate in the initiation and progression of atherosclerosis, at least in part, in a RAGE-dependent manner [39].

It is also well established that cellular proliferation, migration, and expression of extracellular matrix proteins and matrix metalloproteinases contribute to neointimal formation upon vascular injury [159]. In diabetic rats subjected to carotid artery injury induced by balloon angioplasty, the administration of sRAGE resulted in a significantly lower intima-media thickness compared with that seen in diabetic rats treated with vehicle [160]. Our studies have shown that wild-type C57BL/6 mice undergoing arterial endothelial denudation display a striking increase of RAGE in the injured vessel, particularly in activated SMC of the expanding neointima. In parallel, upregulation of AGE and S100/calgranulins is evident in the injured vessel wall [161]. Blockade of RAGE in homozygous RAGE-null mice by soluble truncated receptor or antibodies resulted in significantly decreased neointimal expansion after arterial injury and decreased SMC proliferation, migration, and expression of extracellular matrix proteins. Mice bearing a transgene encoding a RAGE cytosolic tail deletion mutant driven by the SM22a promoter specifically in SMC, demonstrated a critical role for SMC RAGE signaling. Upon arterial injury, neointimal expansion was strikingly suppressed compared with wild-type littermates [161]. These data highlight key roles for RAGE in the modulation of SMC properties in the acutely and chronically injured vessel wall.

Recently, it has been shown that RAGE functions also as an endothelial adhesion receptor promoting leukocyte recruitment by a direct interaction with the leukocyte beta-2-integrin Mac-1 [162]. In an animal model of thioglycollate-induced acute peritonitis, leukocyte recruitment was significantly impaired in RAGE-deficient mice as opposed to wild-type mice. In diabetic wild-type mice, enhanced leukocyte recruitment to the inflamed peritoneum was observed as compared with non-diabetic wild-type mice; this phenomenon was abrogated in the presence of soluble RAGE and was absent in diabetic RAGE-deficient mice [162]. The RAGE–Mac-1 interaction therefore now defines a novel pathway of leukocyte recruitment relevant in inflammatory disorders associated with increased RAGE expression.

While studies in RAGE-deficient mice have confirmed an important role for RAGE as a mediator of diabetic complications and chronic macrovascular disease, it is not yet known which receptors compensate for the absence of RAGE in RAGE-deficient mice, thus ensuring normal development and a normal phenotype in these animals.

AGE, RAGE, and vascular dysfunction in humans: possible therapeutic interventions on AGE formation, AGE cross-linking and AGE–RAGE interaction

There is substantial evidence to support that AGE increase in aging, cardiovascular disease, and diabetes. The plasma levels of AGE correlate with the degree of coronary artery disease in non-diabetic and diabetic human subjects [163–166]. Elevated plasma levels of S100A12 protein, AGE, and CML have been reported in type 2 diabetic patients [167–170]. Using a monoclonal anti-AGE antibody, immunohistochemical analyses of human atherosclerotic lesions have demonstrated diffuse extracellular as well as dense intracellular AGE deposition in macrophages and vascular SMC [72,171,172]. Tissue AGE concentration correlates with the severity of atherosclerotic lesions and the accumulation of plasma proteins, lipoproteins, and lipids in the vessel wall [163,173,174].

Recently, evidence is accumulating to support the hypothesis that RAGE may be a contributing factor in cardiovascular disease, even in the absence of diabetes. Cipollone et al. showed that RAGE was expressed in non-diabetic and diabetic human atherosclerosis and to enhanced degrees in diabetes [175]. RAGE colocalized with cyclooxygenase (COX)-2, type 1/type 2 microsomal prostaglandin (PG) E2, and matrix metalloproteinases (MMP) in the diabetic atherosclerotic plaques [175]. Further, studies on polymorphisms on the RAGE gene have shown that one particular promoter allele (−374A) is associated with a lesser degree of macrovascular disease in diabetic subjects [176,177].

Non-diabetic subjects with the −374T/A or A/A genotypes displayed reduced severity of coronary atherosclerosis [178]. In one smaller study, however, no association between these variants and the incidence of macrovascular disease was found [179].

Targeting of AGE–RAGE system is possible with the use of AGE formation inhibitors, AGE breakers, agents acting against AGE-derived protein cross-linking, and RAGE competitors. The hydrazine compound amino guanidine was the first AGE formation inhibitor discovered [74], and has been by far the most extensively studied compound of this kind thus far. Aminoguanidine has been evaluated in various animal models with different diabetic complications [67,180,181], and is the prototype of a drug class that might eventually find use in the treatment of diabetic complications. Rather than interfering with Amadori's products on proteins, aminoguanidine and other AGE inhibitors likely function as nucleophilic traps for reactive carbonyl intermediates in the formation of AGE [180]. Although encouraging results in animal models of diabetic complications have demonstrated decreased AGE accumulation [83], clinical studies must better define the place of aminoguanidine and other AGE inhibitors [181]. Moreover, clinical trials with aminoguanidine have shown a trend toward reduced renal dysfunction in human diabetic subjects with advanced nephropathy [181]. These findings may provide the first "proof of concept" in man that AGE importantly contribute to the pathogenesis of diabetic complications.

While aminoguanidine prevents AGE formation, it likely will not be effective in patients with a long history of disease and already extensive tissue AGE accumulation. The need to remove irreversibly bound AGE from connective tissues and matrix components has led to the development of AGE-cleaving agents [182]. Studies in animal models and preliminary clinical trials have shown that pimagedine, an AGE inhibitor, and the cross-link breaker ALT-711 can reduce the severity of pathologic lesions associated with AGEs [183,184].

RAGE expression increases in clinical settings characterized by enhanced cellular activation or oxidative stress, such as diabetes, and prolonged exposure of AGE to RAGE-expressing cells determines a chronic state of cellular activation [185].

Interference with the vicious cycle established by RAGE–ligand interaction might interrupt cellular activation and consequently lead to an improvement of various chronic disorders [71,116,186,187]. sRAGE treatment dose-dependently suppress the development of atherosclerosis in animal models, acting as a RAGE competitor in AGE binding, and thereby preventing the AGE–RAGE interactions. Reduced AGE level in sRAGE-treated diabetic mice suggest that sRAGE may enhance the removal of AGE from plasma and tissues [38].

Since endogenous sRAGE does exist in circulating blood, interesting studies on plasma levels of sRAGE further suggest an involvement of RAGE in the pathogenesis/severity of coronary artery disease. In age-matched Italian male subjects without diabetes, endogenously lower levels of plasma sRAGE were associated with enhanced risk of angiographically detected coronary artery disease [188]. When plasma sRAGE levels were divided into quartiles, the lowest levels of sRAGE were associated with the greatest overall risk for disease [188]. Circulating sRAGE levels were significantly lower in type 1 diabetic patients than in non-diabetic subjects and were inversely associated with the severity of some diabetic vascular complications [189].

So far, therefore, AGE have been identified as a main molecular target in diabetic vascular complications; the inhibition of AGE–RAGE interactions and subsequent signal transduction appears to be a promising and rational way for preventing diabetic vascular complications.

Conclusions

The experimental evidence gathered thus far unequivocally demonstrates that AGE can alter vessel wall homeostasis in a pro-atherogenic fashion through multiple mechanisms, i.e., alterations of extracellular matrix permeability, release of inflammatory cytokines and growth factors, alterations of antithrombotic properties of the endothelium and of the vessel wall ability to modulate vascular tone, and the increased expression of adhesion molecules and chemokines by vascular cells. Once initiated, a state of chronic vascular inflammation ensues, sustained by the migration and activation of inflammatory cells – mostly macrophages and T cells – that infiltrate the altered vessel wall. These processes thus trigger a cycle of ongoing cellular injury and vascular dysfunction, in part through the release of inflammatory peptides such as S100/calgranulins and amphoterin, also ligands of RAGE. The pivotal role of RAGE in these processes highlights this ligand–receptor axis as a logical and attractive candidate for therapeutic intervention to limit diabetic vascular damage and its long-term consequences.

References

1 Schwartz CJ, Valente AJ, Sprague EA, et al. Pathogenesis of the atherosclerotic lesion. Implications for diabetes mellitus. *Diabetes Care* 1992;15:1156–1167.

2 Stamler J, Vaccaro O, Neaton JD, et al. other risk factors, and 12-yr cardiovascular mortality for men screened in the Multiple Risk Factor Intervention Trial. *Diabetes Care* 1993;16:434–444.

3 The Diabetes Control and Complications Trial Research Group. The effect of intensive treatment of diabetes on the development and progression of long-term complications in insulin-dependent diabetes mellitus. *N Engl J Med* 1993;329:977–986.

4 Laakso K. Hyperglycemia and cardiovascular disease in type 2 diabetes. *Diabetes* 1999;48:937–942.

5 The Diabetes Control and Complications Trial/Epidemiology of Diabetes Interventions and Complications Research Group. Retinopathy and nephropathy in patients with type 1 diabetes four years after a trial of intensive therapy. *N Engl J Med* 2000;342:381–389.

6 Nathan D. Relationship between metabolic control and long term complications of diabetes. In: Kahn CR, Weir GC, eds. *Joslin's Diabetes Mellitus*. Philadelphia: Lea & Febiger; 1994:620–631.

7 Nathan DM, Lachin J, Cleary P, et al. Intensive diabetes therapy and carotid intima–media thickness in type 1 diabetes mellitus. *N Engl J Med* 2003;348:2294–2303.

8 Kuusisto J, Mykkanen L, Pyorala K, et al. NIDDM and its metabolic control predict heart disease in elderly subjects. *Diabetes* 1994;43:960–967.

9 Kuusisto J, Mykkanen L, Pyorala K, et al. Non-insulin-dependent diabetes and its metabolic control are important predictors of stroke in elderly subjects. *Stroke* 1994;25:1157–1164.

10 Colwell JA. Multifactorial aspects of the treatment of the type II diabetic patient. *Metabolism* 1997;46:1–4.

11 Brownlee M, Cerami A. The biochemistry of the complications of diabetes mellitus. *Annu Rev Biochem* 1981;50:385–432.

12 Nishikawa T, Edelstein D, Du XL, et al. Normalizing mitochondrial superoxide production blocks three pathways of hyperglycaemic damage. *Nature* 2000;404:787–790.

13 Greene DA, Lattimer SA, Sima AA. Sorbitol, phosphoinositides, and sodium–potassium–ATPase in the pathogenesis of diabetic complications. *N Engl J Med* 1987;316:599–606.

14 Wautier JL, Guillausseau PL. Diabetes, advanced glycation end products and vascular disease. *Vasc Med* 1998;3:131–137.

15 Schmidt AM, Yan SD, Wautier JL, et al. Activation of receptor for advanced glycation end products – a mechanism for chronic vascular dysfunction in diabetic vasculopathy and atherosclerosis. *Circ Res* 1999;84:489–497.

16 King GL, Shiba T, Oliver J, et al. Cellular and molecular abnormalities in the vascular endothelium of diabetes mellitus. *Annu Rev Med* 1994;45:179–188.

17 Koya D, King GL. Protein kinase C activation and the development of diabetic complications. *Diabetes* 1998;47:859–866.

18 Lusis AJ. Atherosclerosis. *Nature* 2000;407:233–241.

19 Libby P, Ridker PM, Maseri A. Inflammation and atherosclerosis. *Circulation* 2002;105:1135–1143.

20 Brownlee M, Vlassara H, Cerami A. Nonenzymatic glycosylation products on collagen covalently trap low density lipoprotein. *Diabetes* 1985;34:938–941.

21 Vishwanath V, Frank KE, Elmmets CA, et al. Glycation of skin collagen in type I diabetes mellitus. Correlation with long-term complications. *Diabetes* 1986; 35:916–921.

22 Watanabe J, Wohltmann H, Klein R, et al. Enhancement of platelet aggregation by low density lipoproteins from IDDM patients. *Diabetes* 1988;37:1652–1657.

23 Rosenfield M, Palinski W, Yla-Herttuala S, et al. Distribution of oxidation specific lipid–protein adducts and apolipoprotein B in atherosclerotic lesions of varying severity from WHHL rabbits. *Arteriosclerosis* 1990;10:336–349.

24 Dyer DG, Dunn JA, Thorpe SR, et al. Accumulation of Maillard reaction products in skin collagen in diabetes and aging. *J Clin Invest* 1993;91:2463–2469.

25 Schmidt AM, Hasu M, Popov D, et al. Receptor for advanced glycation end products (AGEs) has a central role in vessel wall interactions and gene activation in response to circulating AGE-proteins. *Proc Natl Acad Sci USA* 1994;91:8807–8811.

26 Tanji N, Markowitz GS, Fu C, et al. Expression of advanced glycation end products and their cellular receptor RAGE in diabetic nephropathy and nondiabetic renal disease. *J Am Soc Nephrol* 2000;11:1656–1666.

27 Hori O, Brett J, Nagashima M, et al. RAGE is a cellular binding site for amphoterin: mediation of neurite outgrowth and co-expression of RAGE and amphoterin in the developing nervous system. *J Biol Chem* 1995;270:25752–25761.

28 Taguchi A, Blood DC, del Toro G, et al. Blockade of amphoterin/RAGE signalling suppresses tumor growth and metastases. *Nature* 2000;405:354–356.

29 Tracey KJ. The inflammatory reflex. *Nature* 2002;420: 853–859.

30 Schmidt AM, Hori O, Chen JX, et al. Advanced glycation endproducts interacting with their endothelial receptor induce expression of vascular cell adhesion molecule-1 (VCAM-1) in cultured human endothelial cells and in mice. A potential mechanism for the accelerated vasculopathy of diabetes. *J Clin Invest* 1995;96:1395–1403.

31 Lander H, Tauras J, Ogiste J, et al. Activation of the receptor for advanced glycation end products triggers a p21ras-dependent mitogen-activated protein kinase pathway regulated by oxidant stress. *J Biol Chem* 1997;272: 17810–17814.

32 Bierhaus A, Chevion S, Chevion M, et al. Advanced glycation end product-induced activation of NF-κB is suppressed by α-lipoic acid in cultured endothelial cells. *Diabetes* 1997;46:1481–1490.

33 Simm A, Munch G, Seif F, et al. Advanced glycation endproducts stimulate the MAP-kinase pathway in tubulus cell line LLC-PK$_1$. *FEBS Lett* 1997;410:481–484.

34 Huttunen HJ, Fages C, Rauvala H. Receptor for advanced glycation endproducts (RAGE)-mediated neurite outgrowth and activation of NF-κB require the cytoplasmic domain of the receptor but different downstream signaling pathways. *J Biol Chem* 1999;274:19919–19924.

35 Treins C, Giorgetti-Peraldi S, Murdaca J, et al. Regulation of vascular endothelial growth factor expression by advanced glycation end products. *J Biol Chem* 2001; 276:43836–43841.

36 Guh JY, Huang JS, Chen HC, et al. Advanced glycation end product-induced proliferation in NRK-49F cells is dependent on the JAK2/STAT5 pathway and cyclin D1. *Am J Kidney Dis* 2001;38:1096–1104.

37 Nakashima Y, Plump A, Raines E, et al. ApoE-deficient mice develop lesions of all phases of atherosclerosis throughout the arterial tree. *Arterioscler Thromb* 1994;141:133–140.

38 Park L, Raman KG, Lee KJ, et al. Suppression of accelerated diabetic atherosclerosis by the soluble receptor for advanced glycation endproducts. *Nat Med* 1998;4: 1025–1031.

39 Bucciarelli LG, Wendt T, Qu W, et al. RAGE blockade stabilizes established atherosclerosis in diabetic apolipoprotein E-null mice. *Circulation* 2002;106:2827–2835.

40 Harding JJ. Nonenzymatic covalent posttranslational modification of proteins *in vivo*. *Adv Protein Chem* 1985;37:247–334.

41 Brownlee M, Cerami A, Vlassara H. Advanced glycosylation end-products in tissue and the biochemical basis of diabetic complications. *N Engl J Med* 1988;318:1315–1321.

42 Higgins PJ, Bunn HF. Kinetic analysis of the nonenzymatic glycosylation of hemoglobin. *J Biol Chem* 1981; 256:5204–5208.

43 Larsen ML, Hørder M, Mogensen EF. Effect of long-term monitoring of glycosylated hemoglobin levels in insulin-dependent diabetes mellitus. *N Engl J Med* 1990; 323:1021–1025.

44 Makita Z, Vlassara H, Rayfield E, et al. Hemoglobin-AGE: a circulating marker of advanced glycosylation. *Science* 1992;258:651–653.

45 Takeuchi M, Yanase Y, Matsuura N, et al. Immunological detection of a novel advanced glycation end-product. *Mol Med* 2001;7:783–791.

46 Thornalley PJ, Langborg A, Minhas HS. Formation of glyoxal, methylglyoxal and 3-deoxyglucosone in the glycation of proteins by glucose. *Biochem J* 1999;344:109–116.

47 Miyata T, Horie K, Ueda Y, et al. Advanced glycation and lipidoxidation of the peritoneal membrane: respective roles of serum and peritoneal fluid reactive carbonyl compounds. *Kidney Int* 2000;58:425–435.

48 Vlassara H, Bucala R, Striker L. Pathogenic effect of advanced glycosylation: biochemical, biologic, and clinical implications for diabetes and aging. *Lab Invest* 1994;2: 138–151.

49 Pongor S, Ulrich PC, Benesath FA, et al. Aging of proteins: isolation and identification of a fluorescent chromophore from the reaction of polypeptides with glucose. *Proc Natl Acad Sci USA* 1984;81:2684–2688.

50 Farmar J, Ulrich P, Cerami A. Novel pyrroles from sulfite-inhibited Maillard reactions, insight into the mechanism of inhibition. *J Org Chem* 1988;53:2346.

51 Ahmed MU, Thorpe SR, Baynes JW. Identification of $N^{ε}$-(carboxymethyl)-lysine as a degradation product of fructoselysine in glycated protein. *J Biol Chem* 1986;261: 4889–4894.

52 Hayase F, Nagaraj RH, Miyata S, et al. Aging of proteins: immunological detection of a glucose-derived pyrrole formed during Maillard reaction *in vivo*. *J Biol Chem* 1989;5:3758–3764.

53 Sell DR, Monnier VM. End-stage renal disease and diabetes catalyze the formation of a pentose-derived crosslink from aging human collagen. *J Clin Invest* 1990;85: 380–384.

54 Beisswenger P, Moore L, Brinck-Johnsen T, et al. Increased collagen-linked pentosidine levels and AGEs in early diabetic nephropathy. *J Clin Invest* 1993;92: 212–217.

55 Reddy S, Bichler J, Wells-Knecht K, et al. N epsilon-(carboxymethyl)lysine is a dominant advanced glycation end product (AGE) antigen in tissue proteins. *Biochemistry* 1995;34:10872–10878.

56 Ikeda K, Higashi T, Sano H, et al. Carboxymethyllysine protein adduct is a major immunological epitope in proteins modified with AGEs of the Maillard reaction. *Biochemistry* 1996;35:8075–8083.

57 Schleicher E, Wagner E, Nerlich A. Increased accumulation of glycoxidation product carboxymethyllysine in human tissues in diabetes and aging. *J Clin Invest* 1997; 99:457–468.

58 Sakata N, Imanaga Y, Meng J, et al. Immunohistochemical localization of different epitopes of advanced glycation end products in human atherosclerotic lesions. *Atherosclerosis* 1998;141:61–75.

59 Degenhardt TP, Thorpe SR, Baynes JW. Chemical modification of proteins by methylglyoxal. *Cell Mol Biol (Noisy-le-grand)* 1998;44:1139–1145.

60 Wells-Knecht KJ, Brinkmann E, Wells-Knecht MC, et al. New biomarkers of Maillard reaction damage to proteins. *Nephrol Dial Transplant* 1996;11:41–47.

61 Niwa T, Katsuzaki T, Miyazaki S, et al. Immunohistochemical detection of imidazolone, a novel advanced glycation end product, in kidneys and aortas of diabetic patients. *J Clin Invest* 1997;99:1272–1280.

62 Ahmed MU, Brinkmann Frye E, Degenhardt TP, et al. N-epsilon-(carboxyethyl)lysine, a product of the chemical modification of proteins by methylglyoxal, increases with age in human lens proteins. *Biochem J* 1997;324:565–570.

63 Odani H, Shinzato T, Usami J, et al. Imidazolium crosslinks derived from reaction of lysine with glyoxal and methylglyoxal are increased in serum proteins of uremic patients: evidence for increased oxidative stress in uremia. *FEBS Lett* 1998;427:381–385.

64 Anderson MM, Hazen SL, Hsu FF, et al. Human neutrophils employ the myeloperoxidase-hydrogen peroxide–chloride system to convert hydroxy-amino acids into glycolaldehyde, 2-hydroxypropanal, and acrolein. A mechanism for the generation of highly reactive alpha-hydroxy and alpha-beta unsaturated aldehydes by phagocytes at sites of inflammation. *J Clin Invest* 1997;99:424–432.

65 Basta G, Lazzerini G, Massaro M, et al. Advanced glycation end products activate endothelium through signal-transduction receptor RAGE: a mechanism for amplification of inflammatory responses. *Circulation* 2002;105:816–822.

66 Sell D, Monnier VM. Structure elucidation of senescence cross-link from human extracellular matrix: implication of pentoses in the aging process. *J Biol Chem* 1989;264:21597–21602.

67 Brownlee M. Advanced glycosylation in diabetes and aging. *Annu Rev Med* 1995;46:223–234.

68 Sugaya K, Fukagawa T, Matsumoto KI, et al. Three genes in the human MHC class III region near the junction with class II: gene for RAGE, PBX2 homeobox gene and a notch homolog, human counterpart of mouse mammary tumor gene int-2. *Genomics* 1994;23:408–419.

69 Ritthaler U, Roth H, Bierhaus A, et al. Expression of RAGE in peripheral occlusive vascular disease. *Am J Pathol* 1995;146:688–694.

70 Miyata T, Hori O, Zhang J, et al. RAGE mediates the interaction of AGE-beta-2-microglobulin with human mononuclear phagocytes via an oxidant-sensitive pathway: implications for the pathogenesis of dialysis-related amyloidosis. *J Clin Invest* 1996;98:1088–1094.

71 Yan SD, Chen X, Fu J, et al. RAGE and amyloid-β peptide neurotoxicity in Alzheimer's disease. *Nature* 1996;382:685–691.

72 Chappey O, Dosquet C, Wautier MP, et al. Advanced glycation end products, oxidant stress and vascular lesions. *Eur J Clin Invest* 1997;27:97–108.

73 Kent MJC, Light ND, Bailey AJ. Evidence for glucose-mediated covalent cross-linking of collagen after glycosylation *in vitro*. *Biochem J* 1985;225:745–752.

74 Brownlee M, Vlassara H, Kooney T, et al. Aminoguanidine prevents diabetes-induced arterial wall protein cross-linking. *Science* 1986;232:1629–1632.

75 Bailey AJ, Paul RG, Knott L. Mechanisms of maturation and ageing of collagen. *Mech Ageing Dev* 1998;106:1–56.

76 Tanaka S, Avigad G, Brodsky B, et al. Glycation induces expansion of the molecular packing of collagen. *J Mol Biol* 1988;203:495–505.

77 Brownlee M, Pongor S, Cerami A. Covalent attachment of soluble proteins by nonenzymatically glycosylated collagen: role in the *in situ* formation of immune complexes. *J Exp Med* 1983;158:1739–1744.

78 Meng J, Sakata N, Takebayashi S, et al. Glycoxidation in aortic collagen from STZ-induced diabetic rats and its relevance to vascular damage. *Atherosclerosis* 1998;136:355–365.

79 Schnider SL, Kohn RR. Effects of age and diabetes mellitus on the solubility and nonenzymatic glucosylation of human skin collagen. *J Clin Invest* 1981;67:1630–1635.

80 Tsilbary EC, Charonis AS, Reger LA, et al. The effect of nonenzymatic glycosylation on the binding of the main noncollagenous NC1 domain to type IV collagen. *J Biol Chem* 1990;263:4302–4308.

81 Charonis AS, Reger LA, Dege JE, et al. Laminin alterations after *in vitro* nonenzymatic glycosylation. *Diabetes* 1988;39:807–814.

82 Cochrane SM, Robinson GB. *In vitro* glycation of a glomerular basement membrane alters its permeability: a possible mechanism in diabetic complications. *FEBS Lett* 1995;375:41–44.

83 Huijberts MSP, Wolffenbuttel BRH, Struijker Boudier HAJ. Aminoguanidine treatment increases elasticity and decreases fluid filtration of large arteries from diabetic rats. *J Clin Invest* 1993;92:1407–1411.

84 Giardino I, Edelstein D, Brownlee M. Nonenzymatic glycosylation *in vitro* and in bovine endothelial cells alters basic fibroblast growth factor activity. *J Clin. Invest* 1994;94:110–117.

85 Bucala R, Makita Z, Koschinsky T, et al. Lipid advanced glycosylation: pathway for lipid oxidation *in vivo*. *Proc Natl Acad Sci USA* 1993;90:6434–6438.

86 Bucala R, Mitchell R, Arnold K, et al. Identification of the major site of apolipoprotein B modification by advanced glycosylation end products blocking uptake by the low density lipoprotein receptor. *J Biol Chem* 1995;270:828–832.

87 Bucala R, Makita Z, Vega G, et al. Modification of low density lipoprotein by advanced glycation end products contributes to the dyslipidemia of diabetes and renal insufficiency. *Proc Natl Acad Sci USA* 1994;91:9441–9445.

88 Loidl-Stahlhofen A, Hannemann K, Spiteller G. Generation of alpha-hydroxyaldehydic compounds in the course of lipid peroxidation. *Biochim Biophys Acta* 1994;1213: 140–148.

89 Glomb MA, Monnier V. Mechanism of protein modifications by glyoxal and glyceraldehyde, reactive intermediates of the Maillard reaction. *J Biol Chem* 1995;270: 10017–10026.

90 Fu MX, Requena JR, Jenkins AJ, et al. The advanced glycation end product, N epsilon-(carboxymethyl)lysine, is a product of both lipid peroxidation and glycoxidation reactions. *J Biol Chem* 1996;271:9982–9986.

91 Steinbrecher UP, Witztum JL. Glucosylation of low-density lipoproteins to an extent comparable to that seen in diabetes slows their catabolism. *Diabetes* 1984; 33:130–134.

92 Klein RL, Laimins M, Lopes-Virella MF. Isolation, characterization, and metabolism of the glycated and nonglycated subfractions of low-density lipoproteins isolated from type I diabetic patients and nondiabetic subjects. *Diabetes* 1995;44:1093–1098.

93 Sobenin IA, Tertov VV, Koschinsky T, et al. Modified low density lipoprotein from diabetic patients causes cholesterol accumulation in human intimal aortic cells. *Atherosclerosis* 1993;100:41–54.

94 Davis JW, Hartman CR, Davis RF, et al. Platelet aggregate ratio in diabetes mellitus. *Acta Haemat* 1982;67: 222–224.

95 Davì G, Rini GB, Averna M. Enhanced platelet release reaction in insulin-dependent and insulin-independent diabetic patients. *Haemostasis* 1982;12:275–281.

96 Sampietro T, Lenzi S, Cecchetti P. Nonenzymatic glycation of human platelet membrane proteins *in vitro* and *in vivo*. *Clin Chem* 1986;32:1328–1331.

97 Yatscoff RW, Mehta A, Gerrard JM. Glycation of platelet protein in diabetes mellitus: lack of correlation with platelet function. *Clin Biochem* 1987;20:359–363.

98 Winocour PD, Watala C, Kinlough-Rathbone Rl. Reduced membrane fluidity and increased glycation of membrane proteins of platelets from diabetic subjects are not associated with increased platelet adherence to glycated collagen. *J Lab Clin Med* 1992;120:921–928.

99 Colwell JA. Vascular thrombosis in Type II diabetes mellitus. *Diabetes* 1993;42:8–11.

100 Jones RL. Fibrinopeptide A in diabetes mellitus: relation to levels of blood glucose, fibrinogen disappearance, and hemodynamic changes. *Diabetes* 1985;34:836–841.

101 Ceriello A, Giugliano D, Quatraro A, et al. Hyperglycemia may determine fibrinopeptide A plasma level increase in humans. *Metabolism* 1989;38:1162–1163.

102 Villanueva GB, Allen N. Demonstration of altered antithrombin III activity due to non enzymatic glycosylation at glucose concentration expected to be encountered in severely diabetic patients. *Diabetes* 1988;37:1103–1107.

103 Gray E, Barrowcliffe TW. Inhibition of antithrombin III by lipid peroxides. *Thromb Res* 1985;37:241–250.

104 Vukovich TC, Schernthaner G. Decreased protein C levels in patients with insulin-dependent type I diabetes mellitus. *Diabetes* 1986;35:617–619.

105 Vlassara H, Brownlee M, Cerami A. High-affinity receptor-mediated uptake and degradation of glucose-modified proteins a potential mechanism for the removal of senescent macromolecules. *Proc Natl Acad Sci USA* 1985;82:5588–5592.

106 Vlassara H, Brownlee M, Cerami A. Novel macrophage receptor for glucose-modified proteins is distinct from previously described scavenger receptors. *J Exp Med* 1986;164:1301–1309.

107 Yang Z, Makita J, Mori Y, et al. Two novel rat liver membrane proteins that bind advanced glycosylation endproducts: relationship to macrophage receptor for glucose-modified proteins. *J Exp Med* 1991;174:515–524.

108 Schmidt AM, Mora R, Cao R, et al. The endothelial cell binding site for advanced glycation endproducts consists of a complex: an integral membrane protein and a lactoferrin-like polypeptide. *J Biol Chem* 1994;269: 9882–9888.

109 Vlassara H, Li Y, Imani F, et al. Galectin-2 as a high affinity binding protein for advanced glycation end products (AGE): a new member of the AGE-receptor complex. *Mol Med* 1995;1:634–646.

110 Kislinger T, Fu C, Huber B, et al. N^{ε} (carboxymethyl) lysine adducts of proteins are ligands for receptor for advanced glycation end products that activate cell signaling pathways and modulate gene expression. *J Biol Chem* 1999;274:31740–31749.

111 Mackic JB, Stins M, McComb JG, et al. Human blood–brain barrier receptors for Alzheimer's amyloid-beta 1–40. Asymmetrical binding, endocytosis, and transcytosis at the apical side of brain microvascular endothelial cell monolayer. *J Clin Invest* 1998;102:734–743.

112 Yan SD, Roher A, Schmidt AM, et al. Cellular cofactors for amyloid beta-peptide-induced cell stress. Moving from cell culture to *in vivo*. *Am J Pathol* 1999;155: 1403–1411.

113 Schmidt AM, Vianna M, Gerlach M, et al. Isolation and characterization of binding proteins for advanced glycosylation endproducts from lung tissue which are present on the endothelial cell surface. *J Biol Chem* 1992;267:14987–14997.

114 Neeper M, Schmidt AM, Brett J, et al. Cloning and expression of a cell surface receptor for advanced glycosylation endproducts of proteins. *J Biol Chem* 1992; 267:14998–15004.

115 Brett J, Schmidt AM, Yan SD, et al. Survey of the distribution of a newly characterized receptor for advanced glycation end products in tissues. *Am J Pathol* 1993; 143:1699–1712.

116 Schmidt AM, Yan SD, Yan SF, et al. The multiligand receptor RAGE as a progression factor amplifying immune and inflammatory responses. *J Clin Invest* 2001;108:949–955.

117 Rong LL, Yan SF, Hans-Wagner D, et al. RAGE-dependent mechanisms accelerate neuronal dysfunction in a murine model of amyotrophic lateral sclerosis. *Society for Neuroscience 32nd Annual Meeting* 2002; 719.2:53.

118 Hofmann MA, Drury S, Fu C, et al. RAGE mediates a novel proinflammatory axis: a central cell surface receptor for S100/calgranulin polypeptides. *Cell* 1999; 97:889–901.

119 Schmidt AM, Hofmann M, Taguchi A, et al. RAGE: a multiligand receptor contributing to the cellular response in diabetic vasculopathy and inflammation. *Semin Thromb Hemost* 2000;26:485–493.

120 Kislinger T, Tanji N, Wendt T, et al. Receptor for advanced glycation end products mediates inflammation and enhanced expression of tissue factor in vasculature of diabetic apolipoprotein E-null mice. *Arterioscler Thromb Vasc Biol* 2001;21:905–910.

121 Wendt T, Bucciarelli L, Qu W, et al. Receptor for advanced glycation endproducts (RAGE) and vascular inflammation: insights into the pathogenesis of macrovascular complications in diabetes. *Curr Atheroscler Rep* 2002;4:228–237.

122 Yan SD, Zhu H, Zhu A, et al. Receptor-dependent cell stress and amyloid accumulation in systemic amyloidosis. *Nat Med* 2000;6:643–651.

123 Schmidt AM, Hori O, Brett J, et al. Cellular receptors for advanced glycation end products: implications for induction of oxidant stress and cellular dysfunction in the pathogenesis of vascular lesions. *Arterioscler Thromb* 1994;14:1521–1528.

124 Yan SD, Schmidt AM, Anderson GM, et al. Enhanced cellular oxidant stress by the interaction of advanced glycation end products with their receptors/binding proteins. *J Biol Chem* 1994;269:9889–9897.

125 Scivittaro V, Ganz MB, Weiss MF. AGEs induce oxidative stress and activate protein kinase C-β_{II} in neonatal mesangial cells. *Am J Physiol Renal Physiol* 2000;278: F676–F683.

126 Wautier MP, Chappey O, Corda S, et al. Activation of NADPH oxidase by AGE links oxidant stress to altered gene expression via RAGE. *Am J Physiol Endocrinol Metab* 2001;280:E685–E694.

127 Basta G, Lazzerini G, Del Turco S, et al. At least 2 distinct pathways generating reactive oxygen species mediate vascular cell adhesion molecule-1 induction by advanced glycation end products. *Arterioscler Thromb Vasc Biol* 2005;25:1401–1407.

128 Siebenlist U, Franzoso G, Brown K. Structure, regulation and function of NF-kappa B. *Annu Rev Cell Biol* 1994;10:405–455.

129 Vlassara H. Receptor-mediated interactions of advanced glycosylation end products with cellular components within diabetic tissues. *Diabetes* 1992;41:52–56.

130 Vlassara H, Brownlee M, Manogue KR, et al. Cachectin/ TNF and IL-1 induced by glucose-modified proteins: role in normal tissue remodeling. *Science* 1988;240: 1546–1548.

131 Kirstein M, Brett J, Radoff S, et al. Advanced protein glycosylation induces transendothelial human monocyte chemotaxis and secretion of platelet-derived growth factor: role in vascular disease of diabetes and aging. *Proc Natl Acad Sci USA* 1990;87:9010–9014.

132 Kirstein M, Aston C, Hintz R, et al. Receptor-specific induction of insulin-like growth factor I (IGF-1) in human monocytes by advanced glycosylation end product-modified proteins. *J Clin Invest* 1992;90: 439–446.

133 Schmidt AM, Yan SD, Brett J, et al. Regulation of human mononuclear phagocyte migration by cell surface-binding proteins for advanced glycation end products. *J Clin Invest* 1993;91:2155–2168.

134 Miyata T, Inagi R, Iida Y, et al. Involvement of beta 2-microglobulin modified with advanced glycation end products in the pathogenesis of hemodialysis-associated amyloidosis. Induction of human monocyte chemotaxis and macrophage secretion of tumor necrosis factor-alpha and interleukin-1. *J Clin Invest* 1994; 93:521–528.

135 Imani F, Horii Y, Suthanthiran M, et al. Advanced glycosylation endproduct-specific receptors on human and rat T-lymphocytes mediate synthesis of interferon gamma: role in tissue remodeling. *J Exp Med* 1993;178: 2165–2172.

136 De Caterina R, Bourcier T, Laufs U, et al. Induction of endothelial–leukocyte interaction by interferon-γ requires coactivation of nuclear factor -κB. *Arterioscler Thromb Vasc Biol* 2001;21:227–232.

137 Libby P, Hansson GK. Involvement of the immune system in human atherogenesis: current knowledge and unanswered questions. *Lab Invest* 1991;64:5–15.

138 Stemme S, Rymo L, Hansson GK. Polyclonal origin of T lymphocytes in human atherosclerotic plaques. *Lab Invest* 1991;65:654–660.

139 Sakata N, Meng J, Takebayashi S. Effects of advanced glycation end products on the proliferation and fibronectin production of smooth muscle cells. *J Atheroscler Thromb* 2000;7:169–176.

140 Esposito C, Gerlach H, Brett J, et al. Endothelial receptor-mediated binding of glucose-modified albumin is

associated with increased monolayer permeability and modulation of cell surface coagulant properties. *J Exp Med* 1989;170:1387–1407.

141 Wautier JL, Zoukourian C, Chappey O, et al. Receptor-mediated endothelial cell dysfunction in diabetic vasculopathy: soluble receptor for advanced glycation end products blocks hyperpermeability in diabetic rats. *J Clin Invest* 1996;97:238–243.

142 Vlassara H, Fuh H, Makita Z, et al. Exogenous advanced glycosylation endproducts induce complex vascular dysfunction in normal animals: a model for diabetic and aging complications. *Proc Natl Acad Sci USA* 1992;89:12043–12047.

143 Bierhaus A, Illmer T, Kasper M, et al. Advanced glycation end product (AGE)-mediated induction of tissue factor in cultured endothelial cells is dependent on RAGE. *Circulation* 1997;96:2262–2271.

144 Emeis JJ, Kooistra T. Interleukin 1 and lipopolysaccharide induce an inhibitor of tissue-type plasminogen activator *in vivo* and in cultured endothelial cells. *J Exp Med* 1986;163:1260–1266.

145 Van Hindsberg VWM, Kooistra T, Van Den Berg EA, et al. Tumour necrosis factor increases the production of plasminogen activator *in vivo* and in cultured endothelial cells. *Blood* 1988;72:1467–1473.

146 Cybulsky MI, Gimbrone Jr MA. Endothelial expression of a mononuclear leukocyte adhesion molecule during atherogenesis. *Science* 1991;251:788–791.

147 Li H, Cybulsky MI, Gimbrone Jr MA, et al. Inducible expression of vascular cell adhesion molecule-1 by vascular smooth muscle cells *in vitro* and within rabbit atheroma. *Am J Pathol* 1993;143:1551–1559.

148 Valencia JV, Mone M, Koehne C, et al. Binding of receptor for advanced glycation end products (RAGE) ligands is not sufficient to induce inflammatory signals: lack of activity of endotoxin-free albumin-derived advanced glycation end products. *Diabetologia* 2004;47:844–852.

149 Bucala R, Tracey J, Cerami A. Advanced glycosylation products quench nitric oxide and mediate defective endothelium-dependent vasodilatation in experimental diabetes. *J Clin Invest* 1991;87:432–438.

150 De Caterina R, Libby P, Peng HB, et al. Nitric oxide decreases cytokine-induced endothelial activation. Nitric oxide selectively reduces endothelial expression of adhesion molecules and proinflammatory cytokines. *J Clin Invest* 1995;96:60–68.

151 Oyama Y, Kawasaki H, Hattori Y, et al. Attenuation of endothelium-dependent relaxation in aorta from diabetic rats. *Eur J Pharmacol* 1986;131:75–78.

152 Brink C, Duncan PG, Douglas JS. Decreased vascular sensitivity to histamine during aging. *Agents Actions* 1984;14:8–10.

153 Ludmer PL, Selwyn A, Shook TL, et al. Paradoxical vasoconstriction produced by acetylcholine in atherosclerotic coronary arteries. *N Engl J Med* 1986;315: 1046–1051.

154 Panza JA, Quyumi AA, Brush JE, et al. Abnormal endothelium-dependent vascular relaxation in patient with essential hypertension. *N Engl J Med* 1990;323:22–27.

155 Quehenberger P, Bierhaus A, Fasching P, et al. Endothelin 1 transcription is controlled by nuclear factor-kappaB in AGE-stimulated cultured endothelial cells. *Diabetes* 2000;49:1561–1570.

156 Vlassara H, Striker LJ, Teichberg S, et al. Advanced glycation endproducts induce glomerular sclerosis and albuminuria in normal rats. *Proc Natl Acad Sci USA* 1994;91:11704–11708.

157 Jensen T, Borch-Johnsen K, Kofoed-Enevoldsen A, et al. Coronary heart disease in young type 1 (insulin-dependent) diabetic patients with and without diabetic nephropathy: incidence and risk factors. *Diabetologia* 1987;30:144–148.

158 Mattock MB, Morrish NJ, Viberti G, et al. Prospective study of microalbuminuria as predictor of mortality in NIDDM. *Diabetes* 1992;41:736–741.

159 Park SH, Marso SP, Zhou Z, et al. Neointimal hyperplasia after arterial injury is increased in a rat model of non-insulin-dependent diabetes mellitus. *Circulation* 2001;104:815–819.

160 Zhou Z, Wang K, Penn MS, et al. Receptor for AGE (RAGE) mediates neointimal formation in response to arterial injury. *Circulation* 2003;107:2238–2243.

161 Sakaguchi T, Yan SF, Yan SD, et al. Central role of RAGE-dependent neointimal expansion in arterial restenosis. *J Clin Invest* 2003;111:959–972.

162 Chavakis T, Bierhaus A, Al-Fakhri N, et al. The pattern recognition receptor (RAGE) is a counterreceptor for leukocyte integrins: a novel pathway for inflammatory cell recruitment. *J Exp Med* 2003;198:1507–1515.

163 Kilhovd BK, Berg TJ, Birkeland KI, et al. Serum levels of advanced glycation end products are increased in patients with type 2 diabetes and coronary heart disease. *Diabetes Care* 1999;22:1543–1548.

164 Aso Y, Inukai T, Tayama K, et al. Serum concentrations of advanced glycation endproducts are associated with the development of atherosclerosis as well as diabetic microangiopathy in patients with type 2 diabetes. *Acta Diabetol* 2000;37:87–92.

165 Kanauchi M, Tsujimoto N, Hashimoto T. Advanced glycation end products in nondiabetic patients with coronary artery disease. *Diabetes Care* 2001;24:1620–1623.

166 Kitauchi T, Yoshida K, Yoneda T, et al. Association between pentosidine and arteriosclerosis in patients receiving hemodialysis. *Clin Exp Nephrol* 2004;8:48–53.

167 Kosaki A, Hasegawa T, Kimura T, et al. Increased plasma S100A12 (EN-RAGE) levels in patients with type 2 diabetes. *J Clin Endocrinol Metab* 2004;89: 5423–5428.

168 Ahmed N, Babaei-Jadidi R, Howell SK, et al. Glycated and oxidized protein degradation products are indicators of fasting and postprandial hyperglycemia in diabetes. *Diabetes Care* 2005;28:2465–2471.

169 Shimada S, Tanaka Y, Ohmura C, et al. *N*-(carboxymethyl)valine residues in hemoglobin (CMV-Hb) reflect accumulation of oxidative stress in diabetic patients. *Diabetes Res Clin Pract* 2005;69:272–278.

170 Kilhovd BK, Giardino I, Torjesen PA, et al. Increased serum levels of the specific AGE-compound methylglyoxal-derived hydroimidazolone in patients with type 2 diabetes. *Metabolism* 2003;52:163–167.

171 Nakamura Y, Horii Y, Nishino T, et al. Immunohistochemical localisation of advanced glycosylation end products in coronary atheroma and cardiac tissue in diabetes mellitus. *Am J Pathol* 1993;143:1649–1656.

172 Vlassara H, Li YM, Imani F, et al. Identification of galectin-3 as a high affinity binding protein for advanced glycation end products (AGEs): a new member of the AGE-receptor complex. *Mol Med* 1996;1:634–646.

173 Monnier VM, Vishwanath V, Frank KE, et al. Relation between complications of type 1 diabetes mellitus and collagen-linked fluorescence. *N Engl J Med* 1986;314:403–408.

174 Sims TJ, Rasmussen LM, Oxlund H, et al. The role of glycation cross-links in diabetic vascular stiffening. *Diabetologia* 1996;39:946–951.

175 Cipollone F, Fazia M, Iezzi A, et al. Suppression of the functionally coupled cyclooxygenase-2/prostaglandin E synthase as a basis of simvastatin-dependent plaque stabilization in humans. *Circulation* 2003;107: 1479–1485.

176 Pettersson-Fernholm K, Forsblom C, Hudson BI, et al. The functional −374 T/A RAGE gene polymorphism is associated with proteinuria and cardiovascular disease in type 1 diabetic patients. *Diabetes* 2003;52:891–894.

177 Falcone C, Campo I, Emanuele E, et al. Relationship between the −374T/A RAGE gene polymorphism and angiographic coronary artery disease. *Int J Mol Med* 2004;14:1061–1064.

178 Falcone C, Campo I, Emanuele E, et al. −374T/A polymorphism of the RAGE gene promoter in relation to severity of coronary atherosclerosis. *Clin Chim Acta* 2005;354:111–116.

179 Kirbis J, Milutinovic A, Steblovnik K, et al. The −429 T/C and − 374 T/A gene polymorphisms of the receptor of advanced glycation end products gene (RAGE) are not risk factors for coronary artery disease in Slovene population with type 2 diabetes. *Collegium Antropol* 2004;28:611–616.

180 Edelstein D, Brownlee M. Mechanistic studies of advanced glycosylation end product inhibition by aminoguanidine. *Diabetes* 1992;41:26–28.

181 Freedman BI, Wuerth JP, Cartwright K, et al. Design and baseline characteristics for the aminoguanidine Clinical Trial in Overt Type 2 Diabetic Nephropathy (ACTION II). *Control Clin Trials* 1999;5:493–510.

182 Vasan S, Zhang X, Zhang X, et al. An agent cleaving glucose-derived protein crosslinks *in vitro* and *in vivo*. *Nature* 1996;382:275–278.

183 Cooper ME, Thallas V, Forbes J, et al. The cross-link breaker, *N*-phenacylthiazolium bromide prevents vascular advanced glycation end-product accumulation. *Diabetologia* 2000;43:660–664.

184 Vasan S, Foiles PG, Founds HW. Therapeutic potential of AGE inhibitors and breakers of AGE protein cross-links. *Expert Opin Investig Drug* 2001;10:1977–1987.

185 Bierhaus A, Schiekofer S, Schwaninger M, et al. Diabetes-associated sustained activation of the transcription factor nuclear factor-kappaB. *Diabetes* 2001;50: 2792–2808.

186 Miyata T, Hori O, Zhang J, et al. The receptor for advanced glycation end products (RAGE) is a central mediator of the interaction of AGE-beta2microglobulin with human mononuclear phagocytes via an oxidant-sensitive pathway. Implications for the pathogenesis of dialysis-related amyloidosis. *J Clin Invest* 1996;98: 1088–1094.

187 Hofmann MA, Drury S, Hudson BI, et al. RAGE and arthritis: the G82S polymorphism amplifies the inflammatory response. *Genes Immun* 2002;3:123–135.

188 Falcone C, Emanuele E, D'Angelo A, et al. Plasma levels of soluble receptor for advanced glycation end products and coronary artery disease in nondiabetic men. *Arterioscler Thromb Vasc Biol* 2005;25:1032–1037.

189 Katakami N, Matsuhisa M, Kaneto H, et al. Decreased endogenous secretory advanced glycation end product receptor in type 1 diabetic patients: its possible association with diabetic vascular complications. *Diabetes Care* 2005;28:2716–2721.

CHAPTER 8

Homocysteine and endothelial dysfunction

Rosalinda Madonna, MD, PhD *& Raffaele De Caterina,* MD, PhD

Introduction

McCully first reported in 1969 that severe hyperhomocysteinemia relates to atherothrombotic vascular disease [1]. Since then, several case–control and prospective studies have found that homocysteine concentration-dependently relates to cardiovascular risk, suggesting a potential causal relationship between plasma homocysteine levels and vascular disease. A recent meta-analysis demonstrated an odds ratio of 1.6–1.8 for vascular disease for a 5 μmol/L increment of homocysteine plasma levels [2]. Many epidemiological studies now show convincingly that severe hyperhomocysteinemia relates to vascular disease, and argue strongly for a causal relationship of severe hyperhomocysteinemia [3,4]. However, the relationship linking the much more common forms of mild hyperhomocysteinemia with vascular disease remains incompletely accepted, and the causality of mild hyperhomocysteinemia for vascular disease is much more questionable. While prospective [5] and cross-sectional studies, [6] as well as more than 20 case–control studies (reviewed in a meta-analysis of 27 studies [2]), have reported an association between mild hyperhomocysteinemia and vascular disease, prospective studies including the North Karelia Project, [7] the Multiple Risk Factor Intervention Trial (MRFIT), [8] the Atherosclerosis Risk in Communities (ARIC) Study, [9] and the Caerphilly Study [10] have not confirmed this association. Table 8.1 summarizes the most significant studies regarding the relationship between plasma homocysteine concentrations and cardiovascular

Table 8.1 Relationship between hyperhomocysteinemia and cardiovascular disease.

Study	Framingham Heart Study	Norway Study	MRFIT	Caerphilly Study	North Karelia Project	ARIC
Design	Cross-sectional	Prospective cohort	Nested case–control	Prospective cohort	Nested case–control	Case–cohort
Endpoint	All-cause and CVD mortality	All-cause and CVD mortality	Nonfatal and fatal MI	Nonfatal and fatal CHD	Nonfatal and fatal MI Stroke	Total mortality Nonfatal and fatal CHD
tHcy range	3.5–66.9	<9–>20	3.7–80.4	7.3–24.5	9.83–10.4	5.3–14.2
OR range	1.0–2.0	1.0–4.5	0.82–1.0	1.0–1.4	1.0–1.10	1.7–3.48
CV risk	Graded increase	Graded increase	No association	No association	No association	Positive graded association in women No association in men
Reference	[6]	[5]	[8]	[10]	[7]	[9]

CVD: cardiovascular disease; MI: myocardial infarction; CHD: coronary heart disease; tHcy: total plasma homocysteine (μmol/L); OR: odds ratio risk. Further doubts arose when another meta-analysis suggested that homozygous carriers of the common 677C→T mutation in the gene encoding a key enzyme (methylene tetrahydrofolate reductase, MTHFR) in homocysteine metabolism appeared to carry no increased risk of vascular disease, despite inducing elevated homocysteine levels [11].

Against this epidemiological background, the present chapter will review the putative mechanisms for homocysteine-mediated vascular injury, with special focus on endothelial dysfunction. For a better understanding of the pathophysiology of homocysteine metabolism, we include a brief review of the biochemistry and physiology of homocysteine and other aminothiols, and then address the question of "desirable" homocysteine plasma levels.

Terminology, biochemistry, distribution, and metabolism of homocysteine

Homocysteine, a thiol(sulfhydryl)-containing amino acid normally present in human plasma and tissues, contributes to the maintenance of intra- and extra-cellular redox homeostasis. Commonly found at relatively low concentrations within cells ($\leqslant 1\,\mu$mol/L) and in the circulation (5–15 μmol/L), homocysteine plays a pivotal intermediary role in the methionine cycle that generates one-carbon methyl groups for transmethylation reactions essential to biological process. Other aminothiols, such as glutathione and cysteine, are more abundant, usually in the 1–10 mmol/L range and 200–300 μmol/L range, respectively [12]. Methionine contains a sulfide sulfur with a general structure designated as R—S—R′, while homocysteine and cysteine are sulfhydryl compounds (R—SH) (Figure 8.1). In the presence of an

electron acceptor such as molecular oxygen, thiols can form oxidized chemical compounds such as disulfides (—S—S—). According to the general reaction

$$2\,RSH + O_2 \rightarrow RSSR + H_2O_2,$$

homocysteine and cysteine undergo auto-oxidation in the presence of molecular oxygen at physiological pH, thus forming homocysteine and cystine, respectively. Oxidation of homocysteine can occur together with that of other thiols, such as cysteine and glutathione, to form mixed disulfides or homocysteine–cysteine mixed disulfides. Transition metals such as copper and cobalt catalyze all oxidizing reactions, and products include mono- or disulfides, as well as hydrogen peroxide and other reactive oxygen species (ROS) [13].

Total plasma homocysteine, termed homocyst(e)ine or total homocysteine (tHcy), includes 85% homocysteine bound to albumin, and the remaining 15%, which is free (not protein bound). The binding of homocysteine to albumin occurs at the level of the free cysteine residue in the N-terminal end of albumin, at position 34 [14]. Thus, albumin appears to be a carrier of homocysteine in the circulation. About 98% of tHcy exists in the oxidized form, as disulfides, while only 2% occurs as the free non-oxidized thiol (Table 8.2) [15]. Because homocysteine lacks a genetic codification, methionine metabolism and dietary uptake through animal proteins determine its plasma and tissue concentrations. The major pathways available for metabolizing homocysteine include remethylation to methionine and transsulfuration to cysteine, and the most important metabolic factors for maintaining homocysteine homeostasis include B-complex vitamins such as folic acid, vitamin B_{12} (cobalamin), and

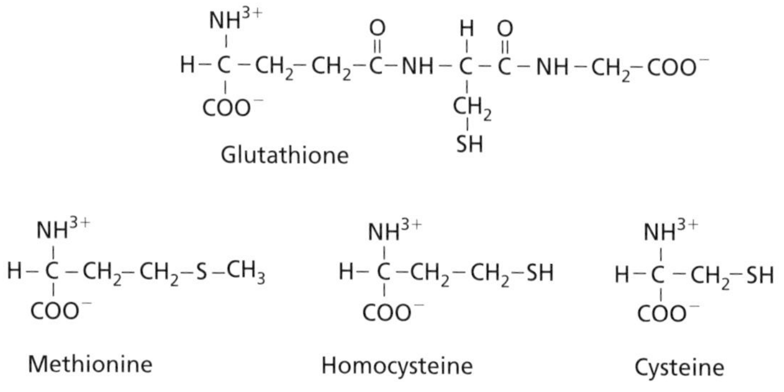

Figure 8.1 Structural formulas of homocysteine and other aminothiols present in normal human plasma and tissues.

vitamin B_6 (pyridoxal phosphate) [16]. The first step of methionine/homocysteine metabolism involves the conversion of dietary methionine to *S*-adenosyl-methionine (SAM, AdoMet), a reaction catalyzed by the vitamin B-independent enzyme methionine-adenosyltransferase. Subsequently, methyl transfer reactions synthesize *S*-adenosylhomocysteine (SAH, AdoHcy), and hydrolysis of SAH leads to homocysteine. Remethylation to methionine, a reaction that requires MTHFR, or transsulfuration to cysteine, which requires cystathionine-β-synthase (CBS), provide two ways of homocysteine disposal, both possibly depending on methionine stores, cofactor availability, and metabolite concentration [17] (Figure 8.2). Homocysteine metabolism undergoes regulation by two mechanisms, i.e., kinetic properties of the key enzymes and variations in the tissue content of these enzymes, ensuring the appropriate distribution of metabolites among the metabolic pathways and preventing the accumulation of homocysteine, SAH and other potentially toxic intermediates. The tissue content of key enzymes such as CBS increases with age, while the activity of methionine synthase and MTHFR declines significantly, thus determining a shift of the metabolic pattern from

methionine conservation to transsulfuration. CBS protein and activity increase with increasing dietary protein intake; in these conditions, methionine synthase decreases markedly, while MTHFR remains the same. Endocrine manipulations of various enzyme activities have been carried out in animal studies: treatments with thyroxine, testosterone, and glucagon all resulted in a reduction of CBS activity [18].

Factors that define the kinetic properties of the enzymes include affinity for substrates, product inhibition, and the allosteric effects of various metabolites. Using these characteristics, we can define two classes of enzymes [19]: "methionine conserving" enzymes such as methionine synthase, which are inhibited by their products and whose sulfur-containing substrates have a relatively low Michaelis constant (K_M); and "methionine catabolyzing" enzymes such as CBS, which conversely have high K_M values and are not inhibited by their products. Additionally, a third mechanism may regulate the distribution of homocysteine between transsulfuration and remethylation. Here, the driving force would involve the differential effects of redox changes in the intracellular environment on methionine synthase and CBS. For example, methionine synthase is vulnerable to oxidation: therefore increased transsulfuration, with a greater production of glutathione, is a metabolic response to oxidative stress [19,20].

Table 8.2 Percent distribution of homocysteine and other aminothiols in normal human plasma.

Aminothiol	Free reduced	Free oxidized	Protein-bound
Homocysteine	2.5	16.7	80.8
Cysteine	3.5	32.3	64.2
Cystienylglycine	10.7	28.6	60.7
Glutathione	75	16.7	8.3

Data from Mansoor et al. [15]

Normal and pathological levels of homocysteine: classification and incidence of hyperhomocysteinemia

In healthy subjects, plasma concentrations of total (reduced and oxidized) homocysteine likely depend

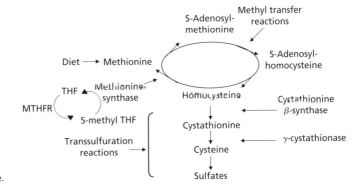

Figure 8.2 Homocysteine metabolism with landmarks to pathways for remethylation and transsulfuration. MTHFR: 5,10-methylene tetrahydrofolate reductase; THF: tetrahydrofolate.

on age and gender, and the range of normal concentrations includes 3–6 μmol/L in newborns and young children; 5–8 μmol/L in adolescents; 5–13 μmol/L in young and middle-age adults; and >10 μmol/L in elderly individuals [21–25]. Concentrations are slightly higher in males than females [21–25]. Pathologically, values of 16–30 and 31–100 μmol/L are classified as moderate and intermediate hyperhomocysteinemia, respectively, whereas fasting plasma homocysteine levels of >100 μmol/L, typically occurring in patients with classic homocystinuria, are classified as severe hyperhomocysteinemia [26,27].

Liver and kidney function, folate and cobalamin status, and to a lesser extent, the redox state of the cell strongly influence plasma homocysteine. Because these factors interrelate differently with drugs and diseases affecting homocysteine metabolism, hyperhomocysteinemia often appears to be the final result of several simultaneous causes (Table 8.3). Elevated levels of homocysteine reflect deficiencies of the various vitamins with functional relevance in its metabolism (vitamin B_6, vitamin B_{12}, and folic acid). Renal function and inborn errors of metabolism contribute importantly to homocysteine homeostasis [28]. Inborn errors of metabolism leading to homocystinuria involve either the transsulfuration or remethylation pathway. Defects in the transsulfuration pathway result from deficiency of CBS, with an incidence of 1:200,000 [29]; defects in remethylation may also result from alterations in the transport or availability of cobalamin or folic acid [30]. In 1969, McCully reported the first case of remethylation disorder in an infant who died at 7 weeks of age. Severe hyperhomocysteinemia and homocystinuria were accompanied by the dislocation of the ocular lens, a marfanoid habitus and other skeletal abnormalities, some degree of mental retardation, and atherothrombotic disease [31]; these are the major hallmarks mostly of CBS deficiency. More rarely, severe MTHFR defects and cobalamin deficiency can cause severe hyperhomocysteinemia and homocystinuria. Several gene mutations can affect MTHFR function, usually accompanied by a residual specific activity of 0–20% and giving rise to symptoms including mental retardation, peripheral neuropathies, and atherothrombosis. While such mutations map to the catalytic domain of MTHFR, they can be divided into several categories on the basis of functional consequences, i.e., defects in the structural stability of the enzyme, defects in the function of catalytic or substrate-binding residues, or defects in the binding of flavin adenine dinucleotide (FAD) [32,33]. Common causes of moderate hyperhomocysteinemia, which occurs in the apparently healthy general population ($\approx$5–7%) and in patients with cardiovascular diseases (15–40%), include deficiencies of folic acid or vitamins B_{12}, and the homozygosity for several mutations in MTHFR, most commonly the substitution of alanine with valine, due to the C677T mutation in exon 4 of the MTHFR gene [33,34] (Table 8.3).

Table 8.3 Factors affecting plasma homocysteine.

Inherited diseases	Acquired diseases	Drugs	Others
CBS deficiency	Deficiency in B-complex vitamins	Phenytoin	Male sex
Methionine synthase deficiency	Vitamin B_6	Methotrexate	Increasing age
MTHRF deficiency	Vitamin B_{12}	Nitrous oxide	Physical inactivity
	Folate	Nicotinic acid	Smoking
	Renal failure	Thiazides	Postmenopausal status
	Proliferating diseases	Lipid-lowering drugs	Increased muscle mass
	Rheumatoid arthritis	Estrogens	Coffee intake
	Hypothyroidism	Insulin	Alcohol consumption
	Hyperthyroidism	Metformin	Down's syndrome
	Diabetes mellitus	Gastric proton pump inhibitors	Gastroplasty
		Vitamin B_6 antagonists	
		L-Dopa	
		Mercaptopurine	

Homocysteine, endothelial dysfunction, and atherosclerosis

Free reduced homocysteine and possibly homocysteine thiolactone (the existence of which *in vivo* has been disputed) are the forms of homocysteine most likely to be atherogenic. The atherogenicity of homocysteine, homocysteine–cysteine mixed disulfide, and protein-bound homocysteine mixed disulfide remains undetermined. A growing body of *in vitro* evidence suggests that homocysteine can mediate endothelial injury through a variety of mechanisms. However, it is not possible to determine with certainty whether similar mechanisms participate importantly in the pathophysiology of hyperhomocysteinemia *in vivo*. The most important *in vitro* results supported by *in vivo* evidence are reviewed below.

Cellular toxicity

Earlier *in vitro* studies suggested that homocysteine may concentration-dependently affect endothelial cell viability, as indicated by 51-chromium release from labeled human endothelial cells [35]. More recently, *in vitro* studies have shown that homocysteine and/or homocysteine thiolactone are cytotoxic for a wide range of cell types through copper-dependent generation of hydrogen peroxide as a product of auto-oxidation [36–38]. Dudman et al. showed that homocysteine and cysteine promote cell detachment in human umbilical artery endothelial cells in culture [39]; because this effect also occurs with cysteine, the significance of such data must be questioned. Furthermore, many earlier *in vitro* cytotoxicity studies used supraphysiological concentrations of homocysteine. Finally, since the metabolic capacity for homocysteine disposal varies widely among different tissues, the presumed cytotoxic effect of homocysteine does not appear to be generalizable to all cell types [19]. For example, cultured vascular smooth muscle cells (VSMC) are extremely resistant upto 40 mmol/L homocysteine, likely because they express an active transsulfuration pathway through the induction of CBS expression and activity [40]. This is not the case for endothelial cells, which use only the folate- and cobalamin-dependent remethylation pathway to dispose of intracellular homocysteine [41]. Consequently, folate and cobalamin deficiency may lead to inefficient homocysteine

remethylation activity in endothelial cells, and thus potentiate homocysteine cytotoxicity.

Impairment of nitric oxide production

Several studies have suggested that even mild hyperhomocysteinemia can impair endothelium-dependent nitric oxide (NO) generation and interfere with NO-dependent responses [42–47]. *In vitro* experiments using isolated rat aortic segments demonstrated that homocysteine (100 μmol/L) inhibits endothelium-dependent relaxation, an effect which is in turn reduced by scavengers of ROS, such as catalase and/or superoxide dismutase (SOD) [48]. *In vitro* experiments using bovine aortic endothelial cells grown in the presence of homocysteine (5 mmol/L for 6 h) demonstrated endothelial inability to inhibit adenosine diphosphate (ADP)-induced platelet aggregation, suggesting that homocysteine treatment suppressed NO production [49]. Subsequent studies on human umbilical vein endothelial cells (HUVEC) in culture demonstrated that homocysteine treatment (5 mmol/L for 4 h) determines the overexpression of endothelial NO synthase (eNOS), with a 58% in steady-state mRNA levels of the enzyme, concordant with reduced bioavailability of NO due to concomitant oxidative stress and peroxynitrite formation [50,51]. An additional mechanism for decreased NO bioavailability was demonstrated by treating endothelial cells with 0.05–1 mmol/L homocysteine for 4 h, leading to concentration-dependent inhibition of intracellular glutathione peroxidase activity and diminished cellular antioxidant defenses [52]. Alternatively, elevated levels of asymmetrical dimethylarginine (ADMA), an endogenous competitive inhibitor of NO synthase, decreased NO bioavailability in monkeys treated with a hyperhomocysteinemic diet [53,54], suggesting an alternative potential mechanism for hyperhomocysteinemia (Figure 8.3). Elevated concentrations of ADMA derive from the increased SAM/SAH ratio consequent to high homocysteine levels (see below) [55].

Impairment of endothelial cell proliferation

Homocysteine is mitogenic for smooth muscle cells (SMC) and anti-mitogenic for vascular endothelial cells [56]. Vascular endothelial cells treated with homocysteine (10–50 μmol/L) were arrested in the

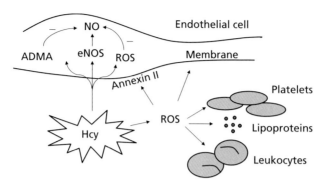

Figure 8.3 Homocysteine and endothelial dysfunction. Oxidation of homocysteine leads to local generation of reactive oxygen species (ROS), with subsequent possible increase in platelet aggregation, leukocyte adhesion, and lipoprotein oxidation. ROS also impair annexin with subsequent inhibition of tissue plasminogen activator (tPA) binding to endothelial cells, and exert direct damage on endothelial cell membrane. Furthermore, extracellular ROS quench nitric oxide (NO) and generate asymmetrical dimethylarginine (ADMA), an endogenous competitive inhibitor of NO synthase. Finally, homocysteine can impair endothelial production of NO and generate ADMA.

G1 phase of the cell cycle [57]. Under these conditions, the intracellular concentrations of *S*-adenosylhomocysteine (SAH) increased and the SAH/*S*-adenosylmethionine (SAM) ratio decreased, adversely affecting the methylation cellular potential and resulting in decreased carboxyl methylation of the *p21ras* carboxy-terminus. In the absence of carboxyl methylation, *p21ras* cannot associate with plasma membrane, resulting in decreased mitogen-activated protein kinase (MAPK) ERK1/2 activity, which participates in cell proliferation, and reduced entry of the cells in the mitotic cycle.

Endothelial and/or leukocyte activation

Low concentrations of homocysteine (25–50 μmol/L) induce the expression of mRNA for monocyte chemoattractant protein (MCP)-1 and interleukin (IL)-8 in a concentration-dependent manner in cultured human aortic endothelial cells [58], but does not affect the expression of other cytokines, including tumor necrosis factor (TNF)-α, granulocyte–macrophage colony-stimulating factor, IL-1β, and transforming growth factor (TGF)-β1. The triggered release of MCP-1 and IL-8 into conditioned medium from homocysteine-treated human aortic endothelial cells renders them chemotactic for U937 monocytoid cells [58]. Co-culture systems of human neutrophils and HUVEC treated with homocysteine (50–400 μmol/L) showed a concentration-dependent increase in adhesion and migration processes [59]. Such studies suggest that homocysteine can enhance leukocyte recruitment onto the vascular endothelium by activating both leukocytes and endothelial cells.

Enhanced oxidative stress

A recent report that examined the ability of antioxidants to block endothelial dysfunction during the transient hyperhomocysteinemia induced by methionine loading suggests that oxidative stress importantly explains endothelial dysfunction in hyperhomocysteinemia [47,60]. In several *in vitro* systems, a number of homocysteine effects on endothelial and SMC results from increased oxidative stress. The basis of the oxidative stress hypothesis relies on the chemical auto-oxidation of homocysteine (2 homocysteine (RSH) + O_2 → homocysteine (RSSR) + $[O_2^{\cdot-}]$ → H_2O_2); the products of such oxidation include homocysteine mono- or disulfides plus hydrogen peroxide and other ROS [13]. Extracellular targets for ROS include cell membranes in platelets and leukocytes as well as lipoproteins; intracellular targets include the endoplasmic reticulum, the Golgi apparatus, and NO.

Many *in vivo* studies have used supraphysiological concentrations (1–10 mmol/L) of homocysteine. Furthermore, the antioxidant defense systems operating *in vivo* do not balance the effects of homocysteine *in vitro*. Generation of oxidative stress through other aminothiols such as cysteine, which has plasma concentrations 25–35 times higher than tHcy, usually does not represent a significant risk factor for cardiovascular disease [61]. Indeed, the daily turnover of plasma homocysteine (1.3 mmol/day in a healthy adult) generates hydrogen peroxide (0.65 mmol/day) [62,63]. Thus, an individual with mild hyperhomocysteinemia, i.e., plasma tHcy ≈ 20 μmol/L, would generate twice that level of hydrogen peroxide (1.88 pmol/min/mL), much less than the oxidative potential of cysteine (see above).

The molecular target hypothesis

The molecular target hypothesis postulates that homocysteine itself may interact either extra- or intra-cellularly with specific molecular targets, thus affecting various cell functions. Homocysteine treatment (0–500 μmol/L) of rat aortic SMC concentration dependently decreases glutathione peroxidase activity and increases SOD activity [64]. In cultured bovine aortic endothelial cells, treatment with homocysteine (50–250 μmol/L) inhibits glutathione peroxidase activity through a direct inactivation of the enzyme and inhibition of protein expression. Indeed, 50 μmol/L homocysteine decreases steady-state mRNA for glutathione peroxidase by 90% [52]. Annexin II, a phospholipid-binding protein expressed on endothelial cells that serves as a docking site for tissue plasminogen activator (tPA), may offer another *in vitro* target for homocysteine. The interaction between homocysteine and annexin inhibits tPA binding to endothelial cells, and consequently blocks the conversion of plasminogen to plasmin, resulting in fibrinolytic defects [65]. Finally, homocysteine forms a mixed disulfide with pro-metalloproteinase-2, thereby activating this protease through a "cysteine switch" mechanism, i.e., the disruption of the critical cysteine-zinc bond that allows the interaction of zinc with a water molecule required for metalloproteinase-2 catalysis [66]. Contrary to the active forms of the enzymes, the propeptide sequences of prometalloproteinases contain a cysteine residue, keeping the enzymes in their latent form by complexing the zinc present in the catalytic domain. The chemical alteration of this bond by homocysteine would cause the activation of metalloproteinase-2 [67] (Figure 8.3).

Evidence for *in vivo* effects of homocysteine

In vivo studies in rabbits, rats, and baboons have shown that parenteral injections of homocysteine may affect vascular endothelium, producing endothelial detachment and subsequent structural changes resembling early atherosclerotic lesions [59,68]. Data obtained in mini-pigs have shown that a methionine-rich diet, consumed for 4 months and able to elevate plasma homocysteine, causes marked structural abnormalities of the abdominal aorta as well as coronary and carotid arteries, including fragmentation of the internal elastic lamina and disruption of elastic fibers and focal areas of SMC hyperplasia [69]. Monkeys that consume methionine-enriched and folate-deficient diets for 4 weeks, capable of producing mild hyperhomocysteinemia (11 μmol/L), show impaired responses to endothelium-dependent vasodilators [70].

Human *in vivo* studies have confirmed the occurrence of endothelial dysfunction in hyperhomocysteinemia. Children with hereditary homocystinuria due to homozygous CBS deficiency showed impaired flow-mediated dilation of the brachial artery after transient vascular occlusion [71], and adult subjects with moderate hyperhomocysteinemia (19–35 μmol/L) showed impaired flow-mediated dilation [42,43]. More recent studies demonstrated that human subjects who were submitted to an acute oral methionine loading experienced impaired endothelium-dependent dilation of resistance arteries within 2 h [44,45,60,72].

Conclusions

Endothelial dysfunction is a key event preceding manifestations of atherothrombotic disease. Results from *in vivo* and *in vitro* studies demonstrate that high levels of homocysteine may induce vascular damage in subjects with severe hyperhomocysteinemia, mainly through endothelial dysfunction. *In vitro* and animal research studies have proposed many pathophysiological mechanisms that may explain the association between hyperhomocysteinemia and endothelial dysfunction, and *in vitro* studies showing that high concentrations of homocysteine reduce bioavailability of NO and enhance SMC proliferation have provided unequivocal and strong evidence for a pro-atherogenic homocysteine action. However, data from clinical and experimental studies remain controversial regarding the potential of mild hyperhomocysteinemia to induce vascular damage *in vivo*. Although the risk of cardiovascular disease concentration-dependently relates to plasma levels of homocysteine, mild hyperhomocysteinemia remains an unproven cause of cardiovascular disease. Current knowledge supports a direct relation between oral folate supplementation and improvement of arterial endothelium-dependent vasodilation in healthy [73] and asymptomatic subjects [74] with mild hyperhomocysteinemia. In healthy subjects with Hcy in the upper normal range (14.9 ± 7.4 µmol/L), folic acid supplementation lowered tHcy and improved endothelium-dependent flow-mediated vasodilation in the brachial artery, an effect largely attributable to NO [73]. In asymptomatic adults with mild hyperhomocysteinemia (8–20 µmol/L), folic acid supplementation resulted in higher serum folate levels, lower tHcy levels (8.1 ± 3 µmol/L), and significantly improved endothelium-dependent dilation compared with placebo [74]. Nevertheless, determining the influence of antioxidant and folate treatments on endothelial dysfunction and vascular outcomes in hyperhomocysteinemic subjects will require well-defined population studies. Indeed, although folate intake effectively lowers tHcy levels [75], the observed beneficial effect on endothelial function may result from an antioxidant activity of folate rather than tHcy lowering. Furthermore, findings about the beneficial effect of folate intake are not univocal, e.g., treatment with folic acid decreased plasma homocysteine levels but did not restore endothelial function or prevent vascular lesion formation and cardiovascular events in some studies in hyperhomocysteinemic animals and hemodialysis patients [76–79]. Indeed, a study in atherosclerotic monkeys with concomitant hypercholesterolemia (12.8 ± 2.8 µmol/L) tested the vasodilatory responses to intra-arterial administration of endothelium-dependent vasodilators such as acetylcholine or ADP, and determined that an atherogenic diet supplemented with vitamin B complex for 6 months decreased plasma homocysteine concentration to 3.5 ± 0.3 µmol/L, but did not prevent progression of atherosclerotic lesions in the carotid artery or restore normal vascular function [76]. Moreover, randomizing hemodialysis patients [77] and patients on peritoneal dialysis [78] (both groups with elevated tHcy at baseline, specifically 42.6 ± 5.8 and 46.9 ± 6.3 µmol/L, respectively), to a 12-week treatment with betaine and/or folic acid did not improve endothelial function, as measured by flow-mediated vasodilation of the brachial artery,

although folic acid supplementation reduced plasma tHcy (to 31.6 ± 4.2 µmol/L). Thus, while defining a "desirable" concentration of plasma homocysteine in the general population might be useful for practical purposes, such definition remains premature. Further studies should clarify the effect of mild hyperhomocysteinemia on endothelial function and the potential of Hcy-lowering treatments in the prevention of vascular disease. Recent observations from the Vitamin Intervention for Stroke Prevention (VISP) randomized controlled trial [80] and The Norwegian Vitamin Trial (NORVIT) study, [81] which both found no effect for folic acid and vitamin B treatment on the risk of reinfarction and stroke, are the first in a series of intervention trials that should clarify the causal role of mild hyperhomocysteinemia in vascular disease.

References

1 McCully KS. Vascular pathology of homocysteinemia: implications for the pathogenesis of arteriosclerosis. *AM J Pathol* 1969;56:111–128.

2 Boushey CJ, Beresford SAA, Omenn GS, et al. A quantitative assessment of plasma homocysteine as a risk for vascular disease. Probable benefits of increasing folic acid intakes. *JAMA* 1995;274:1049–1057.

3 Clarke R, Daly L, Robinson K. Hyperhomocysteinemia: an independent risk factor for vascular disease. *N Engl J Med* 1991;324:1149.

4 Graham IM, Daly L, Refsum H, et al. Plasma Hyperhomocysteine as a risk factor for vascular disease: The European Concerted Action Project. *JAMA* 1997; 277: 1775–1781.

5 Nygard O, Nordrehaug JE, Refsum H, et al. Plasma homocysteine levels and mortality in patients with coronary artery disease. *N Engl J Med* 1997; 337:230–236.

6 Selhub J, Jacques PF, Wilson PWF, et al. Vitamin status and input as primary determinants of homocysteinemia in an elderly population. *JAMA* 1993;270:2693–2698.

7 Alfthan G, Pekkanen J, Jauhiainen M. Relation of serum homocysteinemia and lipoprotein(a) concentrations to atherosclerotic disease in a prospective Finnish population based study. *Atherosclerosis* 1994;106:9–19.

8 Evans R, Shaten J, Hempel J. Homocysteinemia and risk of cardiovascular disease in the Multiple Risk Factor Intervention Trial. *Arterioscler Thromb Vasc Biol* 1997; 17:1947–1953.

9 Folsom A, Nieto J, McGovern P. Prospective study of coronary artery disease incidence in relation to fasting total homocysteine, related genetic polymorphism, and

vitamin B12: the Atherosclerosis Risk in Communities (ARIC) Study. *Circulation* 1998;98:204–210.

10 Ubbink JB, Fehily AM, Pickering J, et al. Homocysteine and ischaemic heart disease in the Caerphilly cohort. *Atherosclerosis* 1998;140:349–356.

11 Brattstrom L, Wilcken D, Ohrvik J, et al. Common methylenetetrahydrofolate reductase gene mutation leads to hyperhomocysteinemia but not to vascular disease. *Circulation* 1998;98:2520–2526.

12 DuVigneaud D, Dyer HM, Harmon J. The growth-promoting properties of homocysteine when added to a cysteine-deficient diet and the proof of the structure of homocysteine. *J Biol Chem* 1993;101:719–726.

13 Kachur AV, Koch CJ, Biaglow JE. Mechanism of copper-catalysed autoxidation of cysteine. *Free Radical Res* 1999;31:23–34.

14 He XM, Carter DC. Atomic structure and chemistry of human serum albumin. *Nature* 1992;358:209–215.

15 Mansoor AM, Svardal AM, Ueland PM. Determination of the *in vivo* redox status of cysteine, cysteinylglycine, homocysteine, and glutathione in human plasma. *Anal Biochem* 1992;200:218–229.

16 Refsum H, Ueland PM, Nygard O, et al. Homocysteine and cardiovascular disease. *Ann Rev Med* 1998;49:31–62.

17 Second International Conference. Homocysteine metabolism. *Neth J Med* 1998;52:S1–S64.

18 Ratnam S, Maclean KN, Jacobs RL, et al. Hormonal regulation of cystathionine beta-synthase expression in liver. *J Biol Chem* 2002;277:42912–42918.

19 Finkelstein JD. Pathways and regulation of homocysteine metabolism in mammals. *Semin Thromb Hemost* 2000;26:219–225.

20 Taoka S, Ohja S, Shan X, et al. Evidence for heme-mediated redox regulation of human cystathionine-beta-synthase activity. *J Biol Chem* 1998;273:25179–25184.

21 Jacobsen DW, Gatautis VJ, Green R. Rapid HPLC determination of total homocysteine and other thiols in serum and plasma: sex differences and correlation with cobalamin and folate concentrations in healthy subjects. *Clin Chem* 1994;40:873–881.

22 Robinson K, Mayer EL, Miller DP, et al. Hyperhomocysteinemia and low pyridoxal phosphate. Common and independent reversible risk factors for coronary artery disease. *Circulation* 1995;92:2825–2830.

23 Vilaseca MA, Moyano D, Ferrer I, et al. Total homocysteine in pediatric patients. *Clin Chem* 1997;43:690–692.

24 Clarke R, Woodhouse P, Ulvik A, et al. Variability and determinants of total homocysteine concentrations in plasma in an elderly population. *Clin Chem* 1998;44:102–107.

25 Hongsprabhas P, Papageorgiou AN, Hoffer LJ. Plasma homocysteine concentrations of preterm infants. *Biol Neonate* 1999;76:65–71.

26 Kang S-S, Wong PWK, Malinow MR. Hyperhomocysteinemia as a risk factor for occlusive vascular disease. *Annu Rev Nutr* 1992;12:279–289.

27 Still R, McDowell I. Clinical implication of plasma homocysteine measurement in cardiovascular disease. *J Clin Pathol* 1998;51:183–188.

28 Fowler B. Genetic defects of folate and cobalamin metabolism. *Eur J Pediatr* 1998;157:S60–S66.

29 Eikelboom JW, Lonn E, Genest JJ, et al. Homocyst(e)ine and cardiovascular disease: a critical review of the epidemiologic evidence. *Ann Intern Med* 1999;131:363–375.

30 Mudd SH, Levy HL, Skovby F. The metabolic and molecular bases if inherited disease. In: Scriver CR, Beaudet AL, Sly WS, Valle D, eds. *The Metabolic Basis of Inherited Disease* New York: McGraw Hill: 1995.

31 Isherwood DM. Homocystinuria. *BMJ* 1996;313.

32 Goyette P, Frosst P, Rosenblatt DS, et al. Seven novel mutations in the methylenetetrahydropholate reductase gene and genotype/phenotype correlations in severe methylenetetrahydropholate reductase deficiency. *Am J Hum Genet* 1995;56:1052–1059.

33 Goyette P, Christensen B, Rosenblatt DS, et al. Severe and mild mutations in cis for the methylenetetrahydrofolate reductase (MTHFR) gene, and description of five novel mutations in MTHFR. *Am J Hum Genet* 1996;59:1268–1275.

34 Frosst P, Blom HJ, Milos R, et al. A candidate genetic risk factor for vascular disease: a common mutation in methylenetetrahydropholate reductase. *Nature Genet* 1995;10:111–113.

35 Wall RT, Harlan JM, Harker LA, et al. Homocysteine-induced endothelial cell injury *in vitro*: a model for the study of vascular injury. *Thromb Res* 1980;18:113–121.

36 Bergmann S, Shatrov V, Ratter F, et al. Adenosine and homocysteine together enhance TNF-mediated cytotoxicity but do not alter activation of nuclear factor-kappa B in L929 cells. *J Immunol* 1994;153:1736–1743.

37 Huang RF, Huang SM, Lin BS, et al. Homocysteine thiolactone induces apoptotic DNA damage mediated by increased intracellular hydrogen peroxide and caspase 3 activation in HL-60 cells. *Life Sci* 2001;68:2799–2811.

38 Sung JJ, Kim HJ, Choi-Kwon S, et al. Homocysteine induces oxidative cytotoxicity in Cu,Zn-superoxide dismutase mutant motor neuronal cell. *Neuroreport* 2002;13:377–381.

39 Dudman NPB, Hicks C, Wang J, et al. Human arterial endothelial cell detachment *in vitro*: its promotion by homocysteine and cysteine. *Atherosclerosis* 1991;91:77–83.

40 Chen P, Poddar R, Tipa EV, et al. Homocysteine metabolism in cardiovascular cells and tissues: implications for hyperhomocysteinemia and cardiovascular disease. *Adv Enzymol Regul* 1999;39:93–109.

41 van der Molen EF, Hiipakka MJ, van Lith-Zanders H, et al. Homocysteine metabolism in endothelial cells of a

patient homozygous for cystathionine beta-synthase (CS) deficiency. *Thromb Haemost* 1997;78:827–833.

42 Tawakol A, Omland T, Gerhard M, et al. Hyperhomocysteinemia is associated with impaired endothelium-dependent vasodilatation in humans. *Circulation* 1997;95:1119–1121.

43 Woo KS, Chook P, Lolin YI, et al. Hyperhomocyst(e)inemia is a risk factor for arterial endothelial dysfunction in human. *Circulation* 1997;96:2542–2544.

44 Bellamy MF, McDowell IFW, Ramsey MW, et al. Hyperhomocysteinemia after an oral methionine load acutely impairs endothelial function in healthy adults. *Circulation* 1998;98:1848–1852.

45 Chambers JC, McGregor A, Jean-Marie J, et al. Acute hyperhomocysteinemia and endothelial dysfunction. *Lancet* 1998;351:36–37.

46 Lambert J, van den Berg M, Steyn M, et al. Familial hyperhomocysteinemia and endothelium-dependent vasodilatation and arterial distensibility of large arteries. *Cardiovasc Res* 1999;42:743–751.

47 Nappo F, De Rosa N, Marfella R, et al. Impairment of endothelial functions by acute hyperhomocysteinemia and reversal by antioxidants vitamins. *JAMA* 1999;281:2113–2118.

48 Emsley AM, Jeremy JY, Gomes GN, et al. Investigation of the inhibitory effect of homocysteine and copper on nitric oxide-mediated relaxation of rat isolated aorta. *Br J Pharmacol* 1999;126:1034–1040.

49 Stamler JS, Osborne JA, Jaraki O, et al. Adverse vascular effects of homocysteine are modulated by endothelium-derived relaxing factor and related oxides of nitrogen. *J Clin Invest* 1993;91:308–318.

50 Upchurch GRJ, Welch JN, Fabian AJ, et al. Stimulation of endothelial nitric oxide production by homocyst(e)ine. *Atherosclerosis* 1997;132:177–185.

51 Zhang X, Li H, Jin H, et al. Effects of homocysteine on endothelial nitric oxide production. *Am J Physiol Renal Physiol* 2000;279:F671–F678.

52 Upchurch GRJ, Welch JN, Fabian AJ, et al. Homocyst(e)ine decreases bioavailable nitric oxide by a mechanism involving glutathione peroxidase. *J Biol Chem* 1997;272:17012–17017.

53 Boger RH, Bode-Boger SM, Sydow K, et al. Plasma concentration of asymmetric dimethylarginine, an endogenous inhibitor of nitric oxide synthase, is elevated in monkeys with hyperhomocyst(e)inemia or hypercholesterolemia. *Arterioscler Thromb Vasc Biol* 2000;20 1557–1564.

54 Boger RH, Lentz SR, Bode-Boger SM, et al. Elevation of asymmetrical dimethylarginine may mediate endothelial dysfunction during experimental hyperhomocysteinemia in humans. *Clin Sci* 2000;100:161–167.

55 Vallance P, Leone A, Calver A, et al. Endogenous dimethylarginine as an inhibitor of nitric oxide synthase. *J Cardiovasc Pharmacol* 1992;20:S60–S62.

56 Tsai J-C, Perrella MA, Yoshizumi M, et al. Promotion of vascular smooth muscle growth by homocysteine: a link to atherosclerosis. *Proc Natl Acad Sci USA* 1994;91: 6369–6373.

57 Wang J, Yoshizumi M, Lai K, et al. Inhibition of growth and p21ras methylation in vascular endothelial cells by homocysteine but not cysteine. *J Biol Chem* 1997;272:25380–25385.

58 Poddar R, Sivasubramanian N, DiBello PM, et al. Homocysteine induces expression and secretion of monocyte chemoattractant protein-1 and interleukin-8 in human aortic endothelial cells: implications for vascular disease. *Circulation.* 2001;103:2717–2723.

59 Dudman NPB, Temple SE, Guo XW, et al. Homocysteine enhances neutrophil-endothelial interactions in both cultured human cells and rats *in vivo. Circ Res* 1999; 84:409–416.

60 Chambers JC, McGregor A, Jean-Marie J, et al. Demonstration of rapid onset vascular endothelial dysfunction after hyperhomocysteinemia: an effect reversible with vitamin C therapy. *Circulation* 1999;99:1156–1160.

61 Raguso CA, Regan MM, Toung VR. Cysteine kinetics and oxidation at different intakes of methionine and cysteine in young adults. *Am J Clin Nutr* 2000;71:491–499.

62 Guttormsen AB, Mansoor AM, Fiskerstrand T, et al. Kinetics of plasma homocysteine in healthy subjects after peroral homocysteine loading. *Clin Chem* 1993;39:980–985.

63 Guttormsen AB, Ueland PM, Svarstad E, et al. Kinetic basis of hyperhomocysteinemia in patients with chronic renal failure. *Kidney Int* 1997;52:495–502.

64 Nishio W, Watanabe Y. Homocysteine as a modulator of platelet-derived growth factor action in vascular smooth muscle cells: a possible role for hydrogen peroxide. *Br J Pharmacol* 1997;122:269–274.

65 Hajjar KA, Mauri L, Jacovina AT, et al. Tissue plasminogen activator binding to the annexin II tail domain: direct modulation by homocysteine. *J Biol Chem* 1998; 273: 9987–9993.

66 Bescond A, Augier T, Chareyre C, et al. Influence of homocysteine on matrix metalloproteinase-2: activation and activity. *Biochem Biophys Res Commun* 1999; 263:498–503.

67 Springman EB, Angleton EL, Birkedal-Hansen H, et al. Multiple modes of activation of latent human fibroblast collagenase: evidence for the role of a Cys73 active-site zinc complex in latency and a "cysteine switch" mechanism for activation. *Proc Natl Acad Sci USA* 1990; 87:364–368.

68 Lang D, Kredan MB, Moat SJ, et al. Homocysteine-induced inhibition of endothelium-dependent relaxation in rabbit aorta: role for superoxide anions. *Arterioscler Thromb Vasc Biol* 2000;20:422–427.

69 Rolland PH, Friggi A, Barlatier A, et al. Hyperhomocysteinemia-induced vascular damage in the

minipigs: captopril-hydrochlorothiazide combination prevents elastic alterations. *Circulation* 1995;91:1161–1174.

70 Lentz SR, Sobey CG, Piegors DJ, et al. Vascular dysfunction in monkeys with diet-induced hyperhomocyst(e)inemia. *J Clin Invest* 1996;98:24–29.

71 Celermajer DS, Sorensen K, Ryalls M, et al. Impaired endothelial function occurs in the systemic arteries of children with homozygous homocystinuria but not in their heterozygous parents. *J Am Coll Cardiol* 1993;22:854–858.

72 Haynes WG, Sinkey CA, Kanani P. Acute methionine loading produces endothelial dysfunction in humans. *J Invest Med* 1997;45:210A.

73 Bellamy MF, McDowell I, Ramsey MW. Oral folate enhances endothelial function in hyperhomocysteinemic subjects. *J Am Coll Cardiol* 1999;34:274–279.

74 Woo KS, Chook P, Lolin YI, et al. Folic acid improves arterial endothelial function in adults with hyperhomocysteinemia. *J Am Coll Cardiol* 1999;34:2002–2006.

75 Homocysteine Lowering Trialists'Collaboration. Lowering blood homocysteine with folic acid based supplements: meta-analysis of randomised trials. *Br Med* 1998;316:894–898.

76 Lentz SR, Malinow MR, Piegors DJ. Consequences of hyperhomocysteinemia on vascular function in atherosclerotic monkeys. *Arterioscler Thromb Vasc Biol* 1997;17:2930–2934.

77 van Gueldner C, Janssen MJFM, Lambert J. No change in impaired endothelial after long-term folic acid therapy of hyperhomocysteinemia in haemodialysis patients. *Nephrol Dial Transplant* 1998;13:106–112.

78 van Gueldner C, Janssen MJFM, Lambert J. Folic acid treatment of hyperhomocysteinemia in peritoneal dialysis patients: no change in endothelial function after long-term therapy. *Perit Dial Int* 1998;18:282–289.

79 Ambrosi P, Rolland PH, Bodard H. Effects of folate supplementation in hyperhomocysteinemic pigs. *J Am Coll Cardiol* 1999;34:274–279.

80 Toole JF, Malinow MR, Chambless LE, et al. Lowering homocysteine in patients with ischemic stroke to prevent recurrent stroke, myocardial infarction, and death: the Vitamin Intervention for Stroke Prevention (VISP) randomized controlled trial. *JAMA.* 2004;291:565–575.

81 Bonaa KH, Njolstad I, Veland PM, et al. Homocysteine lowering and cardiovascular events after acute myocardial infarction. *N Engl J Med.* 2006;354:1578–1588.

CHAPTER 9

Lipoprotein(a) and the artery wall

Angelo M. Scanu, MD *& Marilena Formato,* MD

Introduction

Lipoprotein(a), Lp(a), represents a class of lipoproteins having a protein moiety, apoB100, linked by a single disulfide bond to apolipoprotein(a), apo(a), a highly glycosylated multikringle protein with a high degree of homology with plasminogen. A hallmark of Lp(a) is the marked structural heterogeneity and its ready susceptibility to oxidative, lipolytic, thiolytic, proteolytic, and post-translational modifications. These events, demonstrated *in vitro*, are likely to also occur *in vivo* and, in the artery wall, generate bioactive products with an atherothrombogenic potential.

Heterogeneity of Lp(a) (Figure 9.1)

In normotriglyceridemic plasma, Lp(a) occurs as a low-density lipoprotein (LDL) variant where apoB100 links to apo(a) by a single disulfide bond [1,2]. The LDL of Lp(a) has properties very similar to those of parent LDL, for instance, variability in density, from dense to buoyant, while these two lipoproteins do not differ in terms of apoB100. Regarding apo(a), its heterogeneity is dependent on the number of kringles (K), on the K primary structure, and on the length and degree of glycosylation of the segments joining the kringles. The size of apo(a) is

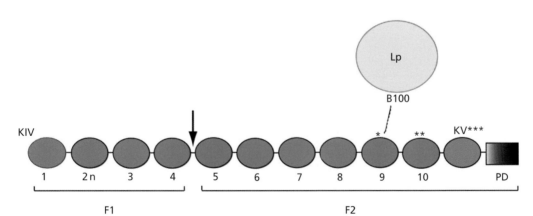

Figure 9.1 Schematic representation of apo(a) showing the 10 types of KIV, one copy of KV and the protease domain (PD). The notation 2n is to indicate that the number of this kringle may vary within and among individuals, accounting for the apo(a) size heterogeneity. The arrow points at the cleavage site in the linker between KIV-4 and KIV-5 caused by enzymes of the elastase and metalloproteinase families, generating two main fragments F1 (N-terminal) and F2 (C-terminal).

*Indicates the kringle involved in disulfide linkage with apoB100-containing lipoproteins (Lp).
**Kringle containing the high-affinity lysine-binding site.
***Kringle containing oxPC adducts.

related to the number of KIV-2 repeats and partially accounts for the plasma levels of Lp(a), with smaller apo(a) size isoforms associating with highest Lp(a) levels. The K primary structure can affect Lp(a) function, e.g., the Trp_{72}–Arg mutation in the lysine-binding site of IV-10 results in a lysine-binding-defective phenotype [3]. Proteolytic cleavage occurs at the linker regions, and O-glycans bound to these linkers may modulate the cleavage [4]. Supporting this hypothesis are the data showing that the linker between KIV-4 and KIV-5, which lack O-glycans, is the preferential site of cleavage by enzymes of the elastase and metalloproteinase families [5].

Lp(a) susceptibility to modification

Oxidation

Like parent LDL, the lipids of the LDL constituent of Lp(a) can undergo oxidative modifications [6]. A recent in vitro study by our group determined that oxidation that causes the breakdown of apoB100 does not affect the integrity of apo(a), although changes detected by intrinsic fluorescence spectroscopy were observed [7]. Oxidation can destabilize Lp(a) and cause aggregation, events that may introduce a confounder when assessing the specificity of oxidized Lp(a) function in biological systems.

Lipolysis

The susceptibility of Lp(a) to the action of enzymes of the phospholipase A_2 (PLA_2) family is well established [8]. Thus modified, Lp(a) has an increased affinity for lysine–sepharose and more readily binds to members of the vascular extracellular matrix (ECM), i.e., laminin, fibronectin, and collagen [9]. Thus, these Lp(a) particles are good candidates for retention in the sub-endothelial intima [10] and, so trapped, are prone to further pro-atherogenic modifications [11].

Thiolysis

In vitro studies have shown that the disulfide bond between apoB100 and apo(a) in Lp(a) can be cleaved under mild reductive conditions, generating free apo(a) and apo(a)-free LDL [1]. The study of these two products have provided valuable information on the structural and functional properties of Lp(a).

The occurrence of a thiolytic event in vivo is suggested by the results of two metabolic studies conducted in humans, showing that 10–20% of the intravenously injected radiolabeled Lp(a) was recovered as an apo(a)-free LDL, suggesting that apo(a) had dissociated from parent Lp(a) [11,12]. The presence of free apo(a) in the arterial wall has also been documented [13].

Proteolysis

Both Lp(a) and free apo(a) can be cleaved by enzymes of the elastase and metalloproteinase families [8]. In each case, under conditions of limited proteolysis, apo(a) is cleaved in the linker region between KIV-4 and KIV-5 (Figure 9.1), the only linker that is free of O-glycans) [5]. Proteolytically derived N- and C-terminal fragments are termed F1 and F2 [1]. In digested Lp(a), F1 no longer attaches to apoB100 and undergoes rapid elimination via the kidney [14]. In turn, F2 remains linked to LDL as a mini-Lp(a) particle that binds to the ECM in vitro more avidly than parent Lp(a) containing the full length apo(a) [15].

Post-translational modification

Recent investigations carried out in our laboratory have shown that some of the lysines of human apo(a) KV, probably lys-12 and lys-42, are chemically linked in a Schiff base to oxidized phosphatidylcholine (oxPC) and suggested, from studies in cultured human macrophages, that these adducts impart pro-inflammatory function to apo(a) [16]. The studies were carried out using Lp(a) preparations from a healthy human donor. It remains to be established whether the number of lysines adducted to oxPC may be affected in high Lp(a) subjects with an established atherosclerotic cardiovascular disease.

Interaction of Lp(a) with the artery wall

Except for one unconfirmed report [17], it is generally accepted that apo(a) immunoreactive material localized in artery wall lesions derives from plasma. Although likely representing a multi-step process, the mechanism or mechanisms underlying this transendothelial transport remain poorly understood.

Endothelium

In vitro studies

Haque et al. [18] demonstrated that apo(a), and, more specifically, its C-terminal domain corresponding to F2, induce the production of chemoattractant CC chemokine I-309 in human umbilical vein endothelial cells (HUVEC). Considering that this chemokine is present in macrophages and co-localizes with apo(a), such production may provide mechanisms for atherogenic action by Lp(a) [18]. Further, Lp(a) and, more efficiently, apo(a), decrease the level of endothelin-1 mRNA and translated protein in HUVEC, but did not affect plasminogen activator inhibitor 1 (PAI-1) [18]. On the other hand, another study reported that Lp(a) may affect genotypic-specific transcriptional regulation of PAI-1 [19, 20], an action also exhibited by very-low-density lipoprotein (VLDL) from hypertriglyceridemic subjects. Additionally, Lp(a) may stimulate expression of vascular adhesion molecule 1 (VCAM-1) and E-selectin in cultured human coronary artery endothelial cells, an effect associated with elevated intracellular free calcium [21]. LDL exhibited the same effect, although to a lesser extent. However, the Lp(a) preparation used in this study was commercial and not adequately characterized. Taken together, discordant findings on this subject may reflect differences in cell culture conditions, as well as differences in Lp(a) preparations and their degree of stability before and after incubation with the cells. A recent study using immunochemical techniques observed apo(a) in endothelial cells of artery lesions, obtained by autopsy, in the circle of Willis [22], suggesting an early involvement of apo(a) in atherosclerosis.

In vivo studies

In vivo models have been used to determine whether Lp(a) might impair endothelial function in the early stage of the atherosclerosis. Schlaich et al. [23] placed a gauge plethysmograph in 57 young white subjects (mean age 37 years) to measure changes in forearm blood flow following infusion of increasing doses of acetylcholine, sodium nitroprusside, and *N*-monomethylarginine (L-NMMA). Neither endothelium-dependent vasodilation (response to acetylcholine) nor endothelium-independent vascular relaxation (response to nitroprusside) correlated with plasma Lp(a) levels, thus excluding a mechanism mediated by nitric oxide (NO). In turn, high plasma Lp(a) levels associated positively with the degree of vasoconstrictive response to L-NMMA, indicating a compensatory increase in the basal production and secretion f NO. However, the potential contribution by an endothelin-mediated mechanism was not ruled out. In apparent conflict with these studies, Tsurumi et al. [24] observed a positive correlation between plasma levels of Lp(a) and endothelium-dependent vasodilation in coronary arteries. However, patients in that investigation were older (mean age 58 years), and also had confounding risk factors. Divergences may also result from different vascular beds, as exemplified by the observations of Sorensen et al. [25], who found an inverse correlation between superficial femoral artery flow-mediated vasodilation and plasma Lp(a) levels in hypercholesterolemic children. Thus, variables like Lp(a) and apo(a) heterogeneity, size and density of LDL as well as high-density lipoprotein (HDL) levels may affect vascular tone, while the effect of Lp(a) remains unclear.

Intima retention

Substantial evidence supports the hypothesis that retention of apoB-containing lipoproteins by the subendothelial intima is a key event in early atherogenesis [10], and that such retention is effected mainly by proteoglycans (PG) [26]. Studies in transgenic mice expressing a human PG-binding defective apoB100 mutant recently showed markedly decreased atherosclerotic lesions compared with control mice expressing wild-type apoB100 [27], thus corroborating the retention hypothesis. Although true for LDL, this mutation may not affect the retention of Lp(a), due to its alternate anchoring capacity via the apo(a)–PG protein core interaction, consistent with the notion that Lp(a) is preferentially retained over LDL (Figure 9.2). Such preferential retention would render Lp(a) relatively more prone to potential modifications (see Table 9.1) that may contribute to the pathogenic action of Lp(a) on plaque formation and progression.

Lp(a) and atherosclerotic plaques

Several studies have demonstrated the presence of apo(a) in human atherosclerotic plaques (see Refs. [2,8] for reviews). By immunochemical criteria, free apo(a) has been described as either intact or

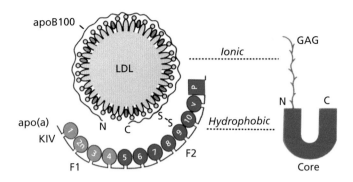

Figure 9.2 Schematic representation of the two-binding modes between Lp(a) and the PO decorin. One-binding mode is electrostatic between apoB100 and the GAG chain of decorin; the other is hydrophobic, between the decorin protein core (brown) and the F2 domain of apo(a), The other kringles are presented in light blue. (Reproduced with permission from Ref. [15]).

Table 9.1 Potential modifiers of Lp(a) structure.

Modifying factors	Outcomes
Oxidation	Generation of O_2 free radicals, particle aggregation, apoB fragmentation
Proteolysis by enzymes of the MMP and serine protease families	Formation of mini-Lp(a), and fragments of apo(a) and apoB
Phospholipases and sphingomyelinases	Particle surface modification, generation of free fatty acids and lyso derivatives
Cleavage of the interchain disulfide bond between apo(a) and apoB by either enzymatic or oxidative processes	Dissociation of apo(a) from the apoB-containing lipoprotein
Oxidation-dependent lysine modification of apo(a)	Formation of adducts between KV of apo(a) and oxPC

The modifications postulated to take place after Lp(a) enters the artery wall are suggested from the results of *in vitro* experiments. MMP: matrix metalloproteinase; s-PLA$_2$: secretory phospholipase A$_2$; SPHases: sphingomyelinases.

fragmented, present at extracellular sites, and co-localized with either apoB, PG, or fibrin. An intracellular localization has also been reported, particularly in foam cells [28]. Some results vary, likely due to the use of fresh surgical specimens in some cases and of autoptic materials in others. Moreover, the sites of sampling, including the abdominal and thoracic aorta, carotid arteries, coronaries, vein grafts, and cerebral vessels, vary at different stages of the disease. Nonetheless, the overall notion is that Lp(a) may undergo modification in the inflammatory atherosclerotic plaque. The presence of free apo(a) indicates a disruption of the disulfide bond between apo(a) and apoB100 via either thiolytic or oxidative events, whereas apo(a) fragments would result from the action of proteolytic enzymes secreted from either activated macrophages, smooth muscle cells, or mast cells. *In vitro* studies suggest that matrix metalloproteinases (MMP) likely play an important role in the fragmentation process. In this context, the activity of macrophage-released sialidases and glycosydases,

able to modify the glycans of the linker regions involved in the cleavage, may aid apo(a) degradation. Apo(a) fragments may be bioactive, and *in vitro* results suggest stronger potency than parent apo(a) in terms of binding to ECM to fibrin [1,8] as well as eliciting a pro-inflammatory response in cultured human macrophages [29].

The issue of plaque stability vs instability has received a limited attention as to Lp(a) and plaque biology. We have approached this issue in a recent study dealing with human carotid plaques obtained by endarterectomy [30]. Plaque instability was defined by the presence of a thin fibrous cap, inflammation, macrophage infiltration, and proximity of the necrotic core to the lumen. Western analyses of plaque extracts showed a marked accumulation of F2, localized immunochemically within the inflamed fibrous cap area with MMP-2 and MMP-9 activity as assessed by *in situ* zymography. In subsequent investigations, we have shown that, compared to stable plaques, human unstable carotid plaques contain an increased concentration of both the inflammatory

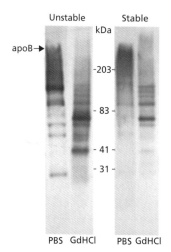

Figure 9.3 Immunoblot analyses on SDS-PAGE, under reducing conditions, of extracts from unstable and stable plaques of human carotid arteries. The gels were probed with a polyclonal antibody specific for human apoB. The arrow indicates the position of intact apoB. The molecular weight markers permit, by extrapolation, to determine the size of the immunodetected apoB fragments. PBS and GdHCl stand for phosphate buffered saline and 6M guanidine hydrochloride extracts, respectively.

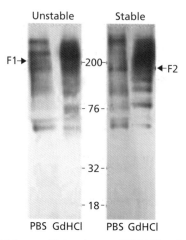

Figure 9.4 Immunoblot analyses on SDS-PAGE under reducing conditions, of extracts from unstable and stable plaques of human carotid arteries. The gels were probed with a polyclonal antibody specific for human apo(a). The arrows indicate the position of F1 and F2. For other details, see Figure 9.3.

chemokines IL-8 and IL-18, and the enzymes MMP-2 and MMP-9 all quantified by ELISA [31]. We also found a correlation between MMP activity and generation of apoB and apo(a) fragments [31] suggesting that the degradation of these two apolipoproteins (Figures 9.3 and 9.4) may serve as a useful biomarker of vessel wall inflammation. In this vein, we observed, within unstable plaques, that areas with a high density of macrophages contain apo(a) that is recognized by T-15, a monoclonal antibody specific for oxPC (Scanu, unpublished observations).

Pleiotropism of the cardiovascular pathogenicity of Lp(a)

Essentially all epidemiological studies that consider age, gender, race, plasma levels of LDL, HDL, and hemostatic factors support the hypothesis of a pathogenic role of Lp(a) levels in plasma as a total particle (see Refs [1,8], for recent reviews). The pathogenic role of Lp(a) may be greater in those particles with small apo(a) size and a small-dense LDL moiety [32]. In the framework of an activated endothelium,

small-dense Lp(a) particles may move more rapidly from plasma to the artery wall than their buoyant counterparts, and may be more prone to modification(s) during the transfer process due to the action of constitutive elements of endothelial cells, e.g., PLA_2 and endothelial lipase. The requirement of activated endothelial cells has been shown in an *in vivo* rabbit model, where the transport of Lp(a) occurred significantly more rapidly in atherosclerotic vessels than controls [33].

Within the intima, the contribution of Lp(a) to early atherogenesis derives from its binding to ECM members. We have shown previously that Lp(a) is well suited for retention, due to its capacity to bind to ECM by both electrostatic and hydrophobic interactions [15]. Once trapped, Lp(a) becomes more susceptible to modifications by one or more of the processes outlined above. Following oxidation, Lp(a) becomes amenable to uptake and degradation by macrophages contributing to foam cell formation. Phospholipolysis enhances the affinity of Lp(a) for ECM, and increased particle retention and proteolysis causes the generation of fragments, the bioactive ones perpetuating the pro-atherothrombogenic action of the parent products. Within this scenario, the enzymes of the MMP family may be viewed as modulators of the pathogenic expression of Lp(a)/apo(a).

Perspectives

While several studies have documented an association between plasma levels and the cardiovascular pathogenicity of Lp(a), a clear understanding of the basic mechanisms underlying this relationship remains unsurprisingly incomplete, considering that Lp(a) is a complex, heterogeneous structure with pleiotropic functions that potentially bridge atherosclerosis and thrombosis. While the LDL component is expected to be a pathogenic contributor [29], much of the specificity of Lp(a) action rests on apo(a) that is itself heterogeneous in kringle number and structure as well as length and degree of glycosylation of the interkringle linkers. The emerging notion that the action of enzymes produced by activated cells of the "inflamed" artery wall can generate bioactive fragments with pathogenic potential opens new horizons for studying the molecular basis for the cardiovascular pathogenicity of Lp(a). Examples of functions where discrete domains do better than the whole apo(a) include those comprising KIV-6 and KIV-7 in the binding to the "foam cell receptor" [28]; KIV-5 to KIV-8 in fibrin binding [34]; KIV-10 in high affinity lysine binding [35]; KV-protease region in fibronectin binding [36]; and KV in the stimulation of IL-8 production by human macrophages [37]. Future studies will likely uncover additional specificities. This new information should increase our understanding of the mechanisms underlying the cardiovascular pathogenicity of Lp(a). Unfortunately, the lack of suitable animal models for studying Lp(a) biology has allowed only limited progress (see Refs [2,8] for reviews). Overall, the information derived from mouse models has been equivocal. However, an important study in apo(a) transgenic mice has provided evidence that fibrinogen deficiency reduces the vascular accumulation of this apolipoprotein and the development of atherosclerosis [38], concordant with previous observations that showed a striking co-localization of apo(a) and fibrin [39] in diseased arteries and the thrombogenic role of fibrin-bound apo(a) [40]. Promising studies have been published recently regarding transgenic rabbits that express human apo(a) on a background of hypercholesterolemia secondary to either high fat diet [41] or LDL receptor deficiency [42]. In either case, introduction of the apo(a) gene enhanced pre-existing atherosclerotic lesions, suggesting that Lp(a) becomes a pathogenic player only in established lesions. However, extrapolating the results of those studies to man is difficult because the apo(a) gene is foreign to the rabbit, and because rabbit apoB, by lacking the unpaired cysteine required to establish a disulfide linkage with apo(a), cannot form a true Lp(a) complex.

Future directions

While several issues remain unresolved, some deserve a higher priority of attention for future research, including:

1 Evolutionary reasons for the obligate transport in the plasma of apo(a) linked to apoB100 lipoproteins.
2 Definition of the factors involved in apo(a)–apoB100 linkage and in the disruption of this linkage at tissue sites.
3 Definition of the physiologic function(s) of Lp(a).
4 In terms of cardiovascular pathogenicity, definition of how much is due to the whole particle and how much to its constituents, apo(a) and LDL, and to derivatives like mini-Lp(a) and fragments.
5 Definition of the importance of density and size of Lp(a) in determining type and extent of modifications of this lipoprotein.
6 Definition of the role of apo(a) size in the pathogenicity of Lp(a).

This list highlights the fact that the solution of the overall cardiovascular pathology will require multidisciplinary approaches, where the human model must play a central role.

Acknowledgments

The original work cited in this review by one of the authors (A.M.S.) was supported by NIH-NHLBI grants # 63115 and 63209. Celina Edelstein provided constructive comments during the preparation of the manuscript.

References

1 Scanu AM, Nakajima K, Edelstein C. Apolipoprotein(a): structure and biology. *Front Biosci* 2001;6:546–554.
2 Hobbs HH, White AL. Lipoprotein(a): intrigues and insights. *Curr Opin Lipidol* 1999;10:225–236.

3 Scanu AM, Edelstein C. Kringle-dependent structural and functional polymorphism of apolipoprotein(a). *Biochim Biophys Acta* 1995;1256:1–12.

4 Garner B, Merry AH, Royle L, et al. Structural elucidation of the *N*- and *O*-glycans of human apolipoprotein(a). Role of *O*-glycans in conferring protease resistance. *J Biol Chem* 2001;276:22200–22208.

5 Scanu AM, Edelstein C. Learning about the structure and biology of human lipoprotein(a) through dissection by enzymes of the elastase family: facts and speculations. *J Lipid Res* 1997;38:2193–2206.

6 Chisolm GM, Penn MS. Oxidized lipoproteins and atherosclerosis. In: Fuster V, Ross R, Topol EJ, eds. *Atherosclerosis and Coronary Artery Disease*. Philadelphia, PA: Lippincott-Raven; 1996:129–149.

7 Edelstein C, Nakajima K, Pfaffinger D, et al. Oxidative events cause degradation of apoB-100 but not of apo [a] and facilitate enzymatic cleavage of both proteins. *J Lipid Res* 2001;42:1664–1670.

8 Scanu AM. Lipoprotein(a) and the atherothrombotic process: mechanistic insights and clinical implications. *Curr Cardiol Rep* 2003;5:106–113.

9 Hoover-Plow J, Khaitan A, Fless GM. Phospholipase A2 modification enhances lipoprotein (a) binding to the subendothelial matrix. *Thromb Haemostasis* 1998;79: 640–648.

10 Williams KJ, Tabas I. The response-to-retention hypothesis of atherogenesis reinforced. *Curr Opin Lipidol* 1998;9:471–474.

11 Knight BL, Perombelon YFN, Soutar AK, et al. Catabolism of lipoprotein(a) in familial hypercholesterolemic subjects. *Atherosclerosis* 1991;87(2–3):227–237.

12 Rader DJ, Mann WA, Cain W, et al. The low density lipoprotein receptor is not required for normal catabolism of Lp(a) in humans. *J Clin Invest* 1995;95:1403–1408.

13 Hoff HF, Oneil J, Smejkal GB, et al. Immunochemically detectable lipid-free apo(a) in plasma and in human atherosclerotic lesions. *Chem Phys Lipids* 1994;67:271–280.

14 Edelstein C, Shapiro SD, Klezovitch O, et al. Macrophage metalloelastase, MMP-12, cleaves human apolipoprotein(a) in the linker region between kringles IV-4 and IV-5. Potential relevance to lipoprotein(a) biology. *J Biol Chem* 1999;274:10019–10023.

15 Scanu AM, Edelstein C, Klezovitch O. Dominant role of the C-terminal domain in the binding of apolipoprotein(a) to the protein core of proteoglycans and other members of the vascular matrix. *Trends Cardiovasc Med* 1999;9:196–199.

16 Edelstein C, Pfaffinger D, Jinman, et al. Lysine-phosphatidylcholine adducts in kringle V impart unique immunological and potential pro-inflammatory properties to human apolipoprotein(a). *J Biol Chem* 2003;278: 52841–52847.

17 Fu L, Jamieson DG, Usher DC, et al. Gene expression of apolipoprotein (a) within the wall of human aorta and carotid arteries. *Atherosclerosis* 2001;158:303–311.

18 Haque NS, Zhang X, French DL, et al. CC chemokine I-309 is the principal monocyte chemoattractant induced by apolipoprotein(a) in human vascular endothelial cells. *Circulation* 2000;102:786–792.

19 Berg KE, Djurovic S, Muller HJ, et al. Studies on effects of Lp(a) lipoprotein on gene expression in endothelial cells *in vitro*. *Clin Genet* 1997;52:314–325.

20 Grenett HE, Benza RI, Fless GM, et al. Genotype-specific transcriptional regulation of PAI-1 gene by insulin hypertriglyceridemic VLDL, and Lp(a) in transfected, cultured human endothelial cells. *Arterioscler Thromb Vasc Biol* 1998;18:1803–1809.

21 Allen S, Khan S, Tam S, et al. Expression of adhesion molecules by Lp(a): a potential novel mechanism for its atherogenicity. *FASEB J* 1998;12:1765–1776.

22 Jamieson DG, Usher DC, Rader DJ, Lavi E. Apolipoprotein(a) deposition in atherosclerotic plaques of cerebral vessels. A potential role for endothelial cells in lesion formation. *Am J Pathol* 1995;147:1567–1574.

23 Schlaich MP, John S, Langenfeld MRW, et al. Does lipoprotein (a) impair endothelial function? *J Am Coll Cardiol* 1998;31:359–365.

24 Tsurumi Y, Nagashima H, Ichikawa KI, et al. Influence of plasma lipoprotein(a) levels on coronary vasomotor response to acetylcholine. *J Am Coll Cardiol* 1995;26: 1242–1250.

25 Sorensen KE, Celermajer DS, Georgakopoulos D, et al. Impairment of endothelium-dependent dilation is an early event in children with familial hypercholesterolemia and is related to the Lp(a) level. *J Clin Invest* 1994;93:50–55.

26 Camejo G, Camejo-Hurt E, Wiklund O, et al. Association of apoB lipoproteins with arterial proteoglycans: pathological significance and molecular basis. *Atherosclerosis* 1998;139:205–222.

27 Skälen K, Gustafsson M, Rydberg EK, et al. Subendothelial retention of atherogenic lipoproteins in early atherosclerosis. *Nature* 2002;417:750.

28 Keesler GA, Gabel BR, Devlin CM, et al. The binding activity of the macrophage lipoprotein(a)/apolipoprotein(a) receptor is induced by cholesterol via a post-translational mechanism and recognized distinct kringle domains of apolipoprotein(a). *J Biol Chem* 1996;271: 32096–32104.

29 Scanu AM. Proteolytic modifications of lipoprotein(a): potential relevance to its postulated athero-thrombogenic role. *J Invest Med* 1998;46:359–363.

30 Fortunato JE, Bassiouny HS, Song RH, et al. Apolipoprotein(a) fragments in relation to human carotid plaque instability. *J Vasc Surg* 2000;32:555–563.

31 Formato M, Farina M, Spirito R. Evidence for a pro-inflammatory and proteolytic environment in plaques from endarterectomy segments of human carotid arteries. *Arterioscler Thromb Vasc Biol* 2004;24:129–135.

32 Nakajima K, Hinman J, Pfaffinger D, et al. Changes in plasma triglyceride levels shift lipoprotein(a) density in parallel with that of low-density lipoprotein independently of apolipoprotein(a) size. *Arterioscler Thromb Vasc Biol* 2001;21:1238–1243.

33 Nielsen LB, Juul K, Nordestgaard BG. Increased degradation of lipoprotein(a) in atherosclerotic compared with nonlesioned aortic intima-inner media of rabbits. *Arterioscler Thromb Vasc Biol* 1998;18:641–649.

34 Klezovitch O, Edelstein C, Scanu AM. Evidence that the fibrinogen binding domain of apo(a) is outside the lysine binding site (LBS) of kringle IV-10. A study involving naturally-occurring lysine binding defective lipoprotein(a) phenotypes. *J Clin Invest* 1996;98: 185–191.

35 Scanu AM, Miles LA, Fless GM, et al. Rhesus monkey lipoprotein(a) binds to lysine–sepharose and u937 monocytoid cells less efficiently than human lipoprotein(a) – evidence for the dominant role of kringle 4–37. *J Clin Invest* 1993;91:283–291.

36 Edelstein C, Yousef M, Scanu AM. Elements in the C-terminus of apolipoprotein(a) responsible for the binding to the tenth type III module of human fibronectin. *J Lipid Res* 2005;46:2673–2680.

37 Klezovitch O, Edelstein C, Scanu AM. Stimulation of interleukin-8 production in human THP-1 macrophages by apolipoprotein(a): evidence for a critical involvement of elements of its C-terminal domain. *J Biol Chem* 2001; 276:46864–46869.

38 Lou XJ, Boonmark NW, Horrigan FT, et al. Fibrinogen deficiency reduces vascular accumulation of apolipoprotein(a) and development of atherosclerosis in apolipoprotein(a) transgenic mice. *Proc Natl Acad Sci USA* 1998; 95:12591–12595.

39 Beisiegel U, Niendorf A, Wolf K, et al. Lipoprotein(a) in the arterial wall. *Eur Heart J* 1990;11(Suppl E):174–183.

40 de la Pena-Diaz A, Izaguirre-Avila R, Angles-Cano E. Lipoprotein Lp(a) and atherothrombotic disease. *Arch Med Res* 2000;31:353–359.

41 Fan J, Shimoyamada H, Sun H, et al. Transgenic rabbits expressing human apolipoprotein(a) develop more extensive atherosclerotic lesions in response to a cholesterol-rich diet. *Arterioscler Thromb Vasc Biol* 2001;21:88–94.

42 Fan J, Sun H, Unoki H, et al. Enhanced atherosclerosis in Lp(a) WHHL transgenic rabbits. *Ann NY Acad Sci* 2001; 947:362–365.

CHAPTER 10

Oxidative stress and vascular disease

Dominik Behrendt, MD *& Peter Ganz,* MD

Oxidative stress

The term oxidative stress implies a condition in which cells are exposed to excessive levels of reactive oxygen species (ROS). High oxidant stress occurs when the formation rate of ROS exceeds the capacity of physiological antioxidant defense mechanisms. Oxidative stress changes the redox state of cells that can be estimated within the cellular environment by measuring the ratio of redox couples. Growing evidence suggests the critical involvement of increased vascular oxidant stress in the pathogenesis of many cardiovascular diseases including atherosclerosis and its risk factors [1] (Figure 10.1). ROS production often begins with reduction of molecular oxygen to superoxide anion (O_2^-) by various oxidases. Superoxide is a source of other oxygen-centered radicals such as hydrogen peroxide (H_2O_2)

and hydroxyl (OH) radicals, which participate in lipid peroxidation. Superoxide has also been implicated in the oxidation of low-density lipoprotein (LDL) cholesterol.

Involvement of ROS in the pathogenesis of vascular disease

ROS serve as second messengers to activate multiple signaling pathways in vascular wall cells. Thus, the abundance of ROS, and particularly excessive generation of O_2^-, potentially alters several important physiological functions including regulation of blood flow, coagulation, inflammation, and cellular growth [2]. Abundant generation of ROS may participate in the pathogenesis of vascular disease, particularly in atherogenesis. Different mechanisms

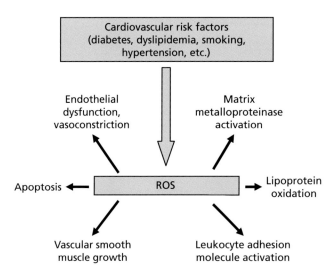

Figure 10.1 Cardiovascular risk factors augment ROS and activate pro-atherogenic pathways. (Adapted from Harrison et al., *Am J Cardiol* 2003;91(Suppl):7A–11A).

for the involvement of oxidative stress in the pathogenesis of vascular disease include promotion of lipid peroxidation, inactivation of vasoprotective substances, and activation of pro-inflammatory and proliferative genes.

Oxidation of LDL

ROS participate in the oxidation of LDL particles, a step critical in the initiation and progression of atherosclerotic lesions. LDL accumulates in the subendothelial space of arteries where it undergoes oxidative modification. Minimally modified LDL, characterized by oxidation principally involving its lipid components and still recognized by LDL receptors, promotes the recruitment of monocytes into the vessel wall and their differentiation into macrophages. Further oxidative modification of minimally oxidized LDL results in fully oxidized LDL, which is recognized by scavenger receptors on macrophages. The oxidation of the LDL particle ignites a number of events that promote the development of atherosclerotic lesions [3]. The receptor-mediated uptake of oxidized LDL by macrophages results in foam cell formation in fatty streaks, the precursors of atheromatous plaques. Furthermore, oxidized LDL promotes leukocyte adhesion to the endothelium, stimulates the release of cytokines from cells within the artery wall, can be directly cytotoxic and causes endothelial dysfunction [4–6]. Superoxide anion importantly mediates LDL oxidation, both as a reactive oxygen radical and as a required substrate or cofactor in the oxidation reactions catalyzed by pro-oxidant enzymes, particularly myeloperoxidase, ceruloplasmin, and lipoxygenases.

Inactivation of other biologically active free radicals

ROS produced by vascular wall cells can directly inactivate other biologically active free radicals, thereby disturbing vascular homeostasis. One major target of ROS, and O_2^- in particular, is endothelium-derived nitric oxide (NO), a key player in the defense against the development of vascular disease. Given the highly reactive and unstable state of both O_2^- and the NO radical, they unsurprisingly react very rapidly to form the major product peroxynitrite. Through this reaction, abundantly produced O_2^- leads to direct inactivation of NO, resulting in loss

of its vasoprotective functions, while the product peroxynitrite is vasotoxic. Under physiological conditions endogenous antioxidant defense mechanisms, including intra- and extracellular forms of superoxide dismutase (SOD), glutathione and glutathione peroxidases, catalase, and antioxidant vitamins C and E, combat oxidant stress. Despite these antioxidant defenses, the degradation of NO by ROS participates prominently in vascular diseases and appears to play a causative role in the impairment of endothelium-dependent vasomotor function.

Activation of pro-inflammatory and proliferative genes

Accumulating evidence suggests that ROS control vascular gene expression [7] through specific redox-sensitive signal transduction pathways. Transcription factors influenced by the cellular redox state include nuclear factor kappa B (NF-κB) and activator protein-1 (AP-1) [7–9]. NF-κB activation participates in the transcription of numerous pro-inflammatory genes, including most cytokine genes. The modulation of pro-inflammatory genes by ROS likely plays a major role in the pathogenesis of vascular disease [10]. For example, the expression of pro-inflammatory adhesion molecules, e.g., vascular cell adhesion molecule 1 (VCAM-1) and intercellular adhesion molecule 1 (ICAM-1), and monocyte chemoattractant protein 1 (MCP-1) occurs through redox-sensitive mechanisms. Underscoring the role of ROS in the signaling pathway, oxidase inhibitors can block cytokine-stimulated VCAM-1 and ICAM-1 gene expression in human aortic endothelial cells (EC). Similarly, oxidase inhibitors also can block angiotensin II (ATII) induced expression of VCAM-1 and MCP-1 [11].

Sources of ROS

Intracellular sources of free radicals and ROS include the NAD(P)H oxidases, nitric oxide synthases (NOS), xanthine oxidoreductase, lipoxygenases, cyclooxygenases, and mitochondrial oxidases (Figure 10.2). NAD(P)H oxidases, endothelial nitric oxide synthase (eNOS), and xanthine oxidoreductase participate importantly in human vessels and are relevant sources of O_2^- overproduction in vascular disease states and atherosclerosis in particular.

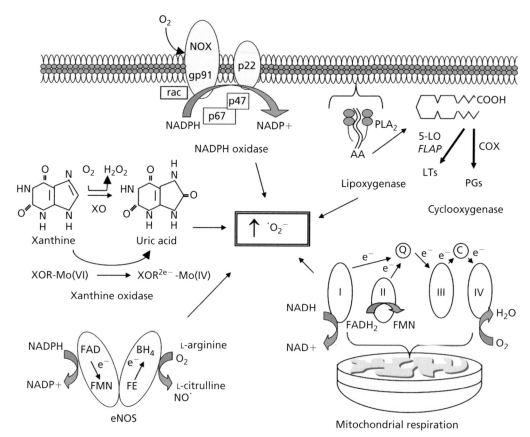

Figure 10.2 Sources of superoxide in the vasculature. NADPH oxidase is activated when the cytoplasmic subunits p67 and p47 and the small G protein rac assemble with the membrane-bound NOX (vascular homolog of gp91^{phox}) and p22^{phox}. The lipoxygenases and COX generate ROS indirectly by promoting formation of inflammatory mediators. Arachidonic acid (AA) that is cleaved from the membrane by phospholipase A$_2$ (PLA$_2$) is then metabolized by 5-lipoxygenase (5-LO) in the presence of its accessory protein (FLAP) to form leukotrienes (LTs). AA is also metabolized by the cyclooxygenases to form members of another family of inflammatory mediators, the prostaglandins (PGs). Mitochondria generate superoxide as electrons are transferred from complex I to complex IV during cellular respiration. XO is an additional source of ROS. Finally, eNOS, when substrate or co-factors are depleted, uncouples to generate superoxide. Q indicates coenzyme Q; C, cytochrome C; FAD, flavin adenine dinucleotide; FMN, flavin mononucleotide; FE, heme iron; BH$_4$, tetrahydrobiopterin. (Reprinted from Leopold et al., *Arterioscler Thromb Vasc Biol* 2005; 25:1332–1340).

NAD(P)H oxidase

Membrane-associated NAD(P)H oxidases, also known as Nox enzymes, are major sources of ROS in vascular tissue [12–14]. At a molecular level, the NAD(P)H oxidases of the vascular tissue appear analogous to the well-characterized phagocytic NAD(P)H oxidase, a protein complex consisting of the protein flavocytochrome b558 formed by the catalytic subunit Nox2 (previously known as gp91 phox), the subunit 22phox and of the cytosolic subunits p47phox, p67phox and G protein rac1 or rac2 [15].

Several Nox proteins (Nox1, Nox3, Nox4) representing molecular homologs of the NAD(P)H oxidase large membrane subunit (Nox2; gp91phox) have been identified [16]. Most cells express multiple differentially regulated Nox subunits. The profile of subunit expression of NAD(P)H oxidases varies both in different vascular beds and in different cell types of the vascular tissue. While Nox2 is expressed in endothelial and adventitial cells of large vessels and in vascular smooth muscle cells (VSMC) of smaller vessels, Nox4 is constitutively expressed in VSMC and EC [17–21]. Pro-atherosclerotic stimuli such as ATII, mechanical stretch, and several pro-inflammatory cytokines stimulate the expression and activity of NAD(P)H oxidases [2].

NAD(P)H oxidases likely play an important role in the oxidative mechanisms involved in hypertension, diabetes and atherosclerosis [22]. Vascular cells and macrophages express NAD(P)H oxidases in atherosclerotic arteries, and some of its subunits have been implicated in atherogenesis.

Increased expression of p22phox mRNA and protein occurs in animal models of atherosclerosis. The subunit p22phox is expressed weakly in non-diseased human coronary arteries, while enhanced expression was detected in neointimal and medial VSMC and infiltrating macrophages in hypercellular regions and at the shoulder region of atherosclerotic lesions [23]. Similarly in experimental models of atherosclerosis, the subunit p47phox increases in diseased compared to non-diseased vessels [24]. p47phox protein has been detected in the adventitia, media, and the neointima, and also in areas of macrophage infiltration. In animals, coronary endothelial cell p47phox participates importantly in increased NAD(P)H oxidase activity in response to agonists such as phorbol ester and tumor necrosis factor alpha (TNF-α) [25]. Disruption of the p47phox gene resulted in decreased vascular superoxide production and inhibited VSMC proliferation. In animal models of atherosclerosis, p47phox gene deficiency resulted in lower levels of aortic superoxide production and reduced atherosclerotic lesion formation in the descending aorta [26]. Such observations support a role for p47phox and NAD(P)H oxidase in atherogenesis.

The subunit Nox2 (gp91phox) may play a role in atherosclerotic lesion development as well. Expressed in intimal VSMC and part of the leukocyte oxidase, Nox2 likely participates in chronic human lesion formation and plaque destabilization [27]. In explanted human atherosclerotic coronary arteries, Nox2 co-localizes with p22phox mainly in plaque macrophages and correlates with plaque macrophage content, whereas Nox4 localizes only in non-phagocytic vascular cells [27]. In directional coronary atherectomy specimens of patients with angina pectoris, ROS generation was higher in unstable vs stable patients and associates closely with the distribution of Nox2 and oxidized LDL [28]. Compared to non-coronary artery disease (non-CAD) patients, coronary arteries from human CAD patients showed increased NAD(P)H oxidase subunit expression, mainly p22phox and Nox2, which correlated in part with higher monocyte/macrophage infiltration, while the level of Nox4 expression correlated most strongly with increased NAD(P)H oxidase activity independent of the presence of CAD [29].

Endothelial nitric oxide synthase

Under certain conditions, the NO producing enzyme eNOS may become a source of ROS. eNOS comprises two globular protein modules, the reductase and oxygenase domain, connected via a flexible protein strand. The reductase domain generates electrons required for NO synthesis by binding NADPH and catalyzing its dehydrogenation. The electrons transfer across the flexible protein strand to the oxygenase domain, which consists of the catalytic center responsible for NO production and binds heme, L-arginine, and tetrahydrobiopterin (BH$_4$) [30], a critical cofactor required for NO synthesis. Depletion of BH$_4$ may result in "uncoupling" of the enzyme eNOS and production of O$_2^-$ instead of NO. Thus, optimal concentration of BH$_4$ is essential for NO production. Through uncoupling of eNOS, deficiency of BH$_4$ may directly contribute to the imbalance between NO and O$_2^-$ production. Peroxynitrite can oxidize BH$_4$, causing its depletion [31]. Protection of BH$_4$ and restoration of eNOS enzymatic activity likely mediates in part the beneficial effect of the antioxidant vitamin C on vascular endothelial function [32]. The critical role of BH$_4$ in NO production is supported by the observation that its replacement partially corrects coronary endothelial dysfunction in patients with CAD [33]. Acute administration of BH$_4$ also improves endothelial function in chronic smokers and patients with hypercholesterolemia [34]. In human diabetic vessels *ex vivo*, dysfunctional eNOS relevantly contributes to the production of vascular O$_2^-$ and NAD(P)H oxidase. Intracellular supplementation of BH$_4$ reduces superoxide production driven by eNOS, supporting the functional role of BH$_4$-dependent eNOS uncoupling in human vessels [35].

Indirect evidence indicates that eNOS uncoupling contributes to endothelial dysfunction and increased production of superoxide anion in hypercholesterolemia [36], hypertension [37], diabetes [38,39], and heart failure [40]. Dysfunctional eNOS may also participate in atherogenesis. While several animal studies have revealed that eNOS gene deficiency results in enhanced atherosclerosis [41,42], other evidence suggests that chronic over-expression of eNOS under certain pathologic conditions does not inhibit, but rather accelerates atherosclerosis [43,44].

Xanthine oxidoreductase

Mammalian xanthine oxidoreductase exists in two interconvertible isoforms, xanthine dehydrogenase (XDH) and xanthine oxidase (XO). XO derives from the initially synthesized XDH, either reversibly by conformational changes or irreversibly by proteolysis. The absolute amount of XO and the ratio of XO to XDH importantly modulate cellular ROS generation. XO is a relevant source of vascular O_2^- production [45–48]. XO metabolizes hypoxanthine, xanthine, and NADH to form O_2 and H_2O_2. XO-generated ROS have been implicated in various clinico-pathologic entities, including ischemia/reperfusion injury, hypercholesterolemia [49], and endothelial dysfunction.

Endothelium-bound XO activity has been shown to be increased in patients with CAD, and associates with impaired radial artery flow-mediated dilation [50]. Orally administered allopurinol rapidly reverses endothelial dysfunction of resistance vessels in smokers, suggesting that XO contributes to endothelial dysfunction caused by cigarette smoking [51]. Similarly, oxypurinol improves brachial artery endothelium-dependent vasomotor responses to acetylcholine (Ach) in hypercholesterolemic patients [52]. In the coronary arteries of CAD patients, electron spin resonance studies showed activation of both NAD(P)H oxidase and XO, and also demonstrated an inverse correlation between endothelial XO activity and the effect of vitamin C on endothelium-dependent vasodilation [50]. In human coronary arteries from CAD patients, the activity and protein expression of XO increased compared to arteries from non-CAD patients, whereas XDH levels remained unchanged [29].

The NAD(P)H oxidase system appears to be critically involved the regulation of XO formation from XDH [53]. H_2O_2 markedly enhances the irreversible conversion of XDH to XO, leading to increased ROS production by XO [54]. By stimulating XDH to XO conversion, the NAD(P)H oxidase system potentially further amplifies the production of ROS.

Vascular endothelium and NO

Abundantly produced ROS target the vascular endothelium and its key mediator, NO. Critically maintaining vascular integrity, vascular endothelium serves not merely as barrier between flowing blood and vascular wall but also uses this strategic location to maintain vascular homeostasis by producing and releasing factors that regulate inflammation, cellular proliferation, and coagulation, and also by modulating vascular tone, caliber, and blood flow in response to numerous humoral, neural, and mechanical stimuli.

NO mediates many of the protective functions of the endothelium. In 1980, Furchgott and Zawadzki [55] demonstrated that isolated arteries relaxed in response to ACh only if the endothelium was intact. In contrast, arteries lacking endothelium constricted in response to ACh. Further studies revealed that ACh stimulated the release of NO, a potent vasodilatory substance, by the endothelium. When NO is lost, e.g., following mechanical denudation of the endothelium or due to pathological disease states affecting the endothelium, a paradoxical vasoconstriction resulting from the direct effect of ACh on vascular smooth muscle replaces the normal vasodilatory response to ACh.

In addition to its potent vasodilating effect, NO counteracts leukocyte adhesion to the endothelium [56,57], vascular smooth muscle proliferation [58], and platelet aggregation [59]. These biological actions of NO render it an important component in the endogenous defense against vascular injury, inflammation, and thrombosis, all key events in vascular diseases including atherosclerosis.

Oxidative stress and endothelial dysfunction

Endothelial dysfunction is a hallmark of many vascular disease states, including hypertension, diabetes mellitus, and atherosclerosis. Accelerated degradation of NO by ROS accounts for a large portion of reduced NO bioavailability and endothelial dysfunction. The EC redox rheostat is primarily regulated by the production of and interaction between NO and O_2^-. Superoxide can inactivate NO directly by reacting very rapidly to form vasoinactive peroxynitrite, a powerful and damaging oxidant more stable than either O_2^- or NO [60,61]. In experimental models of vascular disease, increased O_2^- production participates critically in reduced NO bioactivity and endothelial dysfunction [49]. In human atherosclerotic coronary arteries, p22phox, a subunit of the multi-subunit protein complex NAD(P)H oxidase, increases markedly compared to non-atherosclerotic arteries. Increased superoxide production due to enhanced NAD(P)H activity associates with impaired NO-mediated vasorelaxation in human blood vessels [35]. Scavengers of superoxide restore endothelium-dependent vasomotion in animals and humans with atherosclerosis [62].

Impaired defense mechanisms against oxidant stress can contribute to the detrimental effects of ROS by allowing their unopposed actions on the vessel wall. Under physiological conditions, SOD, a major antioxidant enzyme system of the vessel wall, accelerates the removal of O_2^-. The cytosolic form of SOD permits the release of NO from the endothelium [63–65] and NO-mediated VSMC relaxation [63]. Extracellular SOD likely protects NO during its diffusion from the endothelium to vascular smooth muscle [66]. In patients with CAD, the activity of endothelial SOD diminishes substantially, contributing to coronary endothelial dysfunction [67].

Endothelial vasomotor function

Endothelial dysfunction has several consequences, including impaired endothelium-dependent, NO-mediated vasodilation. Accordingly, testing of endothelium-dependent, NO-mediated vasomotor function has emerged as a useful tool to assess the functional integrity of vascular endothelium *in vivo*. Endothelial function is most commonly measured as the vasomotor response to pharmacological or physical stimuli such as ACh, methacholine, bradykinin, serotonin, substance P, and shear stress [68–72]. The endothelium-dependent vasodilatory response may serve as surrogate for the bioavailability of NO. A well-established technique for the evaluation of coronary endothelial function involves assessment of the change in epicardial diameter in response to graded concentrations of intracoronary ACh using quantitative coronary angiography. Similarly, Doppler flow velocity measurements in response to ACh can assess microvascular endothelial function of the coronary circulation [73–76].

Ludmer and colleagues [68] first showed that ACh infused into the coronary artery causes normal epicardial dilation in patients with angiographically smooth coronary arteries, but causes dose-dependent abnormal constriction in patients with angiographic CAD. Coronary endothelial dysfunction also occurs in angiographically smooth arteries if overt atherosclerosis is present in one or more remaining branches of the coronary artery tree [76]. Cardiovascular risk factors predispose to endothelial dysfunction, even in the absence of atherosclerotic lesions. Abnormal coronary constriction to ACh independently associates with cardiovascular risk factors, and the number of risk factors strongly predicts coronary vasomotor response [69]. Such observations demonstrate that endothelial vasomotor dysfunction can occur well before the structural manifestations of atherosclerosis. Not merely confined to atherosclerotic epicardial vessels, endothelial dysfunction also extends to the coronary microcirculation, where it potentially contributes to myocardial ischemia.

High-resolution ultrasound provides a noninvasive technique to assess endothelium-dependent, flow-mediated dilation of the brachial artery and evaluate endothelial function of the peripheral vascular bed [71,77–81]. This technique employs increased hemodynamic shear stress during reactive hyperemia as a stimulus to provoke the release of NO and induce endothelium-dependent, flow-mediated dilation (FMD) of the brachial artery. Endothelial function of forearm resistance vessels can be assessed by measurement of forearm blood flow (FBF) responses to intra-arterial agonists using strain gauge plethysmography [82–86].

Several studies in patients with atherosclerosis or its risk factors have demonstrated that impaired endothelial function occurs not only in the coronary but also in the peripheral circulation, suggesting that endothelial dysfunction is a generalized, systemic process. Both FMD of the brachial artery [87] and FBF responses to ACh assessed by strain gauge plethysmography [88] are abnormal in hypertensive patients compared to controls. Subjects with type 1 [82] and type 2 [82,84] diabetes mellitus have impaired FBF responses to methacholine, as do patients with dyslipidemia [89]. Advanced age [90] and cigarette smoking [91–93] also associate with reduced endothelial function in the forearm vessels. There is a modest correlation between coronary and brachial artery endothelial function in subjects who undergo both tests [71].

Endothelial vasomotor dysfunction and oxidative stress

Endothelial vasomotor dysfunction has been attributed to reduced bioactivity of NO, and increased vascular oxidant stress is a major cause of loss of NO bioavailability and endothelial dysfunction. In humans, O_2^- production stimulated by NAD(P)H activity correlates with endothelial vasomotor dysfunction and risk factors for atherosclerosis. Inhibition of NAD(P)H oxidases in human blood vessels results in attenuated O_2^- production, enhanced NO bioavailability, and improved endothelial function [94]. In patients with hypercholesterolemia, the endothelium-dependent coronary vasomotor response to ACh associates with susceptibility of LDL to oxidation, underscoring the importance of oxidative stress as a determinant of coronary endothelial dysfunction [72]. Scavenging O_2^- and other oxygen-derived free radicals likely influences NO bioavailability and endothelial vasomotor dysfunction under various pathologic conditions. In patients *in vivo*, intra-arterial delivery of supraphysiological doses of the antioxidant vitamin C can reverse endothelial vasomotor dysfunction. This favorable effect occurs in patients with a variety of risk factors that impair endothelial function, including hypercholesterolemia [95], type 1 and type 2 diabetes mellitus [96,97], smoking [92], and hypertension [98,99]. Thus, supraphysiological doses of the antioxidant vitamin C can acutely improve endothelial function *in vivo*. The magnitude of improvement achieved by acutely administered vitamin C may reflect the magnitude of prevailing vascular oxidant stress. In a longitudinal study, patients with CAD experiencing cardiovascular events had impaired peripheral endothelial vasodilatory function at baseline, but greater benefit from co-administered vitamin C compared with patients without cardiovascular events [86].

Hemodynamic forces and endothelial dysfunction

Hemodynamic forces, including flow-induced shear stress and pressure-generated strain, continuously assault EC that form the interface between flowing blood and vessel wall EC. Currently available evidence suggests that vascular endothelium can discriminate among various fluid mechanical forces generated by pulsatile blood flow and transduce them into regulatory events. Effects of shear stress on the vascular endothelium include modulation of the expression of various genes and the release of endothelium-derived mediators. Additionally, increased blood flow and shear stresses can alter the redox state of EC and redox-sensitive gene expression. Exposure of the endothelium to steady laminar shear stress vs comparable levels of non-laminar, turbulent shear stress results in the upregulation of genes such as eNOS, COX-2, and Mn-SOD, which generally support vasoprotective functions [100]. Current evidence also suggests that ROS can function as second messengers in the effects of hemodynamic shear stress on vascular function. *In vitro*, EC exposed to shear force exhibit increased O_2^- production associated with increased levels of ICAM-1 mRNA. Pretreating EC with antioxidants inhibits shear-induced ICAM-1 expression [101]. In contrast to effects of laminar shear stress that occur only transiently, exposing EC to continuous oscillatory shear results in a sustained increase in NADH oxidase activity, induces the redox-sensitive gene heme oxygenase 1, and increases intracellular O_2^- production [102]. Pulsatility of flow critically determines flow-induced O_2^- production in EC, and EC exposed to both unidirectional and oscillatory shear stress show increased O_2^- production associated with increased mRNA levels of p22phox, suggesting that increased expression of NADH-dependent oxidase mediates flow-induced increase in superoxide anion production [103].

Another hemodynamic force that may promote atherogenesis by inducing oxidative stress in EC involves cyclic strain. In cultured human aortic EC, short-term pulsatile stretch increases O_2^- involving the enzymes NADPH oxidase and eNOS [104]. This oxidative response of EC exposed to cyclic strain involves the protein kinase C pathway and associates with a marked NF-κB activation [105]. Additionally, cyclic strain can induce EC expression of genes such as MCP-1. Cyclic strain inducibility of MCP-1 in EC involves enhanced levels of intracellular ROS, which act as second messengers [106].

Thus, hemodynamic forces contribute to enhanced production of ROS and thereby to endothelial dysfunction. Indeed, regions exposed to disturbed flow, e.g., coronary branch points, are preferred sites for both abnormal endothelium-dependent vasomotor responses [107] and the formation of atherosclerotic lesions, underscoring the relevance of hemodynamic forces in endothelial dysfunction and atherogenesis.

Oxidant stress and inflammation

Inflammatory processes play a central role in various vascular disease states including atherosclerosis. Several markers of inflammation, including cellular adhesion molecules, cytokines, and C-reactive protein (CRP), can predict future cardiovascular events. Activation of the vascular endothelium constitutes the initiating event in vascular inflammation and the development of vascular disease. Once activated, endothelium expresses cellular adhesion molecules and cytokines that work in concert to recruit circulating inflammatory cells into the vessel wall (see Chapter 2). Increased production of ROS is a common mechanism underlying the inflammatory activation of the endothelium. Through the induction of redox-sensitive genes that produce pro-inflammatory mediators and the activation of specific signaling pathways, ROS can directly promote vascular inflammation. For example, superoxide and peroxynitrite can lead to activation of redox-sensitive transcription factors such as NF-κB, a pro-inflammatory transcription factor involved in the transcriptional regulation of genes for most cytokines, and AP-1 in EC, VSMC, and macrophages. Activation of NF-κB associates with endothelial dysfunction and vascular inflammation [108]. ATII-induced inflammatory activation of VSMC associates with NF-κB activation [109]. Moreover, VSMC proliferation requires NF-κB [110]. NF-κB activation in the arterial endothelium shows topographic variation. In experimental models, hypercholesterolemia results in NF-κB activation and increased expression of NF-κB-inducible genes, predominantly in endothelial regions with high probability for atherosclerotic lesion development [111].

Transcription factor AP-1 is activated by H_2O_2, LDL, and oxidized LDL in EC and by H_2O_2 and oxidized LDL in VSMC. The regulation of inflammatory genes MCP-1 and ICAM-1 by H_2O_2 is mediated by AP-1 binding elements in the promoter region of these genes [106,112].

ROS regulate several general classes of genes including adhesion molecules and chemotactic factors such as ICAM-1 and MCP-1. Endothelial adhesion molecules play a crucial role in the interaction between the endothelial surface and circulating leukocytes, and mediate the migration of circulating leukocytes through the endothelial layer and their subsequent accumulation in the intima of the vessel wall [56,113,114]. Several experimental models have demonstrated enhanced recruitment of leukocytes in response to increased oxidant stress. For example, using intravital microscopy, infusion of hypoxanthine/XO into the rat mesenteric circulation increases the number of both rolling and adherent leukocytes [115]. Oxidant-mediated increased adhesion associates with increased ICAM-1 expression. An anti-ICAM-1 antibody can reverse such adhesion, suggesting that increased leukocyte adhesion to vascular endothelium induced by oxidant stress is attributable at least in part to ICAM-1- and (due to other evidence) selectin-dependent mechanisms. The transcription of the ICAM-1 gene in response to cytokines such as TNF-α involves the activation of protein kinase C and, subsequently, the generation of oxidants and activation of NF-κB [116].

The regulation of VCAM-1 expression on vascular EC, another early feature in the pathogenesis of atherosclerosis and other inflammatory diseases, also links to oxidative stress through specific antioxidant sensitive transcriptional regulatory mechanisms [117]. ATII-mediated stimulation of VCAM- expression in EC associates with enhanced ROS production and activation of endothelial NF-κB [118]. ROS also promotes the proliferation of vascular wall cells. Endogenously produced H_2O_2 modulates the proliferation of VSMC [119] and, in low concentrations, H_2O_2 functions as an intracellular signal that triggers a genetic program related to cell growth [120].

Inflammation is an important component in the pathogenesis of vascular disease. In the inflammatory milieu of vascular disease states, cytokines and growth factors promote in turn the generation of

ROS. Cytokines and growth factors such as TNF-α [121], interleukin-1-beta, interferon gamma, and PDGF [122] activate membrane bound NADPH oxidase to produce superoxide in EC. PDGF, thrombin, and TNF-α activate NADH driven superoxide production in VSMC. Thus, the initial inflammatory response ignited by ROS may result in further amplification of vascular oxidant stress, initiating a vicious circle of both oxidative and inflammatory processes critically involved in the development and manifestation of vascular disease.

Oxidant stress and the vulnerable plaque

ROS production in human coronary artery plaques appears to play a role in regulating plaque stability and influencing the occurrence of acute coronary syndromes. Acute coronary syndromes in most cases result from disruption of the atheromatous plaque and exposure of the plaque's thrombogenic lipid core to the bloodstream, resulting in superimposed thrombus formation and partial or complete vessel occlusion. Pathologic and angioscopic examinations have identified ruptured plaques as the responsible lesion in 56–95% of acute coronary syndromes. The majority of myocardial infarctions occur due to the occlusion of coronary segments that contained only mild to moderate (<50%) stenoses in previous coronary angiograms. Thus, infarct-related coronary lesions are not necessarily severely obstructive. In contrast, the functional state of the atheroma – its composition and vulnerability – has emerged as the most important determinant for the occurrence of plaque rupture and its clinical sequelae. The advanced atherosclerotic lesion has a fibrous cap overlying a highly thrombogenic core of lipid and necrotic tissue located within the eccentrically thickened intima. The thickness, the tensile strength and the integrity of the fibrous cap importantly determine plaque stability. The vulnerable plaque typically has a larger lipid core and a thinner more friable fibrous cap than the stable atherosclerotic lesion [123–125]. The fibrous cap consists mainly of extracellular matrix components. Localized inflammation contributes decisively to plaque instability and rupture [126]. By secreting proteolytic enzymes, including members of the matrix metalloproteinases (MMP) family, macrophages can degrade extracellular matrix, weaken the connective-tissue framework of the fibrous cap, and thus increase the risk of plaque rupture. The vulnerable plaque typically contains a prominent accumulation of inflammatory cells including macrophages and T lymphocytes [127–129].

Particularly in areas of high oxidant stress, ROS can actively modulate this process of matrix degradation, thus contributing to the instability of atherosclerotic plaques. Degradation of the extracellular matrix depends on the action of MMPs, particularly MMP-2 and -9. ROS activates the latent proforms of these enzymes (pro-MMP-2 and pro-MMP-9) [130]. Furthermore, superoxide can induce the expression of extracellular matrix-degrading enzymes including MMP-1 and -9 in foam cells, directly contributing to plaque instability. Increased oxidized LDL may further augment plaque instability. Lysophosphatidylcholine, a major component of oxidized LDL, increases the release of MMP-2 by activating endothelial NAD(P)H oxidase [131]. Moreover, oxidized LDL and cytokines potentially promote matrix degradation by inducing membrane type 1-MMP expression [112]. In coronary sections obtained postmortem, the NAD(P)H oxidase subunit p22phox is weakly expressed in non-atherosclerotic coronary arteries, but shows marked expression in atherosclerotic coronary arteries, with intensive immunoreactivity in VSMC, infiltrating macrophages in hypercellular regions and at the shoulder regions of the plaque [23]. ROS production occurs in human coronary plaques obtained from directional coronary atherectomy, and closely associates with the distribution of p22phox, a component of NAD(P)H oxidase, and oxidized LDL. The plaques of patients with unstable angina showed significantly higher ROS generation compared with plaques from patients with stable angina, independent of the degree of coronary stenosis [28].

In coronary artery segments from explanted human hearts, the expression of gp91phox and p22phox mRNA associates with the severity of atherosclerosis. Atherosclerotic coronary arteries show an intense area of superoxide in the plaque shoulder [27].

Oxidative stress and restenosis

Arterial injury induces an immediate and profound increase in vascular oxidative stress, proportional to the degree of injury. Enhanced generation of ROS is mediated in part by the activation of vessel wall NAD(P)H oxidases and associates with induced NF-κB activation [132].

Restenosis following balloon angioplasty, a form of arterial injury, also associates with increased O_2^-, production, a process that likely involves an NAD(P)H oxidase. In the rat carotid artery, increased messenger RNA expression of the p22phox subunit and of homologs of the subunit gp91phox in VSMC, as well as increased gp91phox mRNA in fibroblasts, can occur days after balloon injury [133].

Experimental studies have shown a protective effect of SOD or antioxidants on vasospasm, neo-intimal thickening, or remodeling after balloon injury. The inhibitory effect of antioxidants on smooth muscle cell growth in experiments *in vitro* and *in vivo* suggested a possible beneficial effect on restenosis after coronary angioplasty. In a double-blind randomized trial, treatment of patients with the antioxidant probucol for 4 weeks before and 6 months after coronary angioplasty effectively reduced the rate of restenosis [134]. Assessed by intravascular ultrasound, probucol exerts its anti-restenotic effects predominantly by improving vascular remodeling after angioplasty [135]. In the Probucol Angioplasty Restenosis Trial, treatment of patients with 1000 mg/day of probucol 4 weeks before and until angiographic follow-up 24 weeks later also appeared to reduce restenosis [136].

Clinical outcome studies of antioxidant vitamins

In experimental models, dietary antioxidants such as vitamins C and E can protect against the progression of atherosclerosis. Epidemiological observations suggested an association between diets high in vitamin E or E supplements and decreased rates of cardiovascular disease. However, large-scale intervention studies showed no benefit of vitamin E on cardiovascular events and clinical outcome.

The Gruppo Italiano per lo Studio della Sopravvivenza nell'Infarto (GISSI) Prevenzione Trial, which enrolled 11,000 patients with prior myocardial infarction and randomized them to 300 IU vitamin E vs placebo, found no significant effect of vitamin E during a treatment period of 3.5

years [137]. The HOPE trial [138] randomized 9541 patients in a two-by-two factorial design to receive either 400 IU vitamin E or placebo and either the angiotensin-converting-enzyme inhibitor ramipril or placebo. Over a mean follow-up of 4.5 years, the investigators found no beneficial effect of vitamin E on the primary endpoint, the composite of myocardial infarction, stroke, and death from cardiovascular causes, and also found no significant difference in secondary endpoints including unstable angina, congestive heart failure, revascularization or amputation, death from any cause, complications of diabetes, and cancer. The Study to Evaluate Carotid Ultrasound Changes in Patients Treated with Ramipril [Altace®] and Vitamin E (SECURE) [139] included 732 patients randomized to 2.5 mg/day and 10 mg/day of ramipril or placebo, or to 400 IU of vitamin E or placebo in a factorial design. Carotid ultrasound was used to measure the progression of intimal medial thickening among the groups over 4.5 years of follow up. The progression of carotid thickening was slowed by ramipril, but there was no significant effect of vitamin E. Two trials, the Cambridge Heart Antioxidant Study (CHAOS) and SPACE, that used doses of vitamin E of up to 800 IU reported reduced incidence of cardiovascular events in patients with angiographically proven symptomatic coronary atherosclerosis and in hemodialysis patients with prevalent cardiovascular disease, respectively [140,141].

Taken together, the majority of the performed large scale clinical studies that used antioxidant vitamins at varying concentrations and follow-up times showed no benefit with regard to their respective primary endpoints of clinical outcome and/or progression of atherosclerosis [142]. However, vitamin E may have been used too late in the atherosclerotic process to improve clinical outcome. These trials focused on using antioxidant vitamins to treat late manifestations of atherosclerosis, while oxidant stress may be particularly important in the early stages of this disease [143].

The use of vitamin E as the sole antioxidant may also explain the lack of benefit in these clinical studies. After scavenging a radical, vitamin E becomes a potentially pro-oxidant tocopheroxyl radical, i.e., if it is not recycled back to α-tocopherol by another antioxidant [144,145]. The pro-oxidant potential of antioxidant vitamins, including vitamin E, may have functional relevance *in vivo*. Vitamin C can reduce the vitamin E radical back to vitamin E [146–148]. Therefore, supplementing with a combination of antioxidants, i.e., a "cocktail" of vitamins, may prove more effective than a single antioxidant. Even in a cocktail approach, however, antioxidant vitamins may not be powerful enough or may require a much longer treatment time to show beneficial effects on clinical outcome.

The Heart Protection Study (HPS) [149] randomized 20,536 adults with CAD, other occlusive arterial disease, or diabetes to supplementation with antioxidant vitamins (600 mg vitamin E, 250 mg vitamin C, and 20 mg beta-carotene daily) or matching placebo. Although vitamins substantially increased plasma vitamin concentrations, they did not produce any significant reductions in the 5-year mortality from, or incidence of, any type of vascular disease, cancer, or other major outcome. Investigators found no significant differences in all cause mortality, deaths due to vascular or non-vascular disease, the number non-fatal myocardial infarctions or coronary deaths, stroke, or revascularization. In postmenopausal women with coronary disease, a twice daily combination of 400 IU of vitamin E with 500 mg of vitamin C provided no cardiovascular benefit compared to placebo [150].

Another reason for the observed antioxidant ineffectiveness could relate to the optimum dose and type of antioxidants used. The interpretation of the performed clinical trials is also limited by the lack of assessment of both prevailing oxidant stress and the ability of given antioxidant vitamins to inhibit oxidative injury. The Biomarkers of Oxidative Stress Study (BOSS), which examined the usefulness of quantifying a number of oxidative stress biomarkers, suggested that the F2-isoprostanes offer an accurate quantification of oxidative injury *in vivo* [151]. F2-isoprostanes represent an important biomarker in the assessment of human atherosclerotic cardiovascular disease [152,153]. Biomarkers, which reliably reflect vascular oxidant stress, may be of great value to identify responders and non-responders to antioxidant vitamins in clinical trials.

Given the large body of experimental studies supporting the role of oxidant stress in cardiovascular disease and atherogenesis in particular, the aforementioned negative clinical outcome trials insufficiently refute the "oxidant stress hypothesis" [154,155] but rather indicate that more powerful and more specifically targeted antioxidant regimens may be needed early in the process of vascular dysfunction and disease development to produce a benefit on outcome. For example, a probucol-like potent antioxidant reduced restenosis in patients undergoing percutaneous coronary intervention, most of whom were treated with stents. Interestingly, the antioxidant had a beneficial effect on atherosclerosis in the non-stented reference segments, as evidenced by increase in coronary luminal dimensions [156].

In summary, extensive research has demonstrated a role for ROS and redox-sensitive signaling pathways in several vascular diseases, particularly atherosclerosis. Clinical testing and potential application of these findings will likely require development of novel, potent antioxidants.

References

1 Zalba G, Beaumont J, San Jose G, et al. Vascular oxidant stress: molecular mechanisms and pathophysiological implications. *J Physiol Biochem* 2000;56(1):57–64.

2 Griendling KK, Sorescu D, Ushio-Fukai M. NAD(P)H oxidase: role in cardiovascular biology and disease. *Circ Res* 2000;86(5):494–501.

3 Chisolm GM, Steinberg D. The oxidative modification hypothesis of atherogenesis: an overview. *Free Radical Biol Med* 2000;28(12):1815–1826.

4 Simon BC, Cunningham LD, Cohen RA. Oxidized low density lipoproteins cause contraction and inhibit endothelium-dependent relaxation in the pig coronary artery. *J Clin Invest* 1990;86(1):75–79.

5 Tanner FC, Noll G, Boulanger CM, et al. Oxidized low density lipoproteins inhibit relaxations of porcine coronary arteries. Role of scavenger receptor and endothelium-derived nitric oxide. *Circulation* 1991; 83(6): 2012–2020.

6 Mangin Jr EL, Kugiyama K, Nguy JH, et al. Effects of lysolipids and oxidatively modified low density lipoprotein on endothelium-dependent relaxation of rabbit aorta. *Circ Res* 1993;72(1):161–166.

7 Kunsch C, Medford RM. Oxidative stress as a regulator of gene expression in the vasculature. *Circ Res* 1999;85(8): 753–766.

8 Sun Y, Oberley LW. Redox regulation of transcriptional activators. *Free Radical Biol Med* 1996;21(3):335–348.

9 Winyard PG, Blake DR. Antioxidants, redox-regulated transcription factors, and inflammation. *Adv Pharmacol* 1997;38:403–421.

via nuclear factor-kappaB activation induced by intracellular oxidative stress. *Arterioscler Thromb Vasc Biol* 2000;20(3):645–651.

119 Brown MR, Miller Jr FJ, Li WG, et al. Overexpression of human catalase inhibits proliferation and promotes apoptosis in vascular smooth muscle cells. *Circ Res* 1999;85(6):524–533.

120 Arnold RS, Shi J, Murad E, et al. Hydrogen peroxide mediates the cell growth and transformation caused by the mitogenic oxidase Nox1. *Proc Natl Acad Sci USA* 2001;98(10):5550–5555.

121 De Keulenaer GW, Alexander RW, Ushio-Fukai M, et al. Tumour necrosis factor alpha activates a p22phox based NADH oxidase in vascular smooth muscle. *Biochem J* 1998;329(Pt 3):653–657.

122 Marumo T, Schini-Kerth VB, Fisslthaler B, et al. Platelet-derived growth factor-stimulated superoxide anion production modulates activation of transcription factor NF-kappaB and expression of monocyte chemoattractant protein 1 in human aortic smooth muscle cells. *Circulation* 1997;96(7):2361–2367.

123 Loree HM, Kamm RD, Stringfellow RG, et al. Effects of fibrous cap thickness on peak circumferential stress in model atherosclerotic vessels. *Circ Res* 1992;71(4):850–858.

124 Davies MJ, Richardson PD, Woolf N, et al. Risk of thrombosis in human atherosclerotic plaques: role of extracellular lipid, macrophage, and smooth muscle cell content. *Br Heart J* 1993;69(5):377–381.

125 Felton CV, Crook D, Davies MJ, et al. Relation of plaque lipid composition and morphology to the stability of human aortic plaques. *Arterioscler Thromb Vasc Biol* 1997;17(7):1337–1345.

126 Libby P. Current concepts of the pathogenesis of the acute coronary syndromes. *Circulation* 2001;104(3):365–372.

127 Richardson PD, Davies MJ, Born GV. Influence of plaque configuration and stress distribution on fissuring of coronary atherosclerotic plaques. *Lancet* 1989;2(8669):941–944.

128 Lendon CL, Davies MJ, Born GV, et al. Atherosclerotic plaque caps are locally weakened when macrophages density is increased. *Atherosclerosis* 1991;87(1):87–90.

129 van der Wal AC, Becker AE, van der Loos CM, et al. Site of intimal rupture or erosion of thrombosed coronary atherosclerotic plaques is characterized by an inflammatory process irrespective of the dominant plaque morphology. *Circulation* 1994;89(1):36–44.

130 Rajagopalan S, Meng XP, Ramasamy S, et al. Reactive oxygen species produced by macrophage-derived foam cells regulate the activity of vascular matrix metalloproteinases in vitro. Implications for atherosclerotic plaque stability. *J Clin Invest* 1996;98(11):2572–2579.

131 Inoue N, Takeshita S, Gao D, et al. Lysophosphatidylcholine increases the secretion of matrix metalloproteinase 2 through the activation of NADH/NADPH oxidase in cultured aortic endothelial cells. *Atherosclerosis* 2001;155(1):45–52.

132 Souza HP, Souza LC, Anastacio VM, et al. Vascular oxidant stress early after balloon injury: evidence for increased NAD(P)H oxidoreductase activity. *Free Radical Biol Med* 2000;28(8):1232–1242.

133 Szocs K, Lassegue B, Sorescu D, et al. Upregulation of Nox-based NAD(P)H oxidases in restenosis after carotid injury. *Arterioscler Thromb Vasc Biol* 2002;22(1):21–27.

134 Tardif JC, Cote G, Lesperance J, et al. Probucol and multivitamins in the prevention of restenosis after coronary angioplasty. Multivitamins and Probucol Study Group. *N Engl J Med* 1997;337(6):365–372.

135 Cote G, Tardif JC, Lesperance J, et al. Effects of probucol on vascular remodeling after coronary angioplasty. Multivitamins and Protocol Study Group. *Circulation* 1999;99(1):30–35.

136 Yokoi H, Daida H, Kuwabara Y, et al. Effectiveness of an antioxidant in preventing restenosis after percutaneous transluminal coronary angioplasty: the Probucol Angioplasty Restenosis Trial. *J Am Coll Cardiol* 1997;30(4):855–862.

137 Dietary supplementation with *n*-3 polyunsaturated fatty acids and vitamin E after myocardial infarction: results of the GISSI-Prevenzione trial. Gruppo Italiano per lo Studio della Sopravvivenza nell'Infarto miocardico. *Lancet* 1999;354(9177):447–455.

138 Yusuf S, Dagenais G, Pogue J, et al. Vitamin E supplementation and cardiovascular events in high-risk patients. The Heart Outcomes Prevention Evaluation Study Investigators. *N Engl J Med* 2000;342(3):154–160.

139 Lonn E, Yusuf S, Dzavik V, et al. Effects of ramipril and vitamin E on atherosclerosis: the study to evaluate carotid ultrasound changes in patients treated with ramipril and vitamin E (SECURE). *Circulation* 20 2001;103(7):919–925.

140 Boaz M, Smetana S, Weinstein T, et al. Secondary prevention with antioxidants of cardiovascular disease in endstage renal disease (SPACE): randomised placebo-controlled trial. *Lancet* 2000;356(9237):1213–1218.

141 Stephens NG, Parsons A, Schofield PM, et al. Randomised controlled trial of vitamin E in patients with coronary disease: Cambridge Heart Antioxidant Study (CHAOS). *Lancet* 1996;347(9004):781–786.

142 Jialal I, Devaraj S. Antioxidants and atherosclerosis: don't throw out the baby with the bath water. *Circulation* 2003;107(7):926–928.

143 Lonn E. Do antioxidant vitamins protect against atherosclerosis? The proof is still lacking. *J Am Coll Cardiol* 2001;38(7):1795–1798.

144 Santanam N, Parthasarathy S. Paradoxical actions of antioxidants in the oxidation of low density lipoprotein by peroxidases. *J Clin Invest* 1995;95(6):2594–2600.

145 Landmesser U, Harrison DG. Oxidant stress as a marker for cardiovascular events: Ox marks the spot. *Circulation* 2001;104(22):2638–2640.

146 May JM, Qu ZC, Morrow JD. Interaction of ascorbate and alpha-tocopherol in resealed human erythrocyte ghosts. Transmembrane electron transfer and protection from lipid peroxidation. *J Biol Chem* 1996;271(18): 10577–10582.

147 Packer JE, Slater TF, Willson RL. Direct observation of a free radical interaction between vitamin E and vitamin C. *Nature* 1979;278(5706):737–738.

148 Frei B. Ascorbic acid protects lipids in human plasma and low-density lipoprotein against oxidative damage. *Am J Clin Nutr* 1991;54(6 Suppl):1113S–1118S.

149 MRC/BHF Heart Protection Study of antioxidant vitamin supplementation in 20,536 high-risk individuals: a randomised placebo-controlled trial. *Lancet* 2002; 360(9326):23–33.

150 Waters DD, Alderman EL, Hsia J, et al. Effects of hormone replacement therapy and antioxidant vitamin supplements on coronary atherosclerosis in postmenopausal women: a randomized controlled trial. *JAMA* 2002;288(19):2432–2440.

151 Kadiiska MB, Gladen BC, Baird DD, et al. Biomarkers of oxidative stress study II: are oxidation products of lipids, proteins, and DNA markers of CCl4 poisoning? *Free Radical Biol Med* 2005;38(6):698–710.

152 Milne GL, Musiek ES, Morrow JD. F2-isoprostanes as markers of oxidative stress in vivo: an overview. *Biomarkers* 2005;10(Suppl 1): S10–S23.

153 Morrow JD. Quantification of isoprostanes as indices of oxidant stress and the risk of atherosclerosis in humans. *Arterioscler Thromb Vasc Biol* 2005;25(2):279–286.

154 Witztum JL, Steinberg D. The oxidative modification hypothesis of atherosclerosis: Does it hold for humans? *Trend Cardiovasc Med* 2001;11(3–4):93–102.

155 Steinberg D, Witztum JL. Is the oxidative modification hypothesis relevant to human atherosclerosis? Do the antioxidant trials conducted to date refute the hypothesis? *Circulation* 2002;105(17):2107–2111.

156 Tardif JC, Gregoire J, Schwartz L, et al. Effects of AGI-1067 and probucol after percutaneous coronary interventions. *Circulation* 2003;107(4):552–558.

CHAPTER 11

Infections and vascular disease

Amir Kol, MD, PhD *& Peter Libby,* MD

Introduction

Although atherosclerosis is widely accepted as an inflammatory disease[1], traditional risk factors do not explain fully its progression and varied clinical expressions. Drug trials for hyperlipidemia, long considered an obvious therapeutic target, have shown extraordinary results in primary and secondary prevention in reducing morbidity and mortality in patients with cardiovascular disease. However, not all patients with atherosclerosis have dyslipidemia and not all dyslipidemic subjects develop atherosclerosis. Therefore, recent years have witnessed an increasing search for non-traditional risk factors. Seroepidemiological and experimental research has focused largely on infectious agents including *Herpesviridae* (herpes simplex virus (HSV) and cytomegalovirus (CMV)), *Chlamydia pneumoniae* (*C. pneumoniae*), and, more recently, *Helicobacter pylori* (*H. pylori*). Although clinical trials have not established a benefit for antibiotic treatment in secondary prevention, infectious agents may yet contribute to atheroma formation and evolution in some instances. This chapter will review current knowledge regarding the biological basis of involvement of infectious agents in vascular disease development, the mechanisms that might trigger clinical manifestations and the results of recent clinical trials.

Seroepidemiology and experimental background

Herpesviridae

Prevalent in the general population, HSV and CMV infections are mostly chronic and asymptomatic. Indeed, approximately 80–90% of the adult population have positive antibody titers against HSV-1 [2] and >60% of adults older than 65 years have serologic evidence of previous exposure to CMV [3]. Early studies demonstrated a higher incidence of CMV seropositivity in patients with carotid atherosclerosis compared with control subjects matched for cholesterol levels and other traditional risk factors [4]. In addition, high IgG titers against CMV may indicate increased risk for restenosis 6 months following percutaneous directional coronary atherectomy: the incidence of restenosis was five-fold greater in seropositive patients compared with seronegative patients [5].

Promotion of atherosclerosis in chickens by infecting them with Marek's disease virus, an avian herpes virus, provided the first experimental evidence that *Herpesviridae* might participate directly in the pathogenesis of vascular disease [6]. Since then, improved molecular techniques have detected CMV DNA in the vascular tree (90% of femoral and abdominal arterial samples from patients undergoing vascular surgery vs 53% in a control group) [7]. Because we lack evidence of an active CMV infection in the human vascular tree, and also because of the wide distribution of CMV DNA in the vascular tree [8], the vascular wall might harbor a latent CMV infection that could induce chronic alterations and damage, leading to the development of atherosclerotic lesions [9]. Indeed, the early atherosclerotic lesions found in the coronary arteries of young trauma victims contain genomic sequences and antigens of *Herpesviridae* [10]. More recently, the concept that a chronic latent infection may cause atherosclerosis has focused most often on *C. pneumoniae*.

Chlamydia pneumoniae

Serologic evidence of previous exposure to *C. pneumoniae* increases with age, reaching approximately

40–50% in the middle-aged population [11]. Compared with control subjects, a higher number of patients affected by coronary artery disease and acute myocardial infarction (MI) has antibody titers and specific circulating immune complexes against *C. pneumoniae* [12,13]. In some studies, serologic evidence of previous *C. pneumoniae* infection associates with an approximate two-fold increase in the risk of coronary artery disease [14]. Moreover, elevated antibody titers or immune complexes containing chlamydial lipopolysaccharide (LPS) may confer independent risk for MI [15].

Approximately 50–80% of atherosclerotic coronary artery specimens contain *C. pneumoniae* DNA [16,17]. However, positive tissue samples do not necessarily correlate with antibody titers, thus raising some doubts about the real meaning of seroepidemiological data. As already described for CMV, *C. pneumoniae* DNA seems widely distributed in the human vascular tree [18], and the coronary arteries of young adults who succumb from noncardiac causes contain *C. pnuemoniae* [19]. Therefore, the concept that the vascular wall can harbor a latent infection capable of inducing chronic alterations and damage that lead to the development of atherosclerotic lesions could apply to *C. pneumoniae* as well. In this respect, extensive studies indicate that *Chlamydiae* can achieve a state of chronic, persistent infection, i.e., be present as a viable organism that eludes laboratory culture [20]. In such conditions, *Chlamydiae* express large amounts of heat shock protein (HSP)60, an intracellular protein highly homologous with human HSP60 that likely possesses protective functions during inflammatory conditions. Indeed, our group detected both chlamydial and human HSP60 in the macrophages of human atheroma. Chlamydial HSP60 can induce the secretion of products relevant to the formation and complications of atheroma, i.e., tumor necrosis factor-α (TNF-α) and matrix metalloproteinases [21]. Such experimental data may provide a direct link between chronic latent chlamydial infection and the development of atherosclerosis.

Helicobacter pylori

Serologic positivity for *H. pylori* reaches approximately 40–50% in the general population [22,23]. Although many seroepidemiologic data link H*erpesviridae* and *C. pneumoniae* to atherosclerosis,

the results regarding *H. pylori* have less strength. Some studies suggest a substantial prevalence of *H. pylori* infection (about 65%) in patients with coronary artery disease [22,23] or previous MI [24]. However, the Atherosclerosis Risk in Communities (ARIC) study, a prospective investigation with a median follow-up period of about 3 years, reported that *H. pylori* associates negatively with coronary heart disease events [25].

H. pylori DNA localized in approximately 52% of atherosclerotic plaques obtained from carotid endarterectomy specimens but not in atherosclerosis-free carotid samples obtained at autopsy [26]. In the same study, half of the DNA-positive samples tested positive for morphological and immunohistochemical evidence of *H. pylori* infection. Although an older study reported negative results [27], a study by Farsak et al. identified *H. pylori* DNA in 37% of carotid endarterectomy specimens vs none of the controls [28]. Moreover, *H. pylori*-specific DNA may localize in human coronary artery specimens [29]. Studies examining *H. pylori* in the vascular tree are less extensive than those investigating *Herpesviridae* and *C. pneumoniae*, perhaps because scientific interest in this agent has emerged more recently. However, *H. pylori* DNA may be also widely distributed in the vascular tree. Although *H. pylori* can cause chronic infection of the gastrointestinal tract and no current evidence suggests active infection in the human vascular tree, the concept that the vascular wall may harbor a latent infection that could induce chronic alterations and damage leading to the development of atherosclerotic lesions might apply to *H. pylori* as well.

Infections and clinical manifestations of vascular disease

Despite substantial seroepidemiological and experimental data, the role and the mechanisms of infectious agents in the development and clinical manifestations of vascular disease remain incompletely understood. Table 11.1 provides an overview of possible mechanisms of microbial contribution to the atherosclerotic process.

Infectious agents as direct cause of vascular disease

Do infectious agents directly cause atherosclerosis? Initial studies in chickens infected with Marek's

Table 11.1 Mechanisms of action of infectious agents in atherosclerosis.

Direct infection of vascular cells
Cell lysis
Lipid accumulation
Cytokine production
Adhesion molecules expression
Tissue factor production

Systemic infection
Increased acute-phase protein levels
Promotion of thrombosis
Local activation in response to systemic endotoxemia
    and cytokinemia
Recruitment and activation of leukocytes resident within
    the vessel wall or atheromatous lesions

Adapted from Kol A, Libby P. *Am Heart J* 1999;138: S450–S452.

disease virus [6] generated the illusion that direct viral infection could induce vascular disease. However, the fibrous lesions developed in that experimental situation required a cholesterol-rich diet in order to resemble a true atheroma. More recent animal studies attempted to define the possible role of a direct infection with *C. pneumoniae*. A study on New Zealand White rabbits fed a normal diet and infected by intranasal inoculation showed lesion development resembling the early stages of atheroma (fatty streaks) in a minority of cases; non-infected animals exhibited no lesions [30]. Another group examined C57BL/6J mice infected in the same manner [31]. In that study, the atherosclerotic lesions of apolipoprotein (ApoE)-deficient mice, which develop atherosclerosis spontaneously, showed *C. pneumoniae* for up to 20 weeks after infection, while only a minority of wild-type mice, which do not develop atherosclerosis, showed *C. pneumoniae* in the aortic wall. A more recent study that compared wild-type mice on atherogenic diet with non-infected ApoE-deficient mice found no difference in atherosclerotic lesions between infected and non-infected ApoE-deficient mice [32]. Another recent investigation using wild-type C57BL/6J mice and low-density lipoprotein (LDL)-deficient mice, which develop atherosclerosis only when fed a cholesterol-rich diet [33], determined no difference in the atherosclerotic lesions of cholesterol-fed LDL-deficient mice infected or not infected with *H. pylori*.

Such data indicate in rodents that infectious agents alone cannot directly cause fully developed atherosclerosis, even in a limited number of cases. Indeed, no experimental evidence suggests that atherosclerotic lesions induced by cholesterol-rich diets with a concomitant infection differ histologically from lesions retrieved from non-infected animals. Rather, in order to promote a full expression of vascular disease, it appears that infectious agents may require a permissive hyperlipidemic environment. In this regard, some recent clinical studies suggest that individuals with serologic evidence of chronic *C. pneumoniae* or *H. pylori* infection tend toward a more atherogenic lipid profile, i.e., lower high-density lipoprotein (HDL) and decreased HDL/total cholesterol ratio [34,35].

Effects of infection on vascular cells
Although infectious agents likely do not cause atherosclerosis directly, substantial data indicates that they might influence the progression and clinical expression of vascular disease by infecting vascular cells. The infection and lysis of endothelial and smooth muscle cells, the main constituents of a normal vessel wall, may represent the first step in the alteration of vascular wall homeostasis. Such infection result from either *Herpesviridae* [36,37] or *C. pneumoniae* [38], and *C. pneumoniae* may directly infect macrophages as well [38]. In particular, endothelial cell lysis may allow the migration of leukocytes into the vessel wall and the initiation of an inflammatory process. Additionally, infectious agents may modulate vascular cell activity toward the production of proinflammatory and procoagulant substances. Infectious agents can induce cytokine production by vascular cells. Endothelial cells produce interleukin (IL)-6 in response to CMV infection [39], and IL-6 and -8 in response to infection by *H. pylori* [40]. Monocytes produce TNF-α in response to HSV-1 infection [41], and interferon (IFN)-γ, TNF-α, IL-1β, and IL-6 in response to infection by *C. pneumoniae* [42]. Macrophages produce TNF-α, IL-1β, and colony stimulating factor (CSF) 1 in response to CMV infection [43]. Adhesion molecules expressed on endothelial cells mediate leukocyte-endothelial contact, a fundamental step in the initiation of the inflammatory process of atherogenesis. *Herpesviridae* infection induces one such adhesion molecule, P-selectin, on endothelial

cells [44]. Infection of endothelial cells with *C. pneumoniae* induces expression of E-selectin, intercellular adhesion molecule (ICAM)-1 and vascular adhesion molecule (VCAM)-1 [45], and infection with *H. pylori* provokes increased levels of VCAM-1, ICAM-1, and E-selectin on these same cells [40].

A procoagulant state and the development of a coronary thrombus underlie the acute coronary syndromes. *Herpesviridae* and *C. pneumoniae* modulate procoagulant activity of the infected endothelium. Indeed, infection with HSV-1 augments tissue factor expression [46] and thrombin generation with increased platelet binding [47], and decreases thrombomodulin expression and plasminogen activator inhibitor activity [46,48]. Also, *C. pneumoniae* induces tissue factor expression in endothelial cells [49].

Moreover, systemic infection may induce acute-phase reactants, e.g., C-reactive protein and fibrinogen, that might precipitate or favor thrombosis on an already established atherosclerotic plaque, whereas bacterial endotoxins and cytokines released during bacteremia might activate vascular cells and leukocytes resident within the atheroma, induce local cytokine production or recruit additional leukocytes [50,51].

Effects of chronic latent infection

As discussed earlier, current evidence supports the view of atherosclerosis as a chronic inflammatory disease [1]. It seems unlikely that an acute infection might generate enough inflammation within the vascular wall to trigger atherogenesis. It appears more reasonable that a chronic infection might alter vascular biology by promoting cytokine production and adhesion molecule expression, thereby inducing a chronic local inflammatory state that may favor atherogenesis. Since no evidence suggests active infection in the human vascular tree despite widely distributed DNA of microbial pathogens, the vascular wall may harbor a latent infection that might induce chronic alterations and damage leading to the development of atherosclerotic lesions. In this regard, extensive investigation of the life cycle of *Chlamydiae* indicates that these agents can achieve a state of chronic, persistent infection, wherein the organism neither grows in culture nor replicates, but is viable and metabolically quiescent

[20,52] (Figure 11.1). Several conditions can induce chronic persistent infection, including exposure to IFN-γ, an immune mediator produced by activated T-cells present within atheroma [53]. During this state of infection, as noted above, *Chlamydiae* express large amounts of HSP60. HSP belong to a ubiquitous family of intracellular and highly conserved proteins, whose expression increases during a variety of conditions such as heat shock, nutrient deprivation, infections, and inflammatory reactions, with the function of stabilizing cellular proteins [54]. HSP have high homology across different species and human HSP60 localizes in atherosclerotic lesions [55], raising the possibility that antigenic mimicry, through complement fixation and the generation of a local inflammatory response, may influence atheroma formation and evolution. Indeed, immunization with mycobacterial HSP65 induces arteriosclerosis in normocholesterolemic rabbits [56], and patients with atherosclerotic lesions of the carotid arteries have increased anti-HSP65 serum antibody titers [57]. Human HSP60 expressed by heat-shocked endothelial cells can provoke an autoimmune reaction and mediate endothelial cytotoxicity [58].

Although *C. pneumoniae* can infect most cells present in the atheroma [38], this agent most often occurs in macrophages within human coronary artery lesions [59]. Mediators produced by these phagocytic leukocytes likely contribute importantly to atherogenesis, plaque instability, and thrombosis. Chlamydial HSP60, together with human HSP60, localizes in the macrophages of human atheroma and induces macrophage secretion of TNF-α and matrix metalloproteinases, functions relevant to arterial inflammation and complications of atherosclerosis [21] (Figure 11.2).

C. pneumoniae infection also induces foam cell formation through its LPS [60]. Interestingly, HSP60 activates monocytes, the precursors of macrophages, through CD14 and TLR4, the same receptor pathway utilized by LPS [61].

Cytokine production and adhesion molecule expression comprise essential steps in the inflammatory process of atheroma formation and evolution (see above). Indeed, chlamydial and human HSP60 activate endothelial cells, smooth muscle cells, and macrophages by inducing production of IL-6; they also stimulate the expression of

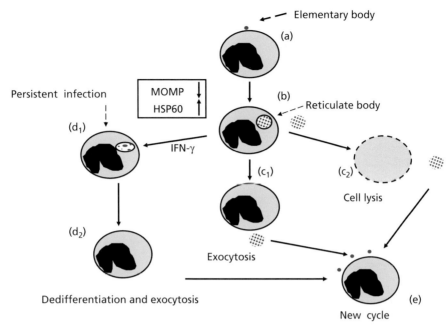

Figure 11.1 *The life cycle of Chlamydiae.* Chlamydiae are obligate intracellular pathogens. The chlamydial life cycle begins when its infectious form, the elementary body (EB, green), enters a host cell, e.g., by phagocytosis (a). The EB, once inside the cell, enlarges to the metabolically active form, the reticulate body (RB) (b). The chlamydial life cycle can then follow two different pathways ($c_{1,2}$ and $d_{1,2}$): (1) the resulting RBs, after undergoing a number of replicative cycles, can assume the form of EBs, and exit the cell by exocytosis (c_1) or through cell lysis (c_2), thereby initiating the next cycle in a new host cell (e); (2) high levels of IFN-γ, antibiotics like penicillin, or lack of nutrients as cysteine might inhibit the replication of RBs, promoting conversion to larger atypical metabolically inactive chlamydial forms which are viable, but not culturable (persistent infection)

(d_1); upon removal of IFN-γ and antibiotics, and restoration of normal levels of cysteine, the atypical forms can dedifferentiate to RBs and complete the life cycle (d_2), becoming ready to begin the next cycle in a new cell (e). During a persistent infection, Chlamydiae reduce the expression of the major outer membrane protein (MOMP) and increase levels of HSP60. Since antibodies to MOMP appear to neutralize Chlamydia infectivity, while HSP60 elicits a local inflammatory response, such a persistent infection might explain why viable Chlamydiae have not been cultured from atherosclerotic tissue and provide a mechanism for a potential link between atherogenesis and chronic latent infections. (Reprinted from Ref. [51], with permission from Elsevier Science).

E-selectin, ICAM-1, and VCAM-1 on endothelial cells [62].

Thus, chlamydial HSP60, a product of chronic persistent infection with *C. pneumoniae*, may influence atherogenesis through antigenic mimicry and activation of vascular cells rather than acting as a protein with protective cellular functions. Serum antibodies against HSP65/60 obtained from subjects with atherosclerosis cross-react with human and chlamydial HSP60 and also mediate endothelial cytotoxicity [63]. Moreover, serum levels of soluble HSP60 increase significantly in subjects with carotid atherosclerosis and correlate with the thickness of the common carotid artery intima/media [64].

Antimicrobial therapy and events

Extensive seroepidemiologic and experimental data linking infectious agents, particularly *C. pneumoniae*, to the development of atheroma and the precipitation of acute vascular events raised hope that antimicrobial therapy might interfere with or prevent these processes.

Generally, physicians treat *Chlamydiae* infections with a class of antibiotics called macrolides. By testing the triple endpoint rate of recurrent ischemia, MI, and ischemic death in unstable angina patients following a 1-month course of oral treatment with roxithromycin, the Roxithromycin Ischemic Syndromes (ROXIS) trial pioneered the

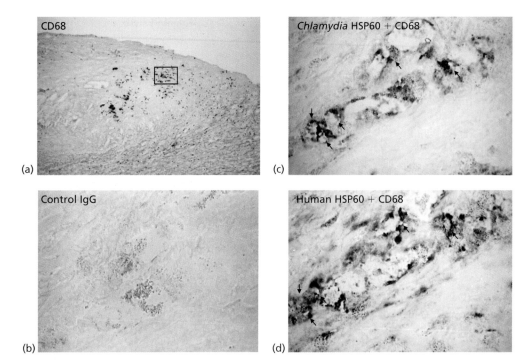

Figure 11.2 Chlamydial HSP60 colocalizes with human HSP60 within atherosclerotic plaque macrophages. Human atherosclerotic plaque (×100) stained for macrophages (CD68, red). The rectangle indicates the macrophage-rich region (intimal plaque shoulder) sampled in high-power views (×400, b, c, and d) of serial sections adjacent to the one depicted in (a). (b) Section stained with mouse IgGs as negative control yielded no staining. (c) Double staining for chlamydial HSP60 (red) and macrophages (CD68, blue). (d) Double staining for human HSP60 (red) and macrophages (CD68, blue). Arrowheads in (c) and (d) indicate macrophages (CD68+) that stain positively for either chlamydial and human HSP60. Analysis of adjacent sections showed that both human and chlamydial HSP60 colocalized within macrophage clusters. The lumen of the artery is at the top of each photomicrograph. Analysis of 7 of 9 samples (77%) showed similar results. (Reprinted from Ref. [21], with permission from Lippincot Williams and Wilkins).

use of macrolides in the secondary prevention of acute coronary events and ischemic death [65]. A significant reduction of ischemic events in treated patients vs the placebo group occurred at day 31 and was reconfirmed at 3 and 6 months [66]. Almost contemporary with the ROXIS trial, another group published similarly encouraging data regarding azithromycin, another macrolide [67]. Among *C. pneumoniae* seropositive survivors of MI treated for 3 or 6 days and followed for a mean period of 18 ± 4 months, the risk of adverse cardiovascular events decreased to the levels of seronegative patients. However, the enthusiasm generated by these initial studies deflated with the preliminary results of the Azithromycin in Coronary Artery Disease: Elimination of Myocardial Infection with Chlamydia (ACADEMIC) trial [68], which treated seropositive patients affected by coronary artery disease with azithromycin or placebo for 3 months and followed them for 2 years. ACADEMIC found no significant difference in the rate of cardiovascular events between the two groups. Nonetheless, a more recent study showed that treatment with roxithromycin for 1 month may prevent the progression of lower limb vascular disease in *C. pneumoniae* seropositive patients [69].

Notably, these preliminary studies were small (about 100 patients in each treatment arm), precluding definitive conclusions about the efficacy of macrolide treatment.

Larger trials have now been published. The Weekly Intervention with Zithromax® Against Atherosclerosis and Related Disorders (WIZARD) trial, which has enrolled 7747 patients with a prior MI randomized to a 3-month course of azithromycin or placebo, determined no benefit of antibiotic therapy

Table 11.2 Main antibiotic trials in patients with coronary artery disease.

Trial	Number of patients	Antibiotic
ROXIS [66], 1999	202	Roxithromycin
ACADEMIC [68], 1999	302	Azithromycin
WIZARD [71], 2003	7722	Azithromycin
ANTIBIO [73], 2003	868	Roxithromycin
AZACS [72], 2003	1439	Azithromycin
ACES [75], 2005	4012	Azithromycin
PROVE-IT [77], 2005	4162	Gatifloxacin

Adapted from Ref. [78].

after a median follow-up of 14 months [70,71]. The Azithromycin in Acute Coronary Syndromes (AZACS) trial enrolled 1439 patients with unstable angina or acute MI. After 6 months of follow-up, AZACS showed that azithromycin treatment for 5 days conferred no benefit [72]. The Antibiotic Therapy in Acute Myocardial Infarction (ANTIBIO) trial, which randomized 868 patients with acute MI to 300 mg of roxithromycin daily or placebo for 6 weeks, showed no benefit for prognosis after a follow-up of 12 months [73]. The Azithromycin and Coronary Events (ACES) trial [74] enrolled 4012 stable coronary artery disease patients randomized to 600 mg of azithromycin weekly or placebo for 1 year and followed-up for 4 years, but no difference was found between the two arms [75]. As part of PROVE-IT TIMI-22, a large trial investigating the beneficial effects of high-dose statin treatment on cardiovascular events [76], 4162 patients hospitalized with an acute coronary syndrome in the preceding 10 days were randomized to 400 mg of gatifloxacin daily or placebo for 10 days a month for 2 years; investigators observed no benefit between the two arms [77]. In addition, a recent meta-analysis of 11 major trials confirmed that antibiotic therapy does not appear to ameliorate prognosis in patients with coronary artery disease [78]. Table 11.2 summarizes major trials of antibiotic therapy in patients with coronary artery disease.

In view of these results, we can hypothesize why macrolide treatment has thus far failed to influence long-term prognosis in patients with vascular disease. Macrolides do not act specifically on C. pneumoniae, although they may target a number of different infectious agents. In the ROXIS trial, titers

of anti-*C. pneumoniae* antibodies in the treatment and placebo groups did not change, while C-reactive protein levels decreased significantly in the treatment arm [66]. Although such findings confirm doubts about the specific effect of roxithromycin on *C. pneumoniae*, they suggest a general decrease of an inflammatory trigger by such antibiotics. As discussed previously, the influence of *C. pneumoniae* on atheroma development seems to require chronic and persistent infection. *C. pneumoniae* localize mainly in the macrophages of human atheroma [21,59]. However, it appears that neither oral azithromycin nor rifampin, an antimicrobial agent of a different class, can eradicate infection from circulating monocytes, the precursors of macrophages [79]. In this setting, the reduced susceptibility of *C. pneumoniae* to antibiotic treatment may render oral therapy useless, and the positive results obtained from earlier small pharmacological trials may result from chance or effects of the tested agents other then anti-chlamydial action. Nonetheless, treatment with macrolides (roxithromycin being the most effective), rifampin, or quinolones may eradicate *C. pneumoniae* from the coronary artery endothelium and smooth muscle cells [80]. In addition, endothelial function in seropositive ischemic patients improves after treatment with azithromycin [81]. Since endothelial and smooth muscle cells infected with *C. pneumoniae* produce adhesion molecules and proinflammatory cytokines [62], the interference of antibiotic treatment with this proinflammatory state may explain, at least in part, the beneficial effects of macrolides observed in some of the earlier trials. Notwithstanding these apparent beneficial effects on the inflammatory burden, the weight of evidence, together with the negative results of the larger trials, suggest that antibiotic treatment, particularly with macrolides, does not modify prognosis in patients with coronary artery disease.

Conclusion

Currently accumulated data reinforce the idea that infectious agents may participate in the pathogenesis of atherosclerosis and the clinical manifestations of vascular disease, particularly in concert with traditional risk factors. Several studies have provided seroepidemiological and experimental data that link *Herpesviridae* and *C. pneumoniae* to atherosclerosis. Available evidence regarding *H. pylori* has less clarity, partly due to a more recent interest in this agent. Infectious agents may influence atherogenesis through a number of mechanisms ranging from cell lysis to stimulation of adhesion molecules expression and cytokine production by infected cells. The development of atherosclerosis after an acute infection seems unlikely. Rather, a chronic and persistent infection may favour, over time, those structural and proinflammatory changes in the vascular wall required for atheroma formation. Preliminary pharmacological trials have suggested that treatment with macrolide antibiotics, particularly roxithromycin, may limit the progression of vascular disease and the recurrence of cardiovascular events, at least in some cases. Nonetheless, large trials have dampened the initial enthusiasm by failing to show that antibiotic treatment modifies prognosis in patients with coronary artery disease. However, antimicrobial drugs do not act specifically against a single infectious agent, and proof of a link between a single infectious agent and vascular disease would require more precise therapeutic agents.

Notwithstanding the negative results of antibiotic trials, the infection hypothesis of atherosclerosis still has interest in view of a large body of accumulated epidemiological, laboratory, and clinical work. The antibiotics evaluated so far may not provide the right means to modify the contribution of chronic infections to the atherosclerotic process. Indeed, infectious agents may combine in some individuals with traditional risk factors, e.g., in the setting of a permissive hyperlipidemic environment, to accelerate atheroma formation and evolution. Moreover, additional infectious agents, acting together, may influence atherosclerosis. Increased infectious burden, represented by the number of infectious agents to which an individual shows seropositivity, correlates with a greater extent of atherosclerosis and a higher cardiovascular mortality rate in some studies [82]. Future experimental and clinical studies should address the many unresolved issues regarding the link between infectious agents and vascular disease.

References

1 Libby P, Ridker PM, Maseri A. Inflammation and atherosclerosis. *Circulation* 2002;105:1135–1143.

2 Visser MR, Vercellotti GM. Herpes simplex virus and atherosclerosis. *Eur Heart J* 1993;14(Suppl K):39–42.

3 Melnick JL, Adam E, Debakey ME. Cytomegalovirus and atherosclerosis. *Eur Heart J* 1993;14(Suppl K): 30–38.

4 Adam E, Melnick JL, Probstfield JL, et al. High levels of cytomegalovirus antibody in patients requiring vascular surgery for atherosclerosis. *Lancet* 1987;2:291–293.

5 Zhou YF, Leon MB, Waclawiw MA, et al. Association between prior cytomegalovirus infection and the risk of restenosis after coronary atherectomy. *N Engl J Med* 1996; 335:624–630.

6 Fabricant CG, Fabricant J, Litrenta MM, et al. Virus-induced atherosclerosis. *J Exp Med* 1978;148:335–340.

7 Hendrix MG, Salimans MM, van Boven CP, et al. High prevalence of latently present cytomegalovirus in arterial walls of patients suffering from grade III atherosclerosis. *Am J Pathol* 1990;136:23–28.

8 Hendrix MG, Daemen M, Bruggeman CA. Cytomegalovirus nucleic acid distribution within the human vascular tree. *Am J Pathol* 1991;138:563–567.

9 Bruggeman CA, van Dam-Mieras MC. The possible role of cytomegalovirus in atherogenesis. *Prog Med Virol* 1991;38:1–26.

10 Yamashiroya HM, Ghosh L, Yang R, et al. Herpesviridae in the coronary arteries and aorta of young trauma victims. *Am J Pathol* 1988;130:71–79.

11 Cook PJ, Honeybourne D. Chlamydia pneumoniae. *J Antimicrob Chemother* 1994;34:859–873.

12 Linnanmaki E, Leinonen M, Mattila K, et al. Chlamydia pneumoniae-specific circulating immune complexes in patients with chronic coronary heart disease. *Circulation* 1993;87:1130–1134.

13 Saikku P, Leinonen M, Mattila K, et al. Serological evidence of an association of a novel Chlamydia, TWAR, with chronic coronary heart disease and acute myocardial infarction. *Lancet* 1988;2:983–986.

14 Thom DH, Wang SP, Grayston JT, et al. Chlamydia pneumoniae strain TWAR antibody and angiographically demonstrated coronary artery disease. *Arterioscler Thromb* 1991;11:547–551.

15 Saikku P. Chlamydia pneumoniae infection as a risk factor in acute myocardial infarction. *Eur Heart J* 1993;14 (Suppl K):62–65.

16 Kuo CC, Shor A, Campbell LA, et al. Demonstration of Chlamydia pneumoniae in atherosclerotic lesions of coronary arteries. *J Infect Dis* 1993;167:841–849.

17 Muhlestein JB, Hammond EH, Carlquist JF, et al. Increased incidence of Chlamydia species within the coronary arteries of patients with symptomatic atherosclerotic versus other forms of cardiovascular disease. *J Am Coll Cardiol* 1996;27:1555–1561.

18 Ong G, Thomas BJ, Mansfield AO, et al. Detection and widespread distribution of Chlamydia pneumoniae in

the vascular system and its possible implications. *J Clin Pathol* 1996;49:102–106.

19 Kuo CC, Grayston JT, Campbell LA, et al. Chlamydia pneumoniae (TWAR) in coronary arteries of young adults (15–34 years old). *Proc Natl Acad Sci USA* 1995;92:6911–6914.

20 Beatty WL, Morrison RP, Byrne GI. Persistent chlamydiae: from cell culture to a paradigm for chlamydial pathogenesis. *Microbiol Rev* 1994;58:686–699.

21 Kol A, Sukhova GK, Lichtman AH, et al. Chlamydial heat shock protein 60 localizes in human atheroma and regulates macrophage tumor necrosis factor-alpha and matrix metalloproteinase expression. *Circulation* 1998; 98:300–307.

22 Ossei-Gerning N, Moayyedi P, Smith S, et al. Helicobacter pylori infection is related to atheroma in patients undergoing coronary angiography. *Cardiovasc Res* 1997;35: 120–124.

23 Pasceri V, Cammarota G, Patti G, et al. Association of virulent Helicobacter pylori strains with ischemic heart disease. *Circulation* 1998;97:1675–1679.

24 Kahan T, Lundman P, Olsson G, et al. Greater than normal prevalence of seropositivity for Helicobacter pylori among patients who have suffered myocardial infarction. *Coron Artery Dis* 2000;11:523–526.

25 Folsom AR, Nieto FJ, Sorlie P, et al. Helicobacter pylori seropositivity and coronary heart disease incidence. Atherosclerosis Risk In Communities (ARIC) Study Investigators. *Circulation* 1998;98:845–850.

26 Ameriso SF, Fridman EA, Leiguarda RC, et al. Detection of Helicobacter pylori in human carotid atherosclerotic plaques. *Stroke* 2001;32:385–391.

27 Blasi F, Ranzi ML, Erba M, et al. No evidence for the presence of Helicobacter pylori in atherosclerotic plaques in abdominal aortic aneurysm specimens. *Atherosclerosis* 1996;126:339–340.

28 Farsak B, Yildirir A, Akyon Y, et al. Detection of Chlamydia pneumoniae and Helicobacter pylori DNA in human atherosclerotic plaques by PCR. *J Clin Microbiol* 2000;38:4408–4411.

29 Kowalski M. Helicobacter pylori (H. pylori) infection in coronary artery disease: influence of H. pylori eradication on coronary artery lumen after percutaneous transluminal coronary angioplasty. The detection of H. pylori specific DNA in human coronary atherosclerotic plaque. *J Physiol Pharmacol* 2001;52:3–31.

30 Fong IW, Chiu B, Viira E, et al. Rabbit model for Chlamydia pneumoniae infection. *J Clin Microbiol* 1997; 35:48–52.

31 Moazed TC, Kuo C, Grayston JT, et al. Murine models of Chlamydia pneumoniae infection and atherosclerosis. *J Infect Dis* 1997;175:883–890.

32 Caligiuri G, Rottenberg M, Nicoletti A, et al. Chlamydia pneumoniae infection does not induce or modify atherosclerosis in mice. *Circulation* 2001;103:2834–2838.

33 Mach F, Sukhova GK, Michetti M, et al. Influence of Helicobacter pylori infection during atherogenesis *in vivo* in mice. *Circ Res* 2002;90:E1–E4.

34 Laurila A, Bloigu A, Nayha S, et al. Chronic Chlamydia pneumoniae infection is associated with a serum lipid profile known to be a risk factor for atherosclerosis. *Arterioscler Thromb Vasc Biol* 1997; 17: 2910–2913.

35 Hoffmeister A, Rothenbacher D, Bode G, et al. Current infection with Helicobacter pylori, but not seropositivity to Chlamydia pneumoniae or cytomegalovirus, is associated with an atherogenic, modified lipid profile. *Arterioscler Thromb Vasc Biol* 2001;21:427–432.

36 Friedman HM, Macarak EJ, MacGregor RR, et al. Virus infection of endothelial cells. *J Infect Dis* 1981; 143:266–273.

37 Tumilowicz JJ, Gawlik ME, Powell BB, et al. Replication of cytomegalovirus in human arterial smooth muscle cells. *J Virol* 1985;56:839–845.

38 Gaydos CA, Summersgill JT, Sahney NN, et al. Replication of Chlamydia pneumoniae *in vitro* in human macrophages, endothelial cells, and aortic artery smooth muscle cells. *Infect Immun* 1996;64: 1614–1620.

39 Almeida GD, Porada CD, St Jeor S, et al. Human cytomegalovirus alters interleukin-6 production by endothelial cells. *Blood* 1994;83:370–376.

40 Innocenti M, Thoreson AC, Ferrero RL, et al. Helicobacter pylori-induced activation of human endothelial cells. *Infect Immun* 2002;70:4581–4590.

41 Gosselin J, Flamand L, D'Addario M, et al. Infection of peripheral blood mononuclear cells by herpes simplex and Epstein-Barr viruses. Differential induction of interleukin 6 and tumor necrosis factor-alpha. *J Clin Invest* 1992;89:1849–1856.

42 Kaukoranta-Tolvanen SS, Teppo AM, et al. Growth of Chlamydia pneumoniae in cultured human peripheral blood mononuclear cells and induction of a cytokine response. *Microb Pathog* 1996;21:215–221.

43 Dudding L, Haskill S, Clark BD, et al. Cytomegalovirus infection stimulates expression of monocyte-associated mediator genes. *J Immunol* 1989;143:3343–3352.

44 Span AH, Van Boven CP, Bruggeman CA. The effect of cytomegalovirus infection on the adherence of polymorphonuclear leucocytes to endothelial cells. *Eur J Clin Invest* 1989;19:542–548.

45 Kaukoranta-Tolvanen SS, Ronni T, Leinonen M, et al. Expression of adhesion molecules on endothelial cells stimulated by Chlamydia pneumoniae. *Microb Pathog* 1996;21:407–411.

46 Key NS, Vercellotti GM, Winkelmann JC, et al. Infection of vascular endothelial cells with herpes simplex virus enhances tissue factor activity and reduces thrombomodulin expression. *Proc Natl Acad Sci USA* 1990;87: 7095–7099.

47 Visser MR, Tracy PB, Vercellotti GM, et al. Enhanced thrombin generation and platelet binding on herpes simplex virus-infected endothelium. *Proc Natl Acad Sci USA* 1988;85:8227–8230.

48 Bok RA, Jacob HS, Balla J, et al. Herpes simplex virus decreases endothelial cell plasminogen activator inhibitor. *Thromb Haemost* 1993;69:253–258.

49 Fryert RH, Schwobe EP, Woods ML, et al. Chlamydia species infect human vascular endothelial cells and induce procoagulant activity. *J Investig Med* 1997;45:168–174.

50 Libby P, Egan D, Skarlatos S. Roles of infectious agents in atherosclerosis and restenosis: an assessment of the evidence and need for future research. *Circulation* 1997;96:4095–4103.

51 Kol A, Libby P. The mechanisms by which infectious agents may contribute to atherosclerosis and its clinical manifestations. *Trends Cardiovasc Med* 1998;8:191–199.

52 Kalayoglu MV, Libby P, Byrne GI. Chlamydia pneumoniae as an emerging risk factor in cardiovascular disease. *J Am Med Assoc* 2002;288:2724–2731.

53 Hansson GK, Holm J, Jonasson L. Detection of activated T lymphocytes in the human atherosclerotic plaque. *Am J Pathol* 1989;135:169–175.

54 Young RA, Elliott TJ. Stress proteins, infection, and immune surveillance. *Cell* 1989;59:5–8.

55 Kleindienst R, Xu Q, Willeit J, et al. Immunology of atherosclerosis. Demonstration of heat shock protein 60 expression and T lymphocytes bearing alpha/beta or gamma/delta receptor in human atherosclerotic lesions. *Am J Pathol* 1993; 142:1927–1937.

56 Xu Q, Dietrich H, Steiner HJ, et al. Induction of arteriosclerosis in normocholesterolemic rabbits by immunization with heat shock protein 65. *Arterioscler Thromb* 1992;12:789–799.

57 Xu Q, Willeit J, Marosi M, et al. Association of serum antibodies to heat-shock protein 65 with carotid atherosclerosis. *Lancet* 1993;341:255–259.

58 Schett G, Xu Q, Amberger A, et al. Autoantibodies against heat shock protein 60 mediate endothelial cytotoxicity. *J Clin Invest* 1995;96:2569–2577.

59 Campbell LA, O'Brien ER, Cappuccio AL, et al. Detection of Chlamydia pneumoniae TWAR in human coronary atherectomy tissues. *J Infect Dis* 1995;172:585–588.

60 Kalayoglu MV, Byrne GI. A Chlamydia pneumoniae component that induces macrophage foam cell formation is chlamydial lipopolysaccharide. *Infect Immun* 1998;66:5067–5072.

61 Kol A, Lichtman AH, Finberg RW, et al. Cutting edge: heat shock protein (HSP) 60 activates the innate immune response: CD14 is an essential receptor for HSP60 activation of mononuclear cells. *J Immunol* 2000;164:13–17.

62 Kol A, Bourcier T, Lichtman AH, et al. Chlamydial and human heat shock protein 60s activate human vascular endothelium, smooth muscle cells, and macrophages. *J Clin Invest* 1999;103:571–577.

63 Mayr M, Metzler B, Kiechl S, et al. Endothelial cytotoxicity mediated by serum antibodies to heat shock proteins of Escherichia coli and Chlamydia pneumoniae: immune reactions to heat shock proteins as a possible link between infection nd atherosclerosis. *Circulation* 1999;99:1560–1566.

64 Xu Q, Schett G, Perschinka H, et al. Serum soluble heat shock protein 60 is elevated in subjects with atherosclerosis in a general population. *Circulation* 2000;102:14–20.

65 Gurfinkel E, Bozovich G, Daroca A, et al. Randomised trial of roxithromycin in non-Q-wave coronary syndromes: ROXIS Pilot Study. ROXIS Study Group. *Lancet* 1997;350:404–407.

66 Gurfinkel E, Bozovich G, Beck E, et al. Treatment with the antibiotic roxithromycin in patients with acute non-Q-wave coronary syndromes. The final report of the ROXIS Study. *Eur Heart J* 1999; 20:121–127.

67 Gupta S, Leatham EW, Carrington D, et al. Elevated Chlamydia pneumoniae antibodies, cardiovascular events, and azithromycin in male survivors of myocardial infarction. *Circulation* 1997;96:404–407.

68 Muhlestein JB, Anderson JL, Carlquist JF, et al. Randomized secondary prevention trial of azithromycin in patients with coronary artery disease: primary clinical results of the ACADEMIC study. *Circulation* 2000;102:1755–1760.

69 Wiesli P, Czerwenka W, Meniconi A, et al. Roxithromycin treatment prevents progression of peripheral arterial occlusive disease in Chlamydia pneumoniae seropositive men: a randomized, double-blind, placebo-controlled trial. *Circulation* 2002;105:2646–2652.

70 Dunne MW. Rationale and design of a secondary prevention trial of antibiotic use in patients after myocardial infarction: the WIZARD (weekly intervention with zithromax [azithromycin] for atherosclerosis and its related disorders) trial. *J Infect Dis* 2000;181(Suppl 3): S572–S578.

71 O'Connor CM, Dunne MW, Pfeffer MA, et al. Azithromycin for the secondary prevention of coronary heart disease events: the WIZARD study: a randomized controlled trial. *J Am Med Assoc* 2003;290:1459–1466.

72 Cercek B, Shah PK, Noc M, et al. Effect of short-term treatment with azithromycin on recurrent ischaemic events in patients with acute coronary syndrome in the Azithromycin in Acute Coronary Syndrome (AZACS) trial: a randomised controlled trial. *Lancet* 2003;361: 809–813.

73 Zahn R, Schneider S, Frilling B, et al. Antibiotic therapy after acute myocardial infarction: a prospective randomized study. *Circulation* 2003;107:1253–1259.

74 Jackson LA. Description and status of the azithromycin and coronary events study (ACES). *J Infect Dis* 2000;181 (Suppl 3):S579–S581.

75 Grayston JT, Kronmal RA, Jackson LA, et al. Azithromycin for the secondary prevention of coronary events. *N Engl J Med* 2005;352:1637–1645.

76 Cannon CP, McCabe CH, Belder R, et al. Design of the Pravastatin or Atorvastatin Evaluation and Infection Therapy (PROVE IT)-TIMI 22 trial. *Am J Cardiol* 2002;89:860–861.

77 Cannon CP, Braunwald E, McCabe CH, et al. Antibiotic treatment of Chlamydia pneumoniae after acute coronary syndrome. *N Engl J Med* 2005;352:1646–1654.

78 Andraws R, Berger JS, Brown DL. Effects of antibiotic therapy on outcomes of patients with coronary artery disease: a meta-analysis of randomized controlled trials. *J Am Med Assoc* 2005;293:2641–2647.

79 Gieffers J, Fullgraf H, Jahn J, et al. Chlamydia pneumoniae infection in circulating human monocytes is refractory to antibiotic treatment. *Circulation* 2001;103:351–356.

80 Gieffers J, Solbach W, Maass M. *In vitro* susceptibility and eradication of Chlamydia pneumoniae cardiovascular strains from coronary artery endothelium and smooth muscle cells. *Cardiovasc Drug Ther* 2001;15:259–262.

81 Parchure N, Zouridakis EG, Kaski JC. Effect of azithromycin treatment on endothelial function in patients with coronary artery disease and evidence of Chlamydia pneumoniae infection. *Circulation* 2002;105: 1298–1303.

82 Espinola-Klein C, Rupprecht HJ, Blankenberg S, et al. Impact of infectious burden on extent and long-term prognosis of atherosclerosis. *Circulation* 2002;105:15–21.

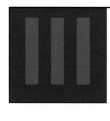

PART III

Diagnostic tools and markers of endothelial functions

CHAPTER 12

Endothelial vasodilatory dysfunction: basic concepts and practical implementation

Scott Kinlay, MBBS *& Peter Ganz,* MD

Introduction

Our understanding of the autocrine and paracrine roles of the endothelium has increased substantially since Furchgott's observation, two decades ago, that relaxation of the rabbit aorta to acetylcholine required an intact endothelium [1], and the subsequent elaboration of nitric oxide (NO) as the predominant endothelium-derived relaxing factor [2,3].

The healthy endothelium responds to a number of stimuli by producing several vasoactive compounds that function to keep shear stress exerted by blood flow within a restricted range [4–6]. Cardiovascular risk factors damage the endothelium and impair this regulatory function, leading to paradoxical vasoconstriction [7–17] and several other adverse inflammatory and thrombotic sequelae that generally promote atherosclerosis [18–20]. This chapter will discuss some of the vasodilatory and vasoconstrictive substances produced by the endothelium, as well as the clinical approaches used to measure these responses.

Basic concepts

Endothelium-derived vasodilators

The principal vasodilators produced by the endothelium include NO, prostacyclin, and endothelium-derived hyperpolarizing factor. Of these, NO plays a central role in mediating many functions of the endothelium beyond vasodilation [6]. As such, the assessment of NO-mediated vasodilation is particularly useful, as it likely reflects the effectiveness of other NO-mediated functions, including its anti-inflammatory and antiproliferative actions and antithrombotic effects at the vessel surface.

Nitric oxide

NO is generated in the endothelium from the amino acid L-arginine by NO synthase (NOS), and several physiological stimuli, including increasing shear stress at the endothelial surface (from blood flow), thrombin, serotonin, and acetylcholine, accelerate its production [21]. Such stimuli activate NOS by several mechanisms including phosphorylation of a specific serine residue in the enzyme (serine 1177 in human cells) [22–24] and by increasing intracellular calcium concentrations and mobilizing calmodulin [25].

NOS associates closely with invaginations in the endothelial luminal surface called *caveolae* [6,26,27], specialized organelles with different concentrations of cholesterol and lipids compared with the remaining cell membrane, and a high concentration of surface receptors and associated G proteins that increase intracellular calcium when activated. A specific caveolar protein, caveolin, binds and inactivates NOS [6,26] and competes with the calcium–calmodulin complex: the former inhibits and the latter activates enzyme activity (Figure 12.1) [6].

NO diffuses through the artery wall to enter vascular smooth muscle cells in the media, where it increases the activity of guanylate cyclase and the concentration of cyclic guanosin monophosphate

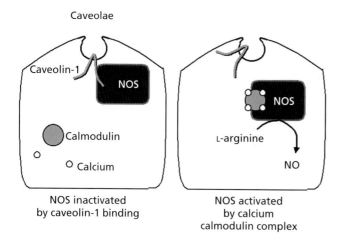

Figure 12.1 Endothelial cells have invaginations, or *caveolae*, closely related to NOS activity. The protein caveolin inactivates NOS, and competes with the calcium–calmodulin complex that activates the enzyme. Reproduced from Ref. [6].

(GMP), thus relaxing vascular smooth muscle and leading to vasodilation [21]. Since shear stress is related to blood velocity, increased blood velocity will augment NO production and cause vasodilation, reducing, in turn, blood velocity toward its original value. In contrast, decreased blood velocity will reduce the stimulus for NO production, promote vasoconstriction, and thereby increase blood velocity toward its original value. In this way, the endothelium regulates vasomotor tone to restore blood velocity and shear stress at the endothelial surface to a narrow range that prevents sluggish blood flow that may promote thrombus formation, or high shear that may injure the arterial intima by predisposing to non-laminar blood flow.

Atherosclerosis and its risk factors impair the normal regulation of vasomotor tone. Under these conditions, pro-oxidant reactive oxygen species increase in the vessel wall. NO is degraded rapidly by oxidant stress, including the very rapid reaction with superoxide anion [28,29] that leads to the formation of the vasoinactive and toxic metabolite peroxynitrite. High concentrations of antioxidant vitamin C, generally achieved only by parenteral administration, can prevent this degradation in experimental studies and in human studies [6,30], supporting the importance of oxidant stress in endothelial dysfunction.

Physiological effects on the endothelium counteract the actions of several agents that constrict vascular smooth muscle cells. For example, activated endothelium generates enough NO to overwhelm the direct effect of acetylcholine, a direct vasoconstrictor, on vascular smooth muscle cells,

resulting in net vasodilation of healthy arteries [1,31]. The vasodilatory action in response to acetylcholine is substantially blocked by inhibitors of NO synthesis such as monomethylarginine [32], suggesting that much of the vasodilation to acetylcholine is indeed mediated by NO. Factors that impair endothelial function lead to less NO generation and ultimately to a net vasoconstrictive response to this agent. Fortunately, acetylcholine delivered as part of a clinical test of endothelial function is rapidly degraded by cholinesterases that are abundant in blood. Thus, the vasoconstrictive response during a clinical test typically reverses within seconds of halting acetylcholine infusion. The wide range in response and the relative safety of acetylcholine have made this agent the stimulus of choice for assessing endothelial vasomotor dysfunction in conduit and resistance arteries. Pharmacological doses of other agents with similar effects on vascular smooth muscle and the endothelium have potential drawbacks, including platelet activation in the case of serotonin, increased risk of ventricular arrhythmias with papaverine, and thrombosis or embolization with thrombin.

Flow-mediated dilation, another commonly used stimulus to assess endothelial vasomotor function [7,33–35], relies on healthy endothelium mediating vasodilation with increasing shear stress from blood flow. Flow-mediated dilation in the conduit arteries can be induced by dilating arteries distal to the study artery. For example, vasodilators delivered distally in the coronary artery will increase blood flow and should promote vasodilation of the more proximal coronary arteries [35]. Similarly, and more commonly exploited clinically, temporary ischemia of a limb will lead to metabolic dilation of the resistance vessels, increasing blood flow velocity and in turn promoting flow-mediated dilation of a conduit artery proximal to the site of ischemia [7,34]. Flow-mediated dilation is also largely a NO-related response, as is blocked by NO inhibitors such as monomethylarginine [36].

Prostacyclin

Prostacyclin, another endothelial product that dilates arteries, is produced from arachidonic acid by cyclo-oxygenases in response to shear stress and a number of factors that also increase NO production. Prostacyclin activates adenylate cyclase to increase cyclic adenosine monophosphate (AMP). In most vascular beds, however, prostacyclin plays only a small role in regulating vasomotor tone compared to NO, but has a greater role in the inhibition of platelet aggregation [37].

Endothelium-derived hyperpolarizing factor

Residual vasodilation to various stimuli after blocking NO and prostacyclin generation supports the likely existence of other endothelium-derived relaxing factors [38]. In isolated artery segments, hyperpolarization of vascular smooth muscle cells occurs without increased cyclic GMP or cyclic AMP typical of NO and prostacyclin-mediated relaxation, suggesting the existence of an endothelium-dependent hyperpolarizing factor (EDHF) [38]. Although the structure of EDHF remains undetermined, EDHF appears more important in small arteries than the large conduit arteries. Recent studies have suggested that one EDHF may be epoxyeicosatrienoic acids (EETs), which are products of cytochrome P450 (CYP) epoxygenase [39,40]. Experimental studies have suggested that EETs possess vasodilatory, anti-inflammatory, anti-proliferative, and fibrinolytic properties [40]. The lack of consistent EDHF inhibitors safe for use in humans has thwarted the clinical study of EDHF.

Endothelium-derived vasoconstrictors

Although several locally produced substances can cause vasoconstriction, most are platelet-derived products, including serotonin and thrombin. However, the endothelium also produces substances that constrict vascular smooth muscle, most importantly, perhaps, endothelin.

Endothelin

Endothelin, one of the most potent vasoconstrictors known, was first discovered as a product secreted by endothelial cells [41]. Endothelin is a peptide generated by successive cleavage of a large polypeptide "big endothelin" within the endothelium [42]. Three isotypes of endothelin have been described (endothelin-1, -2, and -3); however, endothelin-1 is the most abundant in vascular tissue [42]. Activated macrophages and vascular smooth muscle cells also produce endothelin-1, particularly in atherosclerosis [43,44].

Endothelin acts on endothelin-A receptors on vascular smooth muscle to stimulate vasoconstriction and vascular smooth muscle cell proliferation. The maximal vasoconstrictive response *in vivo* takes up to an hour [45–47], in contrast to NO stimulation that can be maximal within seconds. Thus endothelin-1 principally contributes to prolonged changes in basal vascular tone rather than to the minute-by-minute regulation by shear stress or by agonists more characteristic of the shorter-acting NO. Endothelin-B receptors present on the abluminal surface of endothelial cells mediate the increased production of NO in healthy cells [46–48]. Nevertheless, the net action of endothelin-1 is vasoconstriction in most vascular beds, including the coronary arteries, where endothelin-B receptors are particularly sparse or absent on endothelial cells [49,50].

Stimuli for endothelin production include thrombin, angiotensin II, and epinephrine [51,52]. NO inhibits endothelin production; conversely, endothelin inhibits the production of NO [46, 51–53]. Inhibitors of endothelin-A receptors dilate arteries in subjects with atherosclerosis [54–56] or its risk factors compared with healthy subjects [47,57,58], indicating increased bioactivity of endothelin in these conditions. Studies using inhibitors of NO also indicate impaired bioavailability of NO in atherosclerosis and cardiac risk factors (see below). Thus, endothelin and NO participate in a "ying–yang" relationship to regulate vasomotor tone, and net regulatory effect depending on the health of the endothelium.

Methods to measure vasomotor function *in vivo*

Furchgott's original experiment using isolated arterial rings showed paradoxical vasoconstriction of the rings to acetylcholine that resulted from the removal of the endothelium [1]. Many subsequent studies have used acetylcholine or other related analogs to assess endothelial vasomotor function *ex vivo* and *in vivo*.

Methods that measure endothelial vasomotor function *in vivo* are based on physiological or pharmacological stimuli to the endothelium, and use a variety of techniques to assess the resultant vasodilation or vasoconstriction. Endothelium-dependent vasomotor changes are usually compared with baseline or control conditions and also with the effect of endothelium-independent dilators. The latter provide not only evidence that vascular smooth muscle dilatory capacity is intact, but also indicate an upper limit of the vasodilatory response.

The clinical assessment of NO-mediated endothelial function

Physiological techniques to assess conduit artery function

Physiological agents used to study vasomotion in the conduit arteries rely on increasing velocity of blood flow and therefore, shear stress on the endothelium, including exercise and temporary ischemia distal to the studied arterial segment.

Angiography or ultrasound can assess changes in artery size. For example, coronary endothelial function has been assessed by coronary angiography 3–5 min after bicycling on a bicycle ergometer, after a cold pressor test or a mental stress during cardiac catheterization [59,60]. Computerized quantitative angiography uses a known catheter diameter or grid size as a scale to calculate the lumen diameter of the artery. In this manner, changes in conduit artery diameter after physiological stress are compared with baseline diameters. Computerized edge-detection softwares provide reproducible measurements of the lumen of the angiogram in the small ranges of changes observed.

Additionally, ultrasound can non-invasively assess peripheral artery conduit function [7,34,61–63], with the use of two-dimensional ultrasound images of a longitudinal section of an artery [7,34] and wall-tracking methods [62–64] that can measure changes in the lumen diameter of the artery from A-mode echoes.

Both techniques have been used to assess brachial and radial artery function in adults and femoral artery function in children [7,34,61–64] Ultrasound techniques rely on imaging the artery segment at baseline, under resting conditions, followed by imaging the artery after stimulating the endothelium to increase NO production, an action usually achieved by increasing blood flow and shear stress on the endothelium by vasodilating distal resistance vessels (usually by causing 5 min of ischemia from inflating a blood pressure cuff to suprasystolic pressures) [61]. Normal flow-mediated vasodilation peaks at approximately 60–90 s following the release of the blood pressure cuff, and declines to baseline conditions within 10–15 min. The artery segment is also imaged 3–5 min after sublingual nitroglycerin to assess endothelium-independent vasodilation and the capacity of the vascular smooth muscle to dilate.

With two-dimensional ultrasound, the diameter of the artery critically depends on obtaining a good longitudinal section that bisects the artery along its true longitudinal axis. If the ultrasound beam is parallel, but not aligned with the long axis of the artery, a smaller diameter than the true diameter will be measured. To some extent this can be assessed by close inspection of the two-dimensional images at each stage, to check that distinctive features of the artery have been reproduced and that, if possible, a trilaminar appearance of the artery wall is obtained [61].

The diameter of the artery is measured from two-dimensional images off-line and ideally blind to the stage of the study to reduce observer measurement error or bias [61]. Typically, the end-diastolic phase is used to measure diameter, as this is easily identified by the R-wave of the electrocardiogram (ECG) and is less subject to the movement of the artery in the three-dimensional space that may increase variability measurement. More recently, computer programs permit semi-automatic assessment of the lumen diameter, through the use of edge-detection algorithms to identify the lumen borders or the intima–media interface.

The wall-tracking technique uses the A-mode or raw radio frequency data to measure artery diameter [63]. The A-mode yields a strong echo signal at the intima border of the near and far wall of the artery, and the distance between these signals is the artery lumen diameter. The software used in this technique provides the diameter from an average of several cardiac cycles. This technique also uses two-dimensional images to ensure that the ultrasound interrogates the artery dimensions at the true long axis of the artery. Potential errors with wall tracking occur if the ultrasound transducer drifts from the true center of the artery, or with substantial lateral movements in the artery over the cardiac cycle as it particularly occurs in elderly patients. However, both non-invasive techniques avoid the potential risks generally associated with invasive measures, which require the insertion of intra-arterial catheters.

Pharmacological techniques to assess conduit artery function

Infusion of pharmacological agonists for the production of endothelium-dependent NO, including acetylcholine, methacholine, serotonin, and papaverine, can induce alterations in the lumen diameter of conduit arteries that reflect endothelium-dependent vasomotor changes. Due to its rapid onset, short duration of action, and relative safety, acetylcholine is used most commonly.

In our experience assessing coronary endothelial function, the test agents are typically infused into the coronary artery through a small catheter [31]. Compared to delivery of a pharmacological agent as a bolus through a guiding catheter, infusion yields the delivery of a more constant dose to the endothelium, prevents shear stress-related changes in vasomotor tone resulting from the rapid delivery of a bolus, and isolates the action of the agent to one artery, thus limiting any vasoconstriction to a single artery and a single myocardial territory, avoiding vasoconstriction in a larger region that may cause widespread myocardial ischemia. We typically begin with low, graded concentrations of the infused agent, and increase the concentration if visual inspection from the baseline angiogram indicates that the artery has not constricted to >50–70% of the original diameter. Nitroglycerin, given to reverse any vasoconstriction, also assesses the maximum vasodilatory capacity.

Being done with an invasive technique, infusion requires suitable caution in selecting patients with anatomy suitable to be safely studied, and excludes patients with left main stenoses, multivessel surgical disease, severe left ventricular dysfunction, excessive arterial tortuosity, etc. Due to the small but important risks associated with cardiac catheterization, infusion usually assesses coronary endothelial function only in patients undergoing cardiac catheterization for clinical purposes.

Flow-mediated dilation can also assess the function of conduit arteries. Distal infusion of resistance vessel vasodilators, such as adenosine, increases blood flow velocity and acts as a stimulus for endothelium-dependent dilation in the upstream conduit artery [35].

Rarely, the wires and infusion catheters used to deliver the drugs in these invasive tests may themselves cause spasm, invalidating the assessment. In this instance, nitroglycerin is administered and the study is interrupted.

Assessing endothelial function of resistance vessel

Resistance vessels perform an important function as they participate in the regulation of blood flow in response to changes in metabolic needs (metabolic regulation) or to changes in perfusion pressure (autoregulation). In the coronary arteries, the vasomotor function of resistance vessels is assessed by measuring changes in coronary blood flow. Since the tone of resistance vessels critically determines blood flow, altered blood flow without substantial changes in mean blood pressure generally reflects differences in the tone of resistance vessels [65–67].

Following the arterial infusion of endothelium-dependent vasodilators such as acetylcholine, changes in blood flow (usually assessed by changes in diameter and blood flow velocity) document changes in the tone of resistance vessels [65–67]. Doppler flow wires, which send and receive ultrasound signals from a small probe at the end of a 0.014-in.-diameter guidewire, can measure blood flow velocity. The Doppler shift of ultrasound reflected from moving red cells flowing past the wire allows an estimate of blood flow velocity. This technique requires the same precautions and has the same limitations of the invasive assessment of conduit arteries.

Similar considerations in peripheral arteries have led to the widespread use of venous plethysmography to measure changes in forearm blood flow in response to a number of agonists such as acetylcholine or methacholine [68,69]. Forearm blood flow and mean blood pressure provide an estimate of the forearm vascular resistance. Typically, a cuff around the wrist is inflated to suprasystolic pressure, thus separating the forearm from the circulation. In addition, intermittently inflating a second cuff on the upper arm to supravenous pressures, but below arterial pressure, interrupts venous outflow without changing the arterial inflow. During this temporary occlusion, the accumulation of blood per unit of time in the forearm reflects forearm blood flow. Sensitive mercury-in-silastic detectors placed around the forearm expand as the limb increases in size, reducing the diameter of the mercury and changing its conducting properties. Graphing these changes demonstrates that the rate of increase in limb size is proportional to the vasodilation of resistance vessels in the forearm. Increased limb size is measured under baseline conditions with an inactive solution infused into the brachial artery through a small cannula. The measurements are repeated after the infusion of an endothelium-dependent vasodilator, such as acetylcholine or the related agent methacholine, and again after an endothelium-independent dilator such as nitroprusside or a calcium channel blocker. Changes in limb size in response to different concentrations of the endothelium-dependent vasodilator used allow plotting of dose–response curves of dilation in resistance vessels. Simultaneously, similar measurements in the opposite arm submitted to infusion with control saline act as a time control. After controlling for time effects, responses ratios between the studied and control arms can assess vasomotor response to the vasoactive drugs.

Assessing basal endothelium-dependent tone

The healthy endothelium usually generates NO, although at lower levels than stimulated endothelium. This basal production of NO may contribute to regulation of shear stress, and may exert antiplatelet and antiproliferative actions. Such effects can be assessed by blocking NO production with competitive inhibitors of L-arginine such as monomethylarginine [32,36,70]; the subsequent vasoconstriction measures the artery tone related to the basal production of NO.

The clinical assessment of endothelium-derived constricting factors

As noted previously, the endothelium also produces a number of vasoconstrictors, most potently endothelin-1. Specific endothelin antagonists, including bosentan (an endothelin-A and -B receptor blocker), BQ-123 (a specific endothelin-A receptor blocker), and BQ-788 (an endothelin-B receptor blocker), allow investigation of the effects of the basal or constitutive release of endothelin [45–48, 54–56,71,72].

The vascular effects of local (endogenous) endothelin production have been assessed in the coronary and peripheral arteries using these inhibitors. Vascular tone has been assessed using coronary angiography and the plethysmography techniques mentioned above. Endothelin receptor antagonists dilate coronary arteries [54–56] and the pulmonary artery [72]. These studies indicate that a basal production of endothelin contributes to the background vascular tone. The specific endothelin-A receptor antagonist BQ-123 dilates peripheral arteries [45,46], coronary arteries [54,55], particularly those with atherosclerosis, and may be responsible for most of the basal vascular tone at sites of coronary stenoses [54]. The specific endothelin-B receptor antagonist BQ-788 dilates arteries and also indicates a constrictive effect of endothelin-B receptors on vascular smooth muscle predominant over the potential NO-mediated vasorelaxation from the activation of endothelin-B receptors on endothelial cells [46–48].

Drawbacks in assessing endothelium-dependent vasomotion

Vasomotor tone results from the balance of a number of stimuli including the various dilators and constrictors described previously. In addition, sympathetic tone and vasoactive drugs taken by patients accentuate or depress vasomotor responses. Thus, within any individual, variability in vasomotor response likely exists over time. Stopping vasomotor medications for several hours before studying vasomotor function avoids the confounding actions of these drugs on the subtle vasomotor responses elicited by physiological tests. Typically, these involve all long-acting vasodilators such as nitrates, calcium channel blockers, angiotensin-converting enzyme inhibitors, and angiotensin receptor blockers. If it is safe to withhold these medications, they

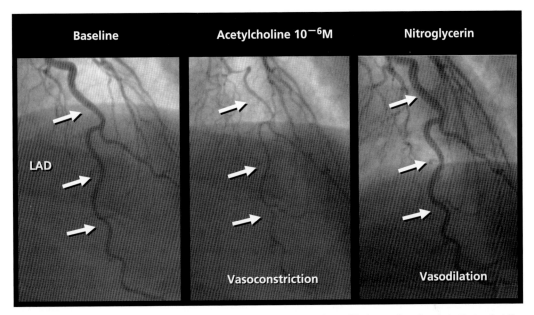

Figure 12.2 An extreme case of endothelial dysfunction, with near occlusion of the left anterior descending artery (LAD) during an intra-arterial infusion of acetylcholine. The normal vasodilation to nitroglycerin indicates that the acetylcholine response is a functional, rather than structural, abnormality.

are usually omitted for at least 12–24 h prior to studying vasomotor function.

In addition to these biological sources of variability in individual subjects, measurement errors may provide random or systematic differences in measurement. Since the changes in endothelium-dependent vasomotion can be very small, measurements blind to treatment stage are preferable.

As a result, the best application of these techniques involves studying changes in groups of patients in response to a factor that may alter endothelium-dependent vasomotor function (e.g., treatment of cardiac risk factors). Such techniques also can test endothelial function in individuals with expected extremes of response, e.g., coronary vasospasm, where complete or near complete occlusion of vessels is evoked (Figure 12.2).

Conclusions

Testing of endothelial function helps us to understand the biological mechanisms that link risk factors to clinical events associated with atherosclerosis, and also how treatment reduces risk. Such responses are subtle, however, and require strict adherence to protocols and methods to reduce

biases and errors that might overwhelm the changes sought by using a variety of techniques. For the most part, these techniques are, at the moment, important research tools that help establishing biological underpinnings of disease and therapy.

References

1 Furchgott RF, Zawadzki JV. The obligatory role of endothelial cells in the relaxation of arterial smooth muscle by acetylcholine. *Nature* 1980;288:373–376.
2 Ignarro LJ, Byrns RE, Buga GM, et al. Endothelium-derived relaxing factor from pulmonary artery and vein possesses pharmacologic and chemical properties identical to those of nitric oxide radical. *Circ Res* 1987;61: 866–879.
3 Palmer RM, Ferrige AG, Moncada S. Nitric oxide release accounts for the biological activity of endothelium-derived relaxing factor. *Nature* 1987;327:524–526.
4 Gimbrone Jr MA, Topper JN, Nagel T, et al. Endothelial dysfunction, hemodynamic forces, and atherogenesis. *Ann NY Acad Sci* 2000;902:230–239; discussion 239–240.
5 Davies PF. Flow-mediated endothelial mechanotransduction. *Physiol Rev* 1995;75:519–560.
6 Kinlay S, Libby P, Ganz P. Endothelial function and coronary artery disease. *Curr Opin Lipidol* 2001;12: 383–389.

7 Celermajer DS, Sorensen KE, Bull C, et al. Endothelium-dependent dilation in the systemic arteries of asymptomatic subjects relates to coronary risk factors and their interaction. *J Am Coll Cardiol* 1994;24:1468–1474.

8 Celermajer DS, Sorensen KE, Spiegelhalter DJ, et al. Aging is associated with endothelial dysfunction in healthy men years before the age-related decline in women. *J Am Coll Cardiol* 1994;24:471–476.

9 Clarkson P, Celermajer DS, Donald AE, et al. Impaired vascular reactivity in insulin-dependent diabetes mellitus is related to disease duration and low density lipoprotein cholesterol levels. *J Am Coll Cardiol* 1996;28:573–579.

10 Heitzer T, Yla-Herttuala S, Luoma J, et al. Cigarette smoking potentiates endothelial dysfunction of forearm resistance vessels in patients with hypercholesterolemia. Role of oxidized LDL. *Circulation* 1996;93:1346–1353.

11 Johnstone MT, Creager SJ, Scales KM, et al. Impaired endothelium-dependent vasodilation in patients with insulin-dependent diabetes mellitus. *Circulation* 1993; 88:2510–2516.

12 Kuhn FE, Mohler ER, Satler LF, et al. Effects of high-density lipoprotein on acetylcholine-induced coronary vasoreactivity. *Am J Cardiol* 1991;68:1425–1430.

13 Seiler C, Hess OM, Buechi M, et al. Influence of serum cholesterol and other coronary risk factors on vasomotion of angiographically normal coronary arteries. *Circulation* 1993;88:2139–2148.

14 Taddei S, Virdis A, Mattei P, et al. Hypertension causes premature aging of endothelial function in humans. *Hypertension* 1997;29:736–743.

15 Vita JA, Treasure CB, Nabel EG, et al. Coronary vasomotor response to acetylcholine relates to risk factors for coronary artery disease. *Circulation* 1990;81:491–497.

16 Vita JA, Treasure CB, Yeung AC, et al. Patients with evidence of coronary endothelial dysfunction as assessed by acetylcholine infusion demonstrate marked increase in sensitivity to constrictor effects of catecholamines. *Circulation* 1992;85:1390–1397.

17 Zeiher AM, Drexler H, Wollschlager H, et al. Modulation of coronary vasomotor tone in humans. Progressive endothelial dysfunction with different early stages of coronary atherosclerosis. *Circulation* 1991;83:391–401.

18 Cigolini M, Targher G, Seidell JC, et al. Relationships of plasminogen activator inhibitor-1 to anthropometry, serum insulin, triglycerides and adipose tissue fatty acids in healthy men. *Atherosclerosis* 1994;106:139–147.

19 Hackman A, Abe Y, Insull Jr W, et al. Levels of soluble cell adhesion molecules in patients with dyslipidemia. *Circulation* 1996;93:1334–1338.

20 Hwang SJ, Ballantyne CM, Sharrett AR, et al. Circulating adhesion molecules VCAM-1, ICAM-1, and E-selectin in carotid atherosclerosis and incident coronary heart disease cases: the Atherosclerosis Risk In Communities (ARIC) study. *Circulation* 1997;96:4219–4225.

21 Kinlay S, Selwyn AP, Delagrange D, et al. Biological mechanisms for the clinical success of lipid-lowering in coronary artery disease and the use of surrogate endpoints. *Curr Opin Lipidol* 1996;7:389–397.

22 Chen ZP, Mitchellhill KI, Michell BJ, et al. AMP-activated protein kinase phosphorylation of endothelial NO synthase. *FEBS Lett* 1999;443:285–289.

23 Dimmeler S, Fleming I, Fisslthaler B, et al. Activation of nitric oxide synthase in endothelial cells by Akt-dependent phosphorylation. *Nature* 1999;399:601–605.

24 Fulton D, Gratton JP, McCabe TJ, et al. Regulation of endothelium-derived nitric oxide production by the protein kinase Akt. *Nature* 1999;399:597–601.

25 Pollock JS, Forstermann U, Mitchell JA, et al. Purification and characterization of particulate endothelium-derived relaxing factor synthase from cultured and native bovine aortic endothelial cells. *Proc Natl Acad Sci USA* 1991; 88:10480–10484.

26 Michel T, Feron O. Nitric oxide synthases: which, where, how, and why? *J Clin Invest* 1997;100:2146–2152.

27 Feron O, Belhassen L, Kobzik L, et al. Endothelial nitric oxide synthase targeting to caveolae. Specific interactions with caveolin isoforms in cardiac myocytes and endothelial cells. *J Biol Chem* 1996;271:22810–22814.

28 Keaney Jr JF, Vita JA. Atherosclerosis, oxidative stress, and antioxidant protection in endothelium-derived relaxing factor action. *Prog Cardiovasc Dis* 1995;38:129–154.

29 Gryglewski RJ, Palmer RM, Moncada S. Superoxide anion is involved in the breakdown of endothelium-derived vascular relaxing factor. *Nature* 1986;320:454–456.

30 Carr AC, Zhu BZ, Frei B. Potential antiatherogenic mechanisms of ascorbate (vitamin C) and alpha-tocopherol (vitamin E). *Circ Res* 2000;87:349–354.

31 Ludmer PL, Selwyn AP, Shook TL, et al. Paradoxical vasoconstriction induced by acetylcholine in atherosclerotic coronary arteries. *N Engl J Med* 1986;315: 1046–1051.

32 Lefroy DC, Crake T, Uren NG, et al. Effect of inhibition of nitric oxide synthesis on epicardial coronary artery caliber and coronary blood flow in humans. *Circulation* 1993;88:43–54.

33 Anderson TJ, Uehata A, Gerhard MD, et al. Close relation of endothelial function in the human coronary and peripheral circulations. *J Am Coll Cardiol* 1995;26: 1235–1241.

34 Lieberman EH, Gerhard MD, Uehata A, et al. Estrogen improves endothelium-dependent, flow-mediated vasodilation in postmenopausal women. *Ann Intern Med* 1994;121:936–941.

35 Cox DA, Vita JA, Treasure CB, et al. Atherosclerosis impairs flow-mediated dilation of coronary arteries in humans. *Circulation* 1989;80:458–465.

36 Lieberman EH, Gerhard MD, Uehata A, et al. Flow-induced vasodilation of the human brachial artery is

impaired in patients 40 years of age with coronary artery disease. *Am J Cardiol* 1996;78:1210–1214.

37 Moncada S, Higgs EA, Vane JR. Human arterial and venous tissues generate prostacyclin (prostaglandin x), a potent inhibitor of platelet aggregation. *Lancet* 1977; 1:18–20.

38 Feletou M, Vanhoutte PM. The alternative: EDHF. *J Mol Cell Cardiol* 1999;31:15–22.

39 Campbell WB, Harder DR. Prologue: EDHF – what is it? *Am J Physiol Heart Circ Physiol* 2001;280:H2413–H2416.

40 Sun J, Sui X, Bradbury JA, et al. Inhibition of vascular smooth muscle cell migration by cytochrome p450 epoxygenase-derived eicosanoids. *Circ Res* 2002;90: 1020–1027.

41 Yanagisawa M, Kurihara H, Kimura S, et al. A novel potent vasoconstrictor peptide produced by vascular endothelial cells. *Nature* 1988;332:411–415.

42 Inoue A, Yanagisawa M, Kimura S, et al. The human endothelin family: three structurally and pharmacologically distinct isopeptides predicted by three separate genes. *Proc Natl Acad Sci USA* 1989;86:2863–2867.

43 Winkles JA, Alberts GF, Brogi E, et al. Endothelin-1 and endothelin receptor mRNA expression in normal and atherosclerotic human arteries. *Biochem Biophys Res Commun* 1993;191:1081–1088.

44 Zeiher AM, Schachlinger V, Hohnloser SH, et al. Coronary atherosclerotic wall thickening and vascular reactivity in humans. Elevated high-density lipoprotein levels ameliorate abnormal vasoconstriction in early atherosclerosis. *Circulation* 1994;89:2525–2532.

45 Haynes WG, Webb DJ. Contribution of endogenous generation of endothelin-1 to basal vascular tone. *Lancet* 1994;344:852–854.

46 Verhaar MC, Strachan FE, Newby DE, et al. Endothelin-A receptor antagonist-mediated vasodilatation is attenuated by inhibition of nitric oxide synthesis and by endothelin-B receptor blockade. *Circulation* 1998;97:752–756.

47 Cardillo C, Kilcoyne CM, Waclawiw M, et al. Role of endothelin in the increased vascular tone of patients with essential hypertension. *Hypertension* 1999;33: 753–758.

48 Strachan FE, Spratt JC, Wilkinson IB, et al. Systemic blockade of the endothelin-B receptor increases peripheral vascular resistance in healthy men. *Hypertension* 1999;33:581–585.

49 Pierre LN, Davenport AP. Relative contribution of endothelin A and endothelin B receptors to vasoconstriction in small arteries from human heart and brain. *J Cardiovasc Pharmacol* 1998;31:S74–S76.

50 Russell FD, Skepper JN, Davenport AP. Detection of endothelin receptors in human coronary artery vascular smooth muscle cells but not endothelial cells by using electron microscope autoradiography. *J Cardiovasc Pharmacol* 1997;29:820–826.

51 Miyauchi T, Masaki T. Pathophysiology of endothelin in the cardiovascular system. *Annu Rev Physiol* 1999;61: 391–415.

52 Ge T, Hughes H, Junquero DC, et al. Endothelium-dependent contractions are associated with both augmented expression of prostaglandin H synthase-1 and hypersensitivity to prostaglandin H2 in the SHR aorta. *Circ Res* 1995;76:1003–1010.

53 Noll G, Buhler FR, Yang Z, et al. Different potency of endothelium-derived relaxing factors against thromboxane, endothelin, and potassium chloride in intramyocardial porcine coronary arteries. *J Cardiovasc Pharmacol* 1991;18:120–126.

54 Kinlay S, Behrendt D, Wainstein M, et al. Role of endothelin-1 in the active constriction of human atherosclerotic coronary arteries. *Circulation* 2001;104:1114–1118.

55 Halcox JP, Nour KR, Zalos G, et al. Coronary vasodilation and improvement in endothelial dysfunction with endothelin ET(A) receptor blockade. *Circ Res* 2001;89:969–976.

56 Wenzel RR, Fleisch M, Shaw S, et al. Hemodynamic and coronary effects of the endothelin antagonist bosentan in patients with coronary artery disease. *Circulation* 1998;98:2235–2240.

57 Cardillo C, Kilcoyne CM, Cannon III RO, et al. Increased activity of endogenous endothelin in patients with hypercholesterolemia. *J Am Coll Cardiol* 2000;36: 1483–1488.

58 Nohria A, Garrett L, Johnson W, et al. Endothelin-1 and vascular tone in subjects with atherogenic risk factors. *Hypertension* 2003;42:43–48.

59 Yeung AC, Vekshtein VI, Krantz DS, et al. The effect of atherosclerosis on the vasomotor response of coronary arteries to mental stress. *N Engl J Med* 1991;325:1551–1556.

60 Nabel EG, Ganz P, Gordon JB, et al. Dilation of normal and constriction of atherosclerotic coronary arteries caused by the cold pressor test. *Circulation* 1988;77:43–52.

61 Corretti MC, Anderson TJ, Benjamin EJ, et al. Guidelines for the ultrasound assessment of endothelial-dependent flow-mediated vasodilation of the brachial artery: a report of the International Brachial Artery Reactivity Task Force. *J Am Coll Cardiol* 2002;39:257–265.

62 Arcaro G, Zenere BM, Travia D, et al. Non-invasive detection of early endothelial dysfunction in hypercholesterolaemic subjects. *Atherosclerosis* 1995;114:247–254.

63 Woodman RJ, Playford DA, Watts GF, et al. Improved analysis of brachial artery ultrasound using a novel edge-detection software system. *J Appl Physiol* 2001;91: 929–937.

64 Joannides R, Bizet-Nafeh C, Costentin A, et al. Chronic ACE inhibition enhances the endothelial control of arterial mechanics and flow-dependent vasodilatation in heart failure. *Hypertension* 2001;38:1446–1450.

65 Lerman A, Burnett Jr JC, Higano ST, et al. Long-term L-arginine supplementation improves small-vessel

coronary endothelial function in humans. *Circulation* 1998;97:2123–2128.

66 Egashira K, Suzuki S, Hirooka Y, et al. Impaired endothelium-dependent vasodilation of large epicardial and resistance coronary arteries in patients with essential hypertension. Different responses to acetylcholine and substance P. *Hypertension* 1995;25:201–206.

67 Drexler H, Fischell TA, Pinto FJ, et al. Effect of L-arginine on coronary endothelial function in cardiac transplant recipients. Relation to vessel wall morphology. *Circulation* 1994;89:1615–1623.

68 Panza JA, Quyyumi AA, Brush Jr JE, et al. Abnormal endothelium-dependent vascular relaxation in patients with essential hypertension. *N Engl J Med* 1990;323:22–27.

69 Creager MA, Cooke JP, Mendelsohn ME, et al. Impaired vasodilation of forearm resistance vessels in hypercholesterolemic humans. *J Clin Invest* 1990;86:228–234.

70 Kinlay S, Creager MA, Fukumoto M, et al. Endothelium-derived nitric oxide regulates arterial elasticity in human arteries *in vivo*. *Hypertension* 2001;38:1049–1053.

71 Krum H, Viskoper RJ, Lacourciere Y, et al. The effect of an endothelin-receptor antagonist, bosentan, on blood pressure in patients with essential hypertension. Bosentan Hypertension Investigators (see comments). *N Engl J Med* 1998;338:784–790.

72 Rubin LJ, Badesch DB, Barst RJ, et al. Bosentan therapy for pulmonary arterial hypertension. *N Engl J Med* 2002; 346:896–903.

CHAPTER 13

Endothelial vasodilatory dysfunction and risk factors in adults

Mark R. Adams, MBBS, PhD, FRACP *&*
David S. Celermajer, MBBS, PhD, FRACP

Arterial endothelial dysfunction, a key early step in the development of atherosclerosis, participates in the pathophysiology of symptomatic coronary artery disease. Endothelial dysfunction may be detected in children and adults many years before the development of clinically apparent or, indeed, even morphologic evidence of atherosclerosis [1,2]. Importantly, dysfunctional endothelium involves the loss of effective nitric oxide (NO) mediated vasodilation in conduit arteries and the microcirculation. In the last 10–15 years, our understanding of the risk factors associated with these changes has increased due to the development of sensitive methods to measure endothelium-dependent vasodilation *in vivo*. Numerous studies have demonstrated that the loss of endothelium-dependent vasodilatory responses relates to the presence of risk factors for atherosclerosis. Multiple risk factors independently associate with impaired endothelium-dependent dilation, and these factors may interact [1,3–5]. Importantly, correction of such risk factors may reverse, partially or completely, the loss of endothelium-dependent dilation [6].

Measuring endothelium-dependent vasodilation in adults

In 1986, Ludmer and colleagues [7] first described *in vivo* measurement of endothelium-dependent vasodilation in conduit arteries, an invasive method, performed at cardiac catheterization, and that involves the infusion of pharmacologic agents directly into the coronary artery being studied. Responses to these agents (in the epicardial coronary arteries) are measured using quantitative coronary angiography. Endothelium-dependent vasodilators such as acetylcholine and substance P produce vasodilation in the presence of normal endothelial function, while substances such as glyceryltrinitrate (GTN) and sodium nitroprusside (SNP) relax smooth muscle cells directly rather than via endothelial NO release, thus producing vasodilation independent of the endothelium. Alternatively, changes in vessel diameter can be measured in response to conditions of hyperemia. Dilator response to these endothelium-dependent vasodilators and physiologic stimuli depend (at least in part) on endothelial production of NO [8,9].

The integrity of endothelium-dependent vasodilation in the coronary *microcirculation* can be assessed in a similar manner, often simultaneously with measurement of large vessel function. In this case, instead of measuring changes in vessel diameter, changes in intracoronary flow velocity or absolute flow are measured in response to infusions of endothelium-dependent vasodilators such as acetylcholine. Such invasive measures provide important insights into the physiologic control of the coronary circulation as well as the abnormalities of function, which occur in disease states and in the presence of risk factors for atherosclerosis. The main disadvantage with these techniques involves their invasive nature, which limits our ability to utilize them in the study of endothelial function in young and asymptomatic subjects, particularly in trials requiring serial measurements.

Minimally invasive techniques are available for measurement of small-vessel endothelium-dependent dilation in the forearm. Such techniques utilize an infusion of an endothelium-dependent vasodilator such as acetylcholine or methacholine into the brachial artery as well as measurement of changes in blood flow in the perfused forearm, as assessed by volume changes, measured by venous occlusion strain gauge plethysmography. In experienced hands, this technique is a sensitive measure of forearm microcirculatory physiology, and has been utilized in many cross-sectional studies and even (more latterly) interventional trials [10].

Our group first described a completely non-invasive technique for assessing forearm brachial artery endothelium-dependent dilation in 1992 [2]. This technique utilizes high-resolution external vascular ultrasound to measure changes in brachial or femoral artery diameter in response to reactive hyperemia (induced by transient distal arm or leg ischemia) and also in response to sublingual GTN. Although vasodilatory response to hyperemia depends mainly on endothelial production of NO, vasodilatory response to nitroglycerin is endothelium independent [11]. Furthermore, such forearm responses correlate with the changes seen in the coronary arteries [12]. Therefore, this technique allows the study of young asymptomatic subjects including children, and also demonstrates impaired endothelium-dependent dilation of the systemic arteries in subjects with risk factors as young as 4 years of age [13].

Dyslipidemia

One of the first risk factors associated with loss of endothelium-dependent dilation was hypercholesterolemia. Vita et al. studied a cohort of subjects with angiographically normal coronary arteries but risk factors for atherosclerosis, and found a highly significant correlation between hypercholesterolemia and abnormal endothelium-dependent dilation to acetylcholine [1]. Other investigators similarly found that hypercholesterolemia associates with abnormal endothelium-dependent dilation even in the absence

of coronary atherosclerosis, and that progressive loss of endothelial function may occur through the early stages of atherosclerosis [3]. The development of a non-invasive ultrasound technique to measure large-vessel endothelial function in the peripheral arterial bed has allowed the assessment of apparently healthy children and adults with hypercholesterolemia, thus demonstrating that endothelium-dependent dilation may be abnormal in the setting of hyperlipidemia, decades before coronary atherosclerosis develops [2]. Further investigation has shown that different atherogenic lipids have varying effects on endothelial function.

Several *in vivo* studies have associated low-density lipoprotein (LDL) cholesterol with reduced endothelium-dependent dilation [1,3]. Although native LDL may participate in this process [14], evidence from animal models and *in vitro* studies suggests that much of the deleterious effect of LDL cholesterol results from oxidatively modified LDL [15–17]. Evidence from these experimental studies also suggests that the formation of reactive hydroxy-fatty acids from polyunsaturated phospholipids and lysophosphatidylcholine may directly impair endothelium-derived dilation [18]. Furthermore, oxidized LDL deleteriously affects endothelial NO production, and directly inactivates NO [19,20]. Oxidized LDL downregulates the transcription of mRNA for NO synthase (NOS), via effects on nuclear factor κB (NF-κB) and protein kinase C (PKC), and directly destabilizes mRNA as well [21]. Oxidized LDL also interferes with normal signal transduction within endothelial cells [22] and may lead to accumulation of competitive inhibitors of NOS such as asymmetric dimethylarginine (ADMA) [23,24].

A relationship between oxidized LDL and impaired endothelial function has also been demonstrated *in vivo* in humans. Anderson and colleagues found that impairment in endothelium-dependent dilation in the coronary circulation associated significantly with the susceptibility of an individual subject's LDL particles to oxidative modification [25]. By promoting oxidative modification of lipids, oxidative stress such as that associated with cigarette smoking may act synergistically with LDL to produce endothelial dysfunction [26]. The morphology of LDL particles also links to their potential for endothelial damage. Small-dense LDL particles, which are more susceptible to oxidation, associate

endothelium-dependent dilation associated with the subsequent risk of clinical events [86]. Suwaidi et al. found that subjects in the worst tertile of coronary endothelium-dependent dilation had a 14% incidence of coronary events over the subsequent 2 years, whilst those in the best tertile of function had a 0% incidence of coronary events [87]. In the forearm circulation, Heitzer and colleagues found a significant difference in coronary event rates between those above and below the median level of microcirculatory endothelium-dependent dilation [88]. Other investigators studying coronary endothelial function have described similar correlations. Impairment of the response to hyperemia associates with cardiovascular risk factors, and the level of impairment may predict future coronary events [89].

Conclusions

The vascular endothelium plays a central role in the regulation of vascular tone, inflammation, thrombosis, and growth. Many of these actions are mediated by the release of NO. In the presence of risk factors for atherosclerosis, endothelial vasodilatory capacity decreases, even in otherwise healthy adults, many years before atherosclerosis becomes clinically apparent. While such changes associate with increased future risk of adverse cardiac events, treatment of risk factors can modify their impact.

References

1 Vita JA, Treasure CB, Nabel EG, et al. Coronary vasomotor response to acetylcholine relates to risk factors for coronary artery disease. *Circulation* 1990;81: 491–497.

2 Celermajer DS, Sorensen KE, Gooch VM, et al. Noninvasive detection of endothelial dysfunction in children and adults at risk of atherosclerosis. *Lancet* 1992; 340:1111–1115.

3 Zeiher AM, Drexler H, Wollschlager H, et al. Modulation of coronary vasomotor tone in humans. Progressive endothelial dysfunction with different early stages of coronary atherosclerosis. *Circulation* 1991; 83:391–401.

4 Yasue H, Matsuyama K, Okumura K, et al. Responses of angiographically normal human coronary arteries to intracoronary injection of acetylcholine by age and segment. Possible role of early coronary atherosclerosis. *Circulation* 1990;81:482–490.

5 Celermajer DS, Sorensen KE, Bull C, et al. Endothelium-dependent dilation in the systemic arteries of asymptomatic subjects relates to coronary risk factors and their interaction. *J Am Coll Cardiol* 1994;24:1468–1474.

6 Ganz P, Creager MA, Fang JC, et al. Pathogenic mechanisms of atherosclerosis: effect of lipid lowering on the biology of atherosclerosis. *Am J Med* 1996; 101: 4A10S–4A16S.

7 Ludmer PL, Selwyn AP, Shook TL, et al. Paradoxical vasoconstriction induced by acetylcholine in atherosclerotic coronary arteries. *N Engl J Med* 1986;315:1046–1051.

8 Hodgson JM, Marshall JJ. Direct vasoconstriction and endothelium-dependent vasodilation. Mechanisms of acetylcholine effects on coronary flow and arterial diameter in patients with nonstenotic coronary arteries. *Circulation* 1989;79:1043–1051.

9 Lefroy DC, Crake T, Uren NG, et al. Effect of inhibition of nitric oxide synthesis on epicardial coronary artery caliber and coronary blood flow in humans. *Circulation* 1993;88:43–54.

10 Calver A, Collier J, Vallance P. Inhibition and stimulation of nitric oxide synthesis in the human forearm arterial bed of patients with insulin-dependent diabetes. *J Clin Invest* 1992;90:2548–2554.

11 Joannides R, Richard V, Haefeli WE, et al. Role of basal and stimulated release of nitric oxide in the regulation of radial artery caliber in humans. *Hypertension* 1995;26:327–331.

12 Anderson TJ, Gerhard MD, Meredith IT, et al. Systemic nature of endothelial dysfunction in atherosclerosis. *Am J Cardiol* 1995;75:71B–74B.

13 Celermajer DS, Sorensen K, Ryalls M, et al. Impaired endothelial function occurs in the systemic arteries of children with homozygous homocystinuria but not in their heterozygous parents. *J Am Coll Cardiol* 1993;22: 854–858.

14 Pritchard Jr KA, Groszek L, Smalley DM, et al. Native low-density lipoprotein increases endothelial cell nitric oxide synthase generation of superoxide anion. *Circ Res* 1995;77:510–518.

15 Simon BC, Cunningham LD, Cohen RA. Oxidized low density lipoproteins cause contraction and inhibit endothelium-dependent relaxation in the pig coronary artery. *J Clin Invest* 1990;86:75–79.

16 Abebe W, Mustafa SJ. Effect of low density lipoprotein on adenosine receptor-mediated coronary vasorelaxation *in vitro*. *J Pharmacol Exp Ther* 1997;282:851–857.

17 Kume N, Cybulsky MI, Gimbrone Jr MA. Lysophosphatidylcholine, a component of atherogenic lipoproteins, induces mononuclear leukocyte adhesion molecules in cultured human and rabbit arterial endothelial cells. *J Clin Invest* 1992;90:1138–1144.

18 Kugiyama K, Kerns SA, Morrisett JD, et al. Impairment of endothelium-dependent arterial relaxation by

lysolecithin in modified low-density lipoproteins. *Nature* 1990;344:160–162.

19 Gryglewski RJ, Palmer RM, Moncada S. Superoxide anion is involved in the breakdown of endothelium-derived vascular relaxing factor. *Nature* 1986;320:454–456.

20 Ohara Y, Peterson TE, Harrison DG. Hypercholesterolemia increases endothelial superoxide anion production. *J Clin Invest* 1993;91:2546–2551.

21 Liao JK, Shin WS, Lee WY, et al. Oxidized low-density lipoprotein decreases the expression of endothelial nitric oxide synthase. *J Biol Chem* 1995;270:319–324.

22 Liao JK, Clark SL. Regulation of G-protein alpha i2 subunit expression by oxidized low-density lipoprotein. *J Clin Invest* 1995;95:1457–1463.

23 Boger RH, Bode-Boger SM, Szuba A, et al. Asymmetric dimethylarginine (ADMA): a novel risk factor for endothelial dysfunction: its role in hypercholesterolemia. *Circulation* 1998;98:1842–1847.

24 Vallance P, Leone A, Calver A, et al. Accumulation of an endogenous inhibitor of nitric oxide synthesis in chronic renal failure. *Lancet* 1992;339:572–575.

25 Anderson TJ, Meredith IT, Charbonneau F, et al. Endothelium-dependent coronary vasomotion relates to the susceptibility of LDL to oxidation in humans. *Circulation* 1996;93:1647–1650.

26 Heitzer T, Yla-Herttuala S, Luoma J, et al. Cigarette smoking potentiates endothelial dysfunction of forearm resistance vessels in patients with hypercholesterolemia. Role of oxidized LDL. *Circulation* 1996;93:1346–1353.

27 Steinberg D, Lewis A. Conner Memorial Lecture. Oxidative modification of LDL and atherogenesis. *Circulation* 1997;95:1062–1071.

28 Sorensen KE, Celermajer DS, Georgakopoulos D, et al. Impairment of endothelium-dependent dilation is an early event in children with familial hypercholesterolemia and is related to the lipoprotein(a) level. *J Clin Invest* 1994;93:50–55.

29 Galle J, Bengen J, Schollmeyer P, et al. Impairment of endothelium-dependent dilation in rabbit renal arteries by oxidized lipoprotein(a). Role of oxygen-derived radicals. *Circulation* 1995;92:1582–1589.

30 Schachinger V, Halle M, Minners J, et al. Lipoprotein(a) selectively impairs receptor-mediated endothelial vasodilator function of the human coronary circulation. *J Am Coll Cardiol* 1997;30:927–934.

31 Raitakari OT, Adams MR, Celermajer DS. Effect of Lp(a) on the early functional and structural changes of atherosclerosis. *Arterioscler Thromb Vasc Biol* 1999;19: 990–995.

32 Matsuda Y, Hirata K, Inoue N, et al. High density lipoprotein reverses inhibitory effect of oxidized low density lipoprotein on endothelium-dependent arterial relaxation. *Circ Res* 1993;72:1103–1109.

33 Takahashi M, Yui Y, Yasumoto H, et al. Lipoproteins are inhibitors of endothelium-dependent relaxation of rabbit aorta. *Am J Physiol* 1990;258:H1–H8.

34 Kuhn FE, Mohler ER, Satler LF, et al. Effects of high-density lipoprotein on acetylcholine-induced coronary vasoreactivity. *Am J Cardiol* 1991;68:1425–1430.

35 Zeiher AM, Schachinger V, Hohnloser SH, et al. Coronary atherosclerotic wall thickening and vascular reactivity in humans. *Circulation* 1994;89:2525–2532.

36 Chowienczyk PJ, Watts GF, Wierzbicki AS, et al. Preserved endothelial function in patients with severe hypertriglyceridemia and low functional lipoprotein lipase activity. *J Am Coll Cardiol* 1997;29:964–968.

37 Lundman P, Tornvall P, Nilsson L, et al. A triglyceride-rich fat emulsion and free fatty acids but not very low density lipoproteins impair endothelium-dependent vasorelaxation. *Atherosclerosis* 2001;159:35–41.

38 Sattar N, Petrie JR, Jaap AJ. The atherogenic lipoprotein phenotype and vascular endothelial dysfunction. *Atherosclerosis* 1998;138:229–235.

39 Inoue T, Saniabadi AR, Matsunaga R, et al. Impaired endothelium-dependent acetylcholine-induced coronary artery relaxation in patients with high serum remnant lipoprotein particles. *Atherosclerosis* 1998;139: 363–367.

40 Vogel RA, Corretti MC, Plotnick GD. Effect of a single high-fat meal on endothelial function in healthy subjects. *Am J Cardiol* 1997;79:350–354.

41 Leung WH, Lau CP, Wong CK. Beneficial effect of cholesterol-lowering therapy on coronary endothelium-dependent relaxation in hypercholesterolaemic patients. *Lancet* 1993;341:1496–1500.

42 Egashira K, Hirooka Y, Kai H, et al. Reduction in serum cholesterol with pravastatin improves endothelium-dependent coronary vasomotion in patients with hypercholesterolemia. *Circulation* 1994;89:2519–2524.

43 Anderson TJ, Meredith IT, Yeung AC, et al. The effect of cholesterol-lowering and antioxidant therapy on endothelium-dependent coronary vasomotion. *N Engl J Med* 1995;332:488–493.

44 Simons LA, Sullivan D, Simons J, et al. Effects of atorvastatin monotherapy and simvastatin plus cholestyramine on arterial endothelial function in patients with severe primary hypercholesterolaemia. *Atherosclerosis* 1998; 137:197–203.

45 O'Driscoll G, Green D, Taylor RR. Simvastatin, an HMG-coenzyme A reductase inhibitor, improves endothelial function within 1 month. *Circulation* 1997;95: 1126–1131.

46 Stroes ES, Koomans HA, de Bruin TW, et al. Vascular function in the forearm of hypercholesterolaemic patients off and on lipid-lowering medication. *Lancet* 1995; 346:467–471.

47 Tamai O, Matsuoka H, Itabe H, et al. Single LDL aphere-sis improves endothelium-dependent vasodilatation in hypercholesterolemic humans. *Circulation* 1997;95: 76–82.

48 Igarashi K, Horimoto M, Takenaka T, et al. Acute choles-terol lowering therapy with LDL-apheresis improves endothelial function of the coronary microcirculation in patients with hypercholesterolemia. *Circulation* 1995;92(Suppl I):452 [Abstract].

49 Clarkson P, Adams MR, Powe AJ, et al. Oral L-arginine improves endothelium-dependent dilation in hypercho-lesterolemic young adults. *J Clin Invest* 1996;97: 1989–1994.

50 Heitzer T, Krohn K, Albers S, et al. Tetrahydrobiopterin improves endothelium-dependent vasodilation by increasing nitric oxide activity in patients with Type II diabetes mellitus. *Diabetologia* 2000;43:1435–1438.

51 Nitenberg A, Antony I, Foult JM. Acetylcholine-induced coronary vasoconstriction in young, heavy smokers with normal coronary angiographic findings. *Am J Med* 1993;95:71–77.

52 Celermajer DS, Sorensen KE, Georgakopoulos D, et al. Cigarette smoking is associated with dose-related and potentially reversible impairment of endothelium-dependent dilation in healthy young adults. *Circulation* 1993;88:2149–2155.

53 Celermajer DS, Adams MR, Clarkson P, et al. Passive smoking and impaired endothelium-dependent arterial dilatation in healthy young adults. *N Engl J Med* 1996;334:150–154.

54 Adams MR, Jessup W, Celermajer DS. Cigarette smoking is associated with increased human monocyte adhesion to endothelial cells: reversibility with oral L-arginine but not vitamin C. *J Am Coll Cardiol* 1997;29:491–497.

55 Blann AD, McCollum CN. Adverse influence of cigarette smoking on the endothelium. *Thromb Haemost* 1993;70: 707–711.

56 Raitakari OT, Adams MR, McCredie RJ, et al. Arterial endothelial dysfunction related to passive smoking is potentially reversible in healthy young adults. *Ann Intern Med* 1999;130:578–581.

57 Williams SB, Goldfine AB, Timimi FK, et al. Acute hyper-glycemia attenuates endothelium-dependent vasodilation in humans *in vivo*. *Circulation* 1998;97:1695–1701.

58 Nitenberg A, Valensi P, Sachs R, et al. Impairment of coronary vascular reserve and ACh-induced vasodilation in diabetic patients with angiographically normal coro-nary arteries and normal left ventricular systolic func-tion. *Diabetes* 1993;43:1017–1025.

59 Johnstone MT, Creager SJ, Scales KM, et al. Impaired endothelium-dependent vasodilation in the human forearm arterial bed of patients with insulin-dependent diabetes mellitus. *Circulation* 1993;88:2510–2526.

60 Clarkson P, Celermajer DS, Donald AE, et al. Impaired vascular reactivity in insulin-dependent diabetes melli-tus is related to disease duration and low density lipoprotein cholesterol levels. *J Am Coll Cardiol* 1996;28: 573–579.

61 Adams MR, Robinson J, McCredie R, et al. Smooth mus-cle dysfunction occurs independently of impaired endothelium-dependent dilation in adults at risk of ath-erosclerosis. *J Am Coll Cardiol* 1998;32:123–127.

62 Takahara N, Kashiwagi A, Nishio Y, et al. Oxidized lipoproteins found in patients with NIDDM stimulate radical-induced monocyte chemoattractant protein-1 mRNA expression in cultured human endothelial cells. *Diabetologia* 1997;40:662–670.

63 Morigi M, Angioletti S, Imberti B, et al. Leukocyte–endothelial interaction is augmented by high glucose con-centrations and hyperglycemia in a NF-kB-dependent fashion. *J Clin Invest* 1998;101:1905–1915.

64 Cardillo C, Nambi SS, Kilcoyne CM, et al. Insulin stimu-lates both endothelin and nitric oxide activity in the human forearm. *Circulation* 1999;100:820–825.

65 Balletshofer BM, Rittig K, Enderle MD, et al. Endothelial dysfunction is detectable in young normotensive first-degree relatives of subjects with type 2 diabetes in association with insulin resistance. *Circulation* 2000;101:1780–1784.

66 Timimi FK, Ting HH, Haley EA, et al. Vitamin C improves endothelium-dependent vasodilation in patients with insulin-dependent diabetes mellitus. *J Am Coll Cardiol* 1998;31:552–557.

67 Mullen MJ, Clarkson P, Donald AE, et al. Effect of enalapril on endothelial function in young insulin-dependent diabetic patients: a randomized, double-blind study. *J Am Coll Cardiol* 1998;31:1330–1335.

68 Zeiher AM, Drexler H, Saurbier B, et al. Endothelium-mediated coronary blood flow modula-tion in humans. Effects of age, atherosclerosis, hypercho-lesterolemia, and hypertension. *J Clin Invest* 1993; 92:652–662.

69 Treasure CB, Manoukian SV, Klein JL, et al. Epicardial coronary artery responses to acetylcholine are impaired in hypertensive patients. *Circ Res* 1992;71:776–781.

70 Cockcroft JR, Chowienczyk PJ, Benjamin N, et al. Preserved endothelium-dependent vasodilatation in patients with essential hypertension. *N Engl J Med* 1994;330:1036–1040.

71 Gardiner HM, Celermajer DS, Sorensen KE, et al. Arterial reactivity is significantly impaired in normoten-sive young adults after successful repair of aortic coarcta-tion in childhood. *Circulation* 1994;89:1745–1750.

72 Perticone F, Ceravolo R, Pujia A, et al. Prognostic signif-icance of endothelial dysfunction in hypertensive patients. *Circulation* 2001;104:191–196.

73 Celermajer DS, Sorensen KE, Spiegelhalter DJ, et al. Aging is associated with endothelial dysfunction in healthy men years before the age-related decline in women. *J Am Coll Cardiol* 1994;24:471–476.

74 McCrohon JA, Adams MR, McCredie RJ, et al. Hormone replacement therapy is associated with improved arterial physiology in healthy post-menopausal women. *Clin Endocrinol (Oxford)* 1996;45:435–441.

75 Lieberman EH, Gerhard MD, Uehata A, et al. Estrogen improves endothelium-dependent, flow-mediated vasodilation in postmenopausal women. *Ann Intern Med* 1994;121:936–941.

76 McCrohon JA, Walters WA, Robinson JT, et al. Arterial reactivity is enhanced in genetic males taking high dose estrogens. *J Am Coll Cardiol* 1997;29:1432–1436.

77 Kushwaha RS. Female sex steroid hormones and lipoprotein metabolism. *Curr Opin Lipidol* 1992;3:167–172.

78 Woo KS, Robinson JT, Chook P, et al. Differences in the effect of cigarette smoking on endothelial function in Chinese and White adults. *Ann Intern Med* 1997;127:372–375.

79 Stamler JS, Osborne JA, Jaraki O, et al. Adverse vascular effects of homocysteine are modulated by endothelium-derived relaxing factor and related oxides of nitrogen. *J Clin Invest* 1993;91:308–318.

80 Tawakol A, Omland T, Gerhard M, et al. Hyperhomocyst(e)inemia is associated with impaired endothelium-dependent vasodilation in humans. *Circulation* 1997;95:1119–1121.

81 Woo KS, Chook P, Chan LL, et al. Long-term improvement in homocysteine levels and arterial endothelial function after 1-year folic acid supplementation. *Am J Med* 2002;112:535–539.

82 Gokce N, Keaney Jr JF, Frei B, et al. Long-term ascorbic acid administration reverses endothelial vasomotor dysfunction in patients with coronary artery disease. *Circulation* 1999;99:3234–3240.

83 Levine GN, Frei B, Koulouris SN, et al. Ascorbic acid reverses endothelial vasomotor dysfunction in patients with coronary artery disease. *Circulation* 1996;93:1107–1113.

84 Raitakari OT, Adams MR, McCredie RJ, et al. Oral vitamin C and endothelial function in smokers: short-term improvement, but no sustained beneficial effect. *J Am Coll Cardiol* 2000;35:1616–1621.

85 Nobuyoshi M, Tanaka M, Nosaka H, et al. Progression of coronary atherosclerosis: is coronary spasm related to progression? *J Am Coll Cardiol* 1991;18:904–910.

86 Murakami T, Mizuno S, Kaku B. Clinical morbidities in subjects with Doppler-evaluated endothelial dysfunction of coronary artery. *J Am Coll Cardiol* 1998;31:341A.

87 Suwaidi JA, Hamasaki S, Higano ST, et al. Long-term follow-up of patients with mild coronary artery disease and endothelial dysfunction. *Circulation* 2000;101:948–954.

88 Heitzer T, Schlinzig T, Krohn K, et al. Endothelial dysfunction, oxidative stress, and risk of cardiovascular events in patients with coronary artery disease. *Circulation* 2001;104:2673–2678.

89 Schachinger V, Zeiher AM. Prognostic implications of endothelial dysfunction: Does it mean anything? *Coronary Artery Dis* 2001;12:435–443.

CHAPTER 14

Endothelial vasodilatory dysfunction in early life

Julian P.J. Halcox, MA, MD, MRCP *& John E. Deanfield,* FRCP

Introduction

Atherosclerosis is the leading killer in the Western world and also much of Asia, with increasing prevalence in developing countries. Currently regarded universally as the critical trigger for the initiation and development of atherosclerotic lesions, endothelial dysfunction likely participates in the pathogenesis of plaque instability and thrombosis that leads to acute complications such as myocardial infarction. Several techniques developed during the past 10–15 years now provide clinical assessment of endothelial function, leading to greatly enhanced appreciation of the role of the vascular endothelium in the pathogenesis of clinical cardiovascular disease. Clearly, endothelial dysfunction develops early in life as a consequence of exposure to conventional as well as novel "cardiac risk factors." This is of key importance, not only to our understanding of the disease process, but also for the development of strategies for the detection and treatment of those at risk for clinical atherosclerotic disease. This chapter describes the non-invasive techniques currently available to assess endothelium-dependent vasodilatory function in young subjects, and also reviews the determinants of endothelial dysfunction in youth. Such data critically increase our understanding of the initiation and progression of cardiovascular disease.

Atherosclerosis in the young

Although clinical consequences of atherosclerosis, such as myocardial infarction and stroke, typically do not manifest until middle and old age, atherogenesis begins early in life. Fatty streaks, the earliest lesions of atherosclerosis, occur even during fetal life, promoted by maternal hypercholesterolemia that increases the number and size of such lesions. In addition, the progression rate of aortic atherosclerotic lesions increases in the children of hypercholesterolemic mothers, suggesting that maternal risk factors during pregnancy participate in the pathogenesis of vascular disease early in life [1,2]. The development of atherosclerosis results from the interaction between intrinsic characteristics as well as exposure to "risk factors." For example, mildly elevated blood pressure in children may accelerate the transition of innocuous childhood fatty streaks to more complex fibrous plaques. Data from the Bogalusa Heart Study and other American populations demonstrate obesity, increased blood pressure, and dyslipidemia among children [3]. A family history of heart disease, insulin resistance, dyslipidemia, excess dietary intake of calories (particularly as saturated fat), cigarette smoking, and physical inactivity foreshadows the development of cardiovascular disease in later life. Cardiovascular risk factors present in youth usually persist into adulthood, promoting atherogenesis from an early age. Indeed, necropsy specimens of young American adults dying of non-cardiac causes show an alarmingly high prevalence of significant coronary atherosclerotic lesions. However, the putative relationship of adult coronary heart disease risk factors to atherosclerotic lesions during childhood is based largely on extrapolation from adult data, illustrated by the association between raised levels of serum cholesterol in early adulthood and increased risk of premature coronary death [4].

Although strategies aimed at detecting and modifying conventional risk factors in early life likely improve long-term outcomes of young subjects at the highest risk of developing atherosclerosis and its complications, including those with diabetes or familial hyperlipidemias, the long natural history and multifactorial nature of atherogenesis make identification and treatment of children at risk a complex but extremely important process.

Endothelial dysfunction and atherogenesis: relevance to youth

The endothelium comprises a single layer of cells that line the luminal surface of blood vessels, acting as a direct functional interface between the components of circulating blood and local tissue. Such cells, which participate in the regulation of multiple local processes in the vasculature, i.e., modulation of vascular tone, cell adhesion, coagulation, inflammation and vascular permeability, are highly susceptible to the stresses of everyday life. By producing and reacting to a number of locally active mediators, particularly nitric oxide (NO), the healthy endothelium acts in a coordinated fashion to balance vasodilatory and vasoconstrictive influences and regulates vascular bed resistance, thus maintaining adequate tissue perfusion [5]. The endothelium also regulates the functions of circulating leukocytes, platelets, and red blood cells. Endothelial dysfunction is associated with reduced anticoagulant properties as well as increased expression on the endothelial surface of molecules that act as attractants and/or receptors for complementary molecules on circulating leukocytes, thus potentially contributing to the early lesions of atherosclerosis [6].

Traditional cardiovascular risk factors, such as hypertension, hyperlipidemia, insulin resistance/diabetes, and tobacco use, are associated with endothelial dysfunction. Experimental studies have shown that reduced bioavailability of NO is a cardinal feature of these conditions. Recent evidence suggests that novel risk factors for atherosclerosis may cause endothelial dysfunction. Indeed, various deleterious and protective environmental and genetic factors likely engender the degree of endothelial dysfunction. Clinical measures of endothelial dysfunction carry long-term prognostic implications for the development of atherosclerosis and its complications [7,8]. Thus, identifying individuals with endothelial dysfunction and monitoring their response to interventions early in the disease process likely will produce beneficial consequences.

Techniques for the measurement of endothelium-dependent vasodilatory function in the young

Techniques in clinical practice focus predominantly on measuring the effects of the endothelium on vascular tone.

Invasive assessment of vascular function

Depending on the question of interest, several different methods can assess endothelium-dependent vasodilatory function. For example, quantitative coronary angiography and Doppler flow wire techniques can measure coronary vascular epicardial and microvascular responses to local infusion of endothelium-dependent pharmacologic probes, such as acetylcholine, bradykinin, and substance P. Similarly, attempts to localize any observed functional vasomotor defect by infusing nitrates, e.g., sodium nitroprusside or nitroglycerin, and subsequent comparison with endothelium-dependent responses can assess the capacity of coronary smooth muscle vasodilators. However, techniques that test coronary endothelial function are highly invasive, expensive, and limited to specialized laboratories. Although such studies provide valuable information, they are not feasible in patients without clinical disease unless coronary angiography is indicated. Thus, children and subjects with preclinical atherosclerosis cannot be studied, repeat procedures are difficult to justify, and for safety reasons such studies are inadvisable in patients with advanced disease.

Invasive testing of peripheral arterial function using similar pharmacologic probes infused via a thin cannula inserted into the brachial or femoral artery allows venous occlusion plethysmography to measure blood flow responses. Although this technique has an excellent safety record and has provided a wealth of information regarding mechanisms of endothelial dysfunction and vascular disease, it is inappropriate for use in children, due to the small but important risk of damaging their arteries.

Considering the ethical and practical limitations of the techniques described above, we clearly need reliable and non-invasive tools to identify and subsequently monitor endothelial dysfunction in humans *in vivo*.

Non-invasive assessment of peripheral vascular function

Principles of flow-mediated dilation

More than a decade ago, our group introduced techniques using high-resolution ultrasound to study the responses of conduit arteries in the systemic circulation to changes in blood flow. In 1980, Furchgott and Zawadzki described the action of a labile substance, termed endothelium-derived relaxing factor (EDRF) that was secreted from endothelial cells and vasodilated rabbit aortic rings [9]. This was subsequently identified as NO, a diatomic molecule produced from L-arginine by the constitutive action of the enzyme endothelial NO synthase (eNOS) [10]. In 1986, Busse and colleagues demonstrated that cultured endothelial cells release EDRF in response to mechanical stress, and Rubanyi confirmed that increased flow conditions also stimulate the release of EDRF, prompting research into the effects of increased vascular shear forces on endothelial function *in vivo* [11,12]. Three years later, Cox et al. demonstrated that epicardial coronary conduit vessels dilate in response to increased blood flow stimulated by the selective infusion of adenosine into the distal vascular bed [13]. Because eNOS inhibition using L-NMMA may suppress vasodilatory responses, such dilation predominantly follows the endothelial release of NO [13–15]. Although the precise mechanisms for the acute detection of shear forces and subsequent signal transduction to modulate vasomotor tone remain incompletely understood, they likely involve the opening of calcium-activated potassium channels, membrane hyperpolarization, and calcium-mediated activation of eNOS. These experimental observations, demonstrating the dependence of arterial tone on the local release of NO in response to shear stress, form the basis of the assessment of flow-mediated endothelium-dependent dilation (FMD) of the brachial artery [16,17]. Such methods rely on measuring changes in vascular diameter that occur in response to reactive hyperemia, induced by inflation of a cuff around a limb.

Methods for assessment of conduit artery FMD [18]

Most studies examine the brachial artery, due to its accessibility, ease of imaging, and the practicality of placing a sphygmomanometer cuff around the forearm. Nevertheless, femoral artery studies may be appropriate in small children due to constraints of vessel size. In our standard protocol, the subject is positioned supine with the arm in a comfortable position, and imaging of the brachial artery, initially acquired at baseline, focuses above the antecubital fossa in the longitudinal plane, using a high-resolution ($\geq 7\,MHz$) linear array vascular ultrasound probe. Doppler indices calculate flow. Inflating a forearm blood pressure cuff to suprasystolic pressure occludes arterial inflow for a standardized time, causing ischemia and the consequent dilation of downstream resistance vessels via autoregulatory mechanisms. The subsequent cuff deflation induces a brief high-flow state through the brachial artery, which can be measured by Doppler analysis after cuff deflation. Such deflation increases shear stress by stimulating brachial artery vasodilation, measured by longitudinal imaging of the artery for 2–5 min after cuff deflation. Following a period of recovery after reactive hyperemia, an exogenous NO donor, e.g., sublingual nitroglycerin ($25–400\,\mu g$), determines the endothelium-independent vasodilatory response, which reflects vascular smooth muscle function. Measures of arterial function vary with duration of blood flow occlusion and nitrate dose (Figure 14.1) [19]. Maximum conduit vessel FMD response usually occurs after 5 min of blood flow occlusion, producing a consistent and reproducible measure of endothelial function. Testing should be performed in a fasting state in a quiet, temperature-controlled room. All vasoactive medications should be withheld for at least four half-lives, and subjects should not exercise or ingest caffeine, high-fat foods or vitamin C prior to the study.

The position of the cuff used to induce the ischemic stimulus may be important. Because upper arm occlusion results in significantly greater hyperemia and vasodilation, and also may better separate subjects with and without coronary risk factors,

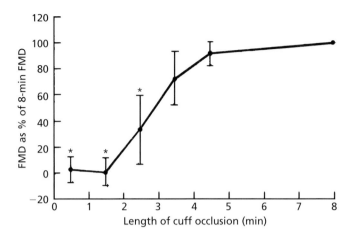

Figure 14.1 Effect of duration of cuff inflation on brachial artery FMD response (*$P < 0.05$ vs %FMD after 8 min). After 4.5 min of occlusion, FMD was mean (SD) 96 (6)% of maximal response and did not increase significantly with longer occlusion times (from Ref. [19]).

some groups prefer this method [20]. However, acquiring accurate data with upper arm occlusion is more challenging technically, due to brachial artery collapse and distorted images caused by shifting soft tissue. Occlusion achieved with a forearm cuff is more reproducible and results in a lower number of uninterpretable scans than upper arm occlusion. Additionally, the relative contribution of endothelium-derived NO to brachial FMD following upper arm cuff occlusion remains unclear. Although we and others confirmed that NO predominantly mediates FMD response following a 4–5-min forearm cuff occlusion, the mechanistic basis of FMD is more complex [21,22]. Different stimuli likely act via differing mechanisms. Similarly, in subjects with hyperlipidemia and healthy controls, inhibiting NO synthesis by administering L-NMMA does not suppress FMD following a more prolonged period of ischemia (15 min) or sustained flow, e.g., hand warming, suggesting that another vasodilatory pathway, e.g., endothelium-derived hyperpolarizing factor (EDHF), mediates FMD response to more intense or persistent shear stresses [22]. Although these recent observations require further study to establish relevant mechanisms and potential clinical implications, they may critically increase our understanding of arterial homeostasis. Such observations also highlight the importance of using the established cuff occlusion/release protocol when assessing NO-dependent responses.

Laboratories throughout the world now measure FMD, and international experts have established guidelines for good practice [18]. Results are reproducible temporally and spatially, and correlate well with coronary vascular endothelial function, at least in adults [23]. Recent studies demonstrate that FMD of the brachial artery independently predicts cardiovascular outcome in adults, consistent with studies of the prognostic value of coronary vascular endothelial function testing [7,24–26]. Although impaired endothelium-dependent vasodilation in childhood likely reflects vascular risk, the long preclinical phase of atherosclerotic disease makes the assessment of the prognostic potential of endothelial function testing in the young logistically challenging.

Laser Doppler flowmetry

Laser Doppler flowmetry can semi-quantitatively assess cutaneous microvascular responses. The laser Doppler technique measures blood flow in the very small blood vessels of the microvasculature, e.g., low-speed flows associated with nutritional blood flow in capillaries close to the skin surface, as well as flow in the underlying arterioles and venules associated with regulation of skin temperature. Measurements achieved by scanning a low-intensity laser beam across the skin surface in a raster fashion, using a moving mirror without direct contact with the skin, offer good temporal and spatial resolution, enabling clinicians to record rapid blood flow changes and also average blood flow measurements over large areas. Testing endothelium-dependent and -independent vasodilatory function involves measuring changes in skin perfusion during local cutaneous delivery of drugs, such as acetylcholine and sodium nitroprusside, by iontophoresis, i.e., inducing the passage of ionic drug solutions into the skin through a small electrical current. This safe method can assess microvascular function in infants and children, although it only allows an assessment of the microvasculature. The relative contribution of NO to the elicited responses remains unclear [27,28].

Assessment of arterial stiffness
Combined with smooth muscle tone and transmural pressure, the structure of the arterial wall, including the relative proportion of collagen and elastin, contributes to large-vessel stiffness. Increased vascular stiffness (reduced compliance) likely reflects relatively stable changes in the arterial wall that result from cumulative vascular injury, e.g., hypercholesterolemia, hypertension, and smoking. Several different methods, including assessment of pulse wave velocity, pulse waveform analysis, and arterial distensibility, allow non-invasive and reproducible measures of arterial stiffness [29]. Measures of stiffness predict cardiovascular outcome [29,30]. Such techniques are eminently suitable for children; indeed, arterial stiffness increases with age [31,32]. Since smooth muscle tone in the arterial wall influences arterial stiffness, locally generated vasoactive substances likely contribute to functional regulation of arterial stiffness. Non-invasive methods currently in development employ measurements of the peripheral arterial waveform to determine the contribution of endothelium-derived NO, released in response to pharmacologic agents, e.g., inhaled β-2 agonists, toward vessel compliance [32,33]. Although promising, the reproducibility, accuracy, and extent of NO dependence of this technique remain incompletely validated.

Non-invasive assessment of coronary vascular function
Using brief infusions of vasodilators such as adenosine or dipyridamole, positron emission tomography (PET) non-invasively assesses coronary flow reserve. In conjunction with PET, cold pressor testing more selectively assesses endothelium-dependent coronary flow responses [34]. Recently, phase-contrast magnetic resonance imaging has shown promise of quantifying coronary blood flow responses [35]. Although technically challenging and time consuming, this non-invasive technique does not require the systemic administration of radioisotopes; thus, it may emerge in the near future as the best means of assessing coronary resistance vessel physiology in children and young adults. However, its widespread application requires further methodological validation. Similarly, magnetic resonance imaging (MRI) evaluation of conduit coronary vessel function will require considerably higher resolution.

Impact of conventional risk factors for atherosclerosis on endothelium-dependent dilation in youth

Non-invasive vascular techniques have enabled studies of the impact of several risk factors on preclinical vascular function in childhood. The deleterious impact of conventional risk factors such as smoking, diabetes, and dyslipidemia, as well as their interactions, on FMD strongly supports a role of endothelial dysfunction in the pathogenesis of early atherosclerosis.

Age and sex
We have long recognized that atherosclerosis is associated with the aging process. Furthermore, clinical manifestations of atherosclerosis occur less commonly in young- and middle-aged women. Using high-resolution ultrasound to assess FMD in 238 healthy individuals between 15 and 72 years of age, we demonstrated that aging is associated with a progressive loss of endothelium-dependent vasodilatory function; this age-related decline in function also occurs later in women [36]. Endothelium-independent responses to sublingual nitroglycerin remain unaffected by aging. Interestingly, FMD was similar in both sexes by the age of 65 years. Such findings reflect and also help to explain the observed age and gender differences in atherosclerosis-related morbidity and mortality. More recent studies have confirmed these observations, demonstrating that aging is associated with impaired NO-mediated endothelium-dependent vasodilatory function, due at least partially to increased oxidative stress [37,38]. Although the forearm microvascular response to acetylcholine diminishes with increasing age, a recent study in healthy young and older men showed preserved responses to bradykinin, substance P, and

isoproterenol [39], suggesting that aging does not universally impair endothelium-dependent vasodilatory responses to different agonists. Further investigation is therefore required to characterize whether this is due to differences in number or sensitivity of receptors, signal-transduction pathways, vasoactive mediators released, or possibly a combination of these factors.

Smoking

Tobacco smoking has long been recognized as a powerful independent risk factor for atherosclerotic vascular disease, and passive smoking has been identified recently as an important risk factor that accounts for up to 20,000 deaths per year in non-smokers in the United States alone. Our group initially showed that cigarette smoking significantly impaired endothelium-dependent vasodilation, measured by FMD, in a dose-related fashion, in young smokers before the development of clinical atherosclerosis [40]. We subsequently showed that endothelial dysfunction also develops following passive exposure to environmental tobacco smoke (Figure 14.2) [41]. Similar to active smokers, the degree of dysfunction is associated with the extent of tobacco exposure, independent of other vascular risk factors. Several potential mechanisms may underpin tobacco smoke-mediated endothelial dysfunction, including direct toxicity to endothelial cells, increased levels of oxidative stress, platelet activation, and relative L-arginine deficiency due to

high levels of endogenous arginine analogs such as asymmetric dimethylarginine [42]. Whatever the specific mechanism, the similar degree of impairment of endothelial vasodilatory function in young individuals exposed passively to significant environmental tobacco smoke as in active smokers has potentially great public health implications. These similarities require attention in the ongoing debate about the acceptability of smoking in the community.

Diabetes

The risk of developing clinical manifestations of atherosclerosis increases several fold in individuals with diabetes. Unsurprisingly, large-vessel endothelial dysfunction occurs early in individuals with insulin-dependent diabetes [43]. The impairment of vascular reactivity likely relates to the duration of diabetes and also to low-density lipoprotein (LDL) cholesterol, even at levels considered acceptable in otherwise healthy individuals. Data demonstrating decreased vascular compliance in young patients with type 1 diabetes support such observations [44]. Children with diabetes have serologic evidence of increased endothelial cell activation (elevation of E-selectin and intercellular adhesion molecule (ICAM)-1 levels), inflammation (elevation of C-reactive protein (CRP) and tumor necrosis factor alpha (TNF-α) levels), and oxidative stress (increased superoxide dismutase, and reduced plasma thiol and red cell glutathione levels), which may be further exacerbated by smoking [45–47].

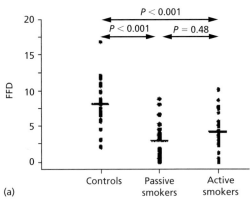
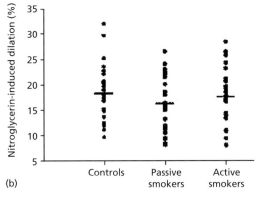

Figure 14.2 Comparison of FMD (a) and nitroglycerin-induced dilation (b) in 26 Controls, 26 Passive Smokers, and 26 Active Smokers. Horizontal lines represent the mean values for each group. FMD was significantly impaired in the passive and active smokers compared with the control subjects, whereas nitroglycerin-induced dilation was similar in all three groups (from Ref. [41]).

These complementary findings help explain the presence of endothelial vasodilatory dysfunction and the propensity to premature atherosclerosis in the diabetic population. Of great current concern is the increasing prevalence of type 2 diabetes in children and young adults, with the attendant adverse consequences on vascular health in the population.

The timing of onset of vascular dysfunction may have important implications for the development of vasculoprotective strategies in diabetes. In a small study investigating the effects of puberty on vascular dysfunction in subjects with diabetes, Elhadd and colleagues demonstrated impaired microvascular function in young adults compared with pre-pubertal children. Compared with adults, adolescents showed higher levels of the adhesion molecules ICAM-1 and E-selectin and lower levels of glutathione, whereas superoxide dismutase levels were lower in pre-pubertal children [48]. Thus, puberty likely modulates endothelial function adversely in diabetes and should be considered in the development of novel investigational and therapeutic approaches to this condition. Thus, our group investigated the effect of a 6-month course of ACE-inhibitor treatment with enalapril on vascular function in 91 young, post-pubertal subjects with diabetes [49]. Unfortunately, we determined no benefit, possibly due to a number of factors including fairly small numbers, the relatively poor tissue specificity of enalapril, and the complex nature of diabetic vasculopathy.

Hypertension

Hypertension in childhood often occurs secondarily to some other pathology; normalizing blood pressure by removing its cause, e.g., renal artery stenosis or pheochromocytoma, suggests that endothelial dysfunction can be reversed in these conditions. Increased plasma levels of the endogenous inhibitors of NO generation, e.g., asymmetric dimethylarginine, occur in children, especially those with secondary hypertension due to renal parenchymal and renovascular disease, which may contribute to hypertension by reducing the glomerular filtration rate that promotes salt and water retention, as well as modulating renin release and inhibiting the release of vascular NO [50]. Familial influences are of well-recognized importance in the development of hypertension. The intriguing observation that

peripheral vascular endothelial dysfunction is present in normotensive first-degree relatives of hypertensive patients and also relates to hyperinsulinemia suggests that insulin resistance may be one of the pathogenic determinants of essential hypertension and its complications [51]. Several genetic factors participate in the pathogenesis of endothelial dysfunction and hypertension in the young (see below).

Dyslipidemia

Hypercholesterolemia predisposes to atherosclerosis in clinical and experimental studies. Adults with elevated levels of serum cholesterol show impaired endothelium-dependent coronary vasodilation, related at least in part to reduced bioavailability of NO [52,53]. We demonstrated impaired FMD in children as young as 7 years of age with familial hypercholesterolemia [16,54]. Notably, the degree of dysfunction in such children was associated with lipoprotein(a) levels [54,55] (see also Chapter 9). A study of over 100 children, which explored the possibility that vascular inflammation underpins the relationship between dyslipidemia and endothelial dysfunction in childhood, showed that elevated serum triglyceride and reduced serum high-density lipoprotein (HDL) levels are associated with increased concentrations of circulating adhesion molecules, thus reflecting endothelial activation [56]. Dietary fat intake appears to have an important acute influence on the vasculature. Although several studies have demonstrated that the postprandial state after a high-fat meal likely induces endothelial dysfunction, probably due to transient oxidative stress, the nature of this effect remains controversial [57,58]. Given the frequency and quantity of fried "fast-foods" currently ingested by children and young adults in Western culture, such data may have important implications for atherosclerosis.

Impact of novel risk factors for atherosclerosis on endothelium-dependent dilation in youth

The risk factor profile associated with initiation and progression of early atherosclerosis differs from that associated with clinical events later in the natural history of the disease.

Obesity and physical activity

Due to changes in dietary habits and reduced physical activity levels, obesity is increasingly prevalent in children and adolescents; in the United States, childhood obesity increased from 5% to 11% over the past three to four decades. Obesity in childhood influences many pathologies including hypertension, type 2 diabetes mellitus, obstructive sleep apnea, dyslipidemia, psychological morbidity, and musculo-skeletal problems. Primary hypertension as well as familial and ethnic predisposition in children increasingly associate with obesity. Indeed, the risk of hypertension is approximately 3-fold higher in obese children. Obesity is associated with over-activity of the sympathetic nervous system (SNS), insulin resistance, and impaired coronary vascular reactivity, explaining in part the adverse cardiovascular prognosis observed in such individuals [59]. Furthermore, obesity is associated with inflammation; i.e., CRP levels rise with increasing fat mass and fall with weight loss. Childhood obesity associates with impaired brachial artery reactivity and decreased vascular compliance, as well as adverse metabolic markers, e.g., insulin resistance, hypo-alphalipoproteinemia, and increased P-selectin and D-dimer [60,61].

Recently, Tounian et al. and our group demonstrated that obesity is linked to arterial stiffness [61,62]. We also showed an association between arterial stiffness and leptin levels over a wide range of body size in adolescents, independent of body mass index and other risk factors for atherosclerosis. Notably, leptin receptors are found on both endothelial and smooth muscle cells. Leptin can induce oxidative stress, enhance sympathetic nervous activity, and increase blood pressure, as well as stimulate smooth muscle migration and proliferation. Thus, leptin appears to mediate vascular dysfunction, and may represent a causal link between obesity and cardiovascular disease.

Somewhat reassuringly, exercise training enhances endothelial function in young men, and even moderate-to-high levels of habitual activity in childhood are significantly correlated with FMD, even after adjustment for other possible cardiovascular risk factors [63,64]. Such findings suggest that exercise programs likely will improve endothelial function and reduce blood pressure in children, and should be coupled with dietary modification for the long-term management of obesity and its potential complications, including hypertension.

Inflammation

In recent years, extensive experimental work has characterized inflammatory processes in the vascular wall that participate in early atherosclerosis and destabilize established plaques. Intriguingly, simple circulating biomarkers of inflammation can be linked with disease activity in clinical studies. For example, the measurement of high-sensitivity CRP independently predicts an adverse cardiovascular prognosis in adults with and without clinical evidence of atherosclerosis [65]. A relationship between inflammation, endothelial dysfunction, and structural vascular disease is apparent at a very early stage in the disease process. A recent study in 79 children demonstrated an inverse relationship between CRP levels and FMD (Figure 14.3), as well as increased carotid intima-media thickness in children with higher CRP levels [66]. suggesting that inflammation is associated with early evidence of structural and functional vascular abnormalities. However, the role of CRP as a marker or active mediator of vascular disease has engendered controversy. Our group developed a *Salmonella typhi* vaccine model, in which a low-grade inflammatory reaction for 48-h post-vaccination associates with temporary but profound dysfunction of the arterial endothelium in resistance and conduit vessels to both physical and pharmacologic dilatory stimuli. Pre-treatment with aspirin can prevent such dysfunction, possibly by modulating the cytokine cascade [67,68]. However, aspirin does not reverse already established vaccine-induced endothelial dysfunction. In keeping with these observations, we and our colleagues showed that prior inflammatory vascular disease has important long-term consequences for vascular health, with evidence of persistent endothelium-dependent vasodilatory dysfunction following Kawasaki disease, and increased arterial stiffness with polyarteritis nodosa [31,69]. Other environmental inflammatory triggers, e.g., childhood infections, likely participate importantly in the development of endothelial dysfunction and atherosclerosis. Indeed, the exposure to an increasing burden of pathogens implicated in atherogenesis independently associates with increased levels of CRP, a greater degree of coronary vascular endothelial

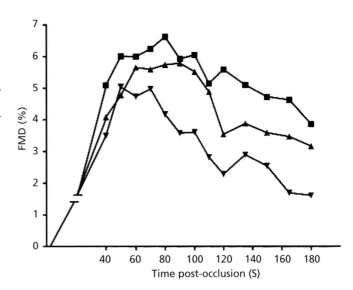

Figure 14.3 Brachial artery FMD responses according to CRP levels: group 1, CRP < 0.1 mg/L (solid squares); group 2, 0.1 mg/L ≤ CRP ≤ 0.7 mg/L (solid triangles); and group 3, CRP > 0.7 mg/L (solid inverted triangles). Mean FMD values are shown at every measurement point between 40 and 180 s after occlusion in each group. The temporal development of FMD responses was similar across CRP groups (effect of time, $P < 0.001$; time × group interaction, $P = 0.5$), but the magnitude of the response was significantly blunted in groups with higher CRP levels (effect of group, $P < 0.05$) (from Ref. [66]).

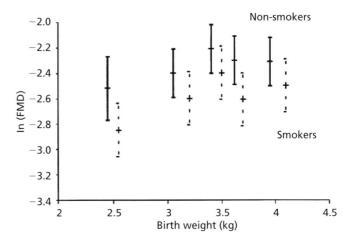

Figure 14.4 Relationship between FMD and birth weight in smokers and non-smokers. There is similar strength of association in both groups, but smokers have lower FMD than non-smokers across birth-weight range (from Ref. [71]).

dysfunction, and angiographic severity of atherosclerosis [70]. Considerable effort is needed to determine how interactions between such inflammatory triggers and genetic factors impact on endothelial function and atherogenesis in early life.

Fetal programming

Many studies have highlighted an independent association between low birth weight and cardiac risk factors such as hypertension and insulin resistance as well as clinical evidence of morbidity and mortality from atherosclerotic disease. We and others demonstrated that a relationship between low birth weight and impaired endothelium-dependent vasodilation was already apparent by the end of the

first decade of life, suggesting vascular programming in the fetus or very early in postnatal life (Figure 14.4) [71,72]. In young adults, the difference in FMD between the top and bottom quintiles of birth weight resembled that observed between smokers and non-smokers; however, an increasing burden of risk factors obscured this relationship. In another study, we found that children with intra-uterine growth retardation had impaired FMD, while children with normal size for their gestational age but low birth weight due to prematurity preserved their endothelial function [73]. These data suggest that the pattern of fetal growth rather than low birth weight *per se* likely primes the vasculature for later dysfunction and atherosclerotic risk. Furthermore, early nutrition and "catch-up" growth during the first few weeks of life appear critically important in programming future growth trajectory and metabolic profile, and may well have critical implications for vascular risk. Ongoing research should further expand our understanding and management of early atherosclerosis risk.

Mental stress

Animal studies have shown that chronic social stress impairs endothelial function by increasing the rate of endothelial cell damage and reducing NO availability in atherosclerotic arteries. In humans, depression is an independent risk factor for the development of coronary artery disease. In patients with established coronary artery disease, mental stress provokes myocardial ischemia and is linked to increased morbidity and mortality. Moreover, chronic stress is associated with accelerated progression of atherogenesis from an early stage. We have demonstrated that acute mental stress, such as that frequently encountered during normal everyday life, transiently impairs endothelium-dependent vasodilatory responses, suggesting an important link between repeated or chronic stress and acceleration of atherosclerosis [74]. The underlying mechanisms remain unclear, but likely are multifactorial, including increased activation of the SNS, increased insulin resistance, oxidative stress, and inflammation. Notably, the endothelin receptor antagonist BQ-123 can attenuate acutely depressed FMD following mental stress, thus implicating endothelin, acting via its ET_A receptor, as a link between mental stress, endothelial dysfunction, and atherosclerosis [75].

Genetics

The important familial contribution to the risk of atherosclerosis has long been recognized. In recent years, extensive work has explored genetic mechanisms involved in the development of endothelial dysfunction and atherogenesis. The technical and ethical problems encountered by *in vivo* studies of gene expression and activity significantly limit their success in humans, particularly children. Therefore, the majority of clinical studies have explored relationships between measures of arterial structure and function and easily identifiable genetic polymorphisms that may influence gene expression/activity. For example, we and others have investigated the

relationship between cardiovascular disease and polymorphisms in the renin–angiotensin system, eNOS, interleukins, NADPH oxidase, and bradykinin and chemokine receptor genes. Problems with such studies include uncertainty regarding the influence of polymorphisms on gene expression/activity *in vivo*, as well as potential interaction with numerous environmental, genetic, and other developmental modifiers. Additionally, very few clinical studies have examined associations between such polymorphisms and functional abnormalities of the endothelium in childhood. By investigating the influence of the eNOS Glu298Asp polymorphism (thought to modulate endothelium-derived NO bioavailability) in 248 young individuals, we demonstrated statistically significant interactions between endothelial function and eNOS genotype, smoking status, and omega-3 fatty acid levels, although the polymorphism considered alone did not appear to influence FMD [76]. Such findings highlight the need to study genetic factors in conjunction with environmental factors that potentially can modify the effects of the gene in question. In order to determine the impact of gene–gene and gene–environment interactions on the development of vascular disease in early life, future studies should include large numbers of young subjects to allow sufficient statistical power.

Other factors

Although the influences of innumerable other factors on endothelial function have been investigated, it is well beyond the scope of this chapter to provide an exhaustive discussion. Our group has investigated endothelial function in children with other conditions that potentially predispose to atherosclerosis, e.g., homocysteine. In addition to its direct toxic effects on the endothelium, homocysteine may increase LDL oxidation, promote smooth muscle proliferation, and potentiate thrombosis. Indeed, early clinical manifestations of atherosclerosis occur in subjects with homocystinuria. We showed impaired FMD of the brachial artery in children with homocystinuria as early as the first decade of life, despite good medical management of the condition [77]; their heterozygote parents, with normal plasma homocysteine levels, had normal FMD. Such findings concur with studies in adults showing that naturally and experimentally elevated homocysteine levels are associated with clinically impaired endothelium-dependent vasodilatory responses.

Chronic renal disease in childhood may predispose to atherosclerosis, possibly due to a combination of factors including blood pressure, dyslipidemia, and other metabolic factors such as increased oxidative stress. Seeking to determine the influence of renal disease and endothelial function independent of the influence of conventional risk factors commonly found in this cohort of patients, we studied 23 children with chronic renal failure but not hypertension, diabetes, or hypercholesterolemia, and not taking vasodilatory medications. We demonstrated impaired FMD in this cohort, as well as elevated levels of dimethylarginines, antibodies to oxidized LDL, and decreased levels of nitrosothiol levels [78]. Such data implicate several mechanisms, including the endogenous inhibition of NO synthesis and increased oxidative stress, in the depressed FMD response that reflects reduced NO bioavailability and the consequent vascular risk in these patients.

Summary

It is increasingly clear that reducing the societal burden of atherosclerosis requires an "investment approach" from an early stage. The study of vascular physiology in children clearly demonstrates that endothelial dysfunction is present from early life, and describes some of the wide range of conditions that associate with clinical evidence of endothelial dysfunction in childhood. Non-invasive techniques permit both cross-sectional and longitudinal studies of populations before clinical disease emerges, and new imaging technologies, such as magnetic resonance imaging and high-resolution computed tomography, should allow more detailed non-invasive assessment of the coronary circulation. In concert with gene-chip technology and new proteomic techniques, data from the Human Genome Project will facilitate research into the nature of gene–gene and gene–environment interactions, and their influences on early vascular health. Finally, a detailed characterization of inflammatory and repair processes in the vasculature likely will enhance our understanding of early atherogenesis, particularly the role of bone-marrow-derived endothelial progenitor cells and other stem cells.

Our ability to study inflammation and vascular dysfunction in the young expands the entire area of preclinical risk stratification and management. Over the next few years, data will emerge from studies prospectively investigating the predictive value of non-invasive measures of endothelial function, coupled with emerging phenotypic and genetic markers of risk. Appreciation of the key role of inflammation and endothelial function should permit us to develop novel protective strategies against atherosclerosis, aimed at protecting the "next generation."

References

1 Napoli C, D'Armiento FP, Mancini FP, et al. Fatty streak formation occurs in human fetal aortas and is greatly enhanced by maternal hypercholesterolemia. Intimal accumulation of low density lipoprotein and its oxidation precede monocyte recruitment into early atherosclerotic lesions. *J Clin Invest* 1997;100: 2680–2690.

2 Napoli C, Glass CK, Witztum JL, et al. Influence of maternal hypercholesterolaemia during pregnancy on progression of early atherosclerotic lesions in childhood: Fate of Early Lesions in Children (FELIC) study. *Lancet* 1999;354 1234–1241.

3 Berenson GS, Srinivasan SR, Bao W, et al. Association between multiple cardiovascular risk factors and atherosclerosis in children and young adults. The Bogalusa Heart Study. *N Engl J Med* 1998;338:1650–1656.

4 Stamler J, Daviglus ML, Garside DB, et al. Relationship of baseline serum cholesterol levels in 3 large cohorts of younger men to long-term coronary, cardiovascular, and all-cause mortality and to longevity. *J Am Med Assoc* 2000;284:311–318.

5 Kharbanda RK, Deanfield JE. Functions of the healthy endothelium. *Coron Artery Dis* 2001;12:485–491.

6 Quyyumi AA. Endothelial function in health and disease: new insights into the genesis of cardiovascular disease. *Am J Med* 1998;105:32S–39S.

7 Halcox JP, Schenke WH, Zalos G, et al. Prognostic value of coronary vascular endothelial dysfunction. *Circulation* 2002;106:653–658.

8 Schachinger V, Zeiher AM. Prognostic implications of endothelial dysfunction: does it mean anything? *Coron Artery Dis* 2001;12:435–443.

9 Furchgott RF, Zawadzki JV. The obligatory role of endothelial cells in the relaxation of arterial smooth muscle by acetylcholine. *Nature* 1980;288:373–376.

10 Fleming I, Busse R. NO: the primary EDRF. *J Mol Cell Cardiol* 1999;31:5–14.

11 Pohl U, Holtz J, Busse R, et al. Crucial role of endothelium in the vasodilator response to increased flow *in vivo*. *Hypertension* 1986;8:37–44.

12 Rubanyi GM, Romero JC, Vanhoutte PM. Flow-induced release of endothelium-derived relaxing factor. *Am J Physiol* 1986;250:H1145–H1149.

13 Cox DA, Vita JA, Treasure CB, et al. Atherosclerosis impairs flow-mediated dilation of coronary arteries in humans. *Circulation* 1989;80:458–465.

14 Nabel EG, Selwyn AP, Ganz P. Large coronary arteries in humans are responsive to changing blood flow: an endothelium-dependent mechanism that fails in patients with atherosclerosis. *J Am Coll Cardiol* 1990;16:349–356.

15 Quyyumi AA, Dakak N, Andrews NP, et al. Contribution of nitric oxide to metabolic coronary vasodilation in the human heart. *Circulation* 1995;92:320–326.

16 Celermajer DS, Sorensen KE, Gooch VM, et al. Noninvasive detection of endothelial dysfunction in children and adults at risk of atherosclerosis. *Lancet* 1992;340:1111–1115.

17 Sorensen KE, Celermajer DS, Spiegelhalter DJ, et al. Noninvasive measurement of human endothelium dependent arterial responses: accuracy and reproducibility. *Br Heart J* 1995;74:247–253.

18 Corretti MC, Anderson TJ, Benjamin EJ, et al. Guidelines for the ultrasound assessment of endothelial-dependent flow-mediated vasodilation of the brachial artery: a report of the International Brachial Artery Reactivity Task Force. *J Am Coll Cardiol* 2002;39:257–265.

19 Leeson P, Thorne S, Donald A, et al. Non-invasive measurement of endothelial function: effect on brachial artery dilatation of graded endothelial dependent and independent stimuli. *Heart* 1997;78:22–27.

20 Vogel RA, Corretti MC, Plotnick GD. A comparison of brachial artery flow-mediated vasodilation using upper and lower arm arterial occlusion in subjects with and without coronary risk factors. *Clin Cardiol* 2000;23:571–575.

21 Joannides R, Haefeli WE, Linder L, et al. Nitric oxide is responsible for flow-dependent dilatation of human peripheral conduit arteries *in vivo*. *Circulation* 1995;91:1314–1319.

22 Mullen MJ, Kharbanda RK, Cross J, et al. Heterogenous nature of flow-mediated dilatation in human conduit arteries *in vivo*: relevance to endothelial dysfunction in hypercholesterolemia. *Circ Res* 2001;88:145–151.

23 Anderson TJ, Uehata A, Gerhard MD, et al. Close relation of endothelial function in the human coronary and peripheral circulations. *J Am Coll Cardiol* 1995;26:1235–1241.

24 Gokce N, Keaney Jr JF, Hunter LM, et al. Risk stratification for postoperative cardiovascular events via noninvasive assessment of endothelial function: a prospective study. *Circulation* 2002;105:1567–1572.

25 Neunteufl T, Heher S, Katzenschlager R, et al. Late prognostic value of flow-mediated dilation in the brachial artery of patients with chest pain. *Am J Cardiol* 2000;86:207–210.

26 Schachinger V, Britten MB, Zeiher AM. Prognostic impact of coronary vasodilator dysfunction on adverse long-term outcome of coronary heart disease. *Circulation* 2000;101:1899–1906.

27 Martin H, Gazelius B, Norman M. Impaired acetylcholine-induced vascular relaxation in low birth weight infants: implications for adult hypertension? *Pediatr Res* 2000;47:457–462.

28 Khan F, Elhadd TA, Greene SA, et al. Impaired skin microvascular function in children, adolescents, and young adults with type 1 diabetes. *Diabetes Care* 2000;23:215–220.

29 Mackenzie IS, Wilkinson IB, Cockcroft JR. Assessment of arterial stiffness in clinical practice. *QJM* 2002;95:67–74.

30 London GM, Cohn JN. Prognostic application of arterial stiffness: task forces. *Am J Hypertens* 2002;15:754–758.

31 Cheung YF, Brogan PA, Pilla CB, et al. Arterial distensibility in children and teenagers: normal evolution and the effect of childhood vasculitis. *Arch Dis Child* 2002;87:348–351.

32 Millasseau SC, Kelly RP, Ritter JM, et al. Determination of age-related increases in large artery stiffness by digital pulse contour analysis. *Clin Sci (Lond)* 2002;103:371–377.

33 Wilkinson IB, Hall IR, MacCallum H, et al. Pulse-wave analysis: clinical evaluation of a noninvasive, widely applicable method for assessing endothelial function. *Arterioscler Thromb Vasc Biol* 2002;22:147–152.

34 Bottcher M, Botker HE, Sonne H, et al. Endothelium-dependent and -independent perfusion reserve and the effect of L-arginine on myocardial perfusion in patients with syndrome X. *Circulation* 1999;99:1795–1801.

35 Panting JR, Gatehouse PD, Yang GZ, et al. Abnormal subendocardial perfusion in cardiac syndrome X detected by cardiovascular magnetic resonance imaging. *N Engl J Med* 2002;346:1948–1953.

36 Celermajer DS, Sorensen KE, Spiegelhalter DJ, et al. Aging is associated with endothelial dysfunction in healthy men years before the age-related decline in women. *J Am Coll Cardiol* 1994;24:471–476.

37 Singh N, Prasad S, Singer DR, et al. Ageing is associated with impairment of nitric oxide and prostanoid dilator pathways in the human forearm. *Clin Sci (Lond)* 2002;102:595–600.

38 Taddei S, Virdis A, Ghiadoni L, et al. Age-related reduction of NO availability and oxidative stress in humans. *Hypertension* 2001;38:274–279.

39 DeSouza CA, Clevenger CM, Greiner JJ, et al. Evidence for agonist-specific endothelial vasodilator dysfunction with ageing in healthy humans. *J Physiol* 2002;542:255–262.

40 Celermajer DS, Sorensen KE, Georgakopoulos D, et al. Cigarette smoking is associated with dose-related and potentially reversible impairment of endothelium-dependent dilation in healthy young adults. *Circulation* 1993;88:2149–2155.

41 Celermajer DS, Adams MR, Clarkson P, et al. Passive smoking and impaired endothelium-dependent arterial dilatation in healthy young adults. *N Engl J Med* 1996;334:150–154.

42 Deanfield J. Passive smoking and early arterial damage. *Eur Heart J* 1996;17:645–646.

43 Clarkson P, Celermajer DS, Donald AE, et al. Impaired vascular reactivity in insulin-dependent diabetes mellitus is related to disease duration and low density lipoprotein cholesterol levels. *J Am Coll Cardiol* 1996;28:573–579.

44 Berry KL, Skyrme-Jones RA, Cameron JD, et al. Systemic arterial compliance is reduced in young patients with IDDM. *Am J Physiol* 1999;276:H1839–H1845.

45 Zoppini G, Targher G, Cacciatori V, et al. Chronic cigarette smoking is associated with increased plasma circulating intercellular adhesion molecule 1 levels in young type 1 diabetic patients. *Diabetes Care* 1999;22:1871–1874.

46 Romano M, Pomilio M, Vigneri S, et al. Endothelial perturbation in children and adolescents with type 1 diabetes: association with markers of the inflammatory reaction. *Diabetes Care* 2001;24:1674–1678.

47 Elhadd TA, Kennedy G, Hill A, et al. Abnormal markers of endothelial cell activation and oxidative stress in children, adolescents and young adults with type 1 diabetes with no clinical vascular disease. *Diabetes Metab Res Rev* 1999;15:405–411.

48 Elhadd TA, Khan F, Kirk G, et al. Influence of puberty on endothelial dysfunction and oxidative stress in young patients with type 1 diabetes. *Diabetes Care* 1998;21:1990–1996.

49 Mullen MJ, Clarkson P, Donald AE, et al. Effect of enalapril on endothelial function in young insulin-dependent diabetic patients: a randomized, double-blind study. *J Am Coll Cardiol* 1998;31:1330–1335.

50 Goonasekera CD, Dillon MJ. Vascular endothelium and nitric oxide in childhood hypertension. *Pediatr Nephrol* 1998;12:676–689.

51 Zizek B, Poredos P. Insulin resistance adds to endothelial dysfunction in hypertensive patients and in normotensive offspring of subjects with essential hypertension. *J Intern Med* 2001;249:189–197.

52 Quyyumi AA, Mulcahy D, Andrews NP, et al. Coronary vascular nitric oxide activity in hypertension and hypercholesterolemia. Comparison of acetylcholine and substance P. *Circulation* 1997;95:104–110.

53 Vita JA, Treasure CB, Nabel EG, et al. Coronary vasomotor response to acetylcholine relates to risk factors for coronary artery disease. *Circulation* 1990;81:491–497.

54 Sorensen KE, Celermajer DS, Georgakopoulos D, et al. Impairment of endothelium-dependent dilation is an early event in children with familial hypercholesterolemia and is related to the lipoprotein(a) level. *J Clin Invest* 1994;93:50–55.

55 Seed M, Hoppichler F, Reaveley D, et al. Relation of serum lipoprotein(a) concentration and apolipoprotein(a) phenotype to coronary heart disease in patients with familial hypercholesterolemia. *N Engl J Med* 1990; 322:1494–1499.

56 Kavazarakis E, Moustaki M, Gourgiotis D, et al. The impact of serum lipid levels on circulating soluble adhesion molecules in childhood. *Pediatr Res* 2002;52:454–458.

57 Williams MJ, Sutherland WH, McCormick MP, et al. Impaired endothelial function following a meal rich in used cooking fat. *J Am Coll Cardiol* 1999;33:1050–1055.

58 Raitakari OT, Lai N, Griffiths K, et al. Enhanced peripheral vasodilation in humans after a fatty meal. *J Am Coll Cardiol* 2000;36:417–422.

59 Sundell J, Laine H, Luotolahti M, et al. Obesity affects myocardial vasoreactivity and coronary flow response to insulin. *Obes Res* 2002;10:617–624.

60 Gallistl S, Sudi KM, Borkenstein M, et al. Correlation between cholesterol, soluble P-selectin, and D-dimer in obese children and adolescents. *Blood Coagul Fibrin* 2000; 11:755–760.

61 Tounian P, Aggoun Y, Dubern B, et al. Presence of increased stiffness of the common carotid artery and endothelial dysfunction in severely obese children: a prospective study. *Lancet* 2001;358:1400–1404.

62 Singhal A, Farooqi IS, Cole TJ, et al. Influence of leptin on arterial distensibility: a novel link between obesity and cardiovascular disease? *Circulation* 2002;106:1919–1924.

63 Clarkson P, Montgomery HE, Mullen MJ, et al. Exercise training enhances endothelial function in young men. *J Am Coll Cardiol* 1999;33:1379–1385.

64 Abbott RA, Harkness MA, Davies PS. Correlation of habitual physical activity levels with flow-mediated dilation of the brachial artery in 5–10 year old children. *Atherosclerosis* 2002;160:233–239.

65 Ridker PM, Cushman M, Stampfer MJ, et al. Inflammation, aspirin, and the risk of cardiovascular disease in apparently healthy men. *N Engl J Med* 1997;336:973–979.

66 Jarvisalo MJ, Harmoinen A, Hakanen M, et al. Elevated serum C-reactive protein levels and early arterial changes in healthy children. *Arterioscler Thromb Vasc Biol* 2002; 22:1323–1328.

67 Hingorani AD, Cross J, Kharbanda RK, et al. Acute systemic inflammation impairs endothelium-dependent dilatation in humans. *Circulation* 2000;102:994–999.

68 Kharbanda RK, Walton B, Allen M, et al. Prevention of inflammation-induced endothelial dysfunction: a novel

vasculo-protective action of aspirin. *Circulation* 2002; 105:2600–2604.

69 Dhillon R, Clarkson P, Donald AE, et al. Endothelial dysfunction late after Kawasaki disease. *Circulation* 1996;94: 2103–2106.

70 Prasad A, Zhu J, Halcox JP, et al. Predisposition to atherosclerosis by infections: role of endothelial dysfunction. *Circulation* 2002;106:184–190.

71 Leeson CP, Kattenhorn M, Morley R, et al. Impact of low birth weight and cardiovascular risk factors on endothelial function in early adult life. *Circulation* 2001;103: 1264–1268.

72 Martin H, Hu J, Gennser G, et al. Impaired endothelial function and increased carotid stiffness in 9-year-old children with low birthweight. *Circulation* 2000;102: 2739–2744.

73 Singhal A, Kattenhorn M, Cole TJ, et al. Preterm birth, vascular function, and risk factors for atherosclerosis. *Lancet* 2001;358:1159–1160.

74 Ghiadoni L, Donald AE, Cropley M, et al. Mental stress induces transient endothelial dysfunction in humans. *Circulation* 2000;102:2473–2478.

75 Spieker LE, Hurlimann D, Ruschitzka F, et al. Mental stress induces prolonged endothelial dysfunction via endothelin-A receptors. *Circulation* 2002;105:2817–2820.

76 Leeson CP, Hingorani AD, Mullen MJ, et al. Glu298Asp endothelial nitric oxide synthase gene polymorphism interacts with environmental and dietary factors to influence endothelial function. *Circ Res* 2002;90: 1153–1158.

77 Celermajer DS, Sorensen K, Ryalls M, et al. Impaired endothelial function occurs in the systemic arteries of children with homozygous homocystinuria but not in their heterozygous parents. *J Am Coll Cardiol* 1993;22: 854–858.

78 Kari JA, Donald AE, Vallance DT, et al. Physiology and biochemistry of endothelial function in children with chronic renal failure. *Kidney Int* 1997;52:468–472.

CHAPTER 15

Endothelial vasodilatory dysfunction in hypertension

Umberto Campia, MD *& Julio A. Panza,* MD

Introduction

Essential hypertension is a highly prevalent disorder and a major cardiovascular risk factor. When a blood pressure threshold value of 140/90 mmHg is used, hypertension occurs in about 25% of the US population, and its prevalence and severity increase with aging [1]. Systolic and diastolic pressures predict the extent of coronary and aortic atherosclerosis in children and young adults [2], and are strongly, significantly, and independently related to the long-term risk of mortality from coronary and all cardiovascular diseases [3]. As shown by the data from the Multiple Risk Factor Intervention Trial (MRFIT) cohort, the risk of cardiovascular mortality rises progressively over the entire range of blood pressures, and no clear threshold between normal and elevated values can be recognized [4].

Despite intense investigation, the mechanisms leading to a persistent elevation of blood pressure and to the vascular complications of hypertension have not been conclusively identified. However, a significant portion of the cardiovascular risk associated with hypertension is secondary to the development of accelerated atherosclerosis and its consequences on the coronary, cerebral, and peripheral circulation. Given the pivotal role of the endothelium in the maintenance and modulation of vascular tone and vessel wall homeostasis, and the association between abnormal endothelium-dependent vasodilatory responses and risk factors for atherosclerosis, research interest has focused on the role of the endothelium in the increased vascular tone of hypertensive states and on the effects of elevated blood pressure levels on endothelial function.

Endothelial cells regulate vascular homeostasis and tone through the synthesis, expression, and release of several factors (Figure 15.1). Physiologically, the endothelium functions in an inhibitory mode, maintaining a relaxed vascular tone and low levels of oxidative stress, and tightly regulating vascular permeability, smooth muscle growth, platelet and leukocyte adhesion and aggregation, and thrombosis [5]. However, in response to a variety of noxious stimuli, the endothelium may undergo phenotypic modulation to a non-adaptive state, a condition commonly named "endothelial dysfunction," characterized by loss or dysregulation of the critical homeostatic mechanisms operative in healthy endothelial cells (see also Chapter 1). This dysfunctional syndrome is associated with a proinflammatory and prothrombotic phenotype, increased oxidative stress, and abnormal modulation of vasoactive pathways, which may lead to different functional manifestations, including, but not limited to, impaired endothelium-dependent vasodilation.

Investigational techniques to assess endothelial function

Studies of endothelial function generally evaluate the vascular responses to endothelium-dependent stimuli (chemical or physical agents that need the presence and the integrity of the endothelium to exert their effects on the smooth muscle) and endothelium-independent stimuli (agents that bypass the endothelium to act directly on the smooth muscle) [6]. Since blood pressure regulation occurs mostly at the level of resistance vessels, an

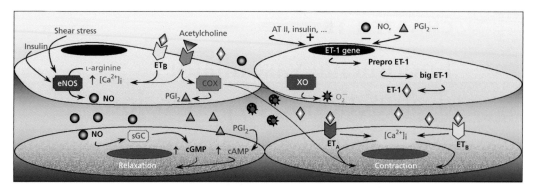

Figure 15.1 Schematic representation of the NO and COX pathways (left side of the figure), and of the ET-1 pathway (right side of the figure). Endothelial cells (represented in green) synthesize and secrete several substances, including NO, O_2^-, PGI_2, and ET-1. NO is produced in response to different biochemical (acetylcholine, insulin, …) and mechanical (shear stress) stimuli, which activate a specific eNOS. NO freely diffuses in the vascular wall, where it is rapidly inactivated by O_2^- produced by XO and other enzymatic sources present in endothelial cells. In the smooth muscle cells (represented in pink), NO activates guanylyl cyclase (sGC), with a consequent increase in intracellular concentrations of cyclic guanosine monophosphate (cGMP) and cell relaxation. PGI_2 is a prostanoid product of the COX cascade, which induces relaxation of smooth muscle cells by augmenting intracellular cyclic adenosine monophosphate (cAMP) concentrations. ET-1 synthesis and secretion are induced by several stimuli, such as AT-II and insulin, and inhibited by NO and PGI_2. ET-1 is secreted in great part towards the smooth muscle cells, on which it exerts vasoconstrictive effects by binding to specific receptors (ET_A and ET_B) and increasing intracellular calcium concentrations ($[Ca^{2+}]_i$). ET-1 also binds on ET_B receptors present on endothelial cells, where it stimulates the release of NO, thereby inducing indirect vasorelaxation. For other abbreviations refer to the text.

appropriate assessment of endothelial function in hypertension should involve the microcirculatory bed, the function of which is reflected in variations of blood flow and vascular resistance. On the other hand, the evaluation of endothelial function of conduit vessel, reflected in changes in arterial diameter, is of value in the investigation of the mechanisms linking hypertension and atherosclerosis.

Various techniques have been devised to study different vascular beds *in vivo*, thus allowing investigation of both resistance and conduit vessels. In particular, the forearm perfusion technique has emerged as a powerful tool for the study of the human microcirculation, since it permits the investigation of the peripheral vascular bed without the confounding effects secondary to the activation of systemic counter-regulatory mechanisms [7]. In this model, drugs are infused directly into the forearm circulation through a catheter placed into the brachial artery, and blood flow is measured non-invasively, by means of strain gauge plethysmography, at various times before and during the infusion of the pharmacologic agents. In recent years, the availability of new investigational drugs for human use has greatly expanded the potential of forearm perfusion studies in the exploration of endothelial function, which has moved from the simple detection of impaired endothelium-dependent vasodilation to more in-depth analysis of the activity of both vasoconstrictive and vasodilatory pathways and their balance in physiologic and pathophysiologic states. Recently, in addition to the forearm perfusion technique, the ultrasonographic assessment of endothelial function has become a standard investigational tool for the non-invasive determination of the effects of essential hypertension and other cardiovascular risk factors on conductance vessels, the site of atherosclerotic plaque formation [8]. With this technique, the endothelium-dependent stimulus is the increased shear stress caused by the rise in blood flow that follows a short period of ischemia, whereas the endothelium-independent stimulus is provided by a systemic dose of a nitrovasodilator. In addition to *in vivo* studies, a significant contribution to our understanding of the role of the endothelium in cardiovascular homeostasis has stemmed from *in vitro* investigations of animal and human vessels. In these procedures, vascular specimens are usually harvested from biopsies of different tissues, mounted in apposite chambers, and studied under a microscope. Then, the responses to various endothelium-dependent and -independent stimuli are evaluated, similar to *in vivo* studies.

Endothelial vasodilatory dysfunction in hypertension and nitric oxide

The pioneering investigations of Furchgott and Zawadski first demonstrated the essential role of the endothelium in the modulation of vascular smooth muscle responses to acetylcholine [9]. Following this seminal observation, intense research efforts have focused on the characterization of the physiologic functions of the endothelium in the regulation of vascular tone and in the maintenance of vessel wall homeostasis, as well as on the potential pathophysiologic role of abnormal endothelial function in cardiovascular disease. Evaluation of vascular responsiveness to acetylcholine and other endothelium-dependent and -independent vasodilators has become a standard test of endothelial function, and an impaired response to different vasoactive agents has been observed in animal models and in humans with various risk factors for atherosclerosis. Over the last decade, our and other laboratories have focused on the assessment of endothelial function in patients with essential hypertension, defined as chronically elevated blood pressure without any apparent underlying cause. Our initial findings showed that, despite similar baseline forearm blood flow (FBF) values between hypertensive patients and normotensive controls, the response to acetylcholine was significantly blunted in subjects with hypertension (Figure 15.2). On the contrary, the response to sodium nitroprusside (SNP), an endothelium-independent agent, did not differ between the two groups, ruling out a decreased responsiveness of vascular smooth muscle to vasodilators as a cause of the observed impairment to acetylcholine stimulation [10]. This evidence was confirmed in subsequent investigations in the peripheral and coronary circulation of essential hypertensive patients [11–14], and then extended to patients with secondary forms of hypertension [15], indicating that endothelial dysfunction is a generalized phenomenon associated with different hypertensive conditions.

Thus, our observations demonstrated the presence of an abnormal microvascular endothelial function

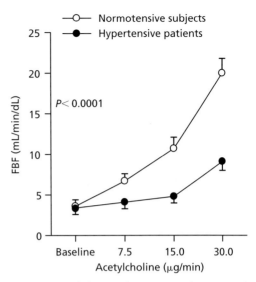

Figure 15.2 Graph showing the responses of FBF to acetylcholine in 18 normal controls (open circles) and 18 hypertensive patients (solid circles). Values are expressed as means and SE. (From Ref [10], with permission from the publisher).

in essential hypertension, and suggested that an endothelial defect may play a pathophysiologic role in the increased vascular resistance characteristic of this condition. However, these findings did not allow a characterization of the mechanisms involved in the abnormal endothelial vasodilatory function observed in the vasculature of hypertensive patients. Since the endothelium exerts its effects on the smooth muscle, and consequently on vascular tone, through the synthesis and release of several vasoactive substances, the next challenge was to identify the mediator(s) involved in the abnormal endothelial function of hypertensive patients. A likely candidate was the endothelium-derived relaxing factor nitric oxide (NO), which is synthesized by the endothelial cells using L-arginine, a non-essential amino acid [16], as a substrate. To test whether NO was involved in the endothelial dysfunction present in the hypertensive vasculature, we and others utilized N^G-monomethyl-L-arginine (L-NMMA), a methylated analog of L-arginine, which allows the functional investigation of NO production [17]. L-NMMA infusion into the brachial artery produced a significant decrease of baseline FBF, and a corresponding increase in vascular resistance, in both hypertensive patients and healthy controls, indicating the existence of a basal release of NO [13,17,18]. However, this effect was significantly blunted in the hypertensive patients compared with control subjects, demonstrating a much lower basal activity of NO in hypertensive vessels [13,18]. During L-NMMA infusion, the vasodilatory response to acetylcholine was significantly diminished in normal subjects, whereas the already blunted response to acetylcholine observed in hypertensive patients did not change to a significant extent [13], suggesting that, in hypertensive vessels, NO contribution to the vasodilatory effect of acetylcholine is reduced. Taken together, these findings indicated that patients with essential hypertension have a defect in the endothelium-derived NO system, which may account, at least in part, for both the increased basal vascular resistance and the abnormal response to acetylcholine present in this condition.

Abnormal NO bioactivity in hypertension: potential mechanisms

Based on the aforementioned results, the ensuing investigational efforts were devoted to the elucidation of the biochemical defect(s) underlying the reduced vascular NO activity observed in essential hypertension. In endothelial cells, NO is synthesized from the amino acid L-arginine by a constitutively expressed isoform of nitric oxide synthase (NOS III or eNOS). NO generation can be stimulated by several endogenous substances (e.g., bradykinin, serotonin), pharmacologic agents (e.g., acetylcholine, substance P), and mechanical forces (e.g., flow-mediated shear stress) acting on the endothelial cells. After its synthesis, NO, a small free radical molecule, freely diffuses in the vascular wall and lumen, where it exerts its numerous effects. Given its high biochemical reactivity, NO is rapidly broken down by other free radicals, in particular superoxide anions, which accounts for its very short biologic half-life (Figure 15.1). One or more abnormalities along the NO pathway could therefore affect NO synthesis and/or degradation, and potentially explain the impaired NO bioactivity present in hypertensive vessels.

Reduced substrate availability
Since NO synthesis involves an enzymatic reaction, a decreased availability of its substrate, L-arginine,

could contribute to a reduced NO bioactivity. To determine whether this mechanism plays a role in essential hypertension, we investigated the effects of L-arginine infusion on basal flow and on the reactivity to acetylcholine of healthy controls and essential hypertensive patients [19]. At baseline, L-arginine did not affect blood flow or vascular resistance in either group. However, the response to acetylcholine was significantly increased during L-arginine infusion in the normotensive subjects. In contrast, in the hypertensive patients, L-arginine did not alter the vasodilatory action of acetylcholine. This effect appeared to be specific to L-arginine, since the administration of its isomer, D-arginine, did not change the response to acetylcholine in normal subjects, and also appeared to be specific to acetylcholine, since the reactivity to SNP was not modified by L-arginine infusion. These findings, therefore, indicated that a decreased availability of L-arginine is not likely a causative mechanism in the decreased NO bioactivity of hypertensive vessels.

Muscarinic receptor defects
As discussed above, the initial studies demonstrating abnormal endothelial function and decreased NO bioactivity in hypertensive patients used muscarinic receptor agonists, typically acetylcholine and metacholine. However, investigations performed in patients with coronary atherosclerosis had shown preserved vasodilatory responses to substance P, a tachykinin receptor agonist, in face of abnormal reactivity to acetylcholine [20,21]. It was therefore hypothesized that, if the defect in vascular NO activity of hypertensive patients were related to an abnormal muscarinic receptor function, the response to substance P would not differ between normotensive controls and hypertensive patients. However, experiments conducted in our laboratory showed significantly blunted reactivity to both acetylcholine and substance P in hypertensive patients compared with healthy controls, with a significant correlation between the responses to the two agents. Furthermore, during L-NMMA infusion, reactivity to substance P was similar between patients and controls, indicating a decreased NO-dependent, substance-P-induced vasodilation in patients with hypertension [22]. Thus, these findings suggested that the abnormal endothelial function in essential hypertension is not limited to a defect at the

muscarinic receptor level, but is likely related to a more generalized biochemical dysregulation of endothelial cells.

Signal-transduction pathways defects

In vitro investigations had shown that endothelial dysfunction in dyslipidemia may progress from a relatively selective abnormality in intracellular signal-transduction pathways to a more generalized impairment of cell function, involving, in an initial phase, only pertussis toxin-sensitive G proteins and, at a later stage, also pertussis toxin-insensitive G proteins [23–25]. On the basis of these findings, we wanted to test whether the reduced NO bioactivity in essential hypertension is due to a defect in a single G-protein-dependent signal-transduction pathway or whether it involves multiple biochemical cascades. To this aim, we compared the vasodilatory responses to *acetylcholine*, which acts on a muscarinic receptor linked to a pertussis toxin-sensitive G protein, and *bradykinin*, a tachykinin receptor/pertussis toxin-insensitive G-protein stimulator, assessing both hypertensive patients and normal controls. Hypertensive patients showed significantly lower reactivity to both acetylcholine and bradykinin compared with healthy individuals [26]. Thus, similar to their responses to acetylcholine and substance P, hypertensive patients had reduced reactivity to bradykinin, suggesting that a defect in a selective G-protein-related pathway is not likely to account for the endothelial dysfunction of hypertensive vessels.

β-adrenergic-dependent NO activity

Previous data from our laboratory had shown a significant contribution of NO to the vasodilation induced by isoproterenol, a β_2-adrenergic receptor agent, in normotensive subjects [27]. Physiologically, β_2-adrenergic agonists stimulate NO synthesis by increasing intracellular cyclic-AMP (cAMP), whereas muscarinic agents activate eNOS through the phosphatidylinositol (PIP)/Ca^{2+} system. To investigate whether the abnormality of the NO pathway present in patients with essential hypertension also affects β_2-adrenergic-dependent NO activity, we infused isoproterenol, alone and in combination with the concomitant administration of L-NMMA, in a group of hypertensive patients and in matched

controls. The vasodilatory effect of isoproterenol was similar between patients with hypertension and normotensive subjects, and was significantly and equally blunted by L-NMMA in both groups [28]. These data indicated a preserved β_2-adrenergic-dependent NO activity in hypertensive patients, and suggest that the endothelial dysfunction in essential hypertension is due to a selective abnormality of NO synthesis, probably related to a defect in the PIP/Ca^{2+} pathway.

NO inactivation by superoxide anions

Physiologically, in the vessel wall, NO undergoes rapid inactivation by reacting with other free radicals produced by different enzymatic systems [29,30] (Figure 15.1). In animal models of hypertension, an increased generation of superoxide anions has been linked to the pathogenesis of the increased vascular tone [31] as well as to the abnormal endothelial reactivity to acetylcholine [32]. Given the availability of scavengers of superoxide anion for human use, studies were conducted to test the hypothesis that an excessive production of these free radicals might contribute to the endothelial dysfunction of hypertensive patients. In a first investigation, the response to acetylcholine before and after the combined infusion of copper–zinc superoxide dismutase (SOD), an extracellular superoxide anion scavenger, was evaluated in normal subjects and in hypertensive patients. The vascular responses to acetylcholine were similar before and after SOD in both patients and controls, providing evidence that the extracellular destruction of NO by superoxide anion does not represent the primary defect in the NO system of hypertensive patients [33]. However, these data did not rule out the possibility of an increased inactivation of NO by intracellular free radicals. An important intracellular source of superoxide radicals is the xanthine oxidase (XO) system, which can be pharmacologically inhibited by oxypurinol. Therefore, to determine whether XO-generated superoxide anions affect NO activity in hypertensive vessels, acetylcholine-induced vasodilation was assessed before and after oxypurinol infusion in patients with essential hypertension [34]. Oxypurinol infusion did not modify the response to acetylcholine, suggesting that XO-generated superoxide anions do not play a significant role in the endothelial dysfunction associated with essential hypertension.

NO and the cyclooxygenase system

The NO system plays a primary role in endothelial physiology. However, other biochemical pathways may exert significant vasoactive actions on the vasculature. In particular, the cyclooxygenase (COX) cascade may lead to the production of several physiologically relevant vasodilatory and vasoconstrictive factors (Figure 15.1). Studies in normal subjects have shown that prostacyclin (PGI$_2$), a vasodilatory prostanoid, contributes to the basal tone in the forearm circulation [35]. Other investigations have suggested that COX activity, either through the production of vasoactive prostanoids [36–38] or through the generation of oxygen free radicals [39,40], may contribute to endothelial dysfunction [41]. The role of COX products in the maintenance of vascular tone and in the endothelium-mediated vasodilation of essential hypertensive and of hypercholesterolemic patients was recently investigated in our laboratory [42]. Intra-arterial aspirin (ASA) reduced basal flow in the three groups to a similar extent, and significantly and equally improved the effect of acetylcholine in healthy controls, in hypertensive patients, and in hypercholesterolemic patients. These findings confirm that, in humans, vasodilatory prostanoids actively contribute to the maintenance of the basal vascular tone, and suggest that COX products do not play a major role in the endothelial dysfunction observed in essential hypertension and in hypercholesterolemia.

The endothelin system: endothelial dysfunction in hypertension extends beyond impaired endothelium-dependent dilation

As previously discussed, the endothelial control of vascular tone is exerted through the release of several vasoactive agents. Together with NO, PGI$_2$, and other vasodilators, endothelial cells synthesize and release constricting factors, which help to maintain and modulate the tone of the vascular bed. Endothelin-1 (ET-1), first isolated in 1988 by Yanagisawa [43], is the most potent known vasoconstrictor produced by the endothelium, and is one of the three members of the endothelin family. ET-1 exerts its biologic activity by binding to two specific endothelin receptor subtypes: endothelin-A (ET$_A$) and endothelin-B (ET$_B$)

[44,45]. In vascular smooth muscle cells, both receptors appear to induce contraction [46,47], whereas, in endothelial cells, the ET$_B$ subtype stimulates the release of NO and PGI$_2$, which cause smooth muscle relaxation [48] (Figure 15.1). Given its powerful and long-lasting vasoconstrictive effects, ET-1 has been considered a likely contributor to the increased vascular tone of hypertensive patients. The initial investigations exploring the potential pathophysiologic role of ET-1 in essential hypertension focused on the measurement of its plasma levels. Although some studies reported modest increases in the concentration of ET-1 in hypertensive patients [49–51], others failed to reproduce these findings [52–54]. However, the pathophysiologic relevance of plasma levels of ET-1 is questionable, since this factor exerts mainly autocrine and paracrine effects, and its secretion by endothelial cells is polarized toward the underlying vascular smooth muscle [55]. Consequently, circulating ET-1 levels likely reflect only the variable spillover of the peptide into the bloodstream, and, therefore, may not necessarily indicate endothelial cell production or its biologic effect on smooth muscle cells. The recent approval of selective and nonselective blockers of the ET$_A$ and ET$_B$ receptors for human use has made available powerful tools to assess the role of ET-1 in cardiovascular homeostasis *in vivo*. In our laboratory, the hypothesis that ET-1 participates in the increased vascular tone of patients with essential hypertension was investigated by comparing vascular responses to ET-1 receptor antagonists in hypertensive patients and normotensive subjects [56]. We infused BQ-123, a selective ET$_A$ receptor antagonist, alone or in combination with BQ-788, a selective ET$_B$ receptor blocker, in the brachial artery of hypertensive patients and of normotensive controls. In healthy subjects, BQ-123 did not affect baseline forearm flow, which remained unaltered also during the combined infusion of BQ-123 and BQ-788. In contrast, in patients with hypertension, BQ-123 caused a significant and progressive increase of forearm flow, which further augmented when BQ-788 was added to the infusion. This response thus indicated that an enhanced vascular ET-1 activity participates in the increased basal vasoconstrictive tone of hypertensive patients (Figure 15.3). To ascertain whether this heightened endothelin-mediated vasoconstrictive tone was related to an increased production or to

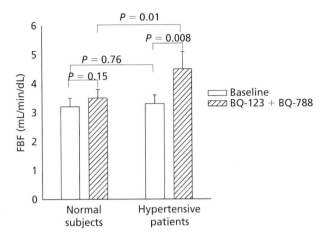

Figure 15.3 Bar graph showing FBF values at baseline (open bars) and after 60 min of intra-arterial infusion of BQ-123 (100 nmol/min) in combination with BQ-788 (50 nmol/min) (hatched bars) in normal subjects (left bars) and hypertensive patients (right bars). Values are expressed as means and SE. (From Ref [59], with permission by the publisher).

a higher sensitivity of the vasculature to the vasoconstrictive effect of the peptide, we also compared the vascular responses to exogenous ET-1 between hypertensive patients and control subjects. The vasoconstrictive effect of ET-1 was higher in hypertensive than in normotensive individuals, suggesting an increased sensitivity of vascular smooth muscle to ET-1 or, alternatively, a decreased production of vasodilatory substances in response to the stimulation of endothelial ET_B receptors. However, our data do not rule out the possibility that an increased ET-1 production might also be involved in the enhanced endothelin-dependent vasoconstrictive tone of hypertensive patients, as suggested by previous *in vitro* investigations [57].

NO and ET-1 interactions in hypertension: endothelial dysfunction at the crossroad of the two systems

The findings of increased ET-1 activity in the vasculature of hypertensive patients [56], together with our data in normotensive subjects demonstrating significant physiologic interactions between ET-1 and NO in the vasculature [58], led us to hypothesize that the enhanced endothelin tone could play a role in the abnormal endothelium-dependent vasodilatory function of hypertensive patients. Therefore, we investigated the effects of ET-1 receptor blockade on the vascular responses to acetylcholine in hypertensive patients and in normotensive subjects [59]. In healthy controls, the combined ET_A and ET_B

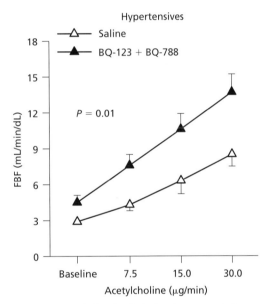

Figure 15.4 Graph showing FBF values in response to the intra-arterial infusion of increasing doses of acetylcholine in hypertensive subjects during infusion of saline (open triangles) and during non-selective $ET_{A/B}$ blockade with BQ-123 (100 nmol/min) in combination with BQ-788 (50 nmol/min) (solid triangles). Values are expressed as means and SE. (From Ref [59], with permission by the publisher).

receptor blockade did not modify acetylcholine-induced vasodilation. In contrast, in hypertensive patients, the combined ET_A and ET_B receptor blockade resulted in a significant potentiation of the vasodilatory response to acetylcholine, thereby suggesting that an increased ET-1 activity may play a role in the abnormal endothelium-dependent dilation observed in essential hypertension (Figure 15.4). These data may have clinically relevant implications. Endothelial dysfunction is increasingly recognized as a therapeutic target to reduce the atherosclerotic potential in hypertension. Therefore, the evidence that endothelin receptor antagonism, in addition to the demonstrated ability to reduce vascular tone and lower blood pressure, improves endothelial function may represent an important therapeutic advantage in the reduction of cardiovascular risk of patients with essential hypertension.

Hypertension, obesity, and the endothelin system

Essential hypertension is a heterogeneous condition, and several mechanisms may contribute to its pathogenesis. Thus, an activation of the ET-1 system might not be present in all hypertensive patients. In support of this view, studies in animal models have indicated that ET-1 activity is predominantly enhanced in low-renin, high-volume forms of experimental hypertension [60] and that an increased renal ET-1 mRNA expression, in conjunction with ET_A/ET_B receptor imbalance, differentiates salt-sensitive from salt-resistant forms of spontaneous hypertension [61] Another condition often associated with activation of the ET-1 system is insulin resistance. Studies in insulin-resistant rats have demonstrated an upregulation of vascular $ET_{A/B}$ receptors, which may contribute to elevated vasoconstrictor responses to ET-1 [62,63]. Since hypertension associated with obesity is commonly characterized by both plasma volume expansion and insulin resistance [64], we investigated the hypothesis that an enhanced ET-1 activity in hypertensive patients is related to increased body mass [65], and we assessed whether differences exist in the activity of the ET-1 system between obese normotensive and hypertensive subjects. To this aim, we infused BQ-123 in the brachial artery of hypertensive patients and of normotensive controls with a range of body mass index (BMI) values. The vasodilatory response to BQ-123 was significantly higher in hypertensive patients than in control subjects. During BQ-123 infusion, a significant increase in FBF from baseline was observed in obese (BMI = $30\,\mathrm{kg/m^2}$) and overweight (BMI, 27–$29.9\,\mathrm{kg/m^2}$) but not in lean (BMI $< 27\,\mathrm{kg/m^2}$) hypertensive patients. In contrast,

no significant change in FBF was observed either in obese, overweight, or lean normotensive subjects. A significant correlation between BMI and the vasodilatory response to ET_A blockade was observed in hypertensive patients but not in control subjects. Thus, our data indicate that, in human hypertension, increased BMI is associated with enhanced ET_A-dependent vasoconstrictive activity, suggesting that this abnormality may play a role in the pathophysiology of obesity-related hypertension and that targeting the ET-1 system may be useful in the treatment of these patients.

Hypertension, ethnicity, and the endothelin system

Epidemiologic data indicate that in African Americans (AA) essential hypertension has higher prevalence, earlier onset, and is associated with more severe end-organ damage, including left ventricular hypertrophy, renal failure, and stroke [66]. Despite intense investigation and the evidence that in AA essential hypertension usually presents with salt-sensitive, low-renin features [67], the pathophysiologic processes underlying this ethnic predisposition have not been fully elucidated [68]. A possible involvement of ET-1 in the development of hypertension and its complications in AA is suggested by the evidence that plasma ET-1 concentrations are increased in hypertensive AA patients compared with Caucasian (CA) patients [69]. We therefore tested the hypothesis that ethnic differences exist in the forearm vascular activity of ET-1 [70] by infusing BQ-123 in AA and CA normotensive subjects and hypertensive patients. BQ-123 did not affect FBF in normotensive subjects, whereas it produced significant vasodilation in hypertensive patients. In the normotensive subgroups, FBF response to BQ-123 was similar between AA and CA. In contrast, in hypertensive patients, the vasodilatory effect of ET_A receptor blockade was significantly higher in AA than in CA. To rule out differences in smooth muscle reactivity, the FBF responses to exogenous ET-1 were analyzed in the hypertensive subgroups. ET-1 induced a significant vasoconstriction in both CA and AA, without differences between them. These data suggest that hypertensive AA have enhanced ET_A-dependent vasoconstrictive tone, probably related to increased production of ET-1. Given the negative vascular effects of ET-1, this abnormality may contribute to the pathogenesis of hypertension and its complications in AA.

Endothelial progenitor cells: a new link between hypertension and endothelial dysfunction?

Besides the phenotypical abnormalities that characterize endothelial dysfunction, acute and chronic injury to the endothelium may lead to endothelial cells apoptosis or necrosis, with loss of continuity of the endothelial layer [71]. Until recently, migration and proliferation of endothelial cells adjacent to the site of injury were considered the main mechanisms of endothelial repair. However, accumulating evidence indicates that peripheral blood contains bone marrow-derived cells, commonly referred to as endothelial progenitor cells (EPCs), that have the potential to proliferate and to differentiate into mature endothelial cells [72] thus providing a circulating pool to repair sites of denuding injury or replace dysfunctional endothelium. Since mobilization of EPCs from the bone marrow is blunted in eNOS deficient mice [73], it is reasonable to speculate that recruitment of EPCs and endothelial repair are impaired in conditions characterized by reduced NO availability such as hypertension [13]. In support of this hypothesis is the evidence that in patients with cardiovascular risk factors and abnormal NO-dependent vasodilation the number of EPCs may represent a surrogate biologic marker for vascular function and cumulative cardiovascular risk [74], and that low levels of circulating EPCs may be associated with the occurrence of cardiovascular events and death from cardiovascular causes [75]. Interestingly, hypertension has emerged as the most important independent predictor of reduced EPCs migration, a marker of functional activity, in patients with cardiovascular risk factors [76]. An increased angiotensin II (AT-II) activity has been considered a likely pathogenetic mechanism of EPC dysfunction in hypertension, since it is associated with a profound downregulation of the endothelial growth factor tissue hepatocyte growth factor [77,78], and with an accelerated senescence of EPCs secondary to increased oxidative stress [79,80]. In keeping with these observations, angiotensin-converting enzyme (ACE) inhibition with ramipril may increase EPCs

number and improve functional parameters in patients with stable CAD [81].

Shear stress and microvascular endothelial function in hypertension

Shear stress acting on the endothelium likely represents the main physiologic stimulus for the release of vasoactive factors and for the regulation of vascular tone [82]. This evidence has been confirmed by investigations conducted in animal vessels, showing that shear stress is a major stimulus for the release of vasoactive factors, including NO, in the microcirculation [83,84]. In humans, however, although several studies had examined the effects of shear stress on endothelium-dependent dilation of conductance vessels in healthy subjects and in patients with risk factors for atherosclerosis [85–88], no investigations had explored the physiologic role of shear stress in the microcirculation, as well as its potential involvement in conditions associated with endothelial dysfunction. Given the lack of physiologic data, we aimed to determine the role of shear stress in the modulation vascular tone of human resistance arteries, and whether this phenomenon is mediated by NO. Furthermore, given the impaired NO-dependent vasodilation in response to pharmacologic agents observed *in vivo* in essential hypertensive and in hypercholesterolemic patients, we also aimed to assess if this mechanism is defective in hypertension and hypercholesterolemia. We therefore investigated the effects of shear stress on arteries isolated from gluteal fat biopsies in normal controls, in hypertensive patients, and in hypercholesterolemic patients [89]. In the arteries from healthy subjects, flow rate-dependent shear stress induced progressive vasodilation, which was blunted during the inhibition of NO synthesis with Nω-nitro-L-arginine (L-NNA), and virtually abolished after mechanical removal of the endothelium. These data indicated that flow-mediated, shear stress-induced vasodilation is operative in the normal human microvasculature, and that this is mediated by NO. In contrast, arteries from hypertensive patients showed significant impairment of flow-mediated dilation compared with those from normal controls, demonstrating that flow-dependent dilation of resistance arteries is impaired in hypertensive patients. Furthermore, flow-mediated dilation was not affected by the inhibition of NO synthesis with L-NNA, indicating that NO activity in response to shear stress is reduced in hypertension and may be responsible for the diminished responses to increases in flow. Of note, arteries from hypercholesterolemic patients had preserved flow-mediated vasodilation compared with those from normal controls. However, in contrast to the response observed in vessels from normal controls, incubation with L-NNA did not significantly affect shear stress-induced dilation of hypercholesterolemic arteries, suggesting the presence of decreased NO synthesis compensated by other endothelial vasodilatory factors. These data are in agreement with the aforementioned *in vivo* observations of impaired endothelium-dependent vasodilation secondary to reduced NO bioactivity in hypertensive patients [10–15], and provide evidence that such abnormality not only affects the response to pharmacologic agonists, but, perhaps more importantly, limits the responses of blood vessels to shear stress, a physiologic mechanism participating in the regulation of microvascular tone. Importantly, impaired shear stress-dependent NO release may contribute to the development and/or the maintenance of increased peripheral resistance in hypertension. Thus, the significant reduction of shear stress-mediated NO-dependent vasodilation could blunt vascular relaxation in response to a variety of other physiologic stimuli, such as exercise, thereby increasing (or preventing the decrease of) vascular resistance, and leading to inappropriate elevations of blood pressure. Moreover, a reduced flow-mediated dilation and a diminished NO activity may be responsible for the structural changes underlying the increased vascular resistance observed in established hypertension [90].

Endothelial dysfunction in hypertension: cause or consequence of elevated blood pressure?

The data from our and other laboratories have clearly demonstrated the presence of impaired endothelium-dependent vasodilation in essential hypertension [10–15,89]. However, whether this abnormality is a primary or secondary phenomenon is still a matter of debate. In support of a primary genesis of endothelial dysfunction is the evidence that normotensive offspring of parents with essential hypertension have depressed endothelium-dependent vasodilation compared with normotensive offspring of normotensive parents [91], and that the bioactivity of NO may be reduced in normotensive individuals with a family history of hypertension [92]. On the other hand, a selective impairment of endothelium-dependent vasodilation after increases in blood pressure has been demonstrated in numerous animal models of induced hypertension [93–95]. Therefore we conducted a study to investigate the effect of increases in intra-arterial pressure on endothelium-dependent vasodilation of small arteries obtained from normotensive individuals [96]. Arteries from subcutaneous gluteal fat were mounted in a vessel chamber and connected at each extremity to a glass microcannula, with a constant internal pressure at baseline of 50 mmHg. The vasodilatory responses to acetylcholine and SNP were assessed at baseline and after increments of internal pressure to 80 and 120 mmHg. A significant reduction in the vasodilatory response to acetylcholine was observed with the progressive increases in intravascular pressure. In contrast, the response to SNP showed a non-significant trend toward vasodilation with the same increments in pressure. Thus, our study demonstrated that short-term increases in intra-arterial pressure directly and significantly depress endothelium-dependent vasodilation of small resistance arteries from normotensive subjects. These study findings have relevant pathophysiologic and clinical implications. First, these data support the notion that hypertension itself can cause endothelial dysfunction in humans. This concept is not necessarily at odds with previous evidence indicating that a reduced NO activity is a primary phenomenon in the pathophysiology of hypertension [91,92]. Indeed, since different mechanisms may underlie the hypertensive process, our findings expand the association between hypertension and endothelial dysfunction to patients in whom a reduction in NO activity may not be the primary cause leading to elevated blood pressure. Second, since an abnormal endothelial function is associated with increased atherosclerotic risk [97], the demonstration that elevated intravascular pressure can directly induce endothelial dysfunction may explain why hypertension represents a risk factor for the development of atherosclerosis, independent of

25 Flavahan NA. Atherosclerotic or lipoprotein-induced endothelial dysfunction: potential mechanisms underlying reduction in EDRF/nitric oxide activity. *Circulation* 1992;85:1927–1938.

26 Panza JA, Garcia CE, Kilcoyne CM, et al. Impaired endothelium-dependent vasodilation in patients with essential hypertension. Evidence that nitric oxide abnormality is not localized to a single signal transduction pathway. *Circulation* 1995;91(6):1732–1738.

27 Cardillo C, Kilcoyne CM, Quyyumi AA, et al. Decreased vasodilator response to isoproterenol during nitric oxide inhibition in humans. *Hypertension* 1997;30(4): 918–921.

28 Cardillo C, Kilcoyne CM, Quyyumi AA, et al. Selective defect in nitric oxide synthesis may explain the impaired endothelium-dependent vasodilation in patients with essential hypertension. *Circulation* 1998;97(9):851–856.

29 Gryglewsky RJ, Palmer RM, Moncada S. Superoxide anion is involved in the breakdown of endothelium-derived vascular relaxing factor. *Nature (London)* 1986;320:454–456.

30 Rubanyi GM, Vanhoutte PM. Oxygen-derived free radicals, endothelium, and responsiveness of vascular smooth muscle. *Am J Physiol* 1986;250:H815–H821.

31 Nakazono K, Watanabe N, Matsuno K, et al. Does superoxide underlie the pathogenesis of hypertension? *Proc Natl Acad Sci USA* 1991;88:1045–1048.

32 Wei EP, Kontos HA, Christman CW, et al. Superoxide generation and reversal of acetylcholine-induced cerebral arteriolar dilatation after acute hypertension. *Circ Res* 1985;57:781–787.

33 Garcia CE, Kilcoyne CM, Cardillo C, et al. Effect of copper–zinc superoxide dismutase on endothelium-dependent vasodilation in patients with essential hypertension. *Hypertension* 1995;26(6 Pt 1):863–868.

34 Cardillo C, Kilcoyne CM, Cannon III RO, et al. Xanthine oxidase inhibition with oxypurinol improves endothelial vasodilator function in hypercholesterolemic but not in hypertensive patients. *Hypertension* 1997;30(1 Pt 1):57–63.

35 Duffy SJ, New G, Tran BT, et al. Relative contribution of vasodilator prostanoids and NO to metabolic vasodilation in the human forearm. *Am J Physiol* 1999;276:H663–H670.

36 Diederich B, Yang ZH, Bühler FR, et al. Impaired endothelium-dependent relaxations in hypertensive resistance arteries involve the COX pathway. *Am J Physiol* 1990;258:H445–H451.

37 Iwama Y, Kato T, Muramatsu M, et al. Correlation with blood pressure of the acetylcholine-induced endothelium-dependent contracting factor in the rat aorta. *Hypertension* 1992;19:326–332.

38 Lüscher TF, Vanhoutte PM. Endothelium-dependent contractions to acetylcholine in the aorta of spontaneously hypertensive rat. *Hypertension* 1986;8:344–348.

39 Vanhoutte PM, Lüscher TF, Graser T. Endothelium-dependent contractions. *Blood Vessels* 1991;28:74–83.

40 Katusic ZS, Vanhoutte PM. Superoxide anion is an endothelium-derived contracting factor. *Am J Physiol* 1989;257:H33–H37.

41 Husain S, Andrews NP, Mulcahy D, et al. Aspirin improves endothelial dysfunction in atherosclerosis. *Circulation* 1998;97:716–720.

42 Campia U, Choucair WK, Bryant MB, et al. Role of cyclooxygenase products in the regulation of vascular tone and in the endothelial vasodilator function of normal, hypertensive, and hypercholesterolemic humans. *Am J Cardiol* 2002;89(3):286–290.

43 Yanagisawa M, Kurihara Kimura S, et al. A novel potent vasoconstrictor peptide produced by vascular endothelial cells. *Nature* 1988;332:411–415.

44 Arai H, Hori S, Aramori I, et al. Cloning and expression of cDNA encoding an endothelin receptor. *Nature* 1990;348:730–732.

45 Sakurai T, Yanagisawa M, Takuwa Y, et al. Cloning of a cDNA encoding a non-isopeptide-selective subtype of the endothelin receptor. *Nature* 1990;348:732–735.

46 Seo B, Oemar BS, Siebenmann R, et al. Both ET$_A$ and ET$_B$ receptors mediate contraction to endothelin-1 in human blood vessels. *Circulation* 1994;89:1203–1208.

47 Haynes WG, Strachan FE, Webb DJ. Endothelin ET$_A$ and ET$_B$ receptors cause vasoconstriction of human resistance and capacitance vessels *in vivo*. *Circulation* 1995;92:357–363.

48 De Nucci G, Thomas R, D'Orleans-Juste P, et al. Pressor effects of circulating endothelin are limited by its removal in the pulmonary circulation and by the release of prostacyclin and endothelium-derived relaxing factor. *Proc Natl Acad Sci USA* 1988;85:9797–9800.

49 Kohno M, Yasumari K, Murakawa K, et al. Plasma immunoreactive endothelin in essential hypertension. *Am J Med* 1990;88:614–618.

50 Shichiri M, Hirata Y, Ando K, et al. Plasma endothelin levels in hypertension and chronic renal failure. *Hypertension* 1990;15:493–496.

51 Saito Y, Nakao K, Mukoyama M, et al. Increased plasma endothelin levels in patients with essential hypertension. *N Engl J Med* 1990;322:205 [Letter].

52 Davenport AP, Ashby MJ, Easton P, et al. A sensitive radioimmunoassay measuring endothelin-like immunoreactivity in human plasma: comparison of levels in patients with essential hypertension and normotensive control subjects. *Clin Sci* 1990;78:261–264.

53 Predel HG, Meyer-Lehnert H, et al. Plasma concentrations of endothelin in patients with abnormal vascular

reactivity: effects of ergometric exercise and acute saline loading. *Life Sci* 1990;47:1837–1843.

54 Schiffrin EL, Thibault G. Plasma endothelin in human essential hypertension. *Am J Hypertens* 1991;4:303–308.

55 Wagner OF, Christ G, Wojta J, et al. Polar secretion of endothelin-l by cultured endothelial cells. *J Biol Chem* 1992;267:16066–16068.

56 Cardillo C, Kilcoyne CM, Waclawiw M, et al. Role of endothelin in the increases vascular tone of patients with essential hypertension. *Hypertension* 1999;33(2): 753–758.

57 Schiffrin EL, Yuan Deng L, Sventek P, et al. Enhanced expression of endothelin-1 gene in resistance arteries in severe human essential hypertension. *J Hypertens* 1997; 15:57–63.

58 Cardillo C, Kilcoyne CM, Cannon III RO, et al. Interactions between nitric oxide and endothelin in the regulation of vascular tone of human resistance vessels *in vivo*. *Hypertension* 2000;35(6)1237–1241.

59 Cardillo C, Campia U, Kilcoyne CM, et al. Improved endothelium-dependent vasodilation after blockade of endothelin receptors in patients with essential hypertension. *Circulation* 2002;105:452–456.

60 Schiffrin EL. Role of endothelin-1 in hypertension. *Hypertension* 1999; 34:876–881.

61 Gariepy CE, Ohuchi T, Williams SC, et al. Salt-sensitive hypertension in endothelin-B receptor-deficient rats. *J Clin Invest* 2000;105:925–933.

62 Katakam PV, Pollock JS, Pollock DM, et al. Enhanced endothelin-1 response and receptor expression in small resistance arteries of insulin-resistant rats. *Am J Physiol* (*Heart Circ Physiol*) 2001;280:H522–H527.

63 Wu SQ, Hopfner RL, McNeill JR, et al. Altered paracrine effect of endothelin in blood vessels of the hyperinsulinemic, insulin resistant obese Zucker rats. *Cardiovasc Res* 2000;45:994–1000.

64 Hall JE, Brands MW, Henegar JR. Mechanisms of hypertension and kidney disease in obesity. *Ann NY Acad Sci* 1999;892:91–107.

65 Cardillo C, Campia U, Iantorno M, et al. Enhanced vascular activity of endogenous endothelin-1 in obese hypertensive patients. *Hypertension* 2004;43:36–40.

66 Cornoni-Huntley J, LaCroix AZ, Havlick RJ. Race and sex differences in the impact of hypertension in the United States. *Arch Int Med* 1989;149:77–88.

67 Weinberger MH, Miller JZ, Luft FC, et al. Definitions and characteristics of sodium sensitivity and blood pressure resistance. *Hypertension* 1986;8(Suppl II):II127–II134.

68 Calhoun DA, Oparil S. Racial differences in the pathogenesis of hypertension. *Am J Med Sci* 1995;310:S86–S90.

69 Ergul S, Parish DC, Puett D, et al. Racial differences in plasma endothelin-1 concentrations in individuals with essential hypertension. *Hypertension* 1996;28: 652–655.

70 Campia U, Cardillo C, Panza JA. Ethnic differences in the vasoconstrictor activity of endogenous endothelin-1 in hypertensive patients. *Circulation* 2004;109:3191–3195.

71 Woywodt A, Bahlmann FH, De Groot K, et al. Circulating endothelial cells: life, death, detachment and repair of the endothelial cell layer. *Nephrol Dial Transplant* 2002; 17:1728–1730.

72 Hristov M, Erl W, Weber PC. Endothelial progenitor cells. Mobilization, differentiation, and homing. *Arterioscl Thromb Vasc Biol* 2003;23:1185–1189.

73 Aicher A, Heeschen C, Mildner-Rihm C, et al. Essential role of endothelial nitric oxide synthase for mobilization of stem and progenitor cells. *Nat Med* 2003;9:1370–1376.

74 Hill JM, Zalos G, Halcox JHP, et al. Circulating endothelial progenitor cells, vascular function, and cardiovascular risk. *N Engl J Med* 2003; 348:593–600.

75 Werner N, Kosiol S, Schiegl T, et al. Circulating endothelial progenitor cells and cardiovascular outcomes. *N Engl J Med* 2005;353:999–1007.

76 Vasa M, Fichtlscherer S, Aicher A, et al. Number and migratory activity of circulating endothelial progenitor cells inversely correlate with risk factors for coronary artery disease. *Circ Res* 2001;89:E1–E7.

77 Van Belle E, Witzenbichler B, Chen D, et al. Potentiated angiogenic effect of scatter factor/hepatocyte growth factor via induction of vascular endothelial growth factor: the case for paracrine amplification of angiogenesis. *Circulation* 1998;97:381–390.

78 Nakano N, Moriguchi A, Morishita R, et al. Role of angiotensin II in the regulation of a novel vascular modulator, hepatocyte growth factor (HGF), in experimental hypertensive rats. *Hypertension* 1997;30:1448–1454.

79 Imanishi T, Moriwaki C, Hano T, et al. Endothelial progenitor cell senescence is accelerated in both experimental hypertensive rats and patients with essential hypertension. *J Hypertens* 2005;23:1831–1837.

80 Imanishi T, Hano T, Nishio I. Angiotensin II accelerates endothelial progenitor cell senescence through induction of oxidative stress. *J Hypertens* 2005;23:97–104.

81 Min TQ, Zhu CJ, Xiang WX, et al. Improvement in endothelial progenitor cells from peripheral blood by ramipril therapy in patients with stable coronary artery disease. *Cardiovasc Drug Ther* 2004;18:203–209.

82 Davies PF. Flow-mediated endothelial mechanotransduction. *Physiol Rev* 1995;75:519–560.

83 Stepp DW, Nishikawa Y, Chilian WM. Regulation of shear stress in the canine coronary microcirculation. *Circulation* 1999;100:1555–1561.

84 Koller A, Sun D, Kaley G. Corelease of nitric oxide and prostaglandins mediates flow-dependent dilation of gracilis muscle arterioles. *Am J Physiol* 1994;267: H326–H332.

85 Celermajer DS, Sorensen KE, Gooch VM, et al. Noninvasive detection of endothelial dysfunction in children

and adults at risk of atherosclerosis. *Lancet* 1992;340: 1111–1115.

86 Joannides R, Haefeli WE, Linder R, et al. Nitric oxide is responsible for flow-dependent dilatation of human peripheral conduit arteries *in vivo. Circulation* 1995;91: 1314–1319.

87 Iiyama K, Nagano M, Yo Y, et al. Impaired endothelial function with essential hypertension assessed by ultrasonography. *Am Heart J* 1996;132:779–782.

88 Duffy SJ, Gokce N, Holbrok M, et al. Effect of ascorbic acid treatment on conduit vessel endothelial dysfunction in patients with hypertension. *Am J Physiol* 2001; 280:H528–H534.

89 Paniagua OA, Bryant MB, Panza JA. Role of endothelial nitric oxide in shear stress-induced vasodilation of human microvasculature. Diminished activity in hypertensive and hypercholesterolemic patients. *Circulation* 2001;103:1752–1758.

90 Ueno H, Kanellakis P, Agrotis A, et al. Blood flow regulates the development of vascular hypertrophy, smooth muscle cell proliferation, and endothelial cell nitric oxide synthase in hypertension. *Hypertension* 2000;36:89–96.

91 Taddei S, Virdis A, Mattei P, et al. Defective L-arginine-nitric oxide pathway in offspring of essential hypertensive patients. *Circulation* 1996;94:1298–1303.

92 Taddei S, Virdis A, Mattei P, et al. Endothelium-dependent forearm vasodilation is reduced in normotensive subjects with family history of hypertension. *J Cardiovasc Pharmacol* 1992;20:S193–S195.

93 Miller MJ, Pinto A, Mullane KM. Impaired endothelium-dependent relaxations in rabbits subjected to aortic coarctation hypertension. *Hypertension* 1987;10:164–170.

94 D'Uscio LV, Barton M, Shaw S, et al. Structure and function of small arteries in salt-induced hypertension. *Hypertension* 1997;30:905–911.

95 DeBruyn VH, Nuno DW, Capelli-Bigazzi M, et al. Effect of acute hypertension in the coronary circulation: role of mechanical factors and oxygen radicals. *J Hypertens* 1994;12:163–172.

96 Paniagua OA, Bryant MB, Panza JA. Transient hypertension directly impairs endothelium-dependent vasodilation of the human microvasculature. *Hypertension* 2000;36:941–944.

97 Biegelsen ES, Loscalzo J. Endothelial function in atherosclerosis. *Coron Artery Dis* 1999;10:241–256.

98 Folkow B. "Structural factor" in primary and secondary hypertension. *Hypertension* 1990:16:89–101.

99 Levy D, Larson MG, Vasan RS, et al. The progression from hypertension to congestive heart failure. *JAMA* 1996;275:1557–1562.

100 Park JB, Charbonneau F, Schiffrin EL. Correlation of endothelial function in large and small arteries in human essential hypertension. *J Hypertens* 2001;19(3):415–420.

101 Irace C, Ceravolo R, Notarangelo L, et al. Comparison of endothelial function evaluated by strain gauge plethysmography and brachial artery ultrasound. *Atherosclerosis* 2001;158(1):53–59.

102 Duffy SJ, Gokce N, Holbrook M, et al. Treatment of hypertension with ascorbic acid. *Lancet* 1999;354: 2048–2049.

103 Duffy SJ, Gokce N, Holbrook M, et al. Effect of ascorbic acid treatment on conduit vessel endothelial function in patients with hypertension. *Am J Physiol Heart Circ Physiol* 2001;280:H528–H534.

104 Jackson TS, Xu A, Vita JA, et al. Ascorbate prevents the interaction of superoxide and nitric oxide only at very high physiological concentrations. *Circ Res* 1998;83:916–922.

105 Ferrannini E, Buzzigoli G, Bonadonna R, et al. Insulin resistance in essential hypertension. *N Engl J Med* 1987;317:350–357.

106 Reaven GM. Insulin resistance and compensatory hyperinsulinemia: role in hypertension, dyslipidemia and coronary heart disease. *Am Heart J* 1991;121: 1283–1288.

107 Pollare T, Lithell H, Berne C. Insulin resistance is a characteristic feature of primary hypertension independent of obesity. *Metabolism* 1990;39(2):167–174.

108 Kaplan NM. The deadly quartet. Upper body obesity, glucose intolerance, hypertriglyceridemia, and hypertension. *Arch Int Med* 1989;149:1514–1520.

109 Desvergne B, Wahli W. Peroxisome proliferator-activated receptors: nuclear control of metabolism. *Endocr Rev* 1999;20:649–688.

110 Marx N, Duez H, Fruchart JC, et al. Peroxisome proliferator activated receptor and atherogenesis: regulator of gene expression in vascular cells. *Circ Res* 2004;94: 1168–1178.

111 Calnek DS, Mazzella L, Roser S, et al. Peroxisome proliferator-activated receptor gamma ligands increase release of nitric oxide from endothelial cells. *Arterioscl Thromb Vasc Biol* 2003;23:52–57.

112 Satoh H, Tsukamoto K, Hashimoto Y, et al. Thiazolidinediones suppress endothelin-1 secretion from bovine vascular endothelial cells: a new possible role of PPARgamma on vascular endothelial function. *Biochem Biophys Res Commun* 1999;254:757–763.

113 Artwohl M, Holzenbein T, Furnsinn C, et al. Thiazolidinediones inhibit apoptosis and heat shock protein 60 expression in human vascular endothelial cells. *Thromb Haemost* 2005;93:810–815.

114 Nakamura Y, Ohya Y, Onaka U, et al. Inhibitory action of insulin-sensitizing agents on calcium channels in smooth muscle cells from resistance arteries of guinea-pig. *Br J Pharmacol* 1998;123:675–682.

115 Takeda K, Ichiki T, Tokunou T, et al. Peroxisome proliferator-activated receptor gamma activators

downregulate angiotensin II type 1 receptor in vascular smooth muscle cells. *Circulation* 2000;102:1834–1839.

116 Barroso I, Gurnell M, Crowley VE, et al. Dominant negative mutations in human PPARgamma associated with severe insulin resistance, diabetes mellitus and hypertension. *Nature* 1999;402:880–883.

117 Campia U, Matuskey LA, Panza JA. Peroxisome proliferator-activated receptor-gamma activation with pioglitazone improves endothelium-dependent dilation in nondiabetic patients with major cardiovascular risk factors. *Circulation* 2006;113:867–875.

118 De Fronzo RA, Cooke CR, Andres R, et al. The effect of insulin on renal handling of sodium, potassium calcium, and phosphate in man. *J Clin Invest* 1975;55:845–855.

119 Scherrer U, Sartori C. Insulin as a vascular and sympathoexcitatory hormone. Implications for blood pressure regulation, insulin sensitivity, and cardiovascular morbidity. *Circulation* 1997;96:4104–4113.

120 Zeng G, Quon MJ. Insulin stimulated production of nitric oxide is inhibited by wortmannin: direct measurement in vascular endothelial cells. *J Clin Invest* 1996; 98:894–898.

121 Zeng G, Nystrom FH, Ravichandran LV, et al. Roles for insulin receptor, PI3 kinase, and Akt in insulin signaling pathways related to production of nitric oxide in human vascular endothelial cells. *Circulation* 2000;101:1539–1545.

122 Cardillo C, Kilcoyne CM, Nambi SS, et al. Vasodilator response to systemic but not to local hyperinsulinemia in the human forearm. *Hypertension* 1998;32:740–745.

123 Cardillo C, Nambi SS, Kilcoyne CM, et al. Insulin stimulates both endothelin and nitric oxide activity in the human forearm. *Circulation* 1999;100:829–825.

124 Steinberg HO, Chaker H, Leaming R, et al. Obesity/insulin resistance is associated with endothelial dysfunction: implications for the syndrome of insulin resistance. *J Clin Invest* 1996;97:2601–2610.

125 Ginsberg HN. Insulin resistance and cardiovascular disease. *J Clin Invest* 2000;106:453–458.

126 Cusi K, Maezono K, Osman A, et al. Insulin differentially affects the PI 3-kinase- and MAP-kinase-mediated signaling in human muscle. *J Clin Invest* 2000;105: 311–320.

127 Cai H, Harrison DG. Endothelial dysfunction in cardiovascular diseases: the role of oxidant stress. *Circ Res* 2000;87:840–844.

128 Barnes PJ, Karin M. Nuclear-factor kappaB: a pivotal transcription factor in chronic inflammatory diseases. *N Engl J Med* 1997;336:1066–1071.

129 Newby DE, Wright RA, Dawson P, et al. The L-arginine/nitric oxide pathway contributes to the acute release of tissue plasminogen activator *in vivo* in man. *Cardiovasc Res* 1998;38:485:492.

130 Newby DE, McLeod AL, Uren NG, et al. Impaired coronary tissue plasminogen activator release is associated with coronary atherosclerosis and cigarette smoking: direct link between endothelial dysfunction and atherothrombosis. *Circulation* 2001;103:1936–1941.

131 Jern S, Wall U, Bergbrant A, et al. Endothelium-dependent vasodilation and tissue-type plasminogen activator release in borderline hypertension. *Arterioscl Thromb Vasc Biol* 1997;17:3376–3383.

132 Yusuf S, Sleight P, Pogue J, et al., for the Heart Outcomes Prevention Evaluation Study Investigators. Effects of an angiotensin-converting-enzyme inhibitor, ramipril, on cardiovascular events in high risk patients. *N Engl J Med* 2000;342:145–153.

133 The Long-Term Intervention with Pravastatin in Ischemic Disease (LIPID) Study Group. Prevention of cardiovascular events and death with pravastatin in patients with coronary heart disease and a broad range of initial cholesterol levels. *N Engl J Med* 1998;339: 1349–1357.

134 Halcox, JPJ, Schenke WH, Zalos G, et al. Prognostic value of coronary vascular endothelial dysfunction. *Circulation* 2002;106:653–658.

135 Suwaidi JA, Hamasaki S, Higano ST, et al. Long-term follow-up of patients with coronary artery disease and endothelial dysfunction. *Circulation* 2000;101:948–954.

136 Schachinger V, Britten MB, Zeiher AM. Prognostic impact of coronary vasodilator dysfunction on adverse long-term outcome of coronary heart disease. *Circulation* 2000;101:1899–1906.

137 Perticone F, Ceravolo R, Pujia A, et al. Prognostic significance of endothelial dysfunction in hypertensive patients. *Circulation* 2001;104:191–196.

138 Panza JA, Quyyumi AA, Callahan T, et al. Effect of antihypertensive treatment on endothelium-dependent vascular relaxation in patients with essential hypertension. *J Am Coll Cardiol* 1993;21:1145–1151.

139 Taddei S, Virdis A, Ghiadoni L, et al. Restoration of nitric oxide availability after calcium antagonist treatment in essential hypertension. *Hypertension* 2001;37:943–948.

140 Taddei S, Virdis A, Ghiadoni L, et al. Lacidipine restores endothelium-dependent vasodilation in essential hypertensive patients. *Hypertension* 1997;30:1606–1612.

141 Taddei S, Virdis A, Ghiadoni L, et al. Effect of calcium antagonist or beta blockade treatment on nitric oxide-dependent vasodilation and oxidative stress in essential hypertensive patients. *J Hypertens* 2001;19:1379–1386.

142 Schiffrin EL, Pu Q, Park JB. Effect of amlodipine compared to atenolol on small arteries of previously untreated essential hypertensive patients. *Am J Hypertens* 2002;15:105–110.

143 Muiesan ML, Salvetti M, Monteduro C, et al. Effect of treatment on flow-dependent vasodilation of the brachial

artery in essential hypertension. *Hypertension* 1999;33: 575–580.

144 Mancini GBJ, Henry GC, Macaya C, et al. Angiotensin-converting enzyme inhibition with quinapril improves endothelial vasomotor dysfunction in patients with coronary artery disease. The TREND (Trial on Reversing ENdothelial Dysfunction) Study. *Circulation* 1996;94:258–265.

145 Taddei S, Virdis A, Ghiadoni L, et al. Effects of angiotensin converting enzyme inhibition on endothelium-dependent vasodilation in essential hypertensive patients. *J Hypertens* 16;16:447–456.

146 Ghiadoni L, Virdis A, Magagna A, et al. Effect of the angiotensin II type 1 receptor blocker candesartan on endothelial function in patients with essential hypertension. *Hypertension* 2000;35:501–506.

CHAPTER 16

Vascular function and diabetes mellitus

Mark A. Creager, MD *& Joshua A. Beckman,* MD

Vascular diseases, including atherosclerosis, medial calcification, and microangiopathy, are prevalent in patients with diabetes mellitus and are the principal causes of death and disability in these individuals. Atherosclerosis occurs earlier in patients with diabetes, frequently with greater severity and more diffuse distribution. Patients with diabetes have an increased prevalence of coronary artery disease, cerebrovascular disease, and peripheral arterial disease, and, as a result, are subject to the fatal and debilitating consequences of myocardial infarction, stroke, and amputation [1,2]. Microvascular disease also contributes importantly to morbidity. Diabetic retinopathy is a leading cause of blindness, and diabetic nephropathy is a major cause of chronic renal failure [3,4]. Diabetes is associated with abnormalities in vascular function and the ensuing morphologic changes associated with atherosclerosis and microvascular diseases. This chapter will review current knowledge regarding the effect of diabetes mellitus on vascular function, and provide a framework for understanding the mechanisms through which vascular disease occurs in patients with diabetes mellitus.

Diabetes and endothelial function

The endothelium plays a pivotal role in maintaining homeostasis of the blood vessels. As discussed elsewhere (see Chapter 1), the endothelium synthesizes biologically active substances that regulate vascular tone, modulate blood cell–vessel wall interaction, prevent thrombosis, and influence smooth muscle growth. Altered levels of endothelium-derived vasoactive substances, such as nitric oxide (NO)

and prostacyclin, occur in diabetes, fostering abnormal leukocyte–vascular wall interaction as well as platelet adhesion and aggregation. Endothelial dysfunction facilitates the diapedesis and activation of macrophages and the expression of endogenous cytokines and mitogens. Such processes contribute to all phases of atherosclerosis, including atherogenesis, intimal proliferation, plaque instability and rupture, and thrombus formation (see Chapters 2 and 3). Therefore, decreased availability of protective endothelial factors may underlie the pathologic changes that occur in patients with diabetes and contribute to the occurrence of vascular events.

Measures of NO bioavailability are useful to assess the health of the endothelium. In response to pharmacologic stimuli such as acetylcholine, histamine, and adenosine diphosphate (ADP) [5–7], endothelium-dependent relaxation provides a surrogate measure of NO bioavailability. This is abnormal in experimental models of diabetes, typically induced by alloxan or streptozotocin [8]. The response to endothelium-independent vasodilators, including exogenous NO donors, is not reduced in the majority of these studies. Observations in patients with diabetes corroborate the animal studies. For example, endothelium-dependent relaxation to acetylcholine is attenuated in the *corpus cavernosum* of diabetic patients when studied *in vitro* [9].

Endothelium-dependent vasodilation to methacholine is decreased in forearm resistance vessels of patients with type 1 diabetes mellitus (Figure 16.1) [10]. In addition, the vasoconstrictive response to N^G-monomethyl-L-arginine, a nitric oxide synthase (NOS) inhibitor, is decreased in patients with type 1 diabetes mellitus, implicating impaired basal release

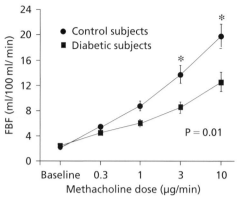

Figure 16.1 Impaired endothelium-dependent vasodilation in patients with type 1 diabetes mellitus. The forearm blood flow response to methacholine, an endothelium-dependent vasodilator, is significantly attenuated in patients with type 1 diabetes mellitus compared with age-matched healthy control subjects. (Reproduced with permission from Ref. [49]).

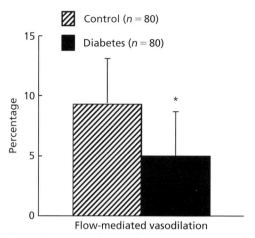

Figure 16.2 Flow-mediated endothelium-dependent vasodilation of the brachial artery in patients with type 1 diabetes mellitus. Endothelium-dependent vasodilation is reduced in this conduit artery in patients with type 1 diabetes compared with healthy control subjects. (Reproduced with permission from Ref. [19]).

of NO from the endothelium [11,12]. However, some studies that excluded patients with diabetes and detectable microalbuminuria, a variable that correlates with the severity of endothelial dysfunction, have not observed defective endothelium-dependent vasodilation in type 1 diabetes mellitus [13,14]. Patients with type 2 diabetes mellitus have impaired vasodilation of resistance vessels to both endogenous and exogenous NO donors. Reduced vasodilation of forearm resistance vessels occurs in type 2 diabetic patients following the intra-arterial administration of endothelium-dependent vasodilators such as acetylcholine or methacholine, and also with endothelium-independent vasodilators such as nitroprusside and nitroglycerin [15,16]. Responsiveness to the calcium channel blocker verapamil remains intact, implicating an abnormal NO signaling pathway [15,16].

Shear stress, induced by increasing flow through a vessel, is a stimulus to assess endothelium-dependent vasodilation in conduit vessels *in vivo* (see also Chapters 12 and 13). In order to assess endothelial function, vascular ultrasonography can evaluate changes that occur, following a flow stimulus, in the diameter of a peripheral conduit artery, such as the brachial artery. Patients with type 1 diabetes mellitus have impaired flow-mediated endothelium-dependent vasodilation in the brachial artery, a non-atherosclerotic peripheral conduit artery

(Figure 16.2) [17–19]. Furthermore, both flow-induced endothelium-dependent and nitroglycerin-induced endothelium-independent vasodilation of peripheral conduit vessels are abnormal in patients with type 2 diabetes mellitus.

Comparable observations have been made in the coronary circulation. Patients with diabetes mellitus studied *in vivo* have impaired endothelium-dependent vasodilation in angiographically normal coronary arteries [20]. In addition, the coronary microvascular responses to cold pressor testing and adenosine, reflecting endothelium-dependent and endothelium-independent vasodilation, respectively, are abnormal in both type 1 and type 2 diabetic patients [21].

Both type 1 and type 2 diabetes mellitus are characterized by hyperglycemia, and type 2 diabetes, in particular, by insulin resistance. Each of these fundamental abnormalities may incite cellular mechanisms that interfere with normal endothelial function. The following sections will discuss the cellular mechanisms whereby hyperglycemia and insulin resistance may cause vascular dysfunction.

Hyperglycemia and endothelial dysfunction

Hyperglycemia *per se* causes endothelial dysfunction. Hyperglycemia attenuates endothelium-dependent vasodilation of normal rat aortas *in vitro* and normal rat arterioles *in vivo* [22,23]. Healthy humans exposed to a hyperglycemic clamp sufficient to increase forearm glucose concentration experience impaired endothelium-dependent vasodilation [24]. Hyperglycemia also decreases flow-mediated endothelium-dependent vasodilation of the brachial artery of healthy subjects [25]. Hyperglycemia may decrease the bioavailability of NO through multiple mechanisms (Figure 16.3). Additionally, hyperglycemia may increase the formation of oxygen-derived free radicals that inactivate NO or cause intracellular signaling disturbances that inhibit NOS activity and thereby reduce NO production [26].

Hyperglycemia is associated with increased oxidative stress. Increased inactivation of NO by oxygen-derived free radicals and decreased production of NO by NOS reduce NO levels in the vascular milieu (see Chapter 10). Cellular sources of oxygen-derived free radicals in hyperglycemic states include the mitochondria, NOS, NADPH oxidase, and cyclooxygenase (COX) (Figure 16.3) [27,28]. Hyperglycemia induces the mitochondrial electron transport chain to generate superoxide anion [28]. Superoxide anion can activate protein kinase C (PKC), which increases the activity of NAD(P)H oxidase, thus increasing production of cytosolic superoxide anion [26]. PKC also upregulates the activity of COX-2 (see below) [29].

Superoxide anion inactivates NO, forming peroxynitrite anion [30]. Both superoxide anion and peroxynitrite uncouple NOS by oxidizing its cofactor tetrahydrobiopterin, shifting the productive capacities of NOS from NO to superoxide anion. The acute administration of tetrahydrobiopterin also improves endothelium-dependent vasodilation in patients with type 2 diabetes [31]. In addition, superoxide anion increases the intracellular production of advanced glycation endproducts (AGE) [28]. Activation of receptors for AGE (RAGE) increases intracellular enzymatic superoxide production [32–34]. Thus, a cascade effect occurs, in which progressive oxidative stress not only inactivates NO but also diminishes its production [35–38].

Proof of principle experiments support these concepts. Oxygen radical scavengers, such as superoxide dismutase, restore the attenuated response to acetylcholine observed in normal rabbit aortic rings or mesenteric vessels incubated in a hyperglycemic medium [23,39]. Scavengers of oxygen radicals restore endothelium-dependent relaxation in aortic rings and mesenteric resistance vessels of diabetic rats *in vitro* and in coronary microvessels *in vivo* [40–42]. Also, α-tocopherol, an anti-oxidant vitamin, improves endothelium-dependent relaxation in diabetic rats [43,44].

Ascorbic acid (vitamin C), an aqueous phase anti-oxidant, can scavenge superoxide anion [45]. The

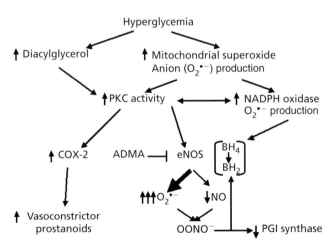

Figure 16.3 Mechanisms through which hyperglycemia decreases the bioavailability of endothelium-derived NO. NADPH: nicotinamide adenine dinucleotide phosphate (reduced form); $O_2^{\bullet-}$: superoxide anion; ADMA: asymmetric dimethylarginine; eNOS: endothelial nitric oxide synthase; BH_4: tetrahydrobiopterin; OONO$^-$: peroxynitrite; PGI: prostacyclin. For other abbreviations refer to text.

acute intra-arterial administration of ascorbic acid improves endothelium-dependent vasodilation in forearm resistance vessels of healthy subjects exposed to hyperglycemic clamp [46]. In addition, the oral administration of vitamin C and vitamin E improves flow-mediated endothelium-dependent vasodilation in the brachial artery of healthy subjects exposed to an acute glucose load [47].

Basic and clinical investigations also support the notion that oxygen-derived free radicals contribute to impaired endothelial function in diabetes. Anti-oxidants also improve endothelium-dependent vasodilation in patients with diabetes. The acute intra-arterial administration of ascorbic acid improves endothelium-dependent vasodilation in forearm resistance vessels of patients with type 1 or type 2 diabetes (Figure 16.4) [48,49]. The chronic administration of anti-oxidant vitamins improves endothelium-dependent vasodilation in patients with type 1 diabetes mellitus [17,50]. Long-term administration of anti-oxidant vitamins to patients with type 2 diabetes improved endothelium-dependent vasodilation in one study, but not in others [17,51,52].

Hyperglycemia also may decrease the synthesis of NO from NOS. Decreased activation of NOS may occur via several mechanisms, including: (1) hyperglycemia-induced alterations in intracellular signaling; (2) oxidation of NOS cofactors; and (3) increased levels of an endogenous antagonist to

L-arginine. Glucose metabolism in hyperglycemic states leads to increased production of diacylglycerol (DAG), which causes membrane translocation and PKC activation [53,54]. Superoxide anion also activates PKC (see above) [28]. Activation of PKC impairs downstream signaling, inhibiting the activity of phosphatidylinositol-3 (PI3) kinase, and thereby reducing activation of the kinase Akt and subsequent phosphorylation of NOS [55,56]. Thus, NO production decreases. Administration of PKC inhibitors improves endothelium-dependent relaxation of rabbit aorta and rat cerebral arterioles exposed to a hyperglycemic milieu [31,57]. Ruboxistaurin, a PKC inhibitor, prevents abnormal endothelium-dependent vasodilation in healthy humans exposed to a hyperglycemic clamp [58]. Thus, compelling evidence suggests that PKC mediates endothelial dysfunction caused by hyperglycemia. In addition, oxidation of tetrahydro-biopterin uncouples the NOS enzyme, resulting in decreased production of NO (see above) [35]. Also, increased activity of the hexosamine pathway inhibits Akt phosphorylation of endothelial NOS (eNOS) [59]. Hyperglycemia is associated with increased levels of asymmetric dimethylarginine (ADMA), a competitive antagonist of NOS that reduces the production of NO from NOS by acting as a competitive antagonist to L-arginine [60]. This appears to be secondary to increased oxidative stress, which impairs the ability of

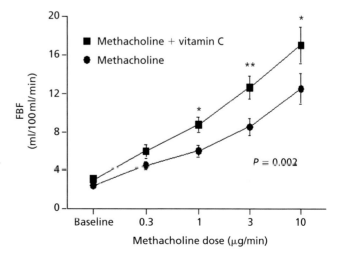

Figure 16.4 The effect of anti-oxidant vitamin C on endothelium-dependent vasodilation in patients with type 2 diabetes mellitus. The forearm blood flow response to methacholine improves significantly during administration of vitamin C. (Reproduced with permission from Ref. [48]).

dimethylarginine dimethylaminohydrolase (DDAH) to metabolize ADMA.

Effects of insulin resistance on endothelial function

Endothelium-dependent vasodilation is impaired in patients with type 2 diabetes and in insulin resistance states other than diabetes, such as obesity and the polycystic ovarian syndrome [15,61,62]. Therapies that enhance insulin sensitivity, such as thiazolidinediones and metformin, improve endothelium-dependent vasodilation [63,64].

Insulin resistance, characterized by abnormalities in insulin signaling that interfere with tissue glucose uptake and subsequent metabolism, impairs the normal vasoactive effects of insulin. Insulin causes vasodilation in healthy subjects exposed to a hyperinsulinemic, euglycemic clamp [65]. This vasodilatory response to insulin is likely mediated by endothelium-derived NO, since it is abrogated by the NOS antagonist, N^G-monomethyl-L-arginine [66]. Molecular and cellular studies have found that insulin stimulates the production of NO from endothelial cells by activating intracellular signaling molecules, including PI3 kinase and, eventually, Akt. This latter activates NOS via phosphorylation of serine$_{1177}$ [55,67–69]. Insulin resistant states show impaired insulin signal transduction via the PI3 kinase pathway, as well as reduced NO synthesis [69,70].

To account for decreased bioavailability of NO and abnormal endothelial function, several relevant mechanisms may operate in states of insulin resistance (Figure 16.5). Patients with insulin resistance have excess liberation of free fatty acids and inflammatory cytokines from the adipose tissue [71]. Administration of free fatty acids to healthy subjects impairs endothelium-dependent vasodilation [72]. Free fatty acids activate PKC and inhibit PI3 kinase, which will further affect downstream targets, particularly NOS (see above) [73,74]. Moreover, free fatty acids may increase the production of reactive oxygen species (ROS) via PKC-dependent activation of NAD(P)H oxidase, thereby ultimately inactivating NO [75]. Dyslipidemia, hypertension, and hyperglycemia frequently accompany states of insulin resistance, each altering endothelial function through distinct mechanisms [24,76–78].

Insulin resistance is associated with elevated serum markers of inflammation such as C-reactive protein (CRP) [79]. Increased release of cytokines such as interleukin-6 (IL-6) and tumor necrosis factor alpha (TNF-α) from the adipose tissues stimulates the hepatic production of CRP. Inflammation impairs endothelium-dependent vasodilation in humans [80,81]. TNF-α inhibits insulin-mediated tyrosine phosphorylation of the insulin receptor and IRS-1 via serine phosphorylation of IRS-1, thereby inhibiting signaling to downstream targets such as PI3 kinase and Akt [82–86]. Administration of TNF-α attenuates

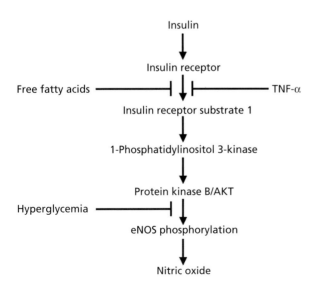

Figure 16.5 The insulin-NO signaling pathway. Insulin stimulates the production of NO via a series of intermediate molecular signals. Relevant mechanisms that may interfere with this pathway in insulin resistant states include excess free fatty acids, inflammatory cytokines, and hyperglycemia.

endothelium-dependent vasodilation in humans [87–89]. Also, co-infusion of TNF-α with insulin inhibits forearm glucose uptake and forearm endothelium-dependent vasodilation [90]. Elevated levels of CRP associate with abnormalities of endothelium-dependent vasodilation, and CRP may interfere directly with NO availability [81,91,92].

Endothelium-derived contracting factors and diabetes

The synthesis and activity of several endothelium-derived contracting factors may increase in diabetes. Several lines of evidence suggest that the contribution of vasoconstrictive prostanoids may have particular relevance to endothelial dysfunction. For example, endothelium-dependent relaxation of rabbit aortae exposed to a hyperglycemic milieu improves following treatment with a COX inhibitor or an antagonist of the receptor for prostaglandin H_2 (PGH_2)/thromboxane A_2 (TXA_2) [22]. Similar observations have been made in aortae excised from diabetic rabbits [93] and cerebral arterioles and arteries of diabetic rats [94]. Human aortic endothelial cells exposed to high glucose selectively augment COX-2, but not COX-1, mRNA, and protein expression [29], an action that is associated with increased thromboxane production and decreased prostacyclin release [29]. These intracellular events may be mediated by PKC, which is activated by hyperglycemia, as discussed previously. Inhibition of PKC reduces glucose-induced upregulation of COX-2 mRNA [29]. Decreased prostacyclin production may result from tyrosine nitration of prostacyclin (PGI_2) synthase, deriving from glucose-induced oxidative stress and the formation of peroxynitrates (see above) [29,95].

Increased production or activity of endothelin also may contribute to abnormal vascular function in patients with diabetes. Experimental models of diabetes and patients with either type 1 or type 2 diabetes show elevated plasma endothelin levels [96–98]. Both glucose and insulin have been implicated as potential stimuli for endothelin production. Elevation of glucose concentration in cultured media increases endothelin release from bovine aortic endothelial cells [99]. In addition, insulin stimulates endothelin gene expression in bovine aortic endothelial cells and endothelin secretion by

human endothelial and vascular smooth muscle cells (SMC) [100–102]. Human investigation has yielded comparable information. A euglycemic hyperinsulinemic clamp increases plasma endothelin levels in normal subjects and in men with type 2 diabetes [101,103]. Blockade of endothelin A and B receptors increases forearm blood flow in humans following the intra-arterial administration of insulin, supporting the concept that insulin stimulates endothelin release [104]. Administration of an endothelin-A receptor antagonist to patients with diabetes increased forearm blood flow in one study, suggesting increased activity of endogenous endothelin-1 [104], refuting observations from another study [105,106].

While increased endogenous activity of endothelin may contribute to vasomotor tone in diabetes, the vasoconstrictive response to exogenous endothelin appears blunted. The maximum response to endothelin is decreased in aortic rings derived from streptozotocin-treated rats [107]. Similarly, the contractile response to endothelin is reduced in subcutaneous small arteries of patients with type 2 diabetes compared with normal subjects when studied by micromyography [108]. Moreover, forearm vasoconstriction to infused endothelin is impaired in patients with type 2 diabetes [109].

The increased activity of angiotensin II that occurs in diabetes may also contribute to altered vasomotor function. In diabetic rats, there is diminished expression of the renin gene, which increases following the administration of insulin [110]. Although activity of the tissue renin–angiotensin system is increased in patients with diabetes, plasma-renin activity often remains low [111]. Glucose increases the expression of the angiotensinogen gene in proximal tubule cells and angiotensin II production in mesangial cells [112]. Also, vascular angiotensin-converting enzyme (ACE) activity increases in experimental models of diabetes [113]. Hyperglycemia potentiates angiotensin II-induced activation of growth-related kinases such as extracellular signal-related kinase (ERK) and mitogen-activated protein kinases (MAPK) [114]. Angiotensin II, which increases oxidative stress via NADPH oxidase and decreases the availability of NO [115], also promotes the migration of monocytes and the growth of vascular SMC, and inhibits vascular SMC apoptosis.

Advanced glycation endproducts

Non-enzymatic glycation of proteins and lipids following the exposure to sugars results in the formation of AGEs, which are prevalent in diabetic vasculature [116]. AGEs contribute to diabetic vascular disease through multiple mechanisms, including the formation of cross-links between molecules in the basement membrane of the extracellular matrix, the production of ROS, and a perturbation of vascular cell structure and function. AGE activation of its receptor, RAGE, stimulates NAD(P)H oxidase and upregulates the transcription factor nuclear factor-κB (NF-κB) and its target genes, including endothelin-1, vascular cell-adhesion molecule-1 (VCAM-1), intercellular adhesion molecule-1 (ICAM-1), E-selectin, tissue factor, and thrombomodulin [117,118]. AGEs reduce endothelial NO bioavailability, both by reducing eNOS activity and by quenching NO (see above) [119].

Treatment of endothelial dysfunction

If decreased bioavailability of NO contributes to vascular disease in diabetes, therapies directed at restoring endothelial function may have beneficial clinical consequences. Several pharmacologic interventions that interfere with the mechanisms underlying endothelial dysfunction in patients with diabetes, including anti-oxidant vitamins, L-arginine, oral hypoglycemic drugs, inhibitors of the renin–angiotensin system, and statins may have beneficial clinical consequences.

Several placebo-controlled studies have evaluated the efficacy of oral anti-oxidant vitamins on endothelial function in diabetes. Evidence suggests that administering vitamin E for 3 months and both vitamin C and vitamin E for 6 months improves flow-mediated vasodilation of the brachial artery in patients with type 1 diabetes [50,120], although the administration of vitamin E for 8 weeks in one study and vitamin C and E for 6 months in another study conferred no benefit on brachial artery endothelial function in patients with type 2 diabetes [52,120]. Long-term administration of anti-oxidant vitamins did not affect the incidence of cardiovascular events in either the Heart Outcomes Prevention and Evaluation (HOPE) study or in a subgroup of patients with diabetes in the Heart Protection Study (HPS) [121]. Thus, despite compelling evidence demonstrating that oxidative stress contributes to endothelial dysfunction in diabetes, clinical studies with anti-oxidant vitamins have been disappointing. These observations should not be interpreted to mean that oxidative stress is not relevant to endothelial dysfunction or to dispute the concept that reduced availability of NO leads to vascular disease. Instead, they point out that oral anti-oxidant vitamins may inadequately scavenge oxidant radicals resident in vascular tissue and emphasize the need to develop more potent anti-oxidant drugs (see also Chapter 22).

Studies on the effect of L-arginine, the precursor of NO, in patients with diabetes have yielded inconsistent data. Oral administration of L-arginine (7 g twice daily) for 6 weeks did not improve endothelium-dependent vasodilation in patients with type 1 diabetes in one study, whereas 9 g per day for 1 week improved endothelium-dependent vasodilation in patients with type 2 diabetes in another study [122,123]. No long-term clinical outcome studies have examined the efficacy of L-arginine in patients with diabetes.

Several trials have examined the effects of oral hypoglycemic drugs on endothelial function. Metformin improves insulin sensitivity and lowers blood glucose in diabetic patients by decreasing hepatic glucose output and increasing peripheral glucose uptake. Compared with placebo, the administration of metformin for 12 weeks improves forearm endothelium-dependent vasodilation to acetylcholine [64]. Members of the thiazolidinedione class of drugs activate peroxisome proliferator-activated receptor (PPAR) γ and lower blood glucose by improving insulin sensitivity. Administration of the thiazolidinedione troglitazone improves endothelium-dependent vasodilation in non-diabetic insulin resistant patients [63,124]. In one study, troglitazone improved endothelium-dependent vasodilation in newly diagnosed patients with type 2 diabetes, but not in patients with long-term diabetes [125]. In the United Kingdom Prospective Diabetes Study (UKPDS), intensive therapy of diabetes with oral hypoglycemic agents, including sulfonylureas and metformin, decreased the incidence of microvascular events, and benefits of macrovascular disease were limited to a marginal effect on the incidence of myocardial infarction. However, in UKPDS, myocardial infarction and mortality decreased significantly (39% and 35%, respectively) among patients receiving metformin alone, but not sulfonylureas [126]. In the PROactive study, the thiazolidinedione pioglitazone did not significantly reduce a composite endpoint of mortality, myocardial infarction, acute coronary syndrome, stroke, coronary or peripheral revascularization, and amputation, though there appeared to be favorable effects on the more limited composite of myocardial infarction, stroke, and death [127].

ACE inhibitors may improve endothelial function through one or two mechanisms. ACE inhibition prevents the degradation of bradykinin by kininase II. Bradykinin causes endothelium-dependent vasodilation by activating NOS. Angiotensin II increases the formation of superoxide anion via NADPH oxidase, which impairs endothelium-dependent vasodilation by scavenging NO (see above) [115]. ACE inhibition prevents the formation of angiotensin, thus reducing oxidant stress. Angiotensin receptor blockade also inhibits superoxide anion formation [128–130]. ACE inhibition and angiotensin II antagonists improved endothelium-dependent vasodilation in patients with diabetes in some studies but not in others [131–134]. Administration of enalapril for 4 weeks improved endothelium-dependent vasodilation of forearm resistance vessels in patients with type 2 diabetes [134], and treatment with losartan, an angiotensin receptor antagonist, yielded similar results after 4 weeks [131,132]. Inhibition of the renin–angiotensin system reduces microvascular complications and atherosclerotic events in patients with diabetes mellitus (see also Chapter 23) [121, 135–137].

Statins may improve the bioavailability of NO by reducing oxidative stress or increasing the activity of NOS [138,139]. Statin therapy improved endothelium-dependent vasodilation in the brachial artery in some, but not all, studies of patients with type 1 or type 2 diabetes [122,140–142]. Indeed, the clinical benefit of statin therapy in patients with diabetes is well established. In the Scandinavian Simvastatin Survival Study (4S) and the Cholesterol and Reduction in Events (CARE) trial, treatment with simvastatin and pravastatin, respectively, decreased the risk of adverse cardiovascular events in patients with coronary artery disease and diabetes [143,144]. Similarly in the HPS, simvastatin reduced the risk of myocardial infarction, stroke, and death in diabetic patients without evident coronary artery disease [145]. Similar observations were made with atorvastatin in the Collaborative Atorvastatin Diabetes Study and the Anglo-Scandinavian Cardiac Outcomes Trial (see also Chapter 21) [146,147].

It therefore appears that most drugs that reduce cardiovascular complications in diabetes associate with improved vasomotor function. Thus, restored endothelial function likely mediates an important component of therapeutic benefit. Future insights will expand our understanding of the precise mechanisms that disturb vascular health in patients with diabetes and will allow development of more specific and targeted therapies to reduce cardiovascular morbidity and mortality.

References

1 Beckman JA, Creager MA, Libby P. Diabetes and atherosclerosis: epidemiology, pathophysiology, and management. *JAMA* 2002;287:2570–2581.

2 Intensive blood-glucose control with sulphonylureas or insulin compared with conventional treatment and risk of complications in patients with type 2 diabetes (UKPDS 33). UK Prospective Diabetes Study (UKPDS) Group. *Lancet* 1998;352:837–853.

3 Merimee TJ. Diabetic retinopathy: a synthesis of perspectives. *N Engl J Med* 1990;322:978–983.

4 Zatz R, Brenner BM. Pathogenesis of diabetic microangiopathy. The hemodynamic view. *Am J Med* 1986; 30:443–453.

5 Meraji S, Jayakody L, Senaratne MP, et al. Endothelium-dependent relaxation in aorta of BB rat. *Diabetes* 1987;36:978–981.

6 Pieper GM, Gross GJ. Oxygen free radicals abolish endothelium-dependent relaxation in diabetic rat aorta. *Am J Physiol* 1988;255:H825–H833.

7 Durante W, Sen AK, Sunahara FA. Impairment of endothelium-dependent relaxation in aortae from spontaneously diabetic rats. *Br J Pharmacol* 1988;94:463–468.

8 De Vriese AS, Verbeuren TJ, Van de Voorde J, et al. Endothelial dysfunction in diabetes. *Br J Pharmacol* 2000;130:963–974.

9 Saenz de Tejada I, Goldstein I, Azodzoi K, et al. Impaired neurogenic and endothelium-mediated relaxation of penile smooth muscle from diabetic men with impotence. *N Engl J Med* 1989;320:1025–1030.

10 Johnstone MT, Creager SJ, Scales KM, et al. Impaired endothelium-dependent vasodilation in patients with insulin-dependent diabetes mellitus. *Circulation* 1993;88:2510–2516.

11 Calver A, Collier J, Vallance P. Inhibition and stimulation of nitric oxide synthesis in the human forearm arterial bed of patients with insulin-dependent diabetes. *J Clin Invest* 1992;90:2548–2554.

12 Elliott TG, Cockcroft JR, Groop PH, et al. Inhibition of nitric oxide synthesis in forearm vasculature of insulin-dependent diabetic patients: blunted vasoconstriction in patients with microalbuminuria. *Clin Sci (Colch)* 1993;85:687–693.

13 Halkin A, Benjamin N, Doktor HS, et al. Vascular responsiveness and cation exchange in insulin-dependent diabetes. *Clin Sci* 1991;81:223–232.

14 Smits P, Kapma JA, Jacobs MC, et al. Endothelium-dependent vascular relaxation in patients with type I diabetes. *Diabetes* 1993;42:148–153.

15 Williams SB, Cusco JA, Roddy M-A, et al. Impaired nitric oxide-mediated vasodilation in patients with non-insulin-dependent diabetes mellitus. *J Am Coll Cardiol* 1996;27:567–574.

16 McVeigh GE, Brennan GM, Johnston GD. Impaired endothelium-dependent and independent vasodilation in patients with type 2 (non-insulin-dependent) diabetes mellitus. *Diabetologia* 1992;35:771–776.

17 Beckman JA, Goldfine AB, Garrett LA, et al. Oral antioxidant therapy improves endothelial function in type 1 but not type 2 subjects with diabetes mellitus. *Am J Cardiol* 2003;285:H2392–H2398.

18 Zenere BM, Arcaro G, Saggiani F, et al. Noninvasive detection of functional alterations of the arterial wall in IDDM patients with and without microalbuminuria. *Diabetes Care* 1995;18:975–982.

19 Clarkson P, Celermajer DS, Donald AE, et al. Impaired vascular reactivity in insulin-dependent diabetes mellitus is related to disease duration and low density lipoprotein cholesterol levels. *J Am Coll Cardiol* 1996; 28:573–579.

20 Nitenberg A, Valensi P, Sachs R, et al. Impairment of coronary vascular reserve and Ach-induced coronary vasodilation in diabetic patients with angiographically normal coronary arteries and normal left ventricular systolic function. *Diabetes* 1993;42:1017–1025.

21 Di Carli MF, Janisse J, Grunberger G, et al. Role of chronic hyperglycemia in the pathogenesis of coronary microvascular dysfunction in diabetes. *J Am Coll Cardiol* 2003;41:1387–1393.

22 Tesfamariam B, Brown ML, Deykin D, et al. Elevated glucose promotes generation of endothelium-derived vasoconstrictor prostanoids in rabbit aorta. *J Clin Invest* 1990;85:929–932.

23 Bohlen HG, Lash JM. Topical hyperglycemia rapidly suppresses EDRF-mediated vasodilation of normal rate arterioles. *Am J Physiol* 1993;265:H219–H225.

24 Williams SB, Goldfine AB, Timimi FK, et al. Acute hyperglycemia attenuates endothelium-dependent vasodilation in humans *in vivo*. *Circulation* 1998;97:1695–1701.

25 Kawano H, Motoyama T, Hirashima O, et al. Hyperglycemia rapidly suppresses flow-mediated endothelium-dependent vasodilation of brachial artery. *J Am Coll Cardiol* 1999;34:146–154.

26 Hink U, Li H, Mollnau H, et al. Mechanisms underlying endothelial dysfunction in diabetes mellitus. *Circ Res* 2001;88:E14–E22.

27 Brownlee M. Biochemistry and molecular cell biology of diabetic complications. *Nature* 2001;414:813–820.

28 Nishikawa T, Edelstein D, Du XL, et al. Normalizing mitochondrial superoxide production blocks three pathways of hyperglycaemic damage. *Nature* 2000;404:787–790.

29 Cosentino F, Eto M, De Paolis P, et al. High glucose causes upregulation of cyclooxygenase-2 and alters prostanoid profile in human endothelial cells: role of protein kinase C and reactive oxygen species. *Circulation* 2003; 107: 1017–1023.

30 Beckman JS, Beckman TW, Chen J, et al. Apparent hydroxyl radical production by peroxynitrite: implications for endothelial injury from nitric oxide and superoxide. *Proc Natl Acad Sci USA* 1990;87:1620–1624.

31 Heitzer T, Krohn K, Albers S, et al. Tetrahydrobiopterin improves endothelium-dependent vasodilation by increasing nitric oxide activity in patients with type II diabetes mellitus. *Diabetologia* 2000; 43:1435–1438.

32 Schmidt AM, Stern D. Atherosclerosis and diabetes: the RAGE connection. *Curr Atheroscler Rep* 2000;2:430–436.

33 Tan KC, Chow WS, Ai VH, et al. Advanced glycation end products and endothelial dysfunction in type 2 diabetes. *Diabetes Care* 2002;25:1055–1059.

34 Wautier MP, Chappey O, Corda S, et al. Activation of NADPH oxidase by AGE links oxidant stress to altered gene expression via RAGE. *Am J Physiol Endocrinol Metab* 2001;280:E685–E694.

35 Milstien S, Katusic Z. Oxidation of tetrahydrobiopterin by peroxynitrite: implications for vascular endothelial function. *Biochem Biophys Res Commun* 1999;263: 681–684.

36 Laursen JB, Somers M, Kurz S, et al. Endothelial regulation of vasomotion in apoE-deficient mice: implications for interactions between peroxynitrite and tetrahydrobiopterin. *Circulation* 2001;103:1282–1288.

37 Guzik TJ, Mussa S, Gastaldi D, et al. Mechanisms of increased vascular superoxide production in human diabetes mellitus: role of NAD(P)H oxidase and endothelial nitric oxide synthase. *Circulation* 2002; 105:1656–1662.

38 Cosentino F, Hishikawa K, Katusic ZS, et al. High glucose increases nitric oxide synthase expression and superoxide anion generation in human aortic endothelial cells. *Circulation* 1997;96:25–28.

39 Tesfamariam B, Cohen RA. Free radicals mediate endothelial cell dysfunction caused by elevated glucose. *Am J Physiol* 1992;236:H321–H326.

40 Hattori Y, Kawasaki H, Abe K, et al. Superoxide dismutase recovers altered endothelium-dependent relaxation in diabetic rat aorta. *Am J Physiol* 1991; 261:H1086–H1094.

41 Langestroer P, Pieper GM. Regulation of spontaneous EDRF release in diabetic rat aorta by oxygen free radicals. *Am J Physiol* 1992;263:H257–H265.

42 Diederich D, Skopec J, Diederich A, et al. Endothelial dysfunction in mesenteric resistance arteries of diabetic rats: role of the free radicals. *Am J Physiol* 1994; 266:H1153–H1161.

43 Keegan A, Walbank H, Cotter MA, et al. Chronic vitamin E treatment prevents defective endothelium-dependent relaxation in diabetic rat aorta. *Diabetologia* 1995; 38:1475–1478.

44 Rösen P, Ballhausen T, Bloch W, et al. Endothelial relaxation is disturbed by oxidative stress in the diabetic rat heart: influence of tocopherol as antioxidant. *Diabetologia* 1995;38:1157–1168.

45 Frei B, England L, Ames BN. Ascorbate is an outstanding antioxidant in human blood plasma. *Proc Natl Acad Sci USA* 1989;86:6377–6381.

46 Beckman JA, Goldfine AB, Gordon MB, et al. Ascorbate restores endothelium-dependent vasodilation impaired by acute hyperglycemia in humans. *Circulation* 2001; 103:1618–1623.

47 Title LM, Cummings PM, Giddens K, et al. Oral glucose loading acutely attenuates endothelium-dependent vasodilation in healthy adults without diabetes: an effect prevented by vitamins C and E. *J Am Coll Cardiol* 2000;36:2185–2191.

48 Ting HH, Timimi FK, Boles KS, et al. Vitamin C improves endothelium-dependent vasodilation in patients with non-insulin-dependent diabetes mellitus. *J Am Coll Cardiol* 1996;97:22–28.

49 Timimi FK, Ting HH, Haley EA, et al. Vitamin C improves endothelium-dependent vasodilation in patients with insulin-dependent diabetes mellitus. *J Am Coll Cardiol* 1998;31:552–557.

50 Skyrme-Jones RA, O'Brien RC, Berry KL, et al. Vitamin E supplementation improves endothelial function in type I diabetes mellitus: a randomized, placebo-controlled study. *J Am Coll Cardiol* 2000; 36:94–102.

51 Paolisso G, Tagliamonte MR, Barbieri M, et al. Chronic vitamin E administration improves brachial reactivity and increases intracellular magnesium concentration in type II diabetic patients. *J Clin Endocrinol Metab* 2000;85:109–115.

52 Gazis A, White DJ, Page SR, et al. Effect of oral vitamin E (alpha-tocopherol) supplementation on vascular endothelial function in type 2 diabetes mellitus. *Diabet Med* 1999;16:304–311.

53 Xia P, Inoguchi T, Kern TS, et al. Characterization of the mechanism for the chronic activation of diacylglycerol-protein kinase C pathway in diabetes and hypergalactosemia. *Diabetes* 1994;43:1122–1129.

54 Inoguchi T, Xia P, Kunisaki M, et al. Insulin's effect on protein kinase C and diacylglycerol induced by diabetes and glucose in vascular tissues. *Am J Physiol* 1994; 267:E369–E379.

55 Kuboki K, Jiang ZY, Takahara N, et al. Regulation of endothelial constitutive nitric oxide synthase gene expression in endothelial cells and *in vivo*: a specific vascular action of insulin. *Circulation* 2000;101: 676–681.

56 Ribiere C, Jaubert AM, Sabourault D, et al. Insulin stimulates nitric oxide production in rat adipocytes. *Biochem Biophys Res Commun* 2002;291:394–399.

57 Tesfamariam B, Brown ML, Cohen RA. Elevated glucose impairs endothelium-dependent relaxation by activating protein kinase C. *J Clin Invest* 1991;87:1643–1648.

58 Beckman JA, Goldfine AB, Gordon MB, et al. Inhibition of protein kinase Cbeta prevents impaired endothelium-dependent vasodilation caused by hyperglycemia in humans. *Circ Res* 2002;90:107–111.

59 Du XL, Edelstein D, Dimmeler S, et al. Hyperglycemia inhibits endothelial nitric oxide synthase activity by post-translational modification at the Akt site. *J Clin Invest* 2001;108:1341–1348.

60 Lin KY, Ito A, Asagami T, et al. Impaired nitric oxide synthase pathway in diabetes mellitus: role of asymmetric dimethylarginine and dimethylarginine dimethylamino-hydrolase. *Circulation* 2002;106:987–992.

61 Laakso M, Edelman SV, Brechtel G, et al. Decreased effect of insulin to stimulate skeletal muscle blood flow in obese man. A novel mechanism for insulin resistance. *J Clin Invest* 1990;85:1844–1852.

62 Paradisi G, Steinberg HO, Hempfling A, et al. Polycystic ovary syndrome is associated with endothelial dysfunction. *Circulation* 2001;103:1410–1415.

63 Watanabe Y, Sunayama S, Shimada K, et al. Troglitazone improves endothelial dysfunction in patients with insulin resistance. *J Atheroscler Thromb* 2000;7:159–163.

64 Mather KJ, Verma S, Anderson TJ. Improved endothelial function with metformin in type 2 diabetes mellitus. *J Am Coll Cardiol* 2001;37:1344–1350.

65 Creager MA, Liang C-S, Coffman JD. Beta adrenergic-mediated vasodilator response to insulin in the human forearm. *J Pharmacol Exp Ther* 1985;235:709–714.

66 Scherrer U, Randin D, Vollenweider P, et al. Nitric oxide release accounts for insulin's vascular effects in humans. *J Clin Invest* 1994;94:2511–2515.

67 Vicent D, Ilany J, Kondo T, et al. The role of endothelial insulin signaling in the regulation of vascular tone and insulin resistance. *J Clin Invest* 2003;111:1373–1380.

68 Zeng G, Quon MJ. Insulin-stimulated production of nitric oxide is inhibited by wortmannin. Direct measurement in vascular endothelial cells. *J Clin Invest* 1996; 98:894–898.

69 Zeng G, Nystrom FH, Ravichandran LV, et al. Roles for insulin receptor, PI3-kinase, and Akt in insulin-signaling pathways related to production of nitric oxide in human vascular endothelial cells. *Circulation* 2000;101:1539–1545.

70 Montagnani M, Golovchenko I, Kim I, et al. Inhibition of phosphatidylinositol 3-kinase enhances mitogenic actions of insulin in endothelial cells. *J Biol Chem* 2002;277:1794–1799.

71 Hennes MM, O'Shaughnessy IM, Kelly TM, et al. Insulin-resistant lipolysis in abdominally obese hypertensive individuals. Role of the renin–angiotensin system. *Hypertension* 1996;28:120–126.

72 Steinberg HO, Tarshoby M, Monestel R, et al. Elevated circulating free fatty acid levels impair endothelium-dependent vasodilation. *J Clin Invest* 1997;100:1230–1239.

73 Dresner A, Laurent D, Marcucci M, et al. Effects of free fatty acids on glucose transport and IRS-1-associated phosphatidylinositol 3-kinase activity. *J Clin Invest* 1999;103:253–259.

74 Griffin ME, Marcucci MJ, Cline GW, et al. Free fatty acid-induced insulin resistance is associated with activation of protein kinase C theta and alterations in the insulin signaling cascade. *Diabetes* 1999;48:1270–1274.

75 Inoguchi T, Li P, Umeda F, et al. High glucose level and free fatty acid stimulate reactive oxygen species production through protein kinase C – dependent activation of NAD(P)H oxidase in cultured vascular cells. *Diabetes* 2000;49:1939–1945.

76 Ting HH, Timimi FK, Haley EA, et al. Vitamin C improves endothelium-dependent vasodilation in forearm resistance vessels of humans with hypercholesterolemia. *Circulation* 1997;95:2617–2622.

77 Creager MA, Cooke JP, Mendelsohn ME, et al. Impaired vasodilation of forearm resistance vessels in hypercholesterolemic humans. *J Clin Invest* 1990;86:228–234.

78 Taddei S, Virdis A, Mattei P, et al. Effect of insulin on acetylcholine-induced vasodilation in normotensive subjects and patients with essential hypertension. *Circulation* 1995;92:2911–2918.

79 Pradhan AD, Cook NR, Buring JE, et al. C-reactive protein is independently associated with fasting insulin in nondiabetic women. *Arterioscler Thromb Vasc Biol* 2003;23:650–655.

80 Hingorani AD, Cross J, Kharbanda RK, et al. Acute systemic inflammation impairs endothelium-dependent dilatation in humans. *Circulation* 2000;102:994–999.

81 Fichtlscherer S, Rosenberger G, Walter DH, et al. Elevated C-reactive protein levels and impaired endothelial vasoreactivity in patients with coronary artery disease. *Circulation* 2000;102:1000–1006.

82 Hotamisligil GS, Budavari A, Murray D, et al. Reduced tyrosine kinase activity of the insulin receptor in obesity–diabetes. Central role of tumor necrosis factor-alpha. *J Clin Invest* 1994;94:1543–1549.

83 Hotamisligil GS, Murray DL, Choy LN, et al. Tumor necrosis factor alpha inhibits signaling from the insulin receptor. *Proc Natl Acad Sci USA* 1994; 91:4854–4858.

84 Hotamisligil GS, Peraldi P, Budavari A, et al. IRS-1-mediated inhibition of insulin receptor tyrosine kinase activity in TNF-alpha- and obesity-induced insulin resistance. *Science* 1996;271:665–668.

85 Rui L, Aguirre V, Kim JK, et al. Insulin/IGF-1 and TNF-alpha stimulate phosphorylation of IRS-1 at inhibitory Ser307 via distinct pathways. *J Clin Invest* 2001; 107:181–189.

86 Kanety H, Feinstein R, Papa MZ, et al. Tumor necrosis factor alpha-induced phosphorylation of insulin receptor substrate-1 (IRS-1). Possible mechanism for suppression of insulin-stimulated tyrosine phosphorylation of IRS-1. *J Biol Chem* 1995;270:23780–23784.

87 Bhagat K, Vallance P. Inflammatory cytokines impair endothelium-dependent dilatation in human veins *in vivo*. *Circulation* 1997;96:3042–3047.

88 Bilsborough W, O'Driscoll G, Stanton K, et al. Effect of lowering tumour necrosis factor-alpha on vascular endothelial function in type II diabetes. *Clin Sci (London)* 2002;103:163–169.

89 Chia S, Qadan M, Newton R, et al. Intra-arterial tumor necrosis factor-{alpha} impairs endothelium-dependent vasodilatation and stimulates local tissue plasminogen activator release in humans. *Arterioscler Thromb Vasc Biol* 2003;23:695–701.

90 Rask-Madsen C, Dominguez H, Ihlemann N, et al. Tumor necrosis factor-alpha inhibits insulin's stimulating effect on glucose uptake and endothelium-dependent vasodilation in humans. *Circulation* 2003; 108:1815–1821.

91 Jarvisalo MJ, Harmoinen A, Hakanen M, et al. Elevated serum C-reactive protein levels and early arterial changes in healthy children. *Arterioscler Thromb Vasc Biol* 2002;22:1323–1328.

92 Venugopal SK, Devaraj S, Yuhanna I, et al. Demonstration that C-reactive protein decreases eNOS expression and bioactivity in human aortic endothelial cells. *Circulation* 2002;106:1439–1441.

93 Tesfamariam B, Jakubowski JA, Cohen RA. Contraction of diabetic rabbit aorta caused by endothelium-derived PGH_2-TxA_2. *Am J Physiol* 1989;257:H1327–H1333.

94 Mayhan WG, Simmons LK, Sharpe GM. Mechanism of impaired responses of cerebral arterioles during diabetes mellitus. *Am J Physiol* 1991;260:H319–H326.

95 Zou M, Martin C, Ullrich V. Tyrosine nitration as a mechanism of selective inactivation of prostacyclin synthase by peroxynitrite. *Biol Chem* 1997;378:707–713.

96 Makino A, Kamata K. Elevated plasma endothelin-1 level in streptozotocin-induced diabetic rats and responsiveness of the mesenteric arterial bed to endothelin-1. *Br J Pharmacol* 1998;123:1065–1072.

97 Sarman B, Farkas K, Toth M, et al. Circulating plasma endothelin-1, plasma lipids and complications in type 1 diabetes mellitus. *Diabetes Nutr Metab* 2000;13:142–148.

98 Laurenti O, Vingolo EM, Desideri GB, et al. Increased levels of plasma endothelin-1 in non-insulin dependent diabetic patients with retinopathy but without other diabetes-related organ damage. *Exp Clin Endocrinol Diabetes* 1997;105(Suppl 2):40–42.

99 Yamauchi T, Ohnaka K, Takayanagi R, et al. Enhanced secretion of endothelin-1 by elevated glucose levels from cultured bovine aortic endothelial cells. *FEBS Lett* 1990;267:16–18.

100 Oliver FJ, de la Rubia G, Feener EP, et al. Stimulation of endothelin-1 gene expression by insulin in endothelial cells. *J Biol Chem* 1991;266:23251–23256.

101 Ferri C, Carlomagno A, Coassin S, et al. Circulating endothelin-1 levels increase during euglycemic hyperinsulinemic clamp in lean NIDDM men. *Diabetes Care* 1995;18:226–233.

102 Anfossi G, Cavalot F, Massucco P, et al. Insulin influences immunoreactive endothelin release by human vascular smooth muscle cells. *Metabolism* 1993;42:1081–1083.

103 Piatti PM, Monti LD, Conti M, et al. Hypertriglyceridemia and hyperinsulinemia are potent inducers of endothelin-1 release in humans. *Diabetes* 1996;45:316–321.

104 Cardillo C, Campia U, Bryant MB, et al. Increased activity of endogenous endothelin in patients with type II diabetes mellitus. *Circulation* 2002;106:1783–1787.

105 McAuley DF, Nugent AG, McGurk C, et al. Vasoconstriction to endogenous endothelin-1 is impaired in patients with type II diabetes mellitus. *Clin Sci (London)* 2000;99:175–179.

106 Nugent AG, McGurk C, Hayes JR, et al. Impaired vasoconstriction to endothelin 1 in patients with NIDDM. *Diabetes* 1996;45:105–107.

107 Fulton DJ, Hodgson WC, Sikorski BW, et al. Attenuated responses to endothelin-1, KCl and $CaCl_2$, but not noradrenaline, of aortae from rats with streptozotocin-induced diabetes mellitus. *Br J Pharmacol* 1991;104:928–932.

108 Rizzoni D, Porteri E, Guelfi D, et al. Structural alterations in subcutaneous small arteries of normotensive and hypertensive patients with non-insulin-dependent diabetes mellitus. *Circulation* 2001;103:1238–1244.

109 McAuley DF, McGurk C, Nugent AG, et al. Vasoconstriction to endothelin-1 is blunted in non-insulin-dependent diabetes: a dose-response study. *J Cardiovasc Pharmacol* 2000;36:203–208.

110 Jaffa AA, Vio C, Velarde V, et al. Induction of renal kallikrein and renin gene expression by insulin and IGF-I in the diabetic rat. *Diabetes* 1997;46:2049–2056.

111 Hsueh WA, Anderson PW. Systemic hypertension and the renin–angiotensin system in diabetic vascular complications. *Am J Cardiol* 1993;72:14H–21H.

112 Leehey DJ, Singh AK, Alavi N, et al. Role of angiotensin II in diabetic nephropathy. *Kidney Int* 2000; 77(Suppl):S93–S98.

113 Crespo MJ, Moreta S, Gonzalez J. Cardiovascular deterioration in STZ-diabetic rats: possible role of vascular RAS. *Pharmacology* 2003;68:1–8.

114 Natarajan R, Scott S, Bai W, et al. Angiotensin II signaling in vascular smooth muscle cells under high glucose conditions. *Hypertension* 1999;33:378–384.

115 Rajagopalan S, Kurz S, Munzel T, et al. Angiotensin II-mediated hypertension in the rat increases vascular superoxide production via membrane NADH/NADPH oxidase activations. Contribution to alterations of vasomotor tone. *J Clin Invest* 1996;97:1916–1923.

116 Brownlee M. Advanced protein glycosylation in diabetes and aging. *Annu Rev Med* 1995;46:223–234.

117 Yan SF, Ramasamy R, Naka Y, et al. Glycation, inflammation, and RAGE: a scaffold for the macrovascular complications of diabetes and beyond. *Circ Res* 2003;93:1159–1169.

118 Naka Y, Bucciarelli LG, Wendt T, et al. RAGE axis: animal models and novel insights into the vascular complications of diabetes. *Arterioscler Thromb Vasc Biol* 2004;24:1342–1349.

119 Bucala R, Tracey KJ, Cerami A. Advanced glycosylation products quench nitric oxide and mediate defective endothelium-dependent vasodilatation in experimental diabetes. *J Clin Invest* 1991;87:432–438.

120 Beckman JA, Goldfine AB, Garrett LA, et al. Oral antioxidant therapy improves endothelial function in type 1 but not type 2 subjects with diabetes mellitus. *Circulation* 2001;104:II327.

121 Effects of ramipril on cardiovascular and microvascular outcomes in people with diabetes mellitus: results of the HOPE study and MICRO-HOPE substudy. Heart Outcomes Prevention Evaluation Study Investigators. *Lancet* 2000;355:253–259.

122 Mullen MJ, Wright D, Donald AE, et al. Atorvastatin but not L-arginine improves endothelial function in type I

diabetes mellitus: a double-blind study. *J Am Coll Cardiol* 2000;36:410–416.

123 Regensteiner JG, Popylisen S, Bauer TA, et al. Oral L-arginine and vitamins E and C improve endothelial function in women with type 2 diabetes. *Vasc Med* 2003;8:169–175.

124 Garg R, Kumbkarni Y, Aljada A, et al. Troglitazone reduces reactive oxygen species generation by leukocytes and lipid peroxidation and improves flow-mediated vasodilatation in obese subjects. *Hypertension* 2000; 36:430–435.

125 Caballero AE, Saouaf R, Lim SC, et al. The effects of troglitazone, an insulin-sensitizing agent, on the endothelial function in early and late type 2 diabetes: a placebo-controlled randomized clinical trial. *Metabolism* 2003;52:173–180.

126 Effect of intensive blood-glucose control with metformin on complications in overweight patients with type 2 diabetes (UKPDS 34). UK Prospective Diabetes Study (UKPDS) Group. *Lancet* 1998;352:854–865.

127 Dormandy JA, Charbonnel B, Eckland DJ, et al. Secondary prevention of macrovascular events in patients with type 2 diabetes in the PROactive Study (PROspective pioglitAzone Clinical Trial In macroVascular Events): a randomised controlled trial. *Lancet* 2005;366:1279–1289.

128 Kintscher U, Wakino S, Kim S, et al. Angiotensin II induces migration and Pyk2/paxillin phosphorylation of human monocytes. *Hypertension* 2001;37:587–593.

129 Xi XP, Graf K, Goetze S, et al. Central role of the MAPK pathway in ang II-mediated DNA synthesis and migration in rat vascular smooth muscle cells. *Arterioscler Thromb Vasc Biol* 1999;19:73–82.

130 Pollman MJ, Yamada T, Horiuchi M, et al. Vasoactive substances regulate vascular smooth muscle cell apoptosis. Countervailing influences of nitric oxide and angiotensin II. *Circ Res* 1996;79:748–756.

131 Cheetham C, O'Driscoll G, Stanton K, et al. Losartan, an angiotensin type I receptor antagonist, improves conduit vessel endothelial function in type II diabetes. *Clin Sci (London)* 2001;100:13–17.

132 Cheetham C, Collis J, O'Driscoll G, et al. Losartan, an angiotensin type 1 receptor antagonist, improves endothelial function in non-insulin-dependent diabetes. *J Am Coll Cardiol* 2000;36:1461–1466.

133 McFarlane R, McCredie RJ, Bonney MA, et al. Angiotensin converting enzyme inhibition and arterial endothelial function in adults with type 1 diabetes mellitus. *Diabet Med* 1999;16:62–66.

134 O'Driscoll G, Green D, Maiorana A, et al. Improvement in endothelial function by angiotensin-converting enzyme inhibition in non-insulin-dependent diabetes mellitus. *J Am Coll Cardiol* 1999;33:1506–1511.

135 Efficacy of atenolol and captopril in reducing risk of macrovascular and microvascular complications in type 2 diabetes: UKPDS 39. UK Prospective Diabetes Study Group. *BMJ* 1998;317:713–720.

136 Tatti P, Pahor M, Byington RP, et al. Outcome results of the Fosinopril versus Amlodipine Cardiovascular Events Randomized Trial (FACET) in patients with hypertension and NIDDM. *Diabetes Care* 1998;21:597–603.

137 Brenner BM, Cooper ME, de Zeeuw D, et al. Effects of losartan on renal and cardiovascular outcomes in patients with type 2 diabetes and nephropathy. *N Engl J Med* 2001;345:861–869.

138 Laufs U, La Fata V, Plutzky J, et al. Upregulation of endothelial nitric oxide synthase by HMG CoA reductase inhibitors. *Circulation* 1998;97:1129–1135.

139 Anderson TJ, Meredith IT, Charbonneau F, et al. Endothelium-dependent coronary vasomotion relates to the susceptibility of LDL to oxidation in humans. *Circulation* 1996;93:1647–1650.

140 Sheu WH, Juang BL, Chen YT, et al. Endothelial dysfunction is not reversed by simvastatin treatment in type 2 diabetic patients with hypercholesterolemia. *Diabetes Care* 1999;22:1224–1225.

141 Tan KC, Chow WS, Tam SC, et al. Atorvastatin lowers C-reactive protein and improves endothelium-dependent vasodilation in type 2 diabetes mellitus. *J Clin Endocrinol Metab* 2002;87:563–568.

142 van Etten RW, de Koning EJ, Honing ML, et al. Intensive lipid lowering by statin therapy does not improve vasoreactivity in patients with type 2 diabetes. *Arterioscler Thromb Vasc Biol* 2002;22:799–804.

143 Pyorala K, Pedersen TR, Kjekshus J, et al. Cholesterol lowering with simvastatin improves prognosis of diabetic patients with coronary heart disease. A subgroup analysis of the Scandinavian Simvastatin Survival Study (4S). *Diabetes Care* 1997;20:614–620.

144 Sacks FM, Pfeffer MA, Moye LA, et al. Cholesterol and Recurrent Events Trial Investigators. The effect of pravastatin on coronary events after myocardial infarction in patients with average cholesterol levels. *N Engl J Med* 1996;335:1001–1009.

145 MRC/BHF Heart Protection Study of cholesterol lowering with simvastatin in 20,536 high-risk individuals: a randomised placebo-controlled trial. *Lancet* 2002;360:7–22.

146 Colhoun HM, Betteridge DJ, Durrington PN, et al. Primary prevention of cardiovascular disease with atorvas-tatin in type 2 diabetes in the Collaborative Atorvastatin Diabetes Study (CARDS): multicentre randomised placebo-controlled trial. *Lancet* 2004; 364:685–696.

147 Sever PS, Poulter NR, Dahlof B, et al. Reduction in cardiovascular events with atorvastatin in 2,532 patients with type 2 diabetes: Anglo-Scandinavian Cardiac Outcomes Trial – lipid-lowering arm (ASCOT-LLA). *Diabetes Care* 2005;28:1151–1157.

CHAPTER 17

Dyslipidemia and endothelial dysfunction: pathophysiology and therapy

*Todd J. Anderson**, MD, FRCPC *& Francois Charbonneau,* MSC, MD

Complications of atherosclerotic vascular disease remain the leading cause of morbidity and mortality in Western society. Atherosclerosis results from a complex interaction between lipids, inflammatory cells, inflammatory mediators, platelets, and the vessel wall. The vascular endothelium plays a key role in vascular homeostasis through the release of a variety of autocrine and paracrine substances, the best characterized being nitric oxide (NO). Endothelial dysfunction is the initial event in atherogenesis and plays a key role in all phases of the disease including acute coronary syndromes (ACS). Attenuation of endothelial function occurs in response to cardiac risk factors, with abnormalities of lipids and lipoproteins being the best characterized.

Much is now known about the pathophysiology of cholesterol metabolism and its subsequent effect on endothelial function. This chapter will outline the relationship between lipid abnormalities and vascular function. There is little doubt that the benefits of lipid lowering on endothelial function and inflammation contribute significantly to the impressive clinical benefits of this therapeutic approach.

Lipids and endothelial function

Endothelial function

The endothelium plays a key role in vascular homeostasis through the release of a variety of autocrine

and paracrine substances [1] (see also Chapter 1). Dysfunction of endothelial cells is a systemic process and the initiating event in atherosclerosis. Broadly speaking, endothelial function refers to a physiological observation resulting from stimulation of vasoactive substances released by or that interact with the vascular endothelium. The most important of the endothelial-derived relaxing factors is NO [2]. NO is synthesized from L-arginine by a family of NO synthases (NOS) [3]. This conversion occurs in response to stimuli such as acetylcholine (Ach) or increased flow and shear stress. Other vasodilating factors include prostacyclin and endothelium-derived hyperpolarizing factor (EDHF). Opposing these are the vasoconstrictive and mitogenic factors that include thromboxane, endothelin-1 (ET-1), and angiotensin II. The balance of these factors determines vasomotor responses and vascular health in general.

In health, the predominant effect of stimulation of the endothelium is vasodilation. While basal and stimulated release of NO have been demonstrated in humans [4,6], anti-inflammatory and antithrombotic properties of the healthy endothelium are equally important.

Lipids and atherosclerosis

The importance of cholesterol in the pathogenesis of atherosclerosis has emerged in the past three decades, due in part to a large body of epidemiological data [7–9]. Refinements in analytical techniques have provided important information about the relative contribution of atherogenic particles,

* Dr. Anderson is a Senior Scholar of the Alberta Heritage Foundation for Medical Research (Edmonton, Alberta).

such as low-density lipoprotein (LDL), triglyceride (TG) rich lipoproteins (TRL), and anti-atherogenic high-density lipoprotein (HDL). Lipid transport via lipoproteins serves to move hydrophobic molecules such as cholesterol, cholesterol ester (CE), phospholipids, and TG from sites of synthesis and absorption to sites of utilization. Lipoproteins contain a bipolar phospholipid shell with associated free cholesterol. At the core are CE and TG, with apolipoproteins providing structural integrity and acting as ligands for various enzymatic reactions [10]. The term dyslipidemia applies to disorders of both lipids and the lipoprotein transport system. In parallel, important discoveries have occurred at the basic science level. Cholesterol is an obligatory component of the atherosclerotic process that includes oxidation, inflammatory and smooth muscle cells, platelets, and a variety of humoral modulators [11,12].

Dyslipidemias and endothelium-dependent vasomotion

In experimental animal models, cholesterol-induced atherosclerosis results in the impairment of endothelium-dependent vasodilation [13]. Ludmer and colleagues were among the first to study this in the human coronary system [5]. While acetylcholine induces NO-dependent epicardial vasodilation in subjects without atherosclerosis, paradoxical vasoconstriction occurs in subjects with atherosclerosis. Subsequent human studies demonstrated similar abnormalities in individuals with hypercholesterolemia without overt signs of atherosclerosis. Such abnormalities occur in both the coronary and peripheral circulation [14–16]. Celermajer et al. reported abnormal endothelial function in young children with familial hypercholesterolemia [17]. These data speak well to the now established notion of endothelial dysfunction as a systemic process more dependent on risk factors than the structural presence of atherosclerosis.

Furthermore, observational human studies have demonstrated a relationship between endothelial function and other lipid subfractions, including HDL and lipoprotein(a) [18–20]. The impact of elevated TG on vascular function remains less clear [21,22]. However, remnant particles of TRL lipolysis likely exert part of their atherogenic potential by attenuating endothelium-dependent vasodilation [23]. Recent studies have demonstrated a relationship between fatty acid composition and vasodilation [24]. A recent study demonstrated a cumulative adverse effect of post-prandial hyperlipidemia and hyperglycemia on peripheral endothelial function [25].

Dyslipidemias and other measures of endothelial function

In addition to vasomotion, the endothelium participates importantly in the interactions between inflammatory leukocytes, platelets, and the vessel wall. Lacoste and colleagues reported an increase in platelet aggregation in blood taken from patients with hypercholesterolemia compared with controls [26]. Many studies have demonstrated adverse effects of hyperlipidemia on the inflammatory cascade [12,27]. Cybulsky and Gimbrone were among the first to demonstrate upregulation of leukocyte adhesion molecules in cholesterol-induced atherogenesis [28]. Similar observations have been made in human endothelial cells [29] and hypercholesterolemic humans [30].

Pathophysiology of lipid-induced endothelial dysfunction

The transduction of an endothelium-dependent signal, e.g., acetylcholine or flow, to the subsequent smooth muscle cell vasodilation involves a number of key processes that can become dysfunctional in response to perturbations in lipid metabolism (Figures 17.1 and 17.2). While cholesterol itself accounts for many of these abnormalities, oxidative modifications of LDL play a key role in the pathogenesis of endothelial dysfunction, leading to either a net decrease in vasodilatory bioactivity (mainly NO) or increased vasoconstrictive activity (Tables 17.1 and 17.2).

Cholesterol and oxidative stress

Oxygen free radicals and oxidized LDL

Several enzyme systems within the vessel wall, including xanthine oxidase, NADH/NADPH oxidase, NOS and cytochrome p450, generate reactive oxygen species such as superoxide anion (O_2^-) and others. Ohara and colleagues made the pivotal discovery that superoxide production from cholesterol-fed rabbits increased dramatically in a xanthine- oxidase-specific process [31]. The source of the excess

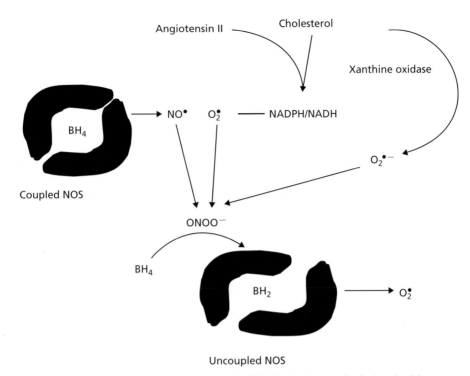

Figure 17.1 Mechanisms producing reactive oxygen species in dyslipidemias (see text for further details).

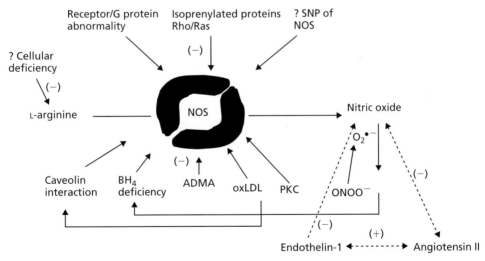

Figure 17.2 Mechanisms of lipid-induced endothelial dysfunction. Attenuation of NO effect results from inadequate substrate, downregulation of NOS, and inactivation of NO. In addition, there is upregulation of the vasoconstrictors ET-1 and angiotensin II.

superoxide was in fact the endothelial cells. Subsequent work by Harrison and others has demonstrated that membrane-bound oxidases, such as NADH/NADPH oxidase, serve as a major source of superoxide, providing substrates for electron transfer to molecular oxygen [32], a system regulated by angiotensin II, shear stress, and other cytokines, with an important interaction between

Table 17.1 Mechanisms of endothelial dysfunction in dyslipidemia.

Enhanced oxidative stress	Cholesterol-induced free radical production
	Lipid peroxidation
	Oxidation of LDL
	PKC activation
	G protein attenuation
Decreased NO production	? Cellular L-arginine deficiency
	Signal-transduction abnormalities
	Caveolin–NOS interactions
Alterations in NOS	Inactivation from ADMA or oxLDL
	Tetrahydrobiopterin deficiency (uncoupled)
	Genetic polymorphisms
NO inactivation	Peroxynitrite production
Upregulation of inflammatory mediators	Upregulation of NF-κB
	Inflammatory cytokine production
	Upregulation of LAMs
	LOX-1 activation
Effects on other vasoactive substances	Increased ET-1 production
	Upregulation of AT-1 receptors
	? Effects on EDHF

ADMA: asymmetric dimethyl arginine; AT-1: angiotensin II receptor (type 1); and LAM: leukocyte adhesion molecules.

Table 17.2 Therapies that improve cholesterol-induced endothelial dysfunction.

Lipid-lowering strategies	HMG CoA reductase inhibition
	Bile-acid resins
	Statins and probucol
	LDL apheresis
	Fibrates
	HDL administration
Antioxidants	Vitamins C and E
	Purple grape juice
	Xanthine oxidase inhibition
NOS augmentation	Tetrahydrobiopterin
	Folic acid

LDL cholesterol and the AT-1 receptor [33]. In segments of the human saphenous vein, hypercholesterolemia is associated with increased NADH oxidase-dependent superoxide production [34].

A major consequence of increased levels of reactive oxygen species involves lipid peroxidation. Steinberg and Witzum have advanced the concept that oxidative modifications of LDL play a central role in the development of atherosclerosis [11,35].

Polyunsaturated fatty acids are especially vulnerable to peroxidation, creating hydroxy fatty acids. Oxidative modifications of LDL occur *in vivo*, and antibodies against circulating oxidized LDL (oxLDL) are associated with atherosclerosis [36]. Indeed, LOX-1, a specific receptor for oxLDL, likely plays a pivotal role in oxidative damage [37].

Mechanisms of oxLDL-induced endothelial dysfunction

Protein kinase C (PKC) inhibitors block the attenuation of endothelium-dependent relaxation by oxLDL [38]. Also, oxidative modifications of lipoprotein phospholipids to lysophosphatidylcholine (lyso-PC) activate PKC in human endothelial cells [39]. A series of studies by Ohara et al. suggest that lyso-PC in oxLDL leads to PKC stimulation and hence to endothelial dysfunction [40]. Further, a recent study demonstrated a beneficial effect of hyperglycemia-induced endothelial dysfunction in subjects treated with PKC inhibitors [41].

oxLDL and endothelial function

Early *in vitro* studies demonstrated that oxidatively modified LDL, but not native LDL, attenuated vasorelaxation of arterial strips to endothelium-dependent agonists [42]. In the human coronary circulation, we previously reported that acetylcholine-mediated vasodilation is associated with LDL susceptibility to oxidation [43]. Subsequent studies confirmed this concept, demonstrating a relationship between endothelium-dependent vasomotion and antibodies directed against oxLDL [44]. In addition, a recent cholesterol-lowering study demonstrated that improved acetylcholine responses correlate closely with oxidative markers [45]. Others have shown parallel changes in oxidative stress and attenuation of endothelial function in post-prandial hyperlipidemic states [25,46]. In a study that examined the relationship between forearm microvascular responses and cardiovascular outcomes, Heitzer et al. demonstrated that peripheral endothelial dysfunction is associated with cardiac events in subjects with coronary artery disease. Moreover, subjects with increased acetylcholine responses to intra-arterial infusion of vitamin C, suggesting increased oxidative stress, had poorer outcomes [47].

Cholesterol, oxidative stress, and NO bioactivity

Much is now known about the processes involved in NO generation via NOS, and the subsequent fate of NO. Indeed, abnormalities in lipoproteins, including oxidation, impair NO bioactivity leading to endothelial dysfunction.

NOS substrate and signal transduction

Since the intracellular levels of L-arginine, a precursor of NO, far exceed the K_m of the NOS enzyme, it would seem unlikely that arginine deficiency should play a major role in determining NO production and therefore NO levels. However, L-arginine beneficially affects endothelial function in hypercholesterolemic patients and the atherosclerosis development in cholesterol-fed rabbits [48]. The mechanism of benefit may involve pathways other than NO. Hyperlipidemia also alters the activation of the NOS enzyme. The relative preservation of the vasodilatory responses to the calcium ionophore A23187 despite attenuation of the responses to other agonists suggests a receptor/secondary messenger abnormality. Cholesterol feeding of pigs produces a defect in endothelium-dependent vasodilation that

resembles the defect produced by pertussis toxin (G protein dependent).

Caveolae, i.e., invaginations of the plasma membrane, participate importantly in cholesterol transport within cells. Recent studies have demonstrated that caveolae contain a regulatory protein, caveolin-1, that interacts with cholesterol, NOS residing within the caveolae, scavenger receptor B1 (SR-B1), and CD36 [49]. Cholesterol-loaded cells demonstrate increased caveolin and decreased eNOS [50,51]. A recent study demonstrated that the ablation of CD36 prevents the negative impact of cholesterol loading on NOS function [52]. oxLDL likely deplete caveolae of cholesterol and prevent agonist stimulation of NOS by disrupting the activation complex.

NOS and tetrahydrobiopterin

NO is synthesized from L-arginine in mammalian cells by a family of three NOS. Endothelial NOS (eNOS, NOS III) is constitutively produced by endothelial cells and encoded by a gene on chromosome 7 [53]. Tetrahydrobiopterin (BH$_4$) is an essential cofactor for the proper flow of electrons to oxidize L-arginine [54]. At suboptimal concentrations of BH$_4$, NOS acts as an NADPH oxidase, in a reaction by which molecular oxygen rather than arginine becomes an electron acceptor, leading to the production of superoxide (O_2^-) and hydrogen peroxide (H_2O_2) rather than NO [55,56]. This has been referred to as the "uncoupling" of the NOS enzyme.

Thus, biopterin metabolism critically regulates NOS activity. In mammalian cells, BH$_4$ is synthesized through two distinct pathways: a *de novo* synthesis that uses GTP as a precursor via GTP cyclohydrolase I and the regeneration of BH$_4$ from a quinonoid form of BH$_2$, through a pterin salvage pathway involving the active form of folate, 5 methyltetrahydrofolate. These pathways depend on a normal cellular redox state, where oxidative stress impairs the recycling of BH$_4$. Peroxynitrite, the product of NO and superoxide, can oxidize BH$_4$, leading to uncoupling of the enzyme [57].

Alterations in NOS activity occur in response to cholesterol or oxLDL. Paradoxically, initial studies demonstrated an increase in total nitrogen oxides produced in response to cholesterol feeding of rabbits [58]. The subsequent observation that superoxide dismutase (SOD) could improve vaso-relaxation in this model supported the concept that enhanced production of superoxide participates importantly in hypercholesterolemia [59]. In contrast to decreased expression of NOS, enzymatic uncoupling determines decreased NO bioactivity. By combining early transcriptional inhibition and post-translational degradation, Liao and others have demonstrated that oxLDL potently affect NOS expression [60].

Inactivation of NO

NO contains an unpaired electron and is hence a free radical itself. It binds superoxide in a reaction 3 times faster than the reaction between superoxide and SOD. In states of free radical excess, such as hypercholesterolemia, NO becomes inactivated, thus contributing to endothelial dysfunction [61]. Numerous human studies have demonstrated the acute improvement in endothelium-dependent vasodilation in response to free radical scavengers such as vitamin C [62,63]. Additionally, lipid radicals induced by LDL oxidation can interact with NO, resulting in its inactivation.

Cholesterol and other vasoactive substances

Impairment of endothelium-dependent vasodilation may also result from increased activity of vasoconstrictors. ET-1 and NO inhibit each other, and ET-1 activity increases in both hypercholesterolemic animals and humans [64,65]. Hypertriglyceridemia and hyperinsulinemia potently induce ET-1 production in the human peripheral circulation [66]. ET-1 also augments pressor responses to angiotensin II [67]; conversely, angiotensin II increases vascular levels of ET-1 [68]. The NOS cofactor BH_4 partially attenuates increased ET-1 induced by cholesterol [69].

Lipids and inflammatory mediators

Loss of anti-inflammatory properties characterizes endothelial dysfunction. While a detailed discussion is beyond the scope of this chapter [12], several important points need to be clarified. In general, NO should be considered an anti-inflammatory molecule that inhibits a number of processes involved in leukocyte adhesion and cytokine formation. Cholesterol induces endothelial cell production of reactive oxygen species leading to oxLDL. In addition to alterations in vasodilation, oxLDL lead to alterations in eNOS, and the accumulation of inflammatory cells via LOX-1 [70]. Inflammatory cells engender more reactive oxygen species that lead, in turn, to the activation of nuclear factor kappa B (NF-κB), a transcription factor that elicits the production of pro-inflammatory mediators, such as leukocyte adhesion molecules, monocyte chemoattractant protein (MCP-1), and interleukins (IL). IL-6 results in C-reactive protein (CRP) generation by the liver. Not only a marker of systemic inflammation [71], CRP induces an inflammatory response in cultured cells [72] and also bind oxLDL [73]. However, more recently, the specificity of these observations has been called in play [74]. Augmented levels of CD40 and its ligand, CD154, occur on the platelets of hypercholesterolemic patients [75], possibly indicating an important interaction between pro-inflammatory and prothrombotic pathways in these subjects.

Beneficial vascular effects of lipid lowering

Lipid-lowering effects

Much has been made of the non-lipid effects of 3-hydroxy-3-methyl glutaryl coenzyme A (HMG CoA reductase) inhibitors (statins) (see Chapter 4). However, many beneficial effects on the vascular wall associate simply with cholesterol lowering. In early studies, animals initially fed an atherogenic diet attained normal endothelial function and normal levels of oxidative stress following consumption of a regression-type diet [76]. Further, recent studies demonstrated that lipid lowering leads to diminished oxLDL accumulation and leukocyte adhesion molecule expression, as well as increased eNOS expression [77].

Pleiotropic effects of statins

Statins possess unique anti-atherogenic properties clearly unrelated to their LDL-lowering effects [78]. The majority of these actions have a direct and positive effect on endothelial function:
(i) Statins stimulate and upregulate NOS [78,79].
(ii) By inhibiting mevalonate synthesis, statins also prevent the synthesis of other important isoprenoid

intermediates of the cholesterol biosynthetic pathway. These intermediates serve as lipid ligands for post-translational alterations of various proteins, including GTP-binding proteins (G proteins). Ras and Rho, small G proteins, play a major role in the pathophysiology of atherosclerosis. Inhibition of Rho by statins mediates the increase in NOS expression [78,80]. A recent study in humans demonstrated attenuation of coronary vasospasm with the Rho kinase inhibitor fasudil [78,81].

(iii) Statins inhibit the upregulation of LOX-1 by oxLDL and the subsequent production of mitogen-activated protein (MAP) kinases [78,82].

(iv) Statins profoundly affect vascular inflammation [10,78].

(v) Statins may stabilize atherosclerotic plaques. Plaque fissuring and rupture are the major cause of ACS. HMG CoA reductase inhibition favorably affects the balance between collagen and inflammatory cells within the plaque [78,83].

(vi) Statins also inhibit platelet function [26,78]. Furthermore, statins inhibit tissue factor expression by macrophages *in vitro*, reducing the thrombotic potential of the vascular wall.

(vii) More recently, statins have been shown to have a favorable effect on the promotion of increased blood levels of endothelial progenitor cells [78,84–86]. This action may be particularly important after an acute myocardial infarction and in vascular repair associated with endothelial dysfunction [87].

Thus, both direct lipid-lowering effects and specific vascular favorable effects likely account for the beneficial effects of statins on endothelial function (see Chapter 4). These observations have been extended to the clinical arena in the last 5 years.

Treatment of lipid-induced endothelial dysfunction in humans

Lipid-lowering strategies

A majority of clinical studies examining potential treatments of endothelial dysfunction occurring in hypercholesterolemia have focused on the stimulation of endothelium-dependent vasomotor responses. Early experimental work clearly demonstrated that changing from a hypercholesterolemic to a normocholesterolemic diet was associated with improved endothelium-dependent arterial relaxation. The first prospective study in humans, published

a decade ago, showed that 6 months of therapy with a low-cholesterol diet and cholestyramine not only decreased total cholesterol by 30%, but also normalized endothelium-dependent epicardial coronary responses to Ach infusion in hypercholesterolemic male subjects with structurally normal arteries [88]. A subsequent study reported a similar effect obtained after 6 months of therapy with lovastatin (40 mg/day), a regimen that also improved vasomotor responses in the coronary microcirculation, where blood flow regulation normally occurs [89]. Subsequently, our group showed that the combination of an HMG CoA reductase inhibitor (lovastatin) and an antioxidant agent (probucol), administered daily for a year, may be more effective than an LDL-reducing regimen (lovastatin and cholestyramine) in improving vasomotor coronary responses when compared with placebo (Figure 17.3) [90]. Interestingly, the improvement in endothelial dysfunction observed in this trial correlated closely with the degree to which LDL particles were resistant to oxidation, independently of cholesterol levels achieved or of treatment allocation, underscoring the important role of increased oxidative stress in hypercholesterolemic endothelial dysfunction.

Contrary to the wealth of studies associating statin therapy with improved endothelium-mediated dilation, fewer studies have examined the effect of fibrates on vasomotor endothelial dysfunction in humans. In a randomized, double-blind, placebo-controlled protocol, Evans et al. studied the effect of ciprofibrate on post-prandial endothelial function in 20 patients with type 2 diabetes. Three months of therapy with ciprofibrate was associated with significantly increased fasting and post-prandial flow-mediated dilation (FMD), whereas no significant improvement occurred in the placebo group [91]. Meco et al. administered bezafibrate (400 mg/day) during 6 months to 16 patients with coronary artery disease, low HDL cholesterol, and impaired FMD (<10%). Associated with increased HDL cholesterol (from 0.79 to 1.0 mM), there was a significant increase in FMD (from 2.5% to 12.3%) [92]. More recent studies have also demonstrated a beneficial effect of therapy with fibrates on vasodilatory responses [93,94].

Aggressive and rapid cholesterol reduction can yield brisk improvement in endothelial dysfunction, thus reducing the probability of cardiovascular events

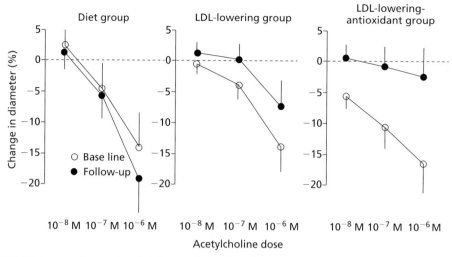

Figure 17.3 LDL lowering (lovastatin and cholestyramine) and LDL-lowering antioxidants (lovastatin and probucol) improve endothelium-dependent vasomotion after 1 year of therapy. Reproduced with permission [90].

in patients at high risk. In the RECIFE study, Dupuis et al. randomized patients admitted for an ACS to pravastatin (40 mg/day) or matching placebo. After only 6 weeks of therapy, patients randomized to the active treatment had significant improvements of endothelium-dependent brachial FMD compared with no change in the placebo group [95]. In patients with severe hypercholesterolemia, simvastatin improved basal NO production in the peripheral circulation within 1 month, whereas a single session of plasmapheresis in patients with familial hypercholesterolemia resulted in significant improvements in endothelium-dependent blood flow responses [96]. A series of recent studies have suggested acute non-lipid-lowering effects of statins on endothelial function. In these investigations, vascular changes were evident as early as 1 day after a single dose of statin with no changes in lipid levels [97–101]. These studies would argue for the possible beneficial pleiotropic effects of the statin class of medications.

This rapid improvement likely plays an important role in the beneficial effect of statin therapy initiated early following an ACS. Indeed, the Myocardial Ischemia Reduction with Aggressive Cholesterol Lowering (MIRACL) trial randomized over 3000 patients admitted for non-Q wave infarction or unstable angina, and prospectively randomized them, in a double-blind fashion within 96 h,

to receive atorvastatin (80 mg/day) or matching placebo for 4 months, resulting in a 16% reduction of the combined endpoint, including death, nonfatal myocardial infarction, resuscitated cardiac arrest, and worsening angina requiring hospital admission [102]. Similarly, the beneficial effects of early and aggressive statin therapy in ACS were confirmed in a more recent trial [103].

The rapid beneficial effects of cholesterol lowering (and more specifically, HMG CoA reductase inhibition) on clinical events are mediated largely through decreased pro-inflammatory endothelial responses characteristic of atherogenesis and its later phase of plaque rupture. Studies by Ridker and Kinlay confirm an anti-inflammatory effect of early statin use [104,105]. Likewise, there are many studies that demonstrate a CRP-lowering effect of statins in stable coronary disease [106]. Some have suggested that the addition of a CRP target of <2 mg/L for lipid lowering might have effects additive to those of the LDL target alone [105,107]. Further studies are required to determine the importance of a CRP-lowering effect with cholesterol-lowering therapy.

Other treatments

As discussed previously, endothelial dysfunction associated with dyslipidemia results from a complex chain of events involving oxygen free radicals, oxidation of key enzymes, and the expression of redox-sensitive genes coding for pro-inflammatory factors. Administration of antioxidants in one form or another has been a focus of attention. For example, the administration of ascorbic acid to hypercholesterolemic subjects improves vasomotor response to Ach infusion in the forearm resistance vessels, as measured using strain gauge plethysmography [63]. Similarly, oxypurinol, a xanthine oxidase inhibitor, improves the blood flow dose–response curve to Ach in hypercholesterolemic subjects [108]. Another study sought to determine whether oxypurinol, the active metabolite of allopurinol, might also improve endothelium-mediated dilation in the same vascular bed, but found no apparent effect, a result attributed to the generation of superoxide radicals associated with the conversion of allo- to oxypurinol [109].

BH_4, a necessary cofactor in the coupling of e-NOS, is particularly vulnerable to oxidation in the presence of excessive production of oxygen free radicals. The effect of supplementing BH_4 on endothelium-mediated dilation is associated with improved endothelium-mediated vasomotor responses, both in the peripheral and the coronary circulation of subjects with either established coronary artery disease or hypercholesterolemia [110]. Folates share a structure similar to biopterins and in addition to lowering homocysteine may prevent oxidation of BH_4 or directly interact with NOS [111,112]. Numerous studies have demonstrated the beneficial effects of folates or methylated folates on hypercholesterolemia-induced endothelial dysfunction [113].

More natural sources of antioxidants have been examined as well. Flavonoid components, i.e., products from red wine and grape juice, possess antioxidant properties and may participate in the putative protective effect of the Mediterranean diet. Stein et al. demonstrated that the ingestion of 7.7 mL/kg/day of purple grape juice is associated with increased resistance of LDL particles to oxidation and a significant improvement in FMD in patients with documented coronary artery disease [114].

Finally, current interest focuses increasingly on the understanding of the potential role of modulating HDL cholesterol levels [115]. Acutely increased HDL cholesterol levels obtained by the infusion of reconstituted HDL particles associate with improved blood flow response to Ach intra-arterial infusion and with increased FMD in hypercholesterolemic men [116]. Similarly, the infusion of apolipoprotein A1 disks has been demonstrated to improve brachial endothelial function [117]. Conventional therapy with HDL raising medications such as niacin has not been well studied [118]. But studies are underway in this area.

Importantly, although many different therapeutic interventions have undisputed beneficial effects on endothelial metabolism and function, only the inhibition of HMG CoA reductase clearly reduces the occurrence of clinical events.

Conclusion

The past two decades have witnessed burgeoning appreciation of the role played by NO, and studies on the endothelium in vascular homeostasis have blossomed. Today, endothelial function can be readily measured in humans, providing a very useful *research* tool to assess the impact of risk factors and their treatment on vascular function. Abnormalities of lipids and lipoproteins adversely affect endothelial function. Importantly, a growing list of therapeutic modalities modulates endothelial dysfunction in this situation. In the past year, several small studies suggested a prognostic role for measures of endothelium-dependent vasomotion. As such, treatments targeted at ameliorating endothelial dysfunction should be undertaken in patients at risk of developing coronary atherosclerosis and its sequelae.

Acknowledgments

The work discussed in this review has been supported in part by the Alberta Heart and Stroke Foundation (Edmonton, Alberta), the Canadian Institutes of Health Research and the Canadian Diabetes Association.

References

1 Verma S, Anderson TJ. Fundamentals of endothelial function for the clinical cardiologist. *Circulation* 2002;105: 546–549.

2 Furchgott RF, Zawadski JV. The obligatory role of endothelial cells in the relaxation of arterial smooth muscle by acetylcholine. *Nature* 1980;288:373–376.

3 Palmer RMJ, Ashton D, Moncada S. Vascular endothelial cells synthesise nitric oxide from L-arginine. *Nature* 1988; 333:664–666.

4 Lefroy DC, Crake T, Uren NG, et al. Effect of inhibition of nitric oxide synthesis on epicardial coronary artery caliber and coronary blood flow in humans. *Circulation* 1993;88:43–54.

5 Ludmer PL, Selwyn AP, Shook TL, et al. Paradoxical vaso-constriction induced by acetylcholine in atherosclerotic coronary arteries. *N Engl J Med* 1986;315:1046–1051.

6 Zeiher AM, Drexler H, Wollschlager H, et al. Modulation of coronary vasomotor tone in humans: progressive endothelial dysfunction with different early stages of coronary atherosclerosis. *Circulation* 1991;83:391–401.

7 Assmann G, Cullen P, Schulte, H. Simple scoring scheme for calculating the risk of acute coronary events based on the 10-year follow-up of the Prospective Cardiovascular Munster (PROCAM) Study. *Circulation* 2002; 105:310–315.

8 Keys A. Coronary heart disease in seven countries. *Nutrition* 1997;13;250–252.

9 Wilson PWF, D'Agostino RB, Levy D, et al. Prediction of coronary heart disease using risk factor categories. *Circulation* 1998;97:1837–1847.

10 Ridker PM, Genest J, Libby, P. Risk factors for atherosclerotic disease. In: Braunwald E, Zipes DP, Libby P, eds. *Heart Disease.* Philadelphia, PA: W.B. Saunders; 2001: 1010–1039.

11 Glass CK, Witztum JL. Atherosclerosis: the road ahead. *Cell* 2001;104:503–516.

12 Libby P, Ridker PM, Maseri A. Inflammation and athero-sclerosis. *Circulation* 2002;105:1135–1143.

13 Heistad DD, Armstrong ML, Marcus ML, et al. Augmented responses to vasoconstrictor stimuli in hypercholesterolemic and atherosclerotic monkeys. *Circ Res* 1984;54:711–716.

14 Creager MA, Cooke JP, Mendelsohn ME, et al. Impaired vasodilation of forearm resistance vessels in hyperchole-sterolemic humans. *J Clin Invest* 1990;86:228–234.

15 Vita JA, Treasure CB, Nabel EG, et al. Coronary vasomo-tor response to acetylcholine relates to risk factors for coronary artery disease. *Circulation* 1990;81:491–497.

16 Zeiher AM, Drexler H, Saurbier B, et al. Endothelium-mediated coronary blood flow modulation in humans: effects of age, atherosclerosis, hypercholesterolemia and hypertension. *J Clin Invest* 1993;92:652–662.

17 Celermajer DS, Sorensen KE, Gooch VM, et al. Non-invasive detection of endothelial dysfunction in children and adults at risk of atherosclerosis. *Lancet* 1992;340: 1111–1115.

18 Kuhn FE, Mohler ER, Satler LF, et al. Effects of high-density lipoprotein on acetylcholine-induced coronary vasoreactivity. *Am J Cardiol* 1991;68:1425–1430.

19 Kuvin JT, Patel AR, Sidhu M, et al. Relation between high-density lipoprotein cholesterol and peripheral vasomotor function. *Am J Cardiol* 2003;92:275–279.

20 Tsurumi Y, Nagashima H, Ichikawa KI, et al. Influence of plasma lipoprotein(a) levels on coronary vasomotor response to acetylcholine. *J Am Coll Cardiol* 1995;26: 1242–1250.

21 Lewis TV, Dart AM, Chin-Dusting JPF. Endothelium-dependent relaxation by acetylcholine is impaired in hypertriglyceridemic humans with normal levels of plasma LDL cholesterol. *J Am Coll Cardiol* 1999;33: 805–812.

22 Schnell G, Robertson A, Malley L, et al. Impaired brachial artery endothelial function is not predicted by elevated triglycerides. *J Am Coll Cardiol* 1999;33:2038–2043.

23 Kugiyama K, Doi H, Motoyama T, et al. Association of remnant lipoprotein levels with impairment of endothelium-dependent vasomotor function in human coronary arteries. *Circulation* 1998;97:2519–2526.

24 Sarabi M, Vessby B, Millgard J, et al. Endothelium-dependent vasodilation is related to the fatty acid compo-sition of serum lipids in healthy subjects. *Atherosclerosis* 2001;156:349–355.

25 Ceriello A, Taboga C, Tonutti L, et al. Evidence for an independent and cumulative effect of postprandial hypertriglyceridemia and hyperglycemia on endothelial dysfunction and oxidative stress generation: effects of short- and long-term simvastatin treatment. *Circulation* 2002;106;1211–1218.

26 Lacoste L, Lam JY, Letchacovski G, et al. Hyperlipidemia and coronary disease: correction of the increased throm-bogenic potential with cholesterol reduction. *Circulation* 1995;92:3172–3177.

27 Libby P, Simon DI. Inflammation and thrombosis: the clot thickens. *Circulation* 2001;103:1718–1720.

28 Cybulsky ML, Gimbrone MA. Endothelial expression of a mononuclear leukocyte adhesion molecule during atherogenesis. *Science* 1991;251:788–791.

29 Haller H, Schaper D, Ziegler W, et al. Low-density lipoprotein induces vascular adhesion molecule expres-sion on human endothelial cells. *Hypertension* 1995;25: 511–516.

30 Davi G, Romano M, Mezzetti A, et al. Increased levels of soluble P-selectin in hypercholesterolemic patients. *Circulation* 1998;97:953–957.

31 Ohara Y, Peterson TE, Harrison DG. Hypercholes-terolemia increases endothelial superoxide anion pro-duction. *J Clin Invest* 1993;91:2546–2551.

32 Harrison, D.G. Cellular and molecular mechanisms of endothelial cell dysfunction. *J Clin Invest* 1997;100: 2153–2157.

33 Warnholtz A, Nickenig G, Schulz E, et al. Increased NADH-oxidase-mediated superoxide production in the early stages of atherosclerosis: evidence for involvement of the renin–angiotensin system. *Circulation* 1999;99: 2027–2033.

34 Guzik TJ, West NE, Black E, et al. Vascular superoxide production by NAD(P)H oxidase: association with endothelial dysfunction and clinical risk factors. *Circ Res* 2000;86:E85–E90.

35 Steinberg D. Oxidative modification of LDL and atherogenesis. *Circulation* 1997;95:1062–1071.

36 Toshima S, Hasegawa A, Kurabayashi M, et al. Circulating oxidized low density lipoprotein levels. A biochemical risk marker for coronary heart disease. *Arterioscler Thromb Vasc Biol* 2000;20:2243–2247.

37 Mehta JL, Li DY. Identification and autoregulation of receptor for Ox-LDL in cultured human coronary artery endothelial cells. *Biophys Res Commun* 1998;248:511–514.

38 Ohgushi M, Kugiyama K, Fukunaga, et al. Protein kinase C inhibitors prevent impairment of endothelium-dependent relaxation by oxidatively modified LDL. *Arterioscler Thromb* 1993;13:1525–1532.

39 Kugiyama K, Ohgushi M, Sugiyama S, et al. Lyso-phosphatidylcholine inhibits surface receptor-mediated intracellular signals in endothelial cells by a pathway involving protein kinase C activation. *Circ Res* 1992;71: 1422–1428.

40 Ohara Y, Sayegh HS, Yamin JJ, et al. Regulation of endothelial constitutive nitric oxide synthase by protein kinase C. *Hypertension* 1995;25:415–420.

41 Beckman JA, Goldfine AB, Gordon MB, et al. Inhibition of protein kinase C beta prevents impaired endothelium-dependent vasodilation caused by hyperglycemia in humans. *Circ Res* 2002;90:107–111.

42 Simon BC, Cunningham LD, Cohen RA. Oxidized low density lipoproteins cause contraction and inhibit endothelium-dependent relaxation in the pig coronary artery. *J Clin Invest* 1990;86:75–79.

43 Anderson TJ, Meredith IT, Charbonneau F, et al. Endothelium-dependent coronary vasomotion relates to the susceptibility of LDL to oxidation in humans. *Circulation* 1996;93:1647–1650.

44 Heitzer T, Yla-Herttuala S, Luoma J, et al. Cigarette smoking potentiates endothelial dysfunction of forearm resistance vessels in patients with hypercholesterolemia: role of oxidized LDL. *Circulation* 1996;93:1346–1353.

45 Penny WF, Ben-Yehada O, Kuroe K, et al. Improvement of coronary artery endothelial dysfunction with lipid-lowering therapy: heterogeneity of segmental response and correlation with plasma-oxidized low density lipoprotein. *J Am Coll Cardiol* 2001;37:766–774.

46 Anderson RA, Evans ML, Ellis GR, et al. The relationships between post-prandial lipaemia, endothelial function and oxidative stress in healthy individuals and patients with type 2 diabetes. *Atherosclerosis* 2001;154: 475–483.

47 Heitzer T, Schlinzig T, Krohn K, et al. Endothelial dysfunction, oxidative stress, and risk of cardiovascular events in patients with coronary artery disease. *Circulation* 2001; 104:2673–2678.

48 Creager MA, Gallagher SJ, Girerd XJ, et al. L-arginine improves endothelium-dependent vasodilation in hypercholesterolemic humans. *J Clin Invest* 1992;90: 1248–1253.

49 Everson WV, Smart EJ. Influence of caveolin, cholesterol, and lipoproteins on nitric oxide synthase: implications for vascular disease. *Trends Cardiovasc Med* 2001; 11:246–250.

50 Feron O, Dessy C, Desager JP, et al. Hydroxy-methylglutaryl-coenzyme A reductase inhibition promotes endothelial nitric oxide synthase activation through a decrease in caveolin abundance. *Circulation* 2001;103:113–118.

51 Feron O, Kelly RA. The caveolar paradox: suppressing, inducing, and terminating eNOS signaling. *Circ Res* 2001;88:129–131.

52 Kincer JF, Uittenbogaard A, Dressman J, et al. Hyper-cholesterolemia promotes a CD36-dependent and endothelial nitric-oxide synthase-mediated vascular dysfunction. *J Biol Chem* 2002;277:23525–23533.

53 Michel T, Feron O. Nitric oxide synthases: Which, where, how and why? *J Clin Invest* 1997;100:2146–2152.

54 Thony B, Auerbach G, Blau N. Tetrahydrobiopterin biosynthesis, regeneration and function. *Biochem J* 2000; 347:1–16.

55 Cosentino F, Katusic ZS. Tetrahydrobiopterin and dysfunction of endothelial nitric oxide synthase in coronary arteries. *Circulation* 1995;91:139–144.

56 Heinzel B, John M, Klatt P, et al. Ca^{2+}/calmodulin-dependent formation of hydrogen peroxide by brain nitric oxide synthase. *Biochem J* 1992;281:627–630.

57 Laursen JB, Somers M, Kurz S, et al. Endothelial regulation of vasomotion in ApoE-deficient mice: implications for interactions between peroxynitrite and tetrahydro-biopterin. *Circulation* 2001;103:1282–1288.

58 Minor RL, Myers PR, Guerra R, et al. Diet induced atherosclerosis increases the release of nitrogen oxides from rabbit aorta. *J Clin Invest* 1990;86:2109–2116.

59 Mugge A, Elwell JH, Peterson TE, et al. Chronic treatment with polyethylene-glycolated superoxide dismutase partially restores endothelium-dependent vascular relaxations in cholesterol-fed rabbits. *Circ Res* 1991; 69:1293–1300.

60 Liao JK, Shin WS, Lee WY, et al. Oxidized low-density lipoprotein decreases the expression of endothelial nitric oxide synthase. *J Biol Chem* 1995;270:319–324.

61 Rubanyi GM, Vanhoutte PM. Superoxide anions and hyperoxia inactivate endothelium-derived relaxing factor. *Am J Physiol* 1986;250:H822–H827.

62 Timimi FK, Ting HH, Haley EA, et al. Vitamin C improves endothelium-dependent vasodilation in patients with

insulin-dependent diabetes mellitus. *J Am Coll Cardiol* 1998;31:552–557.

63 Ting HH, Timimi FK, Haley EA, et al. Vitamin C improves endothelium-dependent vasodilation in forearm resistance vessels of humans with hypercholesterolemia. *Circulation* 1997;95:2617–2622.

64 Cardillo C, Kilcoyne CM, Cannon III RO, et al. Increased activity of endogenous endothelin in patients with hypercholesterolemia. *J Am Coll Cardiol* 2000;36: 1483–1488.

65 Lerman A, Webster MW, Chesebro JH, et al. Circulating and tissue endothelin immunoreactivity in hypercholesterolemic pigs. *Circulation* 1993;88:2923–2928.

66 Piatti PM, Monti LD, Conti M, et al. Hypertriglyceridemia and hyperinsulinemia are potent inducers of endothelin-1 release in humans. *Diabetes* 1996; 45:316–321.

67 Yoshida K, Yasujima M, Kohzuki M, et al. Endothelin-1 augments pressor response to angiotensin II infusion in rats. *Hypertension* 1992;20;292–297.

68 Moreau P, d'Uscio LV, Shaw S, et al. Angiotensin II increases tissue endothelin and induces vascular hypertrophy. *Circulation* 1997;96:1593–1597.

69 Verma S, Dumont AS, Maitland A. Tetrahydrobiopterin attenuates cholesterol induced coronary hyperreactivity to endothelin. *Heart* 2001;86:706–708.

70 Li D, Chen H, Romeo F, et al. Statins modulate oxidized low-density lipoprotein-mediated adhesion molecule expression in human coronary artery endothelial cells: role of LOX-1. *J Pharmacol Exp Ther* 2002;302:601–605.

71 Ridker PM, Stampfer MJ, Rifai N. Novel risk factors for systemic atherosclerosis. *JAMA* 2001;285:2481–2485.

72 Verma S, Li SH, Badiwala MV, et al. Endothelin antagonism and interleukin-6 inhibition attenuate the proatherogenic effects of C-reactive protein. *Circulation* 2002;105:1890–1896.

73 Chang MK, Binder CJ, Torzewski M, et al. C-reactive protein binds to both oxidized LDL and apoptotic cells through recognition of a common ligand: phosphorylcholine of oxidized phospholipids. *Proc Natl Acad Sci USA* 2002;99:13043.

74 Pepys MB. CRP or not CRP? That is the question. *Arterioscler Thromb Vasc Biol* 2005;25:1091–1094.

75 Garlichs CD, John S, Schmeisser A, et al. Upregulation of CD40 and CD40 ligand (CD154) in patients with moderate hypercholesterolemia. *Circulation* 2001;104: 2395–2400.

76 Ohara Y, Peterson TE, Sayegh HS, et al. Dietary correction of hypercholesterolemia in the rabbit normalizes endothelial superoxide anion production. *Circulation* 1995;92:898–903.

77 Aikawa M, Sugiyama S, Hill CC, et al. Lipid lowering reduces oxidative stress and endothelial cell activation in rabbit atheroma. *Circulation* 2002;106:1390–1396.

78 Takemoto M, Liao JK. Pleiotropic effects of 3-hydroxy-3-methylglutaryl coenzyme a reductase inhibitors. *Arterioscler Thromb Vasc Biol* 2001;21:1712–1719.

79 Laufs U, La Fata V, Plutsky J, et al. Upregulation of endothelial nitric oxide synthase by HMG CoA reductase inhibitors. *Circulation* 1998;97:1129–1135.

80 Laufs U, Liao JK. Post-transcriptional regulation of endothelial nitric oxide synthase mRNA stability by Rho GTPase. *J Biol Chem* 1998;273:24266–24271.

81 Masumoto A, Mohri M, Shimokawa H, et al. Suppression of coronary artery spasm by the rho-kinase inhibitor fasudil in patients with vasospastic angina. *Circulation* 2002;105:1545–1547.

82 Mehta JL, Li DY, Chen HJ, et al. Inhibition of LOX-1 by statins may relate to upregulation of eNOS. *Biochem Biophys Res Commun* 2001;289:857–861.

83 Crisby M, Nordin-Fredriksson G, Shah PK, et al. Pravastatin treatment increases collagen content and decreases lipid content, inflammation, metalloproteinases, and cell death in human carotid plaques: implications for plaque stabilization. *Circulation* 2001;103:926–933.

84 Landmesser U, Engberding N, Bahlmann FH, et al. Statin-induced improvement of endothelial progenitor cell mobilization, myocardial neovascularization, left ventricular function, and survival after experimental myocardial infarction requires endothelial nitric oxide synthase. *Circulation* 2004;110:1933–1939.

85 Llevadot J, Murasawa S, Kureishi Y, et al. HMG-CoA reductase inhibitor mobilizes bone marrow-derived endothelial progenitor cells. *J Clin Invest* 2001;108:399–405.

86 Urbich C, Dimmeler S. Endothelial progenitor cells: characterization and role in vascular biology. *Circ Res* 2004;95:343–353.

87 Hill JM, Zalos G, Halcox JP, et al. Circulating endothelial progenitor cells, vascular function, and cardiovascular risk. *N Engl J Med* 2003;348:593–600.

88 Leung WH, Lau CP, Wong CK. Beneficial effect of cholesterol-lowering therapy on coronary endothelium-dependent relaxation in hypercholesterolaemic patients. *Lancet* 1993;341:1496–1500.

89 Egashira K, Hirooka Y, Kai H, et al. Reduction in serum cholesterol with pravastatin improves endothelium-dependent coronary vasomotion in patients with hypercholesterolemia. *Circulation* 1994;89:2519–2524.

90 Anderson TJ, Meredith IT, Yeung AC, et al. The effect of cholesterol-lowering and antioxidant therapy on endothelium-dependent coronary vasomotion. *N Engl J Med* 1995;332:488–493.

91 Evans M, Anderson RA, Graham J, et al. Ciprofibrate therapy improves endothelial function and reduces postprandial lipemia and oxidative stress in type 2 diabetes mellitus. *Circulation* 2000;101:1773–1779.

92 Meco JF, Vila R, Pujol R, et al. Improvement in endothelial dysfunction in patients with hypoalphalipoproteinemia

and coronary artery disease treated with bezafibrate. *J Cardiovasc Pharmacol* 2001;38:250–258.

93 Capell WH, DeSouza CA, Poirier P, et al. Short-term triglyceride lowering with fenofibrate improves vaso-dilator function in subjects with hypertriglyceridemia. *Arterioscler Thromb Vasc Biol* 2003;23:307–313.

94 Kon Koh K, Yeal Ahn J, Hwan Han S, et al. Effects of fenofibrate on lipoproteins, vasomotor function, and serological markers of inflammation, plaque stabiliza-tion, and hemostasis. *Atherosclerosis* 2004;174:379–383.

95 Dupuis J, Tardif JC, Cernacek P, et al. Cholesterol reduc-tion rapidly improves endothelial function after acute coronary syndromes: the RECIFE (reduction of choles-terol in ischemia and function of the endothelium) trial. *Circulation* 1999;99:3227–3233.

96 Tamai O, Matsuoka H, Itabe H, et al. Single LDL apheresis improves endothelium-dependent vasodila-tion in hypercholesterolemic humans. *Circulation* 1997;95:76–82.

97 Beckman JA, Liao JK, Hurley S, et al. Atorvastatin restores endothelial function in normocholesterolemic smokers independent of changes in low-density lipoprotein. *Circ Res* 2004;95:217–223.

98 Wassmann S, Faul A, Hennen B, et al. Rapid effect of 3-hydroxy-3-methylglutaryl coenzyme a reductase inhibition on coronary endothelial function. *Circ Res* 2003;93:e98–e103.

99 Omori H, Nagashima H, Tsurumi Y, et al. Direct *in vivo* evidence of a vascular statin: a single dose of cerivastatin rapidly increases vascular endothelial responsiveness in healthy normocholesterolaemic subjects. *Br J Clin Pharmacol* 2002;54:395–399.

100 Wilson SH, Simari RD, Best PJ, et al. Simvastatin pre-serves coronary endothelial function in hypercholes-terolemia in the absence of lipid lowering. *Arterioscler Thromb Vasc Biol* 2001;21:122–128.

101 Landmesser U, Bahlmann F, Mueller M, et al. Simvastatin versus ezetimibe: pleiotropic and lipid-low-ering effects on endothelial function in humans. *Circulation* 2005;111:2356–2363.

102 Schwartz GG, Olsson AG, Ezekowitz MD, et al. Effects of atorvastatin on early recurrent ischemic events in acute coronary syndromes: the MIRACL study: a randomized controlled trial. *JAMA* 2001;285:1711–1718.

103 Cannon CP, Braunwald E, McCabe CH, et al. Intensive versus moderate lipid lowering with statins after acute coronary syndromes. *N Engl J Med* 2004;350:1495–1504.

104 Kinlay S, Schwartz GG, Olsson AG, et al. High-dose atorvastatin enhances the decline in inflammatory markers in patients with acute coronary syndromes in the MIRACL study. *Circulation* 2003;108:1560–1566.

105 Ridker PM, Cannon CP, Morrow D, et al. C-reactive protein levels and outcomes after statin therapy. *N Engl J Med* 2005;352:20–28.

106 Albert MA, Danielson E, Rifai N, et al. Effect of statin therapy on C-reactive protein levels. *JAMA* 2001;286:64–70.

107 Nissen SE, Tuzcu EM, Schoenhagen P, et al. Statin ther-apy, LDL cholesterol, C-reactive protein, and coronary artery disease. *N Engl J Med* 2005;352:29–38.

108 Cardillo C, Kilcoyne CM, Cannon RO, et al. Xanthine oxidase inhibition with oxypurinol improves endothe-lial vasodilator function in hypercholesterolemic but not in hypertensive patients. *Hypertension* 1997;30:57.

109 O'Driscoll JG, Green DJ, Rankin JM, et al. Nitric oxide-dependent endothelial function is unaffected by allop-urinol in hypercholesterolaemic subjects. *Clin Exp Pharmacol Physiol* 1999;26:779–783.

110 Stroes E, Kastelein J, Cosentino F, et al. Tetrahydro-biopterin restores endothelial function in hypercholes-terolemia. *J Clin Invest* 1997;99:41–46.

111 Hyndman ME, Verma S, Rosenfeld RJ, et al. Interaction of 5-methyltetrahydrofolate and tetrahydrobiopterin on endothelial function. *Am J Physiol Heart Circ Physiol* 2002;282:H2167–H2172.

112 Verhaar MC, Stroes E, Rabelink TJ. Folates and cardio-vascular disease. *Arterioscler Thromb Vasc Biol* 2002;22:6–13.

113 Verhaar MC, Wever RM, Kastelein JJ, et al. 5-Methyltetrahydrofolate, the active form of folic acid restores endothelial function in familial hypercholes-terolemia. *Circulation* 1998;97:237–241.

114 Stein JH, Keevil JG, Wiebe DA, et al. Purple grape juice improves endothelial function and reduces the suscepti-bility of LDL cholesterol to oxidation in patients with coronary artery disease. *Circulation* 1999;100:1050–1055.

115 O'Connell BJ, Genest Jr J. High-density lipoproteins and endothelial function. *Circulation* 2001;104:1978–1983.

116 Spieker LE, Sudano I, Hurlimann D, et al. High-density lipoprotein restores endothelial function in hypercho-lesterolemic men. *Circulation* 2002;105:1399–1402.

117 Bisoendial RJ, Hovingh GK, Levels JH, et al. Restoration of endothelial function by increasing high-density lipoprotein in subjects with isolated low high-density lipoprotein. *Circulation* 2003;107:2944.

118 Kuvin JT, Ramet ME, Patel AR, et al. A novel mechanism for the beneficial vascular effects of high-density lipoprotein cholesterol: enhanced vasorelaxation and increased endothelial nitric oxide synthase expression. *Am Heart J* 2002;144:165–172.

CHAPTER 18

Soluble adhesion molecules as *in vivo* biohumoral markers of vascular cell activation

Jacopo Gianetti, MD, PhD *& Raffaele De Caterina,* MD, PhD

The last two decades have witnessed growing interest in the mechanisms of cell interactions with their surrounding environment, either other cells or components of the extracellular matrix. Most of this knowledge derives from the understanding of structure and function of adhesion molecules, proteins differentiated to permit the large variety and high specificity of all possible cell–cell and cell–matrix interactions. This field of investigation has broad implications for embryogenesis, differentiation, tissue physiology and pathophysiology. In this last context, important processes such as inflammation, atherosclerosis, and immune responses involve the function of adhesion molecules. Consequently, current interest in adhesion molecules importantly permeates vascular biology and cardiology. Methods available today can measure the soluble part of adhesion molecules in biological fluids. Dedicated to the recent evolution of this novel field of vascular biology, this chapter will review the pathophysiological and clinical significance of these measurements.

Adhesion molecules

Adhesion molecules are a heterogeneous class of proteins that mediate the reciprocal adhesion between different cell types, i.e., endothelial cells (EC), monocytes, lymphocytes, platelets and smooth muscle cells (SMC), or between cells and components of the extracellular matrix (Table 18.1). We currently classify six types of adhesion molecules: integrins, selectins, immunoglobulins, cadherins,

proteoglicans, and mucins. Cadherins produce molecular bindings among adjacent cells. Integrins, selectins, and immunoglobulins are the classes most relevant for the measurement of their soluble components. Adhesion molecules may be constitutively expressed on the cell surface, or induced or amplified by stimuli of different nature. We will describe here the pathophysiological relevance of the interactions involving endothelium and circulating leukocytes as well as the most relevant features of integrins, selectins, and their ligands.

Integrins

Integrins are heterodimeric transmembrane proteins composed of two subunits, alpha (α) and beta (β), joined by non-covalent bonds [1,2]. On the basis of common β subunits but variable α subunits, integrins are classified into three subfamilies [3]: the β-1 integrins, also termed *very late appearing antigens* (VLA); the β-2 integrins, or leukocyte integrins; and the β-3 integrins, or cytoadhesins. β-1 integrins bind to a complementary sequence composed of the three amino acids – arginine, glycine, and aspartate (arg-gly-asp, RGD sequence) – present in various components of the extracellular matrix (laminin, collagen, fibronectin) in the basal membrane of epithelial and EC and in the matrix of the vascular *tunica media* and *adventitia* [1,3]. Among these, VLA-4 is the specific ligand for vascular cell adhesion molecule-1 (VCAM-1) [4]. The leukocyte integrins, expressed exclusively on leukocytes [5], bind to other adhesion molecules such as intercellular adhesion molecule-1

Table 18.1 Major types of adhesion molecules of clinical interest, their site of expression, and specific ligands.

Adhesion molecules	Site of expression	Ligands
Selectins		
P-selectin	Activated EC, platelets	Syalyl-Lewis[x] and [a], PSGL-1
L-selectin	Leukocytes (constitutive)	Mucin-like glycoproteins
Immunoglobulins		
ICAM-1	EC	Mac-1, LFA-1
ICAM-2	Activated EC, platelets	LFA-1
VCAM-1	Activated EC	VLA-4
PECAM-1	Activated EC, platelets (constitutive)	
Integrins		
β-1 (VLA)		
VLA-1	Different cell types	Collagen, laminin
VLA-2	Different cell types	Collagen, laminin
VLA-3	Different cell types	Fibronectin–laminin
VLA-4	Different cell types	Fibronectin
VLA-5	Different cell types	Fibronectin
VLA-6	Different cell types	Laminin
β-2 (leukocyte)		
LFA-1 (CD11a)	Leukocytes	ICAM-1, ICAM-2
Mac-1 (CD11b)	Neutrophils, monocytes	ICAM-1, C3b, fibrinogen, factor X
P150/95 (CD11c)	Macrophages	Fibrinogen
β-3 (cytoadhesins)		
GPIIb/IIIa	Platelets–megakaryocytes	Fibrinogen, von Willebrand factor, factor X
VNR	Mesenchymal cells	Vitronectin, fibrinogen, von Willebrand factor, osteopontin

EC: endothelial cells; ICAM: intercellular adhesion molecule; VCAM: vascular cell adhesion molecule; PECAM: platelet endothelial cell adhesion molecule; Mac: Macrophage antigen; LFA: leukocyte function-associated antigen; VLA: very late appearing molecule; VNR: vitronectin receptor; C3: complement component 3; GP: glycoprotein; CD: cluster of differentiation; PSGL-1: P-selectin glycoprotein ligand-1.

(ICAM-1), as is the case for lymphocyte function-associated antigen (LFA) 1 (CD11a/CD18) and Mac1-CD11b/CD18; or ICAM-2, as for LFA-1; or fibrinogen, factor X and C3b inactivated factor, as for Mac-1 [6]. Cytoadhesins, including the platelet receptor glycoprotein (GP)IIb/IIIa and the vitronectin receptor (VNR), bind to fibrinogen, vitronectin, von Willebrand factor, thrombospondin, and osteopontin [1].

Selectins

Selectins form a family of molecules expressed on the plasma membrane of different cell types sharing the common property of binding carbohydrate ligands [7]. Expressed constitutively on all leukocyte classes, leukocyte (L)-selectin is released rapidly in soluble form following cell activation [8]. Cytokines, bacterial endotoxin, or other agonists express endothelial (E)-selectin on EC only after cell activation, a process that requires *de novo* protein synthesis [9]. Conversely,

pre-synthesized platelet (P)-selectin stored in platelet α-granules [10] and Weibel–Palade bodies of EC [11] is expressed rapidly, within seconds, on the cellular surface following activation by thrombin and other non-cytokine mediators [12]. Selectins share a common structure, i.e., a lectin domain with high affinity for carbohydrates, an epithelial growth factor-like region, and a variable number of repetitive structures similar to complement-regulatory proteins [7]. E- and P-selectins bind to carbohydrate structures such as syalyl-Lewis[x] and sulfurated or phosphorylated polysaccharides [11–13], whereas L-selectin binds to mucin-like membrane glycoprotein structures [14]. E-selectin may mediate the adhesion of different leukocyte populations (neutrophils, monocytes, activated T lymphocytes, eosinophils, and basophils) to EC [15,16]. P-selectin recognizes complementary ligands expressed on neutrophils and monocytes [12,17], and L-selectin recognizes, at least in part, inducible receptors on the cell surface of activated EC

[18] and on the vessel wall of high endothelial veins of lymphnodes, thus playing a pivotal role in lymphocyte localization, especially some classes of lymphocytes, in specific sites of the lymphatic tissues [19].

Immunoglobulins

In addition to soluble antibodies, the immunoglobulin superfamily comprises antibody-like T-cell receptors and antigens of the major histocompatibility complex, as well as several proteins that mediate leukocyte adhesion to the endothelial surface, including ICAM-1 and -2, VCAM-1, and platelet endothelial cell adhesion molecule-1 (PECAM-1). The structure of these molecules comprises immunoglobulin-like domains of 90–100 amino acids, organized in a sandwich of two anti-parallel β-sheets stabilized by a disulfide bond [20]. ICAM-1 is expressed constitutively on the cell surface of EC and epithelial and hematopoietic cells as well as fibroblasts, but its expression dramatically increases following stimulation with specific cytokines such as tumor necrosis factor alpha (TNF-α), interleukin (IL) 1α, or 1β and interferon gamma (IFN γ) [21]. ICAM-1 recognizes two leukocyte integrins: LFA-1, also a ligand for ICAM-2 [22], and Mac-1 [23], as specific cognate ligands. VCAM-1, only partially constitutively expressed on the cellular surface of endothelial and SMC [24], is maximally enhanced after stimulation with cytokines [25]. VCAM-1 binds to VLA-4 [26], and can mediate the adhesion of monocytes [27] and most leukocytes and lymphocytes [16] to the endothelium. PECAM-1, which is expressed constitutively on platelets and also on activated EC and leukocytes [28,29], also participates in leukocyte transmigration across the vessel wall; ICAM-1 and VCAM-1 partially control its production [30]. Molecular mechanisms of PECAM-1 activation differ from those of molecules implicated in leukocyte adhesion, since cytokines that usually induce adhesion molecule activation, e.g., TNF-α, inhibit its expression [31].

Role of cell adhesion molecules in atherogenesis and inflammation

(see also Chapters 1 and 2)

Endothelial dysfunction and activation

The endothelium has unique functions controlling (a) hemostasis, including the control of platelet adhesion and activation, coagulation and fibrinolysis; (b) vascular tone; (c) vascular permeability; (d) SMC growth and proliferation and (e) leukocyte adhesion (see, for general overviews [32,33], and Chapters 1–2). Qualitative and quantitative alterations of endothelial functions can lead to decreased antithrombogenic properties of the endothelium and, conversely, to increased vasomotor tone, increased vascular permeability to plasma lipoproteins, increased production of cytokines and growth factors, and hyperadhesiveness toward circulating leukocytes. Overall, such alterations of endothelial functions can be designated as "endothelial dysfunctions" [33] (see Chapter 1). "Endothelial activation" indicates a group of dysfunctions characterized by antigenic changes on the surface of vascular endothelium, particularly occurring in response to inflammatory cytokines and bacterial endotoxin. Such responses modulate the interactions of circulating leukocytes and play a pivotal role in the initiation and progression of atherosclerosis. Through increased expression of tissue factor or cyclooxygenase-2, these changes also induce alterations in vascular thrombogenicity or the production of inflammatory mediators.

Endothelial activation and leukocyte adhesion to the endothelium

Leukocyte adhesion to the endothelium occurs in many inflammatory and immunological processes. For instance, the adhesion of neutrophils to postcapillary venules is typical of acute inflammation. Conversely, monocyte adhesion to the endothelium represents the first event in the pathogenesis of atherosclerosis. Formation of the fatty streak, composed of a focal intra-intimal accumulation of macrophages carrying lipids and surrounded by a loose extracellular matrix and a variable number of lymphocytes, is one of the first events in atherosclerosis, rapidly documented in animals fed a hyperlipidemic diet [1,34]. The adhesion of circulating monocytes to a still morphologically intact endothelium is an obligatory step in this process. Subsequently, monocytes transmigrate into the intima, where monocytes become lipid-laden macrophages (foam cells) peculiar to the fatty streak [35,36]. Molecules of different families mediate the adhesion of leukocytes to EC, epitomized in the "three-step paradigm" documented in other inflammatory processes [37,38]. First, a rolling of monocytes occurs on the endothelial surface, with consistently decreasing velocity. This first event is mediated by the interaction between selectins (E-selectin on EC, L-selectin on leukocytes) and specific ligands expressed on leukocytes and EC, respectively. The initial deceleration allows the leukocytes to recognize the presence of chemotactic factors (second phase: chemoattraction), determining in turn the expression of activated integrin receptors on their surface [39,40]. Such receptors are the ligands for endothelial immunoglobulins [41]. In the third phase, immunoglobulins and integrins interact, and monocytes adhere firmly to EC. Subsequent to adhesion, monocytes transmigrate inside the intima, a phenomenon that also involves the immunoglobulin PECAM-1 [30]. When transformed into foam cells, monocytes contribute to lesion progression via local production of cytokines (IL-1β, TNF-α), platelet-derived growth factor (PDGF), fibroblasts growth factor (FGF), reactive oxygen intermediates, procoagulant factors, and eicosanoids [42], and also propel increased production of matrix components by SMC, which shift their phenotype from contractile to synthetic [43]. The interaction between SMC and components of the extracellular matrix, mediated by receptors of the β-1 integrin family, importantly participates in the migration of SMC inside the intima, contributing to lesion progression [44].

The traditional approach to the study of adhesion molecules involves stimulating a monolayer of EC with inflammatory cytokines. Due to the pleiotropic effects of cytokines, many phenomena occur following such stimulation. Recently, gene transfer techniques, i.e., transfecting EC with complementary DNA (cDNA) for selected adhesion molecules, have demonstrated the physiological role of each molecule. For instance, selective expression of VCAM-1 on the surface sufficiently permits the adhesion of T lymphocytes under conditions of low shear stress [45]. Importantly, this conclusion partially corrects, for the first time, the classical "three-step paradigm," showing the possibility, at least *in vitro*, that some leukocytes may adhere to the endothelium without a previous rolling and without the need of other adhesion molecules.

Secondary interactions involved in leukocyte transmigration

Leukocytes and platelets actively contribute to leukocyte adhesion to an activated endothelium, amplifying cellular responses since the earliest phases. Platelet adhesion promotes EC expression of P-selectin, supporting, through this initial contact, a co-localization of leukocytes, especially in shear stress conditions that normally do not permit adhesion [46]. Platelet-activating factor (PAF) can induce, synergistically with TNF α, the expression of E-selectin and ICAM-1 [47]. Moreover, PAF can induce a blunted vasodilatory response after stimuli such as acetylcholine and 5-hydroxy-tryptamine [48]. Endothelium-platelet binding occurring through PECAM-1 (CD31) partially permits platelet adhesion and aggregation in conditions of endothelial dysfunction or endothelial detachment, as demonstrated by the partial inhibition obtained by adding monoclonal antibodies specific for this molecule [49]. Leukocytes also contribute to the amplification of adhesion contacts since the phase preceding their transmigration into the intima, although their major pro-inflammatory effect occurs when they already are part of the growing atherosclerotic plaque through the secretion of different cytokines and chemoattractants, such as IL-8 [42]. Mast cells sensitive to activation by multiple mechanisms, e.g., pro-oxidant agents, anaphylotoxins, neuropeptides and bacterial products, and highly sensitive to mechanical stimuli also share a potentially pro-atherogenic role. High levels of oxidants, anaphylotoxins, neuropeptides, and bacterial products released in conditions of ischemia–reperfusion, sepsis, and anaphylaxis, can be responsible for mast cell degranulation, consequently promoting further leukocyte adhesion.

Soluble adhesion molecules: nature, potential mechanisms of regulation of the membrane release and pathophysiological role

Soluble adhesion molecules derive from the shedding of transmembrane adhesion molecules, i.e., proteolysis of the extracellular domains. The first observation of these "soluble" adhesion molecules was accomplished *in vitro* by immunoenzymatic measurements in the medium of EC after cytokine activation. In such conditions, levels in the medium were significantly higher compared with the medium of non-activated EC [50]. This finding forms the basis for their use as biohumoral indices of endothelial activation *in vivo*. Since they bind to the same specific ligands as the transmembrane molecules, soluble adhesion molecules continue to be biologically active [51].

Structural features

VCAM-1, the endothelial leukocyte adhesion molecule most relevant for monocyte binding to EC, is initially synthesized as two intracellular precursors of 35 and 37 kDa, the product of two alternatively spliced messenger RNA variants [52]. Following post-translational modifications (N-glycosylation), two transmembrane molecules arise, with a higher molecular weight of 44 and 45 kDa, respectively. Differences of intracellular maturation can be the end-result of the type of stimuli of endothelial activation. For instance, two variants of soluble VCAM-1 occur in mice: the variant with higher molecular weight results from the shedding of the constitutive molecule, while the variant with lower molecular weight only occurs after stimulation with bacterial lipopolysaccharide (LPS) [53]. Soluble L-selectin occurs in two isoforms of 62 and 75 kDa deriving from lymphocytes and neutrophils, respectively [54].

Regulation of shedding from EC

The regulation of adhesion molecule release in the bloodstream remains undetermined, but likely contributes to the modulation of both intercellular communication and gene expression for adhesion molecules, as well as structural and functional alterations of their specific ligands [55]. Several reports indicate that matrix metalloproteinases (MMP) participate in the regulation of adhesion molecule shedding from plasma membranes [56–58]. MMP are Zn^{2+}-endopeptidases that participate importantly in chronic inflammatory diseases of the connective tissue by mediating the destruction of collagen components. EC themselves constitutively express MMP-2 and MMP-3 mRNA, but MMP-3 increases at the mRNA and protein level after TNF-α stimulation, while MMP-9 and MMP-12 mRNA could only be detected in inflammatory conditions [59]. Current knowledge suggests that the release of soluble molecules from cell membranes is proportional

to the expression of transmembrane molecules. Stimuli such as LPS and cytokines initiate a sequence of intracellular events that ultimately increases the expression of genes encoding for adhesion molecules, but simultaneously activate MMP with the subsequent shedding of soluble moieties, as a mechanism of intrinsic downregulation of the activation response. However, already elucidated regulatory mechanisms of shedding also support the hypothesis that the release of soluble adhesion molecules may be partially independent of gene expression, with a possible mismatch between the surface expression and plasma concentration of adhesion molecules. For instance, strong pro-inflammatory stimuli such as phorbol 12-myristate 13-acetate (PMA) and TNF-α significantly increase the shedding of the TNF receptor, although these stimuli have opposite effects on gene expression and surface appearance of the transmembrane molecule (activated by PMA, inhibited by TNF-α) [60]. In lymphocytes, the shedding of L-selectin correlates with activation due to antigen stimulation. Here, the *de novo* expression of the molecule on the cell surface links to antigen detachment from the T-cell receptor [61]. Different stimuli may have different effects on post-translational regulation, such as the glycosylation process and probably also the shedding. For instance, increased concentrations of soluble ICAM-1, apparently in a concentration-dependent manner, occur only after stimulation with TNF and not after other stimuli such as IL-1 and LPS *in vitro* [62].

Mechanisms regulating shedding are specific, at least in part, for the various adhesion molecules. For instance, PMA-induced VCAM-1 shedding results from activation of a specific pathway, since PMA stimulation does not alter generation of soluble forms of three other adhesion molecules, E-selectin, PECAM-1, and ICAM-1 [63]. Using cells derived from genetically deficient mice, the TNF-α-converting enzyme, TACE (also termed ADAM 17) recently has been identified as the protease responsible for PMA-induced VCAM-1 release by murine EC [63]. The authors conclude that TACE-mediated shedding of VCAM-1 may be important for the regulation of VCAM-1 function at the cell surface.

Indeed, a correlation between surface expression and medium concentrations of soluble adhesion molecules remains unconfirmed for the broad range of relevant pathophysiological concentrations of endothelial stimuli. The metabolic disposal and the rate of clearance of soluble adhesion molecules also remains incompletely investigated.

Pathophysiological role of soluble adhesion molecules

Observed therapeutic effects of infused soluble adhesion molecules in *in vivo* models of inflammation underscore their pathophysiological significance. By antagonizing the binding of transmembrane molecules with their specific ligands, soluble forms of these molecules can have broad anti-inflammatory effects, e.g., the administration of soluble P-selectin glycoprotein ligand-1 (PSGL-1) reduced the number of eosinophils and lymphocytes in the bronchoalveolar lavage of a mouse model of asthma [64]. In a murine model of allergy, intravenous infusion of soluble L-selectin diminished leukocyte rolling in a dose-dependent manner, as documented by intravital microscopy [65]. On the other hand, soluble adhesion molecules activate the intracellular cascade ("outside-in signalling"), leading to further inflammation. For instance, soluble VCAM-1 induces chemotaxis of T cells bearing high-affinity VLA-4 in the synovial fluid of patients with rheumatoid arthritis [66].

A recent report described shedding of the integrin LFA-1 (CD11a/CD18) from human leukocytes during the local inflammatory response [67]. Since LFA-1 shed from the endothelium revealed a new ligand-binding conformation, shedding may participate in leukocyte detachment following transendothelial migration and also in the regulation of integrin-dependent outside-in signaling.

In conclusion, soluble forms of adhesion molecules are functional proteins able to interfere with or enhance the inflammatory response, effects possibly dependent on the type of soluble molecules and the functional state of the specific ligand.

Soluble adhesion molecules in clinical settings

Effect of physiological variables on serum concentration of soluble adhesion molecules

The effect of aging on plasma levels of various markers of endothelial dysfunction has been evaluated in healthy subjects by measuring von Willebrand factor, VCAM-1, ICAM-1, E-selectin, P-selectin, and thrombomodulin. The only correlation with age is related to VCAM-1. Levels of thrombomodulin and E-selectin were lower in women. Finally, von Willebrand factor, E-selectin and thrombomodulin showed significant differences according to AB0 erythrocyte antigen groups [68].

Atherosclerotic vascular disease

Soluble adhesion molecules are useful markers of the extension of atherosclerosis, as shown in clinical studies where levels of ICAM-1 and von Willebrand factor were higher in patients with peripheral vascular disease or with ischemic heart disease compared with controls [69]. We also demonstrated that especially VCAM-1, but also ICAM-1, are good markers of the presence atherosclerosis. We studied 11 hypertensive patients with peripheral vascular disease and increased intima–media thickness, 11 subjects with only primary hypertension, and 11 controls, all comparable for age, gender and smoking habits. The mean values of VCAM-1 were 990, 340, and 389 ng/mL in these three groups, respectively. At multivariate analysis, which evaluated the contribution of several potential markers of endothelial activation/dysfunction, only sVCAM-1 remained an independent predictor of intima–media thickness [70]. Another study showed that plasma concentrations of VCAM-1, but not ICAM-1, E-selectin, P-selectin, or thrombomodulin, correlate with the extension of atherosclerosis, as detected by angiography of the aorta, common iliac, femoral, and peripheral arteries [71]. However, in the Atherosclerosis Risk in Communities (ARIC) Study, plasma levels of ICAM-1 and E-selectin, but not VCAM-1, related to the incidence of aortic atherosclerosis and ischemic heart disease [72]. An analysis from the Physicians' Health Study (PHS) cohort confirmed that individuals who subsequently develop symptomatic arterial disease have higher levels of soluble ICAM-1 compared with controls [73]. After adjustment for lipid and non-lipid risk factors, including C-reactive protein (CRP), the odds ratio for the highest quartile of soluble ICAM-1 compared with the lowest quartile was 3.9% (95% confidence interval, 1.7–8.6, $P = 0.001$) [73]. Additionally, the Bezafibrate Infarction Prevention (BIP) Study showed the prognostic value of soluble ICAM-1 by identifying patients with stable coronary artery disease at high risk for subsequent ischemic events [74]. Interpretation of these studies with regard to the importance of ICAM-1 and/or VCAM-1 in various stages or with various extension of atherosclerosis is somewhat precluded by the lack of knowledge of cellular and molecular mechanisms determining the steady-state plasma levels of these molecules [75]. More recently, sICAM-1, similarly to CRP and matrix metallopro-teinase-9, were significantly associated with rapid coronary artery disease progression in chronic patients repeating a coronary angiogram around 6 months later [76].

Diabetes mellitus

E-selectin increases consistently in both type 1 and type 2 diabetic patients compared with controls, and ICAM-1 increases selectively in patients with type 2 diabetes [77]. Plasma levels of E-selectin relate signif-icantly to levels of glycated hemoglobin, suggesting the possibility of using E-selectin as a marker of metabolic compensation. Other recent data confirm that concentrations of soluble E-selectin associate with hyperglycemia, hyperinsulinemia, and insulin resistance [78]. In patients with diabetes, the presence of microalbuminuria, an early index of endothelial dysfunction at least in part secondary to the effect of advanced glycation end products [79], correlated significantly with increased levels of soluble VCAM-1, suggesting that this marker may usefully monitor the efficacy of therapeutic interventions [80]. Such results suggest two distinct phases of the disease, before and after the development of microalbumin-uria, concomitant with the development of micro/macrovascular complications.

Dyslipidemias

Patients with hypertriglyceridemia have higher levels of VCAM-1, and patients with either hypertriglyc-eridemia or hypercholesterolemia show increased levels of ICAM-1 versus controls. Higher concentra-tions of E-selectin were documented in patients with hypercholesterolemia [81], and the effects of an effective triglyceride- or cholesterol-lowering ther-apy on soluble adhesion molecules concentrations appeared restricted to E-selectin [81]. However, another study in a population of patients with famil-ial hypercholesterolemia and higher baseline levels of

low-density lipoprotein (LDL)-cholesterol showed significantly reduced plasma levels of E-selectin and ICAM-1 following LDL apheresis, and a rebound effect occurred at the end of treatment [82]. That study did not measure VCAM-1 concen-trations [82]. In a larger study examining more than 700 patients with documented coronary artery disease and matched with normal controls, levels of ICAM-1 and VCAM-1 related better to the association of LDL and triglycerides (LDL-TG) than to LDL cholesterol alone, suggesting that LDL-TG may better reflect the atherogenic poten-tial of LDL than LDL cholesterol [83].

Hypertension

Systemic hypertension typically associates with endothelial dysfunction. In a study of three patient groups (uncontrolled arterial hypertension, arterial hypertension under pharmacological treatment, and controls), hypertensive patients had higher lev-els of E-selectin compared with normotensive sub-jects, especially in patients with uncontrolled arterial hypertension. The study determined no differences for von Willebrand factor [84]. Investigating the cor-relation between biohumoral markers and func-tional/structural alterations of the vessel walls, the authors measured forearm blood flow in response to acetylcholine (as an endothelial-dependent vaso-dilator) or to nitroprussiate (as an endothelial-independent vasodilator). They also determined minimum vascular resistances, calculated by the ratio of maximal vasodilation after 13 min of ischemia over mean blood pressure [84]. Because E-selectin showed a significant negative correlation with the vascular response to nitroprussiate and a positive correlation with minimal vascular resistances, the authors hypothesized that a significant increase of this biohumoral marker of endothelial activation occurs only in the presence of structural vascular alterations and happens later than functional changes alone.

Ischemic heart disease

Inflammation plays a fundamental role in the pathophysiology of acute ischemic syndromes [85]. Several studies have documented increased levels of inflammatory markers such as CRP [86,87] and IL-6 [88] in patients with unstable angina and acute myocardial infarction. Activated leukocytes were found in both the unstable plaque [89,90] and the microcirculation following ischemia–reperfusion [91]. The presence of activated leukocytes can induce endothelial damage, mediated by the release of oxyradicals [92,93] and lytic enzymes such as elastases, collagenases, and other proteases [94]. The release of other mediators such as PAF, tissue factor, leukotrienes, and IL-1 can amplify platelet aggregation and promote coagulation. The role of adhesion molecules in this pathophysiological process was demonstrated by the finding of increased ICAM-1 and VCAM-1 expression at the level of atherosclerotic plaques [95,96]. Moreover, neutrophils drawn from the coronary sinus in patients with unstable angina showed increased density of CD11b/CD18 compared with stable angina controls or patients without significant lesions in the coronary arteries [97]. Additionally, increased expression of ICAM-1 occurred in the microcirculation following episodes of ischemia–reperfusion [98]. Patients with various manifestations of ischemic heart disease repeatedly show increased levels of soluble adhesion molecules. Compared with controls with "normal" coronary arteries, patients with myocardial infarction, unstable angina, or stable angina showed high levels of soluble ICAM-1 [99]. Compared with subjects with normal coronary arteries, the finding of increased levels of soluble ICAM-1 in patients with myocardial infarction, unstable angina, or stable angina confirms these data [100,101].

An interesting feature in the pathophysiology of acute ischemic syndromes involves the frequent finding of platelet–leukocytes aggregates [102]. *In vitro*, the binding between platelet P-selectin and the Lewis[x] receptor on neutrophils mediates platelet–leukocytes interactions [17,103]; such binding can in turn induce increased expression of CD11b/CD18 on the leukocyte [104] and then stabilize the aggregate by bridging fibrinogen between the neutrophil CD11b/CD18 and the platelet glycoprotein IIb/IIIa [105,106]. Thus, soluble P-selectin might be used as a marker of platelet activation and possibly of the formation of heterotypic neutrophil-platelets aggregates. Indeed, increased levels of soluble P-selectin occurred in patients with unstable angina compared with patients with stable angina or healthy controls, and these levels decreased gradually following resolution of angina [107].

Neutrophil production of superoxide anion decreased following administration of anti-P-selectin or anti-Lewis[x] antibodies, thus supporting the hypothesis that P-selectin mediates the amplification of free radical-induced tissue damage [108]. A consequence of this might also be the increased production of tissue factor, a protein functioning as a cofactor of factor VIIa, by activated monocytes [109]. On the other hand, soluble P-selectin may inhibit the binding of leukocytes to EC, with consequent reduction of the inflammatory response [110] and superoxide anion release [111].

Restenosis following percutaneous coronary interventions

In the era of stents, restenosis following percutaneous coronary interventions (PCI) consists of a complex phenomenon of intimal hyperplasia involving platelet aggregation, activation of the coagulation cascade, inflammation, proliferation, and migration of SMC in the media [112]. While adhesion molecules play an active role in inflammation, mediating the interaction between EC and leukocytes, they also participate in the proliferation of SMC. Antibodies against ICAM-1 or its cognate ligand LFA-1 inhibit intimal hyperplasia in arteries after angioplasty balloon trauma [113]. Therefore, the expression of ICAM-1 on SMC may indicate a major phenotypic alteration of SMC migrating in the media [114]. In addition, selectins likely participate in the pathogenesis of intimal hyperplasia after coronary angioplasty, as indicated by the correlation between basal levels of soluble E-selectin and the ensuing restenosis [115], an observation confirmed by reduced post-PCI intimal hyperplasia after blocking of E- and L-selectin with analogs of Lewis[x] receptor [116]. Levels of soluble adhesion molecules in the systemic circulation directly reflect levels in the coronary circulation, as measured in blood samples drawn from the femoral vein and the coronary sinus, without any acute change after PCI and stenting [117]. Moreover, anti-platelet drugs commonly used after stenting, i.e. aspirin and ticlopidine, can interfere with the expression of leukocyte and platelet adhesion molecules such as L- and P-selectin, whereas E-selectin usually increases for at least 24 h after stenting [118]. We currently have no clear data about the usefulness of soluble adhesion molecules in monitoring restenosis.

Cerebral vascular disorder

Stroke progression involves the activation of EC and platelets. Recently, Kozuka and coworkers measured soluble thrombomodulin and von Willebrand factors as endothelial markers and soluble P- and E-selectin as adhesion molecules during the acute and subacute phases of 52 consecutive patients with acute ischemic stroke and 86 age-matched control subjects [119]. Plasma levels of von Willebrand factor and soluble P- and E-selectins in stroke patients during both acute and subacute phases increased significantly compared with control subjects, and serum levels of soluble thrombomodulin were significantly higher compared with control subjects only during the subacute phase. Compared with lacunar lesions, markers of endothelial injury were high throughout the subacute phase in atherothrombotic infarction, indicating that endothelial damage is maintained for a relatively long time. For this reason, the evaluation of endothelial markers and adhesion molecules might reflect the pathophysiological state of stroke and provide useful information for its treatment. Another study documenting high levels of soluble VCAM-1 in the acute and subacute phase of an ischemic stroke, but not in asymptomatic patients with carotid atherosclerosis, confirmed such observations [120].

Extravascular diseases

Soluble adhesion molecules are under investigation in several other clinical conditions. We report a summary of the main findings in extravascular conditions in Table 18.2.

Areas of clinical investigation and future perspectives

Regulation of leukocyte adhesion molecules, at the background of atherosclerosis, inflammation, vasculitic disorders, and immune phenomena, can occur at the level of gene expression, post-translational modifications, conformational alterations of their complementary ligands, and also at the level of shedding from endothelial surface. Among these, endothelial shedding is less clearly understood, with persistent and considerable uncertainty regarding its pathophysiological role. Therefore, the measurement of sICAM-1, sVCAM-1, and sE-selectin in a large spectrum of disease conditions involving endothelial dysfunctions cannot be interpreted simplistically as due only to surface expression of the transmembrane proteins. Important additional considerations include the inability to measure part of soluble adhesion molecules when already bound to their ligands, and the need to correct plasma levels for the effects of physiological variables such as age, sex and the blood group. Finally, any interpretation regarding the significance of increased plasma concentrations of endothelial adhesion molecules requires an understanding of the metabolic disposition of these molecules. Due to the syaloglycoprotein structure of some endothelial adhesion molecules, the endothelium itself likely plays an active role, through syalidases, on their metabolic disposal. It should be of great interest to test whether metabolic alterations of the clearance of soluble adhesion molecules may occur as a consequence of endothelial dysfunction. Other routes of clearance of adhesion molecules from the circulation

Table 18.2 Soluble adhesion molecules in non-cardiovascular diseases.

Disease	Biohumoral marker	Significant correlation	Reference
Multiple sclerosis	L-selectin	Clinical score, anti-double helix DNA antibodies	[123]
Leukemia	E-Selectin	Leukemic mass	[124]
Autoimmunitary disorders	ICAM-1	AECA, ACL, ANCA	[125]
AIDS	VCAM-1	Lymphocyte count, CD4+	[126]
Hyperthyroidism	ICAM-1	FT3, FT4	[127]
Chronic hepatitis	E-selectin, ICAM-1	–	[128]
Hepatic cirrhosis	VCAM-1, ICAM-1	–	[129]
Idiopathic pulmonary fibrosis	VCAM-1, ICAM-1, E Selectin	Lung capacity	[130]
Allograft rejection	E-Selectin	Obliterative vasculopathy	[131]

AECA: anti-endothelial cell antibodies; ACL: anti-cardiolipin antibodies; ANCA: anti-neutrophil cell antibodies; FT3: free tri-iodotyronine; FT4: free tetra-iodotyronine.

(the kidney?) require further investigation. Currently, a correct and univocal interpretation of the results of immunoenzymatic assays of adhesion molecules remains far from possible. Despite such limitations, measurements of soluble adhesion molecules appear useful in gaining insight to the pathophysiology of diseases and, possibly also clinically, in evaluating disease progression and the efficacy of therapeutic interventions in individual patients. In this regard, we have observed that the beneficial therapeutic effect of prostaglandin (PG) E_1 in patients with peripheral vascular disorders directly correlates with the reduction of soluble adhesion molecule levels [121]. Soluble adhesion molecules also appear useful for assessing patients' prognosis and assisting in risk stratification; the results of at least one prospective study confirm this possibility [122]. Indeed, plasma concentrations of ICAM-1 appear significantly related with the long-term (9-year) risk of acute myocardial infarction in the PHS cohort, particularly in subjects in the highest quartile (>296 ng/mL). Such risk was high for non-smokers as well, ruling out inflammation consequent to smoke as a potential bias. A positive correlation between ICAM-1 and other classic risk factors such as fibrinogen, CRP, cholesterol, and homocysteine was apparent, but adjustment for these variables decreased only slightly the prognostic value of such measurement. Future studies should confirm the independent prognostic ability of these new markers in the long-term prediction of cardiovascular events.

References

1 Ruoslahti F, Pierschbacher MD. New perspectives in cell adhesion: RGD and integrins. *Science* 1987;238:491–497.

2 Hemler ME. VLA proteins in the integrin family: structures, functions, and their role on leukocytes. *Annu Rev Immunol* 1990;8:365–400.

3 Hynes RO. Integrins: a family of cell surface receptors. *Cell* 1987;48:549–554.

4 Osborn L, Hession C, Tizard R, et al. Direct expression cloning of vascular cell adhesion molecule 1, a cytokine-induced endothelial protein that binds to lymphocytes. *Cell* 1989;59:1203–1211.

5 Wright SD, Weitz JI, Huang AJ, et al. Complement receptor type three (CD11b/CD18) of human polymorphonuclear leukocytes recognizes fibrinogen. *Proc Natl Acad Sci USA* 1988;85:7734–7738.

6 Kishimoto TK, Larson RS, Corbi AL, et al. The leukocyte integrins. *Adv Immunol* 1989;46:149–182.

7 Bevilacqua MP, Nelson RM. Selectins. *J Clin Invest* 1993;91:379–387.

8 Kishimoto TK, Jutila MA, Berg EL, et al. Neutrophil Mac-1 and MEL-14 adhesion proteins inversely regulated by chemotactic factors. *Science* 1989;245:1238–1241.

9 Pober JS, Cotran RS. The role of endothelial cells in inflammation. *Transplantation* 1990;50:537–544.

10 Israels SJ, Gerrard JM, Jacques YV, et al. Platelet dense granule membranes contain both granulophysin and P-selectin (GMP-140). *Blood* 1992;80:143–152.

11 Johnston GI, Cook RG, McEver RP. Cloning of GMP-140, a granule membrane protein of platelets and endothelium: sequence similarity to proteins involved in cell adhesion and inflammation. *Cell* 1989;56:1033–1044.

12 Bonfanti R, Furie BC, Furie B, et al. PADGEM (GMP140) is a component of Weibel–Palade bodies of human endothelial cells. *Blood* 1989;73:1109–1112.

13 Lasky LA. Selectins: interpreters of cell-specific carbohydrate information during inflammation. *Science* 1992;258:964–969.

14 Lasky LA, Singer MS, Dowbenko D, et al. An endothelial ligand for L-selectin is a novel mucin-like molecule. *Cell* 1992;69:927–938.

15 Graber N, Gopal TV, Wilson D, et al. T cells bind to cytokine-activated endothelial cells via a novel, inducible sialoglycoprotein and endothelial leukocyte adhesion molecule-1. *J Immunol* 1990;145:819–830.

16 Bochner BS, Luscinskas FW, Gimbrone MA Jr, et al. Adhesion of human basophils, eosinophils, and neutrophils to interleukin 1-activated human vascular endothelial cells: contributions of endothelial cell adhesion molecules. *J Exp Med* 1991;173:1553–1557.

17 Hamburger SA, McEver RP. GMP-140 mediates adhesion of stimulated platelets to neutrophils. *Blood* 1990;75:550–554.

18 Spertini O, Luscinskas FW, Kansas GS, et al. Leukocyte adhesion molecule-1 (LAM-1, L-selectin) interacts with an inducible endothelial cell ligand to support leukocyte adhesion. *J Immunol* 1991;147:2565–2573.

19 Gallatin WM, Weissman IL, Butcher EC. A cell-surface molecule involved in organ-specific homing of lymphocytes. *Nature* 1983;304:30–34.

20 Williams AF, Barclay AN. The immunoglobulin superfamily – domains for cell surface recognition. *Annu Rev Immunol* 1988;6:381–405.

21 Dustin ML, Rothlein R, Bhan AK, et al. Induction by IL 1 and interferon-gamma: tissue distribution, biochemistry, and function of a natural adherence molecule (ICAM-1). *J Immunol* 1986;137:245–254.

22 Dustin ML, Staunton DE, Springer TA. Supergene families meet in the immune system. *Immunol Today* 1988;9:213–215.

23 Carlos TM, Harlan JM. Leukocyte-endothelial adhesion molecules. *Blood* 1994;84:2068–2101.

24 O'Brien KD, Allen MD, McDonald TO, et al. Vascular cell adhesion molecule-1 is expressed in human coronary atherosclerotic plaques. Implications for the mode of progression of advanced coronary atherosclerosis. *J Clin Invest* 1993;92:945–951.

25 Rice GE, Munro JM, Bevilacqua MP. Inducible cell adhesion molecule 110 (INCAM-110) is an endothelial receptor for lymphocytes. A CD11/CD18-independent adhesion mechanism. *J Exp Med* 1990;171:1369–1374.

26 Elices MJ, Osborn L, Takada Y, et al. VCAM-1 on activated endothelium interacts with the leukocyte integrin VLA-4 at a site distinct from the VLA-4/fibronectin binding site. *Cell* 1990;60:577–584.

27 Schleimer RP, Sterbinsky SA, Kaiser J, et al. IL-4 induces adherence of human eosinophils and basophils but not neutrophils to endothelium. Association with expression of VCAM-1. *J Immunol* 1992;148:1086–1092.

28 Albelda SM, Oliver PD, Romer LH, et al. EndoCAM: a novel endothelial cell–cell adhesion molecule. *J Cell Biol.* 1990;110:1227–1237.

29 Newman PJ, Berndt MC, Gorski J, et al. PECAM-1 (CD31) cloning and relation to adhesion molecules of the immunoglobulin gene superfamily. *Science* 1990;247: 1219–1222.

30 Muller WA, Weigl SA, Deng X, et al. PECAM-1 is required for trans migration of leukocytes. *J Exp Med* 1993;178:449–460.

31 Stewart RJ, Kashour TS, Marsden PA. Vascular endothelial platelet endothelial adhesion molecule-1 (PECAM-1) expression is decreased by TNF-alpha and IFN-gamma. Evidence for cytokine-induced destabilization of messenger ribonucleic acid transcripts in bovine endothelial cells. *J Immunol* 1996;156:1221–1228.

32 Gimbrone MA Jr. *Vascular Endothelium in Hemostasis and Thrombosis.* Edinburgh: Churchill Livingstone; 1986.

33 Gimbrone MA Jr, Bevilacqua M. Vascular endothelium: functional modulation at the blood interface. In: Simionescu N, Simionescu M, eds. *Endothelial Cell Biology in Health and Disease.* New York: Plenum Press; 1988:255–273.

34 Rosenfeld ME, Tsukada T, Gown AM, et al. Fatty streak initiation in Watanabe heritable hyperlipemic and comparably hypercholesterolemic fat-fed rabbits. *Arteriosclerosis* 1987;7:9–23.

35 Gerrity RG. The role of the monocyte in atherogenesis: I. Transition of blood-borne monocytes into foam cells in fatty lesions. *Am J Pathol* 1981;103:181–190.

36 Faggiotto A, Ross R, Harker L. Studies of hypercholesterolemia in the nonhuman primate. I. Changes that lead to fatty streak formation. *Arteriosclerosis* 1984;4: 323–340.

37 Springer TA. Traffic signals for lymphocyte recirculation and leukocyte emigration: the multistep paradigm. *Cell* 1994;76:301–314.

38 Luscinskas FW, Gimbrone MA Jr. Endothelial-dependent mechanisms in chronic inflammatory leukocyte recruitment. *Annu Rev Med* 1996;47:413–421.

39 Landis RC, Bennett RI, Hogg N. A novel LFA-1 activation epitope maps to the I domain. *J Cell Biol* 1993;120:1519–1527.

40 Diamond MS, Springer TA. A subpopulation of Mac-1 (CD11b/CD18) molecules mediates neutrophil adhesion to ICAM-1 and fibrinogen. *J Cell Biol.* 1993;120:545–556.

41 Springer TA. Adhesion receptors of the immune system. *Nature* 1990;346:425–434.

42 Clinton SK, Libby P. Cytokines and growth factors in atherogenesis. *Arch Pathol Lab Med* 1992;116:1292–1300.

43 Hedin U, Bottger BA, Forsberg E, et al. Diverse effects of fibronectin and laminin on phenotypic properties of cultured arterial smooth muscle cells. *J Cell Biol* 1988;107:307–319.

44 Thyberg J, Hedin U, Sjolund M, et al. Regulation of differentiated properties and proliferation of arterial smooth muscle cells. *Arteriosclerosis* 1990;10:966–990.

45 Gerszten RE, Luscinskas FW, Ding HT, et al. Adhesion of memory lymphocytes to vascular cell adhesion molecule-1-transduced human vascular endothelial cells under simulated physiological flow conditions *in vitro.* *Circ Res* 1996;79:1205–1215.

46 Kuijper PH, Gallardo Torres HI, et al. Platelet-dependent primary hemostasis promotes selectin- and integrin-mediated neutrophil adhesion to damaged endothelium under flow conditions. *Blood* 1996;87:3271–3281.

47 Sterner-Kock A, Braun RK, Schrenzel MD, et al. Recombinant tumour necrosis factor-alpha and platelet-activating factor synergistically increase intercellular adhesion molecule-1 and E-selectin-dependent neutrophil adherence to endothelium *in vitro.* *Immunology* 1996;87:454–460.

48 DeFily DV, Kuo L, Chilian WM. PAF attenuates endothelium-dependent coronary arteriolar vasodilation. *Am J Physiol* 1996;270:H2094–H2099.

49 Rosenblum WI, Nelson GH, Wormley B, et al. Role of platelet-endothelial cell adhesion molecule (PECAM) in platelet adhesion/aggregation over injured but not denuded endothelium *in vivo* and *ex vivo.* *Stroke* 1996;27:709–711.

50 Pigott R, Dillon LP, Hemingway IH, et al. Soluble forms of E-selectin, ICAM-1 and VCAM-1 are present in the supernatants of cytokine activated cultured endothelial cells. *Biochem Biophys Res Commun* 1992; 187:584–589.

51 Gearing AJ, Newman W. Circulating adhesion molecules in disease. *Immunol Today* 1993;14:506–512.

52 Pirozzi G, Terry RW, Labow MA. Murine vascular cell adhesion molecule-1 (VCAM-1) proteins encoded by alternatively spliced mRNAs are differentially targeted in polarized cells. *Cell Adhes Commun* 1994;2:549–556.

53 Hahne M, Lenter M, Jager U, et al. A novel soluble form of mouse VCAM-1 is generated from a glycolipid-anchored splicing variant. *Eur J Immunol* 1994;24: 421–428.

54 Schleiffenbaum B, Spertini O, Tedder TF. Soluble L-selectin is present in human plasma at high levels and retains functional activity. *J Cell Biol* 1992;119:229–238.

55 Ley K. Molecular mechanisms of leucocyte rolling and adhesion to microvascular endothelium. *Eur Heart J* 1993;14(Suppl I):68–73.

56 Hummel V, Kallmann BA, Wagner S, et al. Production of MMPs in human cerebral endothelial cells and their role in shedding adhesion molecules. *J Neuropathol Exp Neurol* 2001;60:320–327.

57 Ilan N, Mohsenin A, Cheung L, et al. PECAM-1 shedding during apoptosis generates a membrane-anchored truncated molecule with unique signaling characteristics. *FASEB J* 2001;15:362–372.

58 Hattori Y, Kato H, Nitta M, et al. Decrease of L-selectin expression on human CD34 1 cells on freeze-thawing and rapid recovery with short-term incubation. *Exp Hematol* 2001;29:114–122.

59 Galis ZS, Khatri JJ. Matrix metalloproteinases in vascular remodeling and atherogenesis: the good, the bad, and the ugly. *Circ Res* 2002;90:251–262.

60 Nakamura H, Hino T, Kato S, et al. Tumour necrosis factor receptor gene expression and shedding in human whole lung tissue and pulmonary epithelium. *Eur Respir J* 1996;9:1643–1647.

61 Sanchez-Garcia J, Atkins C, Pasvol G, et al. Antigen-driven shedding of L-selectin from human gamma delta T cells. *Immunology* 1996;89:213–219.

62 Sano Y, Hirai S, Katayama M, et al. Immuno-enzymometric analysis for expression and shedding of intercellular adhesion molecule-1 on human endothelial cells stimulated with cytokines or lipopolysaccharide. *Mol Cell Biochem* 1994;139:123–130.

63 Garton KJ, Gough PJ, Philalay J, et al. Stimulated shedding of vascular cell adhesion molecule 1 (VCAM-1) is mediated by tumor necrosis factor-alpha-converting enzyme (ADAM 17). *J Biol Chem* 2003;278: 37459–37464.

64 Borchers MT, Crosby J, Farmer S, et al. Blockade of CD49d inhibits allergic airway pathologies independent of effects on leukocyte recruitment. *Am J Physiol Lung Cell Mol Physiol* 2001;280:L813–L821.

65 Ferri LE, Swartz D, Christou NV. Soluble L-selectin at levels present in septic patients diminishes leukocyte-endothelial cell interactions in mice *in vivo*: a mechanism for decreased leukocyte delivery to remote sites in sepsis. *Crit Care Med* 2001;29:117–22.

66 Kitani A, Nakashima N, Izumihara T, et al. Soluble VCAM-1 induces chemotaxis of Jurkat and synovial fluid T cells bearing high affinity very late antigen-4. *J Immunol* 1998;161:4931–4938.

67 Evans BJ, McDowall A, Taylor PC, et al. Shedding of lymphocyte function-associated antigen (LFA)-1 in a human inflammatory response. *Blood* 2006;107:3593–3599.

68 Blann AD, Daly RJ, Amiral J. The influence of age, gender and ABO blood group on soluble endothelial cell markers and adhesion molecules. *Br J Haematol* 1996;92:498–500.

69 Blann AD, McCollum CN. Circulating endothelial cell/leukocyte adhesion molecules in atherosclerosis. *Thromb Haemostasis* 1994;72:151–154.

70 De Caterina R, Basta G, Lazzerini G, et al. Soluble vascular cell adhesion molecule-1 as a biohumoral correlate of atherosclerosis. *Arterioscler Thromb Vasc Biol* 1997;17:2646–2654.

71 Peter K, Nawroth P, Conradt C, et al. Circulating vascular cell adhesion molecule-1 correlates with the extent of human atherosclerosis in contrast to circulating intercellular adhesion molecule-1, E-selectin, P-selectin, and thrombomodulin. *Arterioscler Thromb Vasc Biol* 1997; 17:505–512.

72 Hwang SJ, Ballantyne CM, Sharrett AR, et al. Circulating adhesion molecules VCAM-1, ICAM-1, and E-selectin in carotid atherosclerosis and incident coronary heart disease cases: the Atherosclerosis Risk In Communities (ARIC) study. *Circulation* 1997;96:4219–4225.

73 Ridker PM, Hennekens CH, Roitman-Johnson B, et al. Plasma concentration of soluble intercellular adhesion molecule 1 and risks of future myocardial infarction in apparently healthy men. *Lancet* 1998;351:88–92.

74 Haim M, Tanne D, Boyko V, et al. Soluble intercellular adhesion molecule-1 and long-term risk of acute coronary events in patients with chronic coronary heart disease. Data from the Bezafibrate Infarction Prevention (BIP) Study. *J Am Coll Cardiol* 2002;39:1133–1138.

75 Ballantyne CM, Entman ML. Soluble adhesion molecules and the search for biomarkers for atherosclerosis. *Circulation* 2002;106:766–767.

76 Zouridakis E, Avanzas P, Arroyo-Espliguero R, et al. Markers of inflammation and rapid coronary artery disease progression in patients with stable angina pectoris. *Circulation* 2004;110:1747–1753.

77 Cominacini L, Fratta Pasini A, Garbin U, et al. Elevated levels of soluble E-selectin in patients with IDDM and NIDDM: relation to metabolic control. *Diabetologia* 1995;38:1122–1124.

78 Bluher M, Unger R, Rassoul F, et al. Relation between glycaemic control, hyperinsulinaemia and plasma concentrations of soluble adhesion molecules in patients with impaired glucose tolerance or Type II diabetes. *Diabetologia* 2002;45:210–216.

79 Basta G, Lazzerini G, Massaro M, et al. Advanced glycation end products (AGEs) activate endothelium via RAGE: a mechanism for amplification of inflammatory responses. *Circulation* 2002;105:816–822.

80 Schmidt AM, Crandall J, Hori O, et al. Elevated plasma levels of vascular cell adhesion molecule-1 (VCAM-1) in diabetic patients with microalbuminuria: a marker of vascular dysfunction and progressive vascular disease. *Br J Haematol* 1996;92:747–750.

81 Sampietro T, Tuoni M, Ferdeghini M, et al. Plasma cholesterol regulates soluble cell adhesion molecule expression in familial hypercholesterolemia. *Circulation* 1997;96:1381–1385.

82 Blann AD, Tse W, Maxwell SJ, et al. Increased levels of the soluble adhesion molecule E-selectin in essential hypertension. *J Hypertens* 1994;12:925–928.

83 Marz W, Scharnagl H, Winkler K, et al. Low-density lipoprotein triglycerides associated with low-grade systemic inflammation, adhesion molecules, and angiographic coronary artery disease: the Ludwigshafen Risk and Cardiovascular Health study. *Circulation* 2004;110: 3068–3074.

84 De Caterina R, Ghiadoni L, Taddei S, et al. Soluble E-selectin in essential hypertension – a correlate of vascular structural changes. *Am J Hypertens* 2001;14:259–266.

85 Entman ML, Ballantyne CM. Inflammation in acute coronary syndromes. *Circulation* 1993;88:800–803.

86 Berk BC, Weintraub WS, Alexander RW. Elevation of C-reactive protein in "active" coronary artery disease. *Am J Cardiol* 1990;65:168–172.

87 Liuzzo G, Biasucci LM, Gallimore JR, et al. The prognostic value of C-reactive protein and serum amyloid a protein in severe unstable angina. *N Engl J Med* 1994;331:417–424.

88 Plutzky J. Inflammatory pathways in atherosclerosis and acute coronary syndromes. *Am J Cardiol* 2001; 88:10K–15K.

89 Neri-Serneri GG, Abbate R, Gori AM, et al. Transient intermittent lymphocyte activation is responsible for the instability of angina. *Circulation* 1992;86:790–797.

90 Jude B, Agraou B, McFadden EP, et al. Evidence for time-dependent activation of monocytes in the systemic circulation in unstable angina but not in acute myocardial infarction or in stable angina. *Circulation* 1994;90:1662–1668.

91 Hansen PR. Role of neutrophils in myocardial ischemia and reperfusion. *Circulation* 1995;91:1872–1885.

92 Badwey JA, Karnovsky ML. Active oxygen species and the functions of phagocytic leukocytes. *Annu Rev Biochem* 1980;49:695–726.

93 Weiss SJ. Tissue destruction by neutrophils. *N Engl J Med* 1989;320:365–376.

94 Henson PM, Johnston Jr RB. Tissue injury in inflammation. Oxidants, proteinases, and cationic proteins. *J Clin Invest* 1987;79:669–674.

95 Printseva O, Peclo MM, Gown AM. Various cell types in human atherosclerotic lesions express ICAM-1. Further immunocytochemical and immunochemical studies employing monoclonal antibody 10F3. *Am J Pathol* 1992;140:889–896.

96 Poston RN, Haskard DO, Coucher JR, et al. Expression of intercellular adhesion molecule-1 in atherosclerotic plaques. *Am J Pathol* 1992;140:665–673.

97 Mazzone A, De Servi S, Ricevuti G, et al. Increased expression of neutrophil and monocyte adhesion molecules in unstable coronary artery disease. *Circulation* 1993;88:358–363.

98 Kukielka GL, Hawkins HK, Michael L, et al. Regulation of intercellular adhesion molecule-1 (ICAM-1) in ischemic and reperfused canine myocardium. *J Clin Invest* 1993;92:1504–1516.

99 Blann AD, Amiral J, McCollum CN. Circulating endothelial cell/leucocyte adhesion molecules in ischaemic heart disease. *Br J Haematol* 1996; 95: 263–265.

100 Shyu KG, Chang H, Lin CC, et al. Circulating intercellular adhesion molecule-1 and E-selectin in patients with acute coronary syndrome. *Chest* 1996;109: 1627–1630.

101 Haught WH, Mansour M, Rothlein R, et al. Alterations in circulating intercellular adhesion molecule-1 and L-selectin: further evidence for chronic inflammation in ischemic heart disease. *Am Heart J* 1996;132:1–8.

102 Ott I, Neumann FJ, Gawaz M, et al. Increased neutrophil-platelet adhesion in patients with unstable angina. *Circulation* 1996;94:1239–1246.

103 Larsen E, Palabrica T, Sajer S, et al. PADGEM-dependent adhesion of platelets to monocytes and neutrophils is mediated by a lineage-specific carbohydrate, LNF III (CD15). *Cell* 1990;63:467–474.

104 Dore M, Simon SI, Hughes BJ, et al. P-selectin- and CD18-mediated recruitment of canine neutrophils under conditions of shear stress. *Vet Pathol* 1995; 32:258–268.

105 Gawaz MP, Loftus JC, Bajt ML, et al. Ligand bridging mediates integrin alpha IIb beta 3 (platelet GPIIB-IIIA) dependent homotypic and heterotypic cell–cell interactions. *J Clin Invest* 1991;88:1128–1134.

106 Spangenberg P, Redlich H, Bergmann I, et al. The platelet glycoprotein IIb/IIIa complex is involved in the adhesion of activated platelets to leukocytes. *Thromb Haemostasis* 1993;70:514–521.

107 Ikeda H, Takajo Y, Ichiki K, et al. Increased soluble form of P-selectin in patients with unstable angina. *Circulation* 1995;92:1693–1696.

108 Nagata K, Tsuji T, Todoroki N, et al. Activated platelets induce superoxide anion release by monocytes and neutrophils through P-selectin (CD62). *J Immunol* 1993;151:3267–3273.

109 Celi A, Pellegrini G, Lorenzet R, et al. P-selectin induces the expression of tissue factor on monocytes. *Proc Natl Acad Sci USA* 1994;91:8767–8771.

110 Gamble JR, Skinner MP, Berndt MC, et al. Prevention of activated neutrophil adhesion to endothelium by soluble adhesion protein GMP140. *Science* 1990;249:414–417.

111 Wong CS, Gamble JR, Skinner MP, et al. Adhesion protein GMP140 inhibits superoxide anion release by human neutrophils. *Proc Natl Acad Sci USA* 1991; 88:2397–2401.

112 Libby P, Schwartz D, Brogi E, et al. A cascade model for restenosis: a special case of atherosclerosis progression. *Circulation* 1992;86(Suppl III):47–52.

113 Yasukawa H, Imaizumi T, Matsuoka H, et al. Inhibition of intimal hyperplasia after balloon injury by antibodies to intercellular adhesion molecule-1 and lymphocyte function-associated antigen-1. *Circulation* 1997;95: 1515–1522.

114 Tanaka H, Suzuki A, Schwartz D, et al. Activation of smooth muscle and endothelial cells following balloon injury. *Ann NY Acad Sci* 1995;748:526–529.

115 Belch JJ, Shaw JW, Kirk G, et al. The white blood cell adhesion molecule E-selectin predicts restenosis in patients with intermittent claudication undergoing percutaneous transluminal angioplasty. *Circulation* 1997;95:2027–2031.

116 Barron MK, Lake RS, Buda AJ, et al. Intimal hyperplasia after balloon injury is attenuated by blocking selectins. *Circulation* 1997;96:3587–3592.

117 Mulvihill NT, Foley JB, Walsh MA, et al. Relationship between intracoronary and peripheral expression of soluble cell adhesion molecules. *Int J Cardiol* 2001;77:223–229.

118 Atalar E, Aytemir K, Haznedaroglu I, et al. Platelet and leukocyte deactivation after intracoronary stent placement in patients receiving combined antiplatelet therapy. *Clin Appl Thromb Hemost* 2001;7:116–121.

119 Kozuka K, Kohriyama T, Nomura E, et al. Endothelial markers and adhesion molecules in acute ischemic stroke – sequential change and differences in stroke subtype. *Atherosclerosis* 2002;161:161–168.

120 Blann A, Kumar P, Krupinski J, et al. Soluble intercellular adhesion molecule-1, E-selectin, vascular cell adhesion molecule-1 and von Willebrand factor in stroke. *Blood Coagul Fibrinol* 1999;10:277–284.

121 Gianetti J, De Caterina M, De Cristofaro T, et al. Intravenous prostaglandin E1 reduces soluble vascular cell adhesion molecule-1 in peripheral arterial obstructive disease. *Am Heart J* 2001;142:733–739.

122 Pradhan AD, Rifai N, Ridker PM. Soluble intercellular adhesion molecule-1, soluble vascular adhesion molecule-1, and the development of symptomatic peripheral arterial disease in men. *Circulation* 2002;106:820–825.

123 Mossner R, Fassbender K, Kuhnen J, et al. Circulating L-selectin in multiple sclerosis patients with active, gadolinium-enhancing brain plaques. *J Neuroimmunol* 1996;65:61–65.

124 Sudhoff T, Wehmeier A, Kliche KO, et al. Levels of circulating endothelial adhesion molecules (sE-selectin and sVCAM-1) in adult patients with acute leukemia. *Leukemia* 1996;10:682–686.

125 Coll-Vinent B, Grau JM, Lopez-Soto A, et al. Circulating soluble adhesion molecules in patients with classical polyarteritis nodosa. *Br J Rheumatol* 1997;36:1178–1183.

126 Gattegno L, Bentata-Peyssare M, Gronowski S, et al. Elevated concentrations of circulating intercellular adhesion molecule 1 (ICAM-1) and of vascular cell adhesion molecule 1 (VCAM-1) in HIV-1 infection. *Cell Adhes Commun* 1995;3:179–185.

127 Wenisch C, Myskiw D, Gessl A, et al. Circulating selectins, intercellular adhesion molecule-1, and vascular cell adhesion molecule-1 in hyperthyroidism. *J Clin Endocrinol Metab* 1995;80:2122–2126.

128 Kaplanski G, Farnarier C, Payan MJ, et al. Increased levels of soluble adhesion molecules in the serum of patients with hepatitis C. Correlation with cytokine concentrations and liver inflammation and fibrosis. *Digest Dis Sci* 1997;42:2277–2284.

129 Marui A, Fukuda Y, Koyama Y, et al. Serum levels of soluble intercellular adhesion molecule-1 and soluble vascular cell adhesion molecule-1 in liver disease, and their changes by treatment with interferon. *J Int Med Res* 1996;24:258–265.

130 Ashitani J, Mukae H, Ihiboshi H, et al. [Serum-soluble adhesion molecules in patients with idiopathic pulmonary fibrosis and acute respiratory distress syndrome]. *Nihon Kyobu Shikkan Gakkai Zasshi* 1997;35:942–947.

131 Shreeniwas R, Schulman LL, Narasimhan M, et al. Adhesion molecules (E-selectin and ICAM-1) in pulmonary allograft rejection. *Chest* 1996;110:1143–1149.

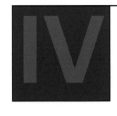

PART IV
Endothelium-directed prevention and therapy

CHAPTER 19

Hormone replacement therapy and cardiovascular disease

Tommaso Simoncini, MD, PhD

Cardiovascular risk in women before and after the menopause

Cardiovascular disease (CVD) represents the leading cause of morbidity and mortality in Western countries in women [1]. A rapid increase in CVD risk can be observed in the first years after the menopause, when the relative hazard is heightened by the combined actions of aging and ovarian hormones depletion. This identifies the climacteric as a gender-specific condition of increased CVD risk, so much so that menopause has been proposed as an independent cardiovascular risk factor [2]. Data from the *European Cardiovascular Disease Statistics* indicate that in the European Union about 46% of women die due to CVD, vs 38% of men [3]. Similar data are found in the USA [1]. The exact figures of the burden of CVD with aging and with the menopausal transition can be estimated as follows: before age 65 CVD causes 25% of deaths in men and only 18% of deaths in women, while if the population between 65 and 75 is also included in the estimate, the percentages become 31% of men's deaths and 29% of females' deaths caused by CVD [1]. Coronary heart disease alone is the first reason of death in women of less than 75 years, explaining 12% of deaths vs 8% of deaths due to breast cancer, the most common female cancer in this age range [1].

CVD has different symptoms and prognosis in women as compared to men, resulting in different morbidity and mortality rates. The *Global Use of Strategies to Open Occluded Coronary Arteries in Acute Coronary Syndromes Trial* (GUSTO IIb) indicates that women admitted to hospital due to acute coronary syndromes are older than men and have significantly higher rates of diabetes, hypertension, and prior heart failure [4]. At the same time, they have significantly lower rates of prior myocardial infarction (MI) and are less likely ever to have smoked [4]. ECG signs of myocardial ischemia are frequently different in the two sexes, and women are more likely to have unstable angina and acute coronary syndromes in the absence of severe coronary stenosis at coronary angiography as opposed to men [4]. Women have also higher rates of complications after acute coronary syndromes and are more likely to die after hospital admission than men [4]. Indeed a retrospective analysis on a large population from the *National Registry for Myocardial Infarction*, in the USA, indicates that women have an in-hospital mortality rate of 16.7%, compared to 11.5% for men, with the difference being maximal for the younger population (less than 70 years) [5].

Effects of the climacteric transition on cardiovascular risk

The climacteric transition is associated with a variety of metabolic modifications that follow the failure of ovarian hormonal synthesis, many of which have an impact on cardiovascular risk.

The lipid profile is considerably worsened in postmenopausal women as compared to fertile ones. Total cholesterol concentration increases significantly, mainly due to increased levels of low-density lipoprotein cholesterol (LDL-C) and very low-density lipoprotein cholesterol (VLDL-C) [6]. Lipoprotein(a) (Lp(a)) also shows an upward trend, as well as serum triglycerides [6]. At the same time, high-density lipoprotein cholesterol (HDL-C) is generally decreased after the menopause, although the extent of this change is variable [6]. These modifications are largely due to the climacteric hormonal milieu, but other factors have a significant influence, such as the increased body weight and fat/lean body mass ratio, as well as the change of the body fat toward an android distribution [6].

The postmenopausal woman is also characterized by a different hemostatic/fibrinolytic profile as compared to the fertile years, with opposing increases of procoagulant factors (such as factor VII or fibrinogen) as well as of profibrynolitic molecules (such as antithrombin III and plasminogen) [6]. Peripheral insulin sensitivity progressively decreases during the climacterium, due to the changes in the body composition and body fat distribution [6]. This is particularly true in overweight women, but *de novo* reduced carbohydrate tolerance is also seen in nonobese, healthy postmenopausal women [6].

Finally, the menopause is accompanied by a decreased vascular reactivity, as shown by decreased prostacyclin and nitric oxide (NO) and increased endothelin production, leading to impaired endothelium-dependent vasodilation [6]. Increases in diastolic and, mostly, systolic blood pressure are recorded early in the climacterium, which add to the age-related changes [6]. The increase in blood pressure seems to be associated with the changes in body composition and is not clearly linked to sex steroid depletion [6].

The relevance of the modifications of CVD risk factors seen after the menopause may be different than estimated in men. Indeed, there is evidence that CVD risk factors have a gender-specific weight. For instance, while increases in LDL-C are strongly associated with increased cardiovascular risk in men, low HDL and raised triglycerides seem to better estimators of risk in women [6].

Sex steroid hormones and the cardiovascular system

The epidemiological association between impaired ovarian function and increased risk of cardiovascular events led several years ago to the hypothesis of a protective role of sex steroid hormones on the cardiovascular system. Since then, a multitude of studies have been performed, unveiling a series of possible targets for sex hormones at the cardiovascular level.

Estrogen receptors in the cardiovascular system

Estrogen actions are exerted through specific receptors, that can act as transcription factors, regulating gene expression, or can alternatively induce rapid signaling independently by the transcription machinery [7]. The presence and action of these receptors in the human cardiovascular system sets the basis for the gender-related differences in the function and dysfunction of vascular cells [8].

Currently, two subtypes of the human estrogen receptor (ER) have been identified, ERα [9] and ERβ [10]. ERα is expressed in the human vasculature, both in endothelial and in smooth muscle cells (SMC) [11]. ERβ distribution in vascular tissues is less characterized, but human endothelial cells synthesize ERβ, and blood vessels of non-human primates, mice, and rats [11] express this receptor subtype as well. In vascular tissues, ERα seems to be predominant in the endothelial cell population, while ERβ is mainly expressed by SMC and pericytes [12,13]. In the heart, both ERα and ERβ are expressed [14]. The two receptor isoforms seem to have different roles at the vascular level. In fact, ERα-deficient mice are not protected by estrogen treatment from balloon vascular injury [15], while ERβ knockouts are still protected [16]. In agreement with the suggested role for ERα in mediating anti-atherogenic actions, a male patient carrying a mutated ERα showed early atherosclerotic degeneration [17,18].

Sex steroids and atherosclerosis

Sex steroids regulate vessel wall function, controlling the proliferation, survival and migration of endothelial, smooth muscle, stromal cells, and leukocytes [11,19]. Endothelial cell proliferation after injury is enhanced by estrogens [11,19] and the apoptotic process of endothelial cells is blocked by female sex steroids [20], as well. In agreement, estrogen treatment has anti-atherogenic effects *in vivo* [21,22].

Atherosclerosis shares several analogies with inflammatory processes [22]. Various atherogenic stimuli, such as modified LDL, oxidative free radicals, homocysteine, and infectious agents, lead to endothelial dysfunction [22] and promote monocyte adhesion and accumulation to the vessel wall [23]. Estrogens have anti-inflammatory effects on the vascular endothelium, where they reduce endothelial leukocyte adhesion molecule expression induced by inflammatory cytokines [23], therefore inhibiting leukocyte adhesion to endothelial cells. This direct anti-inflammatory action is shared also by some selective estrogen receptor modulators (SERMs), such as raloxifene [24] and by synthetic steroids like tibolone [25].

Sex steroids and vascular tone

Some of the actions exerted by estrogens on the vessel wall are induced via transcriptional regulation of target genes, but others are independent by such mechanisms, and have thus been indicated as "non-genomic." One of these actions is vasodilation, which occurs in a matter of seconds to minutes [26]. This acute effect results from the regulation of ion fluxes and of vasoactive molecules on endothelial and SMC. Regulation of NO synthesis is a major target of estrogens at the endothelial level. Estrogen-induced endothelium-dependent vasodilation *in vivo* depends on NO production, and estrogens regulate NO release by several means [27]. The principal mechanism is the rapid activation of the endothelial nitric oxide synthase (eNOS). ERα is involved in this process, which is in part due to activation of MAP kinases (MAPK) [7]. Additionally, ERα rapidly activates eNOS through the PI3K/Akt pathway [7,27–29]. Another possible mechanism of regulation of eNOS by estrogens may involve the chaperone protein heat shock protein 90 (Hsp90), which dissociates from ER upon binding with the ligand. Indeed, Hsp90 interacts with eNOS and regulates its enzymatic activity [30]. Additional mechanisms for non-genomic estrogen-induced vasodilation are the rapid regulation of Ca^{++} mobilization and the control of cell membrane K^+ channels [31] in vascular SMC, that produces vessel relaxation. The vasodilatory effects of estrogens have been also found to be shared by progesterone [31].

Beyond being rapidly regulated, eNOS is also transcriptionally induced by estrogens [27]. Other genes involved in vascular tone regulation are also under estrogen control, and these include cyclooxygenase-1, prostaglandin H synthase and endothelin-1 [6]. These transcriptional effects, may be important for the improvement of vascular reactivity seen in

postmenopausal women receiving estrogen treatment for long time [6].

Hormone replacement therapy and CVD

Since the early 1990s, a number of studies have been performed with the aim of understanding the clinical effects of re-establishing pre-menopausal estrogen levels during the climacterium. However, despite the enormous amount of data available nowadays, this topic remains one of the more controversial in modern medicine, and deserves a thorough discussion.

Hormone replacement therapy and markers of cardiovascular risk

While lipid profile worsens after the menopause, administration of hormone replacement therapy (HRT) is associated with improved lipid profile. The various hormones and routes of administration used have different effects. Oral estrogens, alone or combined with progestins, reduce total and LDL-C, slightly increasing HDL-C and triglycerides, while transdermal estrogens have a lesser impact on lipid profile [6]. Carbohydrate metabolism is improved during estrogen replacement therapies. Peripheral insulin sensitivity is enhanced in women taking estrogens, but the addition of a progestin blunts this action [6]. However, the data are limited, and the type, the dose and the route of administration of the progestin may be important to overcome this negative effect. In addition, there is evidence that HRTs have positive effects in postmenopausal women with type 2 diabetes, improving glucose tolerance and cholesterol levels [32,33].

HRTs have complex effects on hemostasis, the overall balance being neutral or even favorable, with a profibrynolitic shift [34]. The users of HRT studied by the *Atherosclerosis Risk in Communities (ARIC) Study* showed marked reductions of fibrinogen and antithrombin III levels, together with increases of factor VII, and protein C concentrations [35]. Moreover, the administration of combined estro-progestin therapy induces a 50% decrease of plasminogen activator inhibitor-1 (PAI-1) circulating levels, with an activation of fibrinolysis [6]. However, the impact of hormone replacement on hemostasis is also largely dependent on the way of administration, and sex steroids are virtually neutral on hemostatic parameters when given transdermally [36–38].

HRT is neutral on blood pressure in postmenopausal women [6], but hormone therapies counteract the increase in body weight and the shift toward an android distribution of body fat in climacteric women [6]. HRT actions on body weight may thus help prevent obesity-related diseases, such as glucose intolerance, high blood pressure, and CVD. Vascular reactivity is improved in postmenopausal women receiving estrogens. Both the peripheral as well as the coronary districts are sensitive to sex steroids, and respond to estrogens with rapid endothelium-dependent vasodilation [39,40].

In agreement with *in vitro* and animal studies, the literature indicates that HRTs have an impact on markers of vascular inflammation [41–44]. Indeed, clinical studies show that estrogen treatments in postmenopausal women [45] lower the levels of soluble endothelial adhesion molecules in the bloodstream. Recent studies assessed that circulating adhesion molecule level is a marker of vascular atherosclerotic disease extension [46] as well as a predictor of future cardiovascular events [47]. While this would represent an anti-atherogenic action, HRT has been indicated to be pro-inflammatory due to the recorded increases in circulating levels of C-reactive protein (CRP) [48,49]. Elevated baseline CRP levels are associated with increased cardiovascular risk [47], but there is no evidence that slight CRP increases starting from normal values indicate a worsened cardiovascular prognosis [50]. In addition, HRT is associated with increases of CRP, but not of interleukin-6 (IL-6), which controls CRP production in the liver [51], this would suggest that increased CRP concentrations may not indicate a pro-inflammatory action on the vessels of HRT.

HRT and CVD: major clinical trials

A variety of high-quality observational studies have been performed in the past, indicating that users of HRT are significantly protected from cardiovascular events. The follow-up of the *Nurses' Health Study* cohort indicates a reduction in the incidence of major coronary events between 40% and 60% in postmenopausal women receiving estrogens alone or with added progestins as compared to controls [52,53]. The estimated benefit lasts up to 4–5 years after the cessation of the therapy. Moreover, women who use HRT have a reduced risk of dying for any cause, and the mortality reduction is maximal in those at higher risk for cardiovascular events [52,53]. An extensive meta-analysis using only high-quality trials recently provided a similar estimate of the extent of cardiovascular protection in postmenopausal women receiving HRT [54]. Despite these data, the clinical value of HRTs for the prevention of CVD in postmenopausal women is not definitely ascertained, and doubts have been shed on this issue after the recent publication of large prospective interventional trials.

The first to be published has been the *Heart and Estrogen/Progestin Replacement Study* (HERS) [55]. The HERS is a secondary prevention trial that enrolled 2763 postmenopausal women with established coronary artery disease. After the qualifying coronary event, patients were initiated on placebo or conjugated equine estrogens (CEE 0.625 mg/day) combined with medroxyprogesterone acetate (MPA 2.5 mg/day) in a continuous/combined fashion, for a median of 4.1 years. The main result of the HERS trial was that the initiation of HRT did not prevent the recurrence of coronary events. Available results show that the women enrolled in the active treatment arm had an excess of death in the first year after the initiation of HRT, but showed thereafter a progressive reduction of cardiovascular events incidence over the next 4 years, with a significant trend [55]. Although the HERS has raised a hot public and scientific debate, the clinical relevance of this trial is limited. The mean age of the HERS participants was advanced (67 years), there was a high prevalence of overweight women, and hypertension, dyslipidemia, and diabetes were very common. In current clinical practice, it is extremely uncommon to put such women in the late menopause with a recent heart attack on a full-dose HRT, such as the one used in HERS. Indeed, a retrospective study conducted in an Italian menopause clinic showed that, by checking 1459 consecutive women, only 0.4% matched the entry criteria of HERS [56]. Additionally, it is well possible that the use of such a high dose of CEE may have caused the excess of cardiovascular events seen in the first year due to thrombosis, that were more common in the active treatment group [55].

The results of the *Estrogen Replacement and Atherosclerosis* (ERA) trial [57] support the HERS data. The ERA study analyzed, in a prospective and randomized fashion, a cohort of 309 women with angiographically determined coronary lesions. The participants were given placebo or CEE alone or in association with MPA, at the same dose as in the HERS. The cohort was reevaluated with coronary angiography after 3 years, with the primary aim of determining the evolution of coronary plaques. At the follow-up angiography, the plaques were not significantly evolved in any arm, and the women receiving HRT did not have an advantage compared with their controls [57].

These landmark studies have led to the hurried conclusion that sex steroid hormones have no role in the treatment of acute coronary syndromes or in the prevention of the development of established atherosclerosis. Such conclusion leaves the relevant issue of understanding whether estrogens may instead protect normal vessels from the development of atherosclerosis and eventually reduce the incidence of heart disease in healthy patients in the long term [58], as suggested by the wealth of basic and animal studies, unanswered.

HRT and CVD: primary prevention trials

Two large interventional trials in the setting of primary prevention of CVD with HRT have been attempted in the recent past: the *Women's Health Initiative* (WHI) trial in the USA and the *Women's International Study of long Duration Oestrogen after Menopause* (WISDOM) in Europe. However, only the first trial has been published, as the latter has been interrupted after the publication of the results of the WHI [59].

The WHI was planned in the early 1990s under the auspices of the US National Institute of Health, and was intended to determine the impact of different strategies of intervention in postmenopausal women on the future incidence of CVD, osteoporosis and bone fractures, mammary and colon cancer (in addition to other major endpoints). Between 1993 and 1998, the WHI enrolled 161,809 postmenopausal women aged 50–79, who were randomized to five different intervention arms (placebo, CEE 0.625 mg/die + MPA 2.5 mg/die, CEE 0.625 mg/die, vitamin D + calcium, diet + physical exercise). In March 2002 the CEE + MPA arm was prematurely interrupted, based on the evaluation of a global risk/benefit index used by

the trial's Drug Safety Monitoring Board [60]. The premature discontinuation of the CEE + MPA arm was motivated by an apparent increase of breast cancer in the treated women that exceeded the boundaries established at the beginning of the trial, therefore indicating that women receiving CEE + MPA were exposed to an unfavorable risk/benefit balance. From the cardiovascular standpoint, women receiving hormone replacement tended to develop more coronary heart disease as compared with their controls, but the trend was not significant [61]. In agreement with previous observations from the *Nurses' Health Study* as well as from the HERS trial, the likelihood of having a coronary event during hormone administration decreased with time [61], which may indicate either that only a subset of women can benefit from hormone replacement, and that the beneficial effects might become visible only after a sufficient length of exposure.

More recently, the arm of the WHI trial investigating the effects of unopposed estrogen on postmenopausal women without a uterus has been published, and the results indicate striking differences compared with the CEE + MPA arm [62]. Indeed, while overall no excess of coronary heart disease has been found in the intervention group, a trend toward a protective effect of estrogen administration has been found in younger postmenopausal women [62], providing an indication that the addition of MPA to CEE might hamper the positive effects of estrogens on the vessels. Basic studies on the effects of different progestogenic compounds on endothelial cells confirm the existence of differences in the signaling events elicited by natural progesterone compared with synthetic progestins, which may well have an impact on vascular function [63].

After years during which the public perception on the effects of hormonal replacement after the menopause had been entirely negative, and after the endorsement of more restrictive guidelines and limitations for the use of these therapies in postmenopausal individuals by scientific societies and health authorities, this publication has reopened the debate, and new and more careful analyses are currently ongoing with the aim of reconciling the apparent discrepancy between the WHI results and previous observational trials [64].

Indeed, as the previous secondary prevention trials, the WHI study is biased by important pitfalls that severely limit its application in clinical practice. Indeed, the WHI cannot be strictly considered a primary prevention trial, since the mean age at the enrollment in the CEE + MPA arm was 63.3 years, and was 63.6 years in the CEE-only arm [60,62]. This means that the WHI population does not represent the average woman who is generally referred to HRT, i.e., the early, healthy postmenopausal woman [56]. Moreover, while the study was meant to be a primary prevention trial, the participating women turned out to be largely unhealthy at the enrollment. Indeed, the vast majority of the participants were overweight or overtly obese, hypertensive and hypercholesterolemic, with a large fraction of them being on active pharmacological treatments due to concurrent diseases [60,62]. Therefore, these women cannot be considered free of atherosclerosis at the beginning of the trial, and this makes this population unfit to test the hypothesis that sex steroids may prevent the development of atherosclerosis in non-diseased vessels [65].

Another important issue raised by the large trials on HRT and CVD is the possible role of alternative hormonal regimens and the possible different impact of HRTs in non-US women. Indeed, these large trials have all been performed on women residing in North America, who had been prescribed the most popular combination of estrogen plus progestin on this market, i.e., the continuous–combined combination of CEE and MPA. Although there is no indication that a different regimen may have produced different effects, there is a wealth of evidence that the biological effects of oral CEE are different from those of transdermal estradiol, and, mostly, that the different synthetic progestins have very distinct characteristics [63]. Besides opening a new debate on the best estrogen or progestin for the long-term postmenopausal HRT, these trial are also pushing the discussion on the role of other molecules, such as SERMs or synthetic tissue-specific steroids, as possible (and perhaps safer) alternatives to standard HRTs.

HRT and cardiovascular risk: future perspectives to prevent CVD

Given the apparent presence of subpopulations of women in the clinical trials who develop adverse events after initiation of HRT, a great effort has recently been dedicated to the identification of women at higher risk, and a particular attention has been given to the thrombotic predisposition.

A population-based, case–control study conducted in Seattle, enrolling 232 postmenopausal women with a previous MI and 723 control women without previous MI, evaluated the risk of a first nonfatal MI based on current use of HRT and the presence or absence of prothrombotic mutations such as the coagulation factor V Leiden and prothrombin 20210 G→A variants [66]. Among hypertensive women, the prothrombin variant was a risk factor for MI, and there was also a significant interaction between the use of HRT and the presence of the prothrombin variant on the risk of MI. Indeed, compared with non-users of HRT with wild-type genotype, women who were current users and who had the prothrombin variant had a nearly 11-fold increase in the risk of a nonfatal MI [66]. On the opposite, no interaction was found for factor V Leiden in either hypertensive or non-hypertensive women [66]. However, a case–control study conducted among women with established coronary disease enrolled in the HERS and in the ERA trials showed that the Leiden mutation was present in 16.7% women with venous thromboembolism (VTE) as compared with only 6.3% controls [67]. In women without the factor V Leiden mutation, risk associated with HRT use was significantly increased (OR 3.7), but in women with the Leiden mutation, the estimated risk associated with HRT was increased nearly 6-fold [67]. The OR for women with the Leiden mutation who were assigned to HRT compared with wild-type women assigned to placebo was 14.1, and the estimated absolute incidence of VTE was 15.4/1000 per year compared with 2.0/1000 per year in women without the mutation who were taking a placebo [67]. If these findings will be confirmed in other studies, the screening for the prothrombin 20210 G→A variant, factor V Leiden, as well as for other markers of thrombotic risk may permit a better assessment of the risks and benefits associated with HRT in postmenopausal women.

Additional indications for the relevance of the genetic asset for the responses to HRT come from studies investigating the differential responses to HRT depending on different ERα polymorphisms.

Indeed, in a postmenopausal population of women with established coronary artery disease, nearly 20% of the women who had the IVS1-401 C/C genotype had an increase in the HDL-C level with HRT that was more than twice the increase observed in the other women [68,69]. This effect was specific for changes in the HDL subfraction 3 (HDL3), and similar patterns of response were observed for 3 other highly linked ERα intron 1 polymorphisms [68,69]. The pattern of increased response of HDL-C in women with the IVS1-401 C/C genotype was evident in both the women receiving estrogens and those receiving estrogens plus progestins [68,69]. In addition, women with the ERα IVS1-401 C/C genotype receiving HRT had nearly a 2-fold greater reduction in E-selectin compared with C/T or T/T women [68,69], while there was no augmentation of the HRT-associated increase in CRP among the C/C women compared with C/T or T/T women [68,69]. The full characterization of the interaction between the genetic status and the outcome of hormone administration seems therefore to be important, and may open a new avenue of investigations that will hopefully allow to select women who will benefit more from the cardiovascular effects of HRT, and to eventually exclude others who may be at increased risk of complications.

HRT and CVD: recent advances

In addition to the various issues discussed, evidence is growing that the cardioprotective effects of hormonal replacement may be dependent on its use during a very specific "window of opportunity." Particularly, it seems both biologically conceivable and consistent with the available clinical evidence that the alleged positive effects of sex steroids is limited to the perimenopausal period, and that when their administration is initiated later in life this therapy could instead be either ineffective or even associated with adverse effects. This concept is not based solely on a biological rationale, but also on the re-analysis of the effects of hormonal therapies on the younger subgroups of women in the large clinical trials. Recent data from the *Nurses' Health Study* confirms that the timing of the initiation of hormonal replacement is critical for obtaining heart protection. Indeed, in women that begin this therapy at the time of their menopause, a 45%

reduction of coronary events is seen, while no effects are seen in women that start later in life or with physical and demographic characteristics similar to those of the women enrolled in the WHI trial [70]. A similar re-analysis has been announced on the WHI cohorts, but is not yet published at this time. When available, these results may have a major impact on clinical practice, that may reopen the debate on the opportunity to use steroid hormones to prevent heart disease in young, healthy postmenopausal women [64].

Alternatives to standard HRTs

In the search for molecules with a different and possibly more favorable profile for the long-term hormonal treatment of women after the menopause, the pharmacological research in the past 15 years has led to the identification of compounds which modulate the receptors for estrogens in new and different ways. The SERMs and the tissue-specific steroid tibolone are examples of these alternative possibilities.

SERMs act through binding to ERα and β and inducing specific conformational shifts, different from the ones induced by 17β-estradiol [71]. Tibolone is a synthetic steroid i.e., rapidly metabolized to a 3α-OH and a 3β-OH metabolite, characterized by high estrogen agonistic activity, and to a Δ^4-isomer, with mixed progestogenic and androgenic action [72]. Both SERMs and tibolone, upon binding to estrogen receptors, activate genomic as well as non-genomic signaling machineries in vascular cells [19,25,73,74].

Among these molecules, the SERM raloxifene is perhaps the best characterized in relation to cardiovascular actions. The *Multiple Outcomes of Raloxifene Evaluation* (MORE) is a randomized, placebo-controlled trial, started in 1994 and enrolling 7705 postmenopausal women, who were followed for 36 months, after which a significant reduction of vertebral fractures was found in women receiving raloxifene compared with controls [75]. Among the secondary endpoints evaluated, the study also indicated a positive effect for the prevention of cardiovascular events [76]. The administration of raloxifene to postmenopausal women is associated with an improvement of the lipid profile and of hemostatic parameters [77]. Recent data also indicate that raloxifene induces a reduction of serum homocysteine levels [78]. Moreover, no increases in circulating concentrations of CRP are found during raloxifene administration, as opposed to what is found during standard HRTs [78].

Like natural estrogens, SERMs exert direct actions on the vascular wall [19]. *In vitro* studies indicate that SERMs decrease the expression of endothelial leukocyte adhesion molecules [24] and stimulate the synthesis and release of NO in endothelial cells [73]. Similar to 17β-estradiol, NO induction is due to rapid activation of eNOS [74], which requires an ER-dependent recruitment of the MAPK and PI3K/Akt pathways. The activation of these non-genomic pathways by SERMs may be pathophysiologically important, since, through the activation of these pathways, estrogens exert vascular anti-inflammatory effects *in vivo* [28] and glucocorticoids reduce the area of ischemia in an animal model of MI [79]. In agreement, the administration of raloxifene to ovariectomized rabbits prevents aortic cholesterol accumulation and the worsening of arterial dilatory function due to hormonal deprivation [80]. The vasodilatory actions of raloxifene have been confirmed in *ex vivo* experiments using isolated vessel rings from rabbits [81], where raloxifene actions depend on NO release.

While the available data on SERMs indicate that these molecules are a safe alternative to standard HRTs for the long-term treatment of postmenopausal women, the evidence on the long-term effects on the cardiovascular system is missing, and specific trials are needed to address this issue. In particular, important information will derive from the ongoing *Raloxifene Use for The Heart* (RUTH) trial. RUTH is a prospective, double-blind, randomized study enrolling 10,101 women at high cardiovascular risk, with a programmed duration of 5 years. This trial will soon provide evidence on the impact of raloxifene administration after the menopause on the incidence of major cardiovascular events and of breast cancer.

Conclusions

HRTs are effective tools for the prevention of the acute and long-term complications of the climacterium. Although for many years hormone replacement after the menopause has been considered an effective treatment to decrease the incidence of CVD, this indication is now under close scrutiny, and certainly more caution is required. While the recent clinical studies apparently do not support such a role for HRTs in CVD prevention, the vast evidence coming from basic research as well as from previous observational trials should not be quickly dismissed and disregarded. On the contrary, these discrepancies should foster new research. In addition, clinical evidence has been recently presented indicating that steroid hormones may indeed protect from CVD provided that they are given at the right time and in the appropriate formulations. Understanding how to select the individuals who likely benefit from HRT, identifying those who may develop complications, as well as finding and using new molecules are important avenues for future research and, eventually, for a better treatment of these women.

References

1 Thom T, Haase N, Rosamond W, et al. Heart disease and stroke statistics – 2006 update. A Report From the American Heart Association Statistics Committee and Stroke Statistics Subcommittee. *Circulation* 2006.

2 Braunwald E. Shattuck lecture – cardiovascular medicine at the turn of the millennium: triumphs, concerns, and opportunities. *N Engl J Med* 1997;337:1360–1369.

3 Petersen S, Peto V, Scarborough P, et al. for the British Heart Foundation Health Promotion Research Group. Coronary heart disease statistics 2005 edition. In: British Heart Foundation, ed. Coronary Heart Disease Statistics. Oxford: British Heart Foundation Health Promotion Research Group, Department of Public Health, University of Oxford; 2005.

4 Hochman JS, Tamis JE, Thompson TD, et al. Sex, clinical presentation, and outcome in patients with acute coronary syndromes. Global Use of Strategies to Open Occluded Coronary Arteries in Acute Coronary Syndromes IIb Investigators. *N Engl J Med* 1999;341:226–232.

5 Vaccarino V, Parsons L, Every NR, et al. Sex-based differences in early mortality after myocardial infarction. National Registry of Myocardial Infarction 2 Participants. *N Engl J Med* 1999;341:217–225.

6 Genazzani AR, Gambacciani M. Cardiovascular disease and hormone replacement therapy. Position Paper from the International Menopause Society Expert Workshop. *Climacteric* 2000;3:233–240.

7 Simoncini T, Genazzani AR. Non-genomic actions of sex steroid hormones. *Eur J Endocrinol* 2003;148:281–292.

8 Mendelsohn ME, Karas RH. Molecular and cellular basis of cardiovascular gender differences. *Science* 2005;308: 1583–1587.

9 Green S, Walter P, Kumar V, et al. Human oestrogen receptor cDNA: sequence, expression and homology to v-erb-A. *Nature* 1986;320:134–139.

10 Mosselman S, Polman J, Dijkema R. ER beta: identification and characterization of a novel human estrogen receptor. *FEBS Lett* 1996;392:49–53.

11 Mendelsohn ME, Karas RH. The protective effects of estrogen on the cardiovascular system. *N Engl J Med* 1999;340:1801–1811.

12 Karas RH, Patterson BL, Mendelsohn ME. Human vascular smooth muscle cells contain functional estrogen receptor. *Circulation* 1994;89:1943–1950.

13 Register TC, Adams MR. Coronary artery and cultured aortic smooth muscle cells express mRNA for both the classical estrogen receptor and the newly described estrogen receptor beta. *J Steroid Biochem Mol Biol* 1998; 64:187–191.

14 Grohe C, Kahlert S, Lobbert K, et al. Cardiac myocytes and fibroblasts contain functional estrogen receptors. *FEBS Lett* 1997;416:107–112.

15 Karas RH, Hodgin JB, Kwoun M, et al. Estrogen inhibits the vascular injury response in estrogen receptor beta-deficient female mice. *Proc Natl Acad Sci USA* 1999; 96:15133–15136.

16 Pare G, Krust A, Karas RH, et al. Estrogen receptor-alpha mediates the protective effects of estrogen against vascular injury. *Circ Res* 2002;90:1087–1092.

17 Sudhir K, Chou TM, Chatterjee K, et al. Premature coronary artery disease associated with a disruptive mutation in the estrogen receptor gene in a man. *Circulation* 1997; 96:3774–3777.

18 Sudhir K, Chou TM, Messina LM, et al. Endothelial dysfunction in a man with disruptive mutation in oestrogen-receptor gene. *Lancet* 1997;349:1146–1147.

19 Simoncini T, Genazzani AR. Direct vascular effects of estrogens and selective estrogen receptor modulators. *Curr Opin Obstet Gynecol* 2000;12:181–187.

20 Adams MR, Kaplan JR, Manuck SB, et al. Inhibition of coronary artery atherosclerosis by 17-beta estradiol in ovariectomized monkeys. Lack of an effect of added progesterone. *Arteriosclerosis* 1990;10:1051–1057.

21 Arnal JF, Gourdy P, Elhage R, et al. Estrogens and atherosclerosis. *Eur J Endocrinol* 2004;150:113–117.

22 Hansson GK. Inflammation, atherosclerosis, and coronary artery disease. *N Engl J Med* 2005;352:1685–1695.

23 Simoncini T, Maffei S, Basta G, et al. Estrogens and glucocorticoids inhibit endothelial vascular cell adhesion molecule-1 expression by different transcriptional mechanisms. *Circ Res* 2000;87:19–25.

24 Simoncini T, De Caterina R, Genazzani AR. Selective estrogen receptor modulators: different actions on

vascular cell adhesion molecule-1 (VCAM-1) expression in human endothelial cells. *J Clin Endocrinol Metab* 1999; 84:815–818.

25 Simoncini T, Genazzani AR. Tibolone inhibits leukocyte adhesion molecule expression in human endothelial cells. *Mol Cell Endocrinol* 2000;162:87–94.

26 Gilligan DM, Badar DM, Panza JA, et al. Acute vascular effects of estrogen in postmenopausal women. *Circulation* 1994;90:786–791.

27 Chambliss KL, Shaul PW. Estrogen modulation of endothelial nitric oxide synthase. *Endocr Rev* 2002;23: 665–686.

28 Simoncini T, Hafezi-Moghadam A, Brazil DP, et al. Interaction of oestrogen receptor with the regulatory subunit of phosphatidylinositol-3-OH kinase. *Nature* 2000;407:538–541.

29 Simoncini T, Rabkin E, Liao JK. Molecular basis of cell membrane estrogen receptor interaction with phosphatidylinositol 3-kinase in endothelial cells. *Arterioscler Thromb Vasc Biol* 2003;23:198–203.

30 Garcia-Cardena G, Fan R, Shah V, et al. Dynamic activation of endothelial nitric oxide synthase by Hsp90. *Nature* 1998;392:821–824.

31 White MM, Zamudio S, Stevens T, et al. Estrogen, progesterone, and vascular reactivity: potential cellular mechanisms. *Endocr Rev* 1995;16:739–751.

32 Wilson PW. Lower diabetes risk with hormone replacement therapy: an encore for estrogen? *Ann Intern Med* 2003;138:69–70.

33 Bonds DE, Lasser N, Qi L, et al. The effect of conjugated equine oestrogen on diabetes incidence: the Women's Health Initiative randomised trial. *Diabetologia* 2006: 1–10.

34 Koh KK, Mincemoyer R, Bui MN, et al. Effects of hormone-replacement therapy on fibrinolysis in postmenopausal women. *N Engl J Med* 1997;336:683–690.

35 Nabulsi AA, Folsom AR, White A, et al. Association of hormone-replacement therapy with various cardiovascular risk factors in postmenopausal women. The Atherosclerosis Risk in Communities Study Investigators. *N Engl J Med.* 1993;328:1069–1075.

36 Straczek C, Oger E, Yon de Jonage-Canonico MB, et al. for the Estrogen and Thromboembolism Risk (ESTHER) Study Group. Prothrombotic mutations, hormone therapy, and venous thromboembolism among postmenopausal women: impact of the route of estrogen administration. *Circulation* 2005;112:3495–3500.

37 Scarabin PY, Oger E, Plu-Bureau G. Differential association of oral and transdermal oestrogen-replacement therapy with venous thromboembolism risk. *Lancet* 2003;362: 428–432.

38 Straczek C, Alhenc-Gelas M, Aubry ML, et al. Genetic variation at the estrogen receptor alpha locus in relation to venous thromboembolism risk among

postmenopausal women. *J Thromb Haemost* 2005;3: 1535–1537.

39 Rosano GM, Sarrel PM, Poole-Wilson PA, et al. Beneficial effect of oestrogen on exercise-induced myocardial ischaemia in women with coronary artery disease. *Lancet* 1993;342:133–136.

40 Rosano GM, Caixeta AM, Chierchia S, et al. Short-term anti-ischemic effect of 17beta-estradiol in postmenopausal women with coronary artery disease. *Circulation* 1997;96:2837–2841.

41 van Baal WM, Kenemans P, Emeis JJ, et al. Long-term effects of combined hormone replacement therapy on markers of endothelial function and inflammatory activity in healthy postmenopausal women. *Fertil Steril* 1999; 71:663–670.

42 Koh KK, Blum A, Hathaway L, et al. Vascular effects of estrogen and vitamin E therapies in postmenopausal women. *Circulation* 1999;100:1851–1857.

43 Koh KK, Bui MN, Mincemoyer R, et al. Effects of hormone therapy on inflammatory cell adhesion molecules in postmenopausal healthy women. *Am J Cardiol* 1997;80:1505–1507.

44 Scarabin PY, Alhenc-Gelas M, Oger E, et al. Hormone replacement therapy and circulating ICAM-1 in postmenopausal women – a randomised controlled trial. *Thromb Haemost* 1999;81:673–675.

45 Caulin-Glaser T, Farrell WJ, Pfau SE, et al. Modulation of circulating cellular adhesion molecules in postmenopausal women with coronary artery disease. *J Am Coll Cardiol* 1998;31:1555–1560.

46 De Caterina R, Basta G, Lazzerini G, et al. Soluble vascular cell adhesion molecule-1 as a biohumoral correlate of atherosclerosis. *Arterioscler Thromb Vasc Biol* 1997;17: 2646–2654.

47 Ridker PM, Hennekens CH, Roitman-Johnson B, et al. Plasma concentration of soluble intercellular adhesion molecule 1 and risks of future myocardial infarction in apparently healthy men. *Lancet* 1998;351:88–92.

48 Bermudez EA, Rifai N, Buring J, et al. Interrelationships among circulating interleukin-6, C-reactive protein, and traditional cardiovascular risk factors in women. *Arterioscler Thromb Vasc Biol* 2002;22:1668–1673.

49 Lakoski SG, Herrington DM. Effects of hormone therapy on C-reactive protein and IL-6 in postmenopausal women: a review article. *Climacteric* 2005;8:317–326.

50 Pradhan AD, Manson JE, Rossouw JE, et al. Inflammatory biomarkers, hormone replacement therapy, and incident coronary heart disease: prospective analysis from the Women's Health Initiative observational study. *JAMA* 2002;288:980–987.

51 Vitale C, Gebara O, Mercuro G, et al. Value of C-reactive protein levels and IL-6 in predicting events levels in women at increased cardiovascular risk. *Maturitas* 2005; 50:239–246.

52 Grodstein F, Stampfer MJ, Manson J, et al. Postmenopausal estrogen and progestin use and the risk of cardiovascular disease. *N Engl J Med* 1996;335: 453–461.

53 Grodstein F, Stampfer MJ, Colditz GA, et al. Postmenopausal hormone therapy and mortality. *N Engl J Med* 1997;336:1769–1775.

54 Nelson HD. Assessing benefits and harms of hormone replacement therapy: clinical applications. *JAMA* 2002; 288:882–884.

55 Hulley S, Grady D, Bush T, et al. Randomized trial of estrogen plus progestin for secondary prevention of coronary heart disease in postmenopausal women. Heart and Estrogen/Progestin Replacement Study (HERS) Research Group. *JAMA* 1998;280:605–613.

56 Gambacciani M, Rosano G, Monteleone P, et al. Clinical relevance of the HERS trial. *Lancet* 2002;360:641.

57 Herrington DM, Reboussin DM, Brosnihan KB, et al. Effects of estrogen replacement on the progression of coronary-artery atherosclerosis. *N Engl J Med* 2000;343: 522–529.

58 Genazzani AR, Gambacciani M, Simoncini T. Estrogens and women's health: a scary or a fairy tale? *Gynecol Endocrinol* 2004;18:175–178.

59 Vickers M, Meade T, Darbyshire J. WISDOM: history and early demise – was it inevitable? *Climacteric* 2002; 5:317–325.

60 The Writing Group for the Women's Health Initiative Investigators. Risks and benefits of estrogen plus progestin in healthy postmenopausal women: principal results from the Women's Health Initiative randomized controlled trial. *JAMA* 2002;288:321–333.

61 Manson JE, Hsia J, Johnson KC, et al. the Women's Health Initiative Investigators. Estrogen plus progestin and the risk of coronary heart disease. *N Engl J Med* 2003;349:523–534.

62 The Women's Health Initiative Steering Committee. Effects of Conjugated Equine Estrogen in Postmenopausal Women With Hysterectomy: The Women's Health Initiative Randomized Controlled Trial. *JAMA* 2004;291: 1701–1712.

63 Simoncini T, Mannella P, Fornari L, et al. Differential signal transduction of progesterone and medroxyprogesterone acetate in human endothelial cells. *Endocrinology* 2004;145:5745–5756.

64 Mandavilli A. News feature: hormone in the hot seat. *Nat Med* 2006;12:8–9.

65 Grodstein F, Clarkson TB, Manson JE. Understanding the divergent data on postmenopausal hormone therapy. *N Engl J Med* 2003;348:645–650.

66 Psaty BM, Smith NL, Lemaitre RN, et al. Hormone replacement therapy, prothrombotic mutations, and the risk of incident nonfatal myocardial infarction in postmenopausal women. *JAMA* 2001;285:906–913.

67 Herrington DM, Vittinghoff E, Howard TD, et al. Factor V Leiden, hormone replacement therapy, and risk of venous thromboembolic events in women with coronary disease. *Arterioscler Thromb Vasc Biol* 2002;22:1012–1017.

68 Herrington DM, Howard TD, Brosnihan KB, et al. Common estrogen receptor polymorphism augments effects of hormone replacement therapy on E-selectin but not C-reactive protein. *Circulation* 2002;105:1879–1882.

69 Herrington DM, Howard TD, Hawkins GA, et al. Estrogen-receptor polymorphisms and effects of estrogen replacement on high-density lipoprotein cholesterol in women with coronary disease. *N Engl J Med* 2002;346: 967–974.

70 Grodstein F, Manson JE, Stampfer MJ. Hormone therapy and coronary heart disease: the role of time since menopause and age at hormone initiation. *J Women's Health* 2006;15:35–44.

71 Riggs BL, Hartmann LC. Selective estrogen-receptor modulators – mechanisms of action and application to clinical practice. *N Engl J Med* 2003;348:618–629.

72 Kenemans P, Speroff L. Tibolone: clinical recommendations and practical guidelines. A report of the International Tibolone Consensus Group. *Maturitas* 2005;51: 21–28.

73 Simoncini T, Genazzani AR. Raloxifene acutely stimulates nitric oxide release from human endothelial cells via an activation of endothelial nitric oxide synthase. *J Clin Endocrinol Metab* 2000;85:2966–2969.

74 Simoncini T, Genazzani AR, Liao JK. Nongenomic mechanisms of endothelial nitric oxide synthase activation by the selective estrogen receptor modulator raloxifene. *Circulation* 2002;105:1368–1373.

75 Ettinger B, Black DM, Mitlak BH, et al. Reduction of vertebral fracture risk in postmenopausal women with osteoporosis treated with raloxifene: results from a 3-year randomized clinical trial. Multiple Outcomes of Raloxifene Evaluation (MORE) Investigators. *JAMA* 1999;282:637–645.

76 Barrett-Connor E, Grady D, Sashegyi A, et al. Raloxifene and cardiovascular events in osteoporotic postmenopausal women: four-year results from the MORE (Multiple Outcomes of Raloxifene Evaluation) randomized trial. *JAMA* 2002;287:847–857.

77 Delmas PD, Bjarnason NH, Mitlak BH, et al. Effects of raloxifene on bone mineral density, serum cholesterol concentrations, and uterine endometrium in postmenopausal women. *N Engl J Med* 1997;337:1641–1647.

78 Walsh BW, Paul S, Wild RA, et al. The effects of hormone replacement therapy and raloxifene on C-reactive protein and homocysteine in healthy postmenopausal women: a randomized, controlled trial. *J Clin Endocrinol Metab* 2000;85:214–218.

79 Hafezi-Moghadam A, Simoncini T, Yang E, et al. Acute cardiovascular protective effects of corticosteroids are mediated by non-transcriptional activation of endothelial nitric oxide synthase. *Nat Med* 2002;8:473–479.

80 Bjarnason NH, Haarbo J, Byrjalsen I, et al. Raloxifene inhibits aortic accumulation of cholesterol in ovariectomized, cholesterol-fed rabbits. *Circulation* 1997;96: 1964–1969.

81 Figtree GA, Lu Y, Webb CM, et al. Raloxifene acutely relaxes rabbit coronary arteries *in vitro* by an estrogen receptor-dependent and nitric oxide-dependent mechanism. *Circulation* 1999;100:1095–1101.

CHAPTER 20

Anti-atherogenic effects of omega-3 fatty acids

Antonella Zampolli, DBiol, PhD, *Erling Falk,* MD, *&*
Raffaele De Caterina, MD, PhD

Introduction

n-3 (omega-3) (polyunsaturated) fatty acids, mostly eicosapentaenoic acid (EPA) and docosahexaenoic acid (DHA), feature a variety of beneficial effects ranging from fetal development to cancer prevention [1]. However, the original biochemical interest in such compounds was originally spurred by clues suggesting cardiovascular protective effects. Bang and Dyerberg, who first hypothesized an epidemiologic association between dietary consumption of n-3 fatty acids and cardiovascular protection [2,3], identified high consumption of fish and fish oil-derived n-3 fatty acids as the likely explanation for the strikingly low rate of coronary heart disease events reported in the Inuit population [2,3]. Since their initial reports, parallel research has provided further evidence for this cardioprotection and deeper understanding of its underlying mechanisms. Current knowledge suggests that decreased atherogenesis is involved, at least in part, in cardiovascular protection by n-3 fatty acids. This chapter summarizes the evidence for such a claim and describes the mechanisms putatively involved.

Evidence for anti-atherogenic effects of n-3 fatty acids

Effects of n-3 fatty acid in animal models of atherosclerosis

Although extensively documented in humans, the hypotriglyceridemic action of n-3 fatty acid, associated with reduced very-low-density lipoproteins

(VLDL) plasma levels, eludes routine observation in animal models compared to consistent reports of reduced high-density lipoprotein (HDL) cholesterol [4]. Anti-atherogenic effects of n-3 fatty acids in animal models are thus usually not associated with the favorable effects on serum lipids that occur in humans (see below). Despite this n-3 fatty acids lessen the development of atherosclerotic lesions in several animal models, although results have not been unequivocal, likely due to differences between species chosen and variations in study design. n-3 fatty acids were usually supplemented as fish oils. Studies in non-human primates, pigs, rabbits, and mice sought to determine the effect of n-3 fatty acids on atherogenesis or lesion regression. The design of most such studies has been criticized for a variety of reasons. In most studies, fish oil supplementation reached extremely high levels – between 10% and 40% of total energy intake as n-3 fatty acids – while "realistic" values should be 1–2% [4]. Many studies lacked an appropriate control: some simply substituted fish oils for saturated fats, and the control oil in others had a different polyunsaturated/saturated (P/S) ratio, a variable that might influence lesion development [5,6]. Moreover, the choice of endpoint parameters and relative methods in the evaluation of atherosclerosis varied greatly. Different experimental models resulted in different outcomes: in some cases, drastic dietary changes induced atherogenesis, quite different from the pathophysiologic conditions that occur in humans. Ideally, studies should use animal models with inception and progression of atherosclerosis similar to that occurring in humans, and control oil should be carefully chosen [4]. Most experimental studies available in the literature do not meet these criteria.

Studies in non-human primates

Several studies used monkeys to determine the effects of n-3 fatty acid on lipoprotein cholesterol and triglycerides plasma levels [7–10] and on atherosclerosis development [11–13]. Metabolic differences between species and different study designs have made it difficult to compare such studies. Because studies usually substituted n-3 fatty acids for fat in high amounts, experimental results can be attributed either to n-3 fatty acid or the removal of hyperlipidemic (saturated) fatty acids. Monkey studies consistently show decreased levels of plasma HDL cholesterol, an effect often observed in other species [4], but, despite this, the development of atherosclerosis in general appears retarded or diminished [11,12]. Such results were obtained by concomitantly removing saturated fats from the diet and replacing them with high amounts of fish oil, without balancing the saturated/unsaturated ratio. Additionally, studies aimed at demonstrating the effect of alpha-linolenic acid (ALA) on atherogenesis support a protective effect for this specific n-3 fatty acid [14,15]. One regression study that used sunflower oil as a control, supplementing atherogenic and therapeutic diets with a relatively low dose of fish oil (2.5% of total energy intake), resulted in increased levels of cholesterol and phospholipid in the aortic intima and no changes in atherosclerosis [13]. In an *in vivo* baboon model, high doses of fish oil vs olive oil supplementation prevented platelet deposition on a plastic vascular shunt and vascular lesion formation in response to mechanical vascular injury in endarterectomized carotids and uninjured aortas [16]. Recently, in a macaque model, the effect of fish oil on the long-term occlusive tendency of aorto-coronary vein bypass grafts was evaluated and these compounds were found ineffective compared with olive oil [17].

Studies in swine

Pigs have been used widely in studies of lipoprotein metabolism, which appears similar to humans, and also for the study of the effects of a variety of compounds on atherosclerosis, since spontaneous atherogenesis occurs in this species with an early spontaneous beginning. However, native lesion development in pigs is slow, and requires acceleration by high-fat diet, cholesterol, and bile acids supplementation. Although fish oils in swine usually decrease triglycerides and HDL cholesterol [4], their effect on atherosclerosis vary. Mechanically abraded vessels sometimes show significant dose-dependent reductions in the extent of aortic and coronary luminal encroachment, while non-abraded arteries show no progression of atherosclerosis [18–21]. However, one set of studies demonstrated no reduction in aortic lesion area [18 21]. The same studies specifically addressed the question of lesion regression. Following a period of atherosclerosis induced by an atherogenic diet, fish oil supplementation favorably affected atherosclerosis, and regression was more evident with low levels of plasma cholesterol. However, these studies used either no control oil or a control oil with a Polyunsaturated/saturated (P/S) fatty acid ratio that differed from fish oil [22,23]. Compared with a control oil with a matching P/S fatty acid ratio, fish oil increased low-density lipoproteins (LDL), decreased HDL, increased susceptibility of LDL to oxidation, but overall did not induce lesion regression [24,25].

Studies in rabbits

A cholesterol-rich or a casein-based, fat-free diet induces atherosclerosis in rabbits easily and quickly, providing a convenient study model. Watanabe heritable hyperlipidemic rabbits (WHHL), which lack functional native LDL receptors, thereby promoting atherosclerosis resembling one type of human inheritable atherosclerosis, provide a well-established model for atherosclerosis. However, lipoprotein metabolism differs in rabbits and humans. In rabbits, increased dietary cholesterol does not result in elevated LDL, but rather elevates β-VLDL. Thus, changes in lipoprotein levels in rabbits may not be relevant to humans. Studies seeking to verify the effect of n-3 fatty acids in rabbit atherosclerosis models are inconsistent regarding lipoproteins and triglyceride/cholesterol concentrations [4]. More important, however, even results of n-3 fatty acid supplementation on atherosclerosis in this species disagree, and most studies lack an adequate control. Fish oils were found to inhibit atherosclerosis development in cholesterol-fed rabbits [26–28], to enhance lesion formation [29,30], or to have no effect [31,32]. However, fish oils reduced intimal proliferation in arteries following balloon injury [33,34], an effect inversely related to serum cholesterol values and in agreement with data obtained in porcine models [22,35]. Further, vitamin E supplementation apparently enhanced the efficacy of fish oil in rabbits [28].

Initial reports in WHHL rabbits suggested that n-3 fatty acids had either no effect on plasma lipids and aortic lesion size [36] or lowered triglycerides, total lipoproteins, and cholesterol in female rabbits, and also did not affect lesion size of treated vs untreated controls [37]. A similar experimental protocol with different criteria for lesion evaluations showed that fish oil reduced triglyceride and cholesterol levels and aortic lesions [38]. Recently, a direct comparison of fish oil vs olive oil treatment confirmed a hypolipidemic effect of fish oil in this species; these findings also associated with slowed development of atherosclerosis in young WHHL rabbits [39].

Studies in mouse models

Studies in mouse models are scarce. Reiner et al. by comparing saturated fatty acid- and fish oil-supplemented diets, evaluated the effect of n-3 fatty acids on the development of atherosclerosis and on the secretory activity of peritoneal macrophages in C57BL/6J mice, an atherosclerosis-susceptible strain [40]. Here fish oils diminished lesion size. Macrophages displayed a decreased ability to produce tumor necrosis factor alpha (TNF-α), both basally and after induction by lipopolysaccharide (LPS); hampered production of interleukin 1 beta (IL-1β); reduced lipoprotein lipase expression; and enhanced nitrate synthesis, an index of nitric oxide production. A recent study on murine macrophages determined that fish oil reduced the expression of intercellular adhesion molecule 1 (ICAM-1) and scavenger receptor A type I and II [41], suggesting that n-3 fatty acids affect macrophage phenotype and the role of macrophages in lesion formation.

Recently, transgenic mouse models of atherosclerosis have been introduced [42]. The LDL receptor-deficient (LDLR$^{-/-}$) mouse develops atherosclerosis after consuming a Western-type, high-fat diet [43]. In this model, LDL are not efficiently cleared from plasma, and hypercholesterolemia and atherogenesis proceed with a pattern similar to humans.

Atherosclerosis proceeds spontaneously and very rapidly, without diet modification, in apoE-deficient mice, another model of atherogenesis [44,45]. However, since apoE is a constituent of all lipoproteins except LDL, and serves as a ligand for receptors involved in the clearance of chylomicrons and VLDL remnants, the serum lipid profile of such mice differs significantly from humans. The only human counterpart of this animal model involves the genetic defect of apoE, a rare clinical condition that leads to severe atherosclerosis.

In both LDL receptor- and apoE-knockout models, atherosclerotic lesions begin to spread from the abdominal aorta to the whole aorta and its main branches, predominantly at bifurcation sites. The pattern of lesion formation is similar in both models [46]. Although gender influence is controversial, actively produced estrogens seem protective.

While the effect of n-3 fatty acid in the LDL receptor model had not been the object of any published work until recently, studies of n-3 fatty acid in the apoE$^{-/-}$ mice have been done. Calleja et al. fed ApoE$^{-/-}$ mice diets enriched with different oils commonly used in human nutrition, without adding cholesterol [47]. Following evaluation of lesion area, male animals appeared to respond to sunflower oil, rich in n-6 polyunsaturated fatty acids, while females responded to palm oil and elevated concentrations of olive oil, rich in mono-unsaturated fatty acids. Adan et al. recently fed 7-week-old apoE-deficient mice an atherogenic diet in the presence or absence of DHA supplementation (1% final concentration) for 8 weeks [48a], and observed no effect of DHA on atherosclerosis: size and extension of lesions in the aortic arch and the thoracic and abdominal aorta were similar in both experimental groups. Cholesterol and cholate in the diet might have influenced these results. We have recently evaluated the effects of n-3 (in the form of fish oil) compared with n-6 fatty acids (in the form of corn oil) in both the apoE- and the LDL receptor-knockout models. Both n-3 and n-6 polyunsaturated fatty acid supplementation retarded the development of atherosclerosis in LDLR$^{-/-}$ mice, with a stronger effect seen with n-3 polyunsaturated fatty acid especially in the regions (such as the aortic arch) more susceptible to lesion development. There was an important strain-dependence of the effect, with no protection

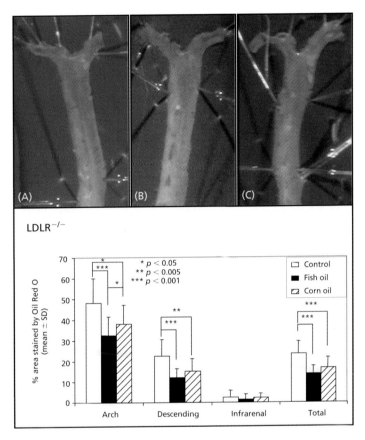

Figure 20.1 The effect of omega-6 (corn oil) and omega-3 polyunsaturated fatty acids (fish oil) on the aortic plaque burden in LDLR$^{-/-}$ mice. Representative en face staining with Oil Red O of aortas excised from LDLR$^{-/-}$ mice fed a Western-type diet supplemented with (A) 1% fish oil, (B) 1% corn oil, (C) unsupplemented. The reduction in the atherosclerotic burden due to both classes of polyunsaturated fatty acids is especially evident in the aortic arch and in the descending aorta and is greater for the fish oil group. (D) The difference between the fish oil and the corn oil group is significant in the arch region ($P < 0.05$ by t-test). (Unpublished data in the context of Ref. [48b]).

against atherosclerosis in apoE$^{-/-}$ mice [48b] (Figure 20.1).

In summary, differences in study design and species hamper animal experimental studies with n-3 fatty acid. Although most studies suggest the existence of anti-atherogenic effects, no definite claim in this direction can be universally made.

Studies in humans

A 30-year follow-up study in men free of overt cardiovascular disease at baseline who consumed up to 35 g fish per day recently confirmed that nutritional intake of n-3 fatty acids likely leads to cardioprotection [49]. Additionally, a nested-case study conducted on healthy subjects from the Physicians' Health Study cohort recently associated baseline blood values of long-chain n-3 polyunsaturated fatty acids with reduced risk of sudden death [50]. The American Heart Association has recently recommended that all adults eat fish twice a week as a means of preventing coronary heart disease [51].

However, gathering evidence regarding the true anti-atherogenic effect of n-3 fatty acid in humans remains difficult, largely due to the multifactorial nature of ischemic heart disease. Autopsy studies in Alaskan natives, who consumed high amounts of fish-derived products, and non-natives, who mostly consumed Western-type diets, provide circumstantial evidence about a lesser extent of atherosclerosis in populations exposed to high nutritional intake of n-3 fatty acids. Newman and coworkers reported a decreased percent of intima covering with fatty streaks and raised lesions in Alaskan natives who consumed a high n-3 fatty acid diet [52] vs non-natives [53]. The magnitude of difference in fatty streak development appeared larger in younger age groups [53] (Figure 20.2), suggesting the effect of diet mainly on early events leading to fully developed atherosclerotic lesions. Prospective studies in humans, although scant, most point to the occurrence of such effects. A study of the effect of high-dose n-3 fatty acid supplementation on coronary

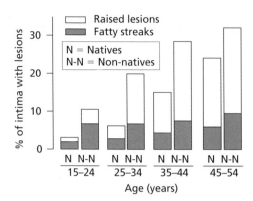

Figure 20.2 Percent of coverage of the aorta with fatty streaks (open areas) and raised plaques (cross-hatched areas) in Alaskan natives vs non-natives, divided by age. Notice the larger difference, attributable to the prevalence of fatty streaks, in younger age groups. (Redrawn, modified, from Ref. [53]).

artery disease regression, evaluated by angiography, was negative [54], but a subsequent well-controlled study (the Study on prevention of Coronary atherosclerosis by Intervention with Marine Omega-3 fatty acids (SCIMO)) showed slowed lesion progression in subjects supplemented with lower doses (1.65 g/day of EPA + DHA) [55]. Interestingly, the same authors recently reported that, in the very same subjects, the same treatment had no effect on carotid intima–media thickness, as evaluated by carotid ultrasound [56], indicating some district specificity for fish oil in humans. Some have speculated that daily intake of n-3 fatty acids (0.5 to 2.0 g) may reduce clinical endpoints [57]. By contrast, higher doses yield no effect [54]. However, this contention is based on a small number of studies that examined the effects of n-3 fatty acids on true atherogenesis, and not on a mixed endpoint. One study following coronary bypass surgery indicates that n-3 fatty acids significantly reduce vein graft stenosis [58], a process regarded as an accelerated form of atherosclerosis. While studies on restenosis following percutaneous coronary angioplasty are contradictory and largely inconclusive [59–70], issues of study design still leave the door open to the possibility that n-3 fatty acids may effect restenosis [71a]. However, restenosis following percutaneous interventions results from mechanical injury to an already diseased vessel wall; thus, its relevance to native atherosclerosis is controversial.

Very recently, the results of a large Japanese study (the Japan EPA Lipid Intervention Study (JELIS)) in over 20,000 Japanese subjects (overall with a high baseline intake of n-3 fatty acids compared to Western populations) were presented. Subjects were treated with either a relatively high dose of EPA (1800 mg/day) or nothing, against the background of optimal medical therapy. The study examined whether the administration of EPA, in both a primary and a secondary prevention setting, could reduce major coronary events, including sudden cardiac death, fatal and nonfatal myocardial infarction (MI), unstable angina and the number of cases of angioplasty/ stenting or coronary bypass grafting, in a prospective, double-blind open-label study with blinded adjudications of endpoints [71b]. In an average follow-up of 4.6 years, the study found a significant (19%, $P = 0.01$) reduction in the combined primary endpoint, which was due to a reduction in myocardial infarction and unstable angina but not, at variance from previous studies, in sudden cardiac death. This reduction appeared to be totally independent from any change in serum cholesterol [71c]. These results are important indirect evidence in humans for a reduction in either the progression of atherosclerosis or its propensity to acute complications, such as plaque rupture and coronary thrombosis.

In summary, based on at least one placebo-controlled prospective study in native atherosclerosis in the coronary arteries, a placebo-controlled prospective study in coronary bypass surgery grafts, and a recent large-scale study on coronary events, human studies provide stronger evidence of an anti-atherogenic effect of n-3 fatty acids than do animal studies.

Interference of n-3 fatty acids with atherogenesis: putative mechanisms

Molecular mechanisms in atherogenesis

The initial event in the development of atherosclerosis involves endothelial dysfunction that precedes any morphologic evidence of endothelial damage [72]. A number of different stimuli, including toxins, shear stress, cigarette smoking, and high cholesterol levels, can trigger endothelial dysfunction. One

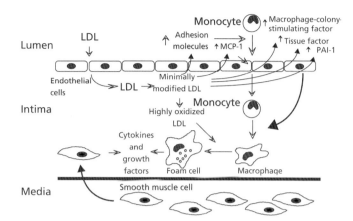

Figure 20.3 A scheme of the modifications of the arterial intima occurring in early atherogenesis. (Reproduced with permission from Ref. [94]).

type of endothelial dysfunction, termed endothelial "activation," involves endothelium that modifies its phenotype in a pro-adhesive direction, triggering increased adhesion of circulating monocytes, whose subsequent infiltration in the arterial intima is one of the first visible findings in atherosclerosis. In the intima, monocytes become activated and begin to incorporate circulating LDL oxidized through exposure to reactive oxygen species of both endothelial and macrophagic origin, thus initiating fatty streak formation (Figure 20.3) (see Chapters 1 and 2) [73].

Atherosclerosis and inflammation share similar basic mechanisms involving early phase adhesion of leukocytes to vascular endothelium. Multiple protein families, each with a distinct function, provide "traffic signals" for leukocytes, including: (a) the "selectin" family of adhesion molecules; (b) chemoattractants, comprised of "classical" chemoattractants such as N-formyl peptides, complement components, leukotriene B4 and platelet-activating factor (which act broadly on neutrophils, eosinophils, basophils and monocytes) and "chemokines" such as monocyte chemoattractant protein 1 (MCP-1), and IL-8 (which have selectivity for leukocyte subsets); and (c) the immunoglobulin superfamily members such as ICAM-1, ICAM-2, ICAM-3, and vascular cell adhesion molecule 1 (VCAM-1), which recognize "integrin" ligands on the leukocyte surface.

For neutrophil and, probably, lymphocyte adhesion, selectins mediate the initial tethering of the circulating leukocyte, allowing it to roll over the endothelium, considerably slowing its speed and allowing leukocytes to "sense" the presence of chemotactic gradients. Final firm attachment of leukocytes to the endothelium requires interaction between integrin ligands on the leukocyte surface and immunoglobulin superfamily members expressed on the endothelium, such as ICAM-1, ICAM-2, and VCAM-1. The multiple molecular choices available for each of these ligand–ligand interactions provide great diversity in signal combinations, allowing selective responses of different leukocyte classes to inflammatory agents, preferential recirculation patterns of lymphocyte subpopulations, or the selective binding of monocytes to arterial endothelium during early phases of atherogenesis.

Compared with other forms of leukocyte–endothelial interactions, monocyte recruitment into the intima of large arteries is specific for atherosclerosis. Thus, these localized monocyte–endothelium interactions may reflect specific molecular changes in the adhesive properties of the endothelial surface, leading to surface expression of "athero-ELAMs", i.e., endothelium–leukocyte adhesion molecules (ELAMs) expressed in the early phases of atherosclerosis. The first such protein, originally identified in the rabbit hypercholesterolemic model, is VCAM-1, a member of the immunoglobulin superfamily expressed on human vascular endothelium in at least two molecular forms. Both forms bind a heterodimeric integrin receptor, VLA4, whose leukocyte selectivity of expression on monocytes and lymphocytes, but not on neutrophils, can explain the selectivity of monocyte recruitment in early atherogenesis [74]. In cholesterol-fed rabbits, endothelial cells express VCAM-1 early, before macrophages/foam cells appear in a temporal pattern consistent with its pathogenetic role in lesion development in the intima of the developing fatty streak. Pathophysiologically relevant stimuli for VCAM-1 expression in atherogenesis could include minimally oxidized LDL or β-VLDL in the rabbit, the advanced glycosylation end products (AGEs) associated with diabetes or uremia, lipoprotein (Lp(a)), or perhaps homocysteine, elevated in homocysteinuria and in subtler forms of congenital or acquired enzyme defects in its biosynthetic pathway. In addition to these humoral stimuli, VCAM-1 endothelial gene expression also responds to hemodynamic forces, thus potentially explaining the localization of atherosclerosis in particular points of the arterial vasculature. (For a general review on these issues, see Ref. [74]; see also Chapters 1 and 2.)

The progression from fatty streak to atheroma is driven by the production of cytokines and chemoattractants that determine the intimal accumulation of leukocytes, smooth muscle cells and fibroblasts, as well as platelet adhesion. The thin-capped, lipid-rich atheromatous plaques have a strong tendency to rupture and are at risk of complicating with thrombosis, which is usually the ultimate event leading to unstable angina and myocardial infarction [75]. Thus, n-3 fatty acids may theoretically act on atherogenesis at several potential points, as discussed briefly below.

Effects of n-3 fatty acids on plasma lipids

In humans, n-3 fatty acids decrease serum triglycerides. In marked hypertriglyceridemia, VLDL cholesterol decreases and LDL cholesterol increases or remains unchanged [76,77]. In patients with mixed hyperlipidemia and in marked hypertriglyceridemia, n-3 fatty acids highly effectively reduce both triglyceride and VLDL levels. Thus, n-3 fatty acids appear to reduce one of the atherogenic triggers.

Effects of n-3 fatty acids on cellular responses to atherogenic triggers

Dietary consumption of n-3 fatty acids such as EPA and DHA allows their incorporation in the phospholipids of cell membranes, replacing arachidonic acid (AA). Originally, the beneficial effects of n-3 fatty acids on the cardiovascular system were attributed to their substitution of AA. Metabolites that derive from n-3 fatty acid enzymatic metabolization (through cyclooxygenase, lipoxygenase, and cytochrome P450 monoxygenase) are less prothrombotic and vasoconstrictive compared with

the corresponding AA derivatives. DHA and EPA both appear active, possibly with more prominent effects by DHA. Since DHA, at variance from EPA, is a poor substrate for metabolization into eicosanoids, effects of n-3 fatty acids other than generation of eicosanoids likely play a greater role in preventing atherogenesis.

In these last years, direct effects on endothelial activation have been demonstrated, including: reduced production of cytokines such as IL-1 and TNF in LPS-stimulated monocytes [78]; the reduced production of the mitogen and smooth muscle cell attractant platelet-derived growth factor (PDGF-A and -B) protein and mRNA [79,80]; the reduced expression of tissue factor by monocytes [81]; increased bioavailability of endothelial nitric oxide [82]; the specific downregulation of gene expression for MCP-1 [83]; and the reduced expression of endothelial adhesion molecules, essential for monocyte adhesion to sites of inflammation and dysfunctional endothelium [84].

Modulation of endothelial–leukocyte interactions by n-3 fatty acids

To assess the effects of various fatty acids on the surface expression of endothelial–leukocyte adhesion molecules and characterize the mechanisms and functional relevance of such effects, we used human adult saphenous vein endothelial cells activated by cytokines in an *in vitro* model of the early steps in atherogenesis. When added to cultured endothelial cells hours to days before the stimulation with cytokines, i.e., early enough to allow a significant incorporation in cell membrane phospholipids, the n-3 fatty acid DHA significantly inhibited events involving endothelial activation, including the expression of adhesion molecules such as VCAM-1, E-selectin, and, to a lesser extent, ICAM-1, after stimulation with virtually any stimulus able to elicit the coordinated expression of such genes [84,85]. Thus, such inhibition could be demonstrated with IL-1α and IL-1β, TNF-α, IL-4, and LPS (Figure 20.4). Inhibition of adhesion molecule expression occurred in a range of DHA concentrations compatible with its nutritional supplementation in normal Western diets. Additionally, such inhibition occurred at any time point after the appearance of cytokine effect, modifying the specific kinetics of surface expression of adhesion molecules, and was strictly related in its

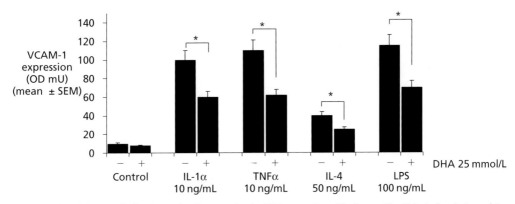

Figure 20.4 The inhibition of adhesion molecule expression by DHA, occurring with diverse stimuli, including IL-1α and IL-1β, TNF-α, IL-4, and LPS. Asterisks denote significant differences at $P < 0.01$. (From De Caterina et al., unpublished).

magnitude to the extent of incorporation into total cell lipids. Indeed, the extent of VCAM-1 inhibitory effect paralleled the incorporation of DHA and the overall increased incorporation of n-3 fatty acids, and related inversely to the content of n-6 fatty acids. Following the fate of ^{14}C-labeled DHA into cell phospholipids, we demonstrated significant incorporation of DHA into the phosphatidyl ethanolamine pool. This pool is not the most abundant phospholipid pool, and is located in the inner leaflet of plasma membrane, possibly in a strategic position for influencing intracellular signal-transduction pathways. Not limited to the expression of transmembrane molecules involved in leukocyte recruitment, this effect occurs also for other cytokine-activated products, such as the soluble proteins IL-6 and IL-8, involved in either the amplification of the inflammatory response (IL-6) or in the specific chemoattraction for granulocytes (IL-8). A functional counterpart also accompanied this effect, i.e., reduced monocyte or monocytoid cell adhesion to cytokine-activated endothelium. Compared to DHA, EPA was weaker in inhibiting the expression of these molecules as well as monocyte adhesion, although still more potently than other fatty acids. We also showed that parallel reductions in VCAM-1 mRNA steady state levels, as assessed by Northern analysis, accompany DHA's effects on VCAM-1 expression [84,85]. While Weber et al. reported comparable results in experiments with remarkably similar design [86], they also demonstrated that DHA inhibits activation of the nuclear factor kappa B (NF-κB) system of transcription factors [86], which controls the coordinated expression of adhesion

molecules and of leukocyte-specific chemoattractants upon cytokine stimulation [87,88].

We further analyzed endothelial effects of various fatty acids differing in chain length, number, position (n-3 vs n-6 vs n-9), and *cis/trans* configuration of the double bonds. Using VCAM-1 surface expression as a readout, we concluded that saturated fatty acids are inactive; potency of polyunsaturated fatty acids increases with the number of unsaturations; potency does not depend on chain length; the single double bond present in the monounsaturated fatty acid, oleic acid, is indeed sufficient to produce all the effects obtainable with higher unsaturated fatty acids, albeit at higher concentrations; finally, for such an effect to occur, even the configuration (*cis* vs *trans*) of the double bond does not really matter, since oleic acid (19:1 n-9 *cis*) and its *trans* stereoisomer elaidic acid are of equal potency [89]. Indeed, we also inhibited NF-κB activation by incubating endothelial cells with oleic acid [90].

Inhibiting endothelial activation with unsaturated fatty acids: possible molecular mechanisms

To identify mechanisms for these effects, we demonstrated inhibition of NF-κB activation by DHA (the most potent fatty acid inhibitor of endothelial activation) in parallel with measurements of production of hydrogen peroxide by cultured endothelial cells. This reactive oxygen species (or one of more of its downstream unstable products) is likely a critical mediator of NF-κB activation (Figure 20.5). Indeed, we showed previously that treatment of endothelial cells with polyethylene glycol (PEG) complexed

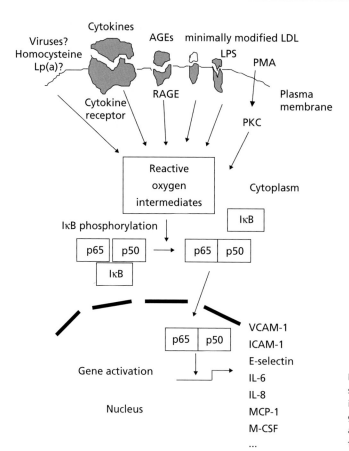

Figure 20.5 A scheme of the intracellular signal-transduction pathways leading to increased gene expression of target genes upon endothelial cell exposure to atherogenic triggers. (Redrawn, modified, from Ref. [87]).

superoxide dismutase (a cell membrane-permeable form of this enzyme, which catalyzes the conversion of superoxide anion to hydrogen peroxide) has little affect on VCAM-1 mRNA production. In contrast, treating endothelial cells with PEG catalase, which acts by accelerating the degradation of hydrogen peroxide, quenches endothelial activation [91], suggesting that hydrogen peroxide (or some of its downstream products) more relevantly activates NF-κB than do upstream products (e.g., superoxide anion). We also assessed the production of intracellular hydrogen peroxide (and/or its downstream products) by the dichloro-fluoresceine method before or after stimulation with IL-1 or TNF. In both experimental systems, we could document (unpublished results) decreased baseline production of reactive oxygen species after enriching cell membranes with DHA, and an even more pronounced dampening of the increase produced by stimulation with cytokines. Saturated fatty acids served as a

negative control in these experiments. Therefore, our current understanding of these phenomena suggests that a property related to fatty acid peroxidability (the presence of multiple double bonds), usually regarded as a detrimental consequence of polyunsaturated fatty acid enrichment of cell membranes, directly associates with this putatively favorable outcome (Figure 20.6).

Such results have spurred reappraisal of how the action of fatty acids on endothelial cells may modulate not only general phenomena such as atherogenesis but also, potentially, inflammation or some immune responses. Since all these effects occurred even in the presence of inhibitors of metabolic conversion of fatty acids to eicosanoids, they provide a novel explanation for the modulating effect of n-3 fatty acids in atherogenesis, distinct from the now outdated hypothesis of substrate substitution [92]. The results with oleic acid also might partially explain the beneficial effects of olive-oil-rich

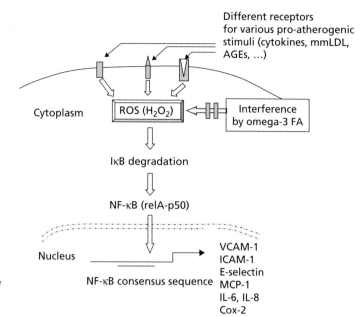

Figure 20.6 A scheme of the putative site of action of n-3 fatty acids on endothelial activation.

("Mediterranean") diets on atherogenesis. Notably, incorporation of oleic acid likely occurred at the expense of saturated fatty acids, thus disclosing the potentially additive effects of n-3 fatty acids, which mostly substitute less unsaturated fatty acids in the membrane phospholipid pools. If extended to cell types different from endothelial cells such as the monocyte–macrophage that also undergo the "activation" phenomena when stimulated by cytokines or LPS, such effects may provide a coherent explanation for several previous observations such as the inhibition of cytokine formation by LPS-activated macrophages [78]. Such effects might associate closely with the peroxidability of polyunsaturated fatty acid.

Future research will further elucidate molecular aspects of these phenomena [93] and expand the greater scope of this research line to explain the many biological effects of unsaturated fatty acids as modulators of biological responses to cytokines.

References

1 Connor WE. Importance of n-3 fatty acids in health and disease. *Am J Clin Nutr* 2000;71(Suppl):171S–175S.

2 Bang HO, Dyerberg J. The composition of food consumed by Greenlandic Eskimos. *Acta Med Scand* 1973;200:69–73.

3 Dyerberg J, Bang HO. Hemostatic function and platelet polyunsaturated fatty acids in Eskimos. *Lancet* 1979;2:433–435.

4 Harris WS. n-3 Fatty acids and serum lipoproteins: animal studies. *Am J Clin Nutr* 1997;65:1611S–1616S.

5 Goodnight SH, Harris WS, Connor WE, et al. Polyunsaturated fatty, hyperlipidemia and thrombosis. *Arteriosclerosis* 1982;2:87–113.

6 Kim DN, Schmee J, Lee KT, et al. Hypoatherogenic effect of dietary corn oil exceeds hypocholesterolemic effect in swine. *Atherosclerosis* 1984;52: 101–113.

7 Ward M, Clarksob TB. The effect of menhaden oil-containing diet on hemostatic and lipid parameters of nonhuman primates with atherosclerosis. *Arteriosclerosis* 1985;57:325–335.

8 Parks JS, Wilson MD, Johnson FL, et al. Fish oil decreases hepatic cholesteryl ester secretion but not apoB secretion in African Green Monkeys. *J Lipid Res* 1989;30: 1535–1544.

9 Parks JS, Gebre AK. Studies on the effect of dietary fish oil on the physical and chemical properties of low density lipoproteins in cynomolgus monkeys. *J Lipid Res* 1991;32: 305–315.

10 Abbey M, Clifton P, McMurchie EJ, et al. Effect of a high fat/cholesterol diet with or without eicosapentaenoic acid on plasma lipid, lipoproteins and lipid transferase activity in the marmoset. *Arteriosclerosis* 1990;81:163–174.

11 Davies HR, Bridenstine RT, Vesselinovitch D, et al. Fish oil inhibits development of atherosclerosis in Rhesus monkeys. *Arteriosclerosis* 1987;7:441–449.

12 Parks JS, Kadick-Sawyer J, Bullock BC, et al. Effect of dietary fish oil on coronary artery and aortic atherosclerosis in African Green monkeys. *Arteriosclerosis* 1990;10: 1102–1112.

13 Smuts C, Kruger M, van Jaarsveld P, et al. The influence of fish oil supplementation on plasma lipoproteins and arterial lipids in Vervet monkeys with established atherosclerosis. *Prostag Leukot Essent Fatty Acids* 1992;47:129–138.

14 Wolfe MS, Sawter JK, Morgan TM, et al. Dietary polyunsaturated fat decreases coronary artery atherosclerosis in a pediatric-aged population of African Green monkeys. *Arterioscler Thromb* 1994;4:587–597.

15 Rudel LL, Johnson FL, Sawyer JK, et al. Dietary polyunsaturated fat modified low density lipoproteins and reduces atherosclerosis of non-human primates. *Am J Clin Nutr* 1995;62(Suppl):463S–470S.

16 Harker LA, Kelley AB, Hanson SR, et al. Interruption of vascular thrombus formation and vascular lesion formation by dietary n-3 fatty acids in fish oils in non human primates. *Circulation* 1993;87:1017–1029.

17 Boerboom LE, Olinger GN, Almassi GH, et al. Both fish oil supplementation and aspirin fail to inhibit atherosclerosis in long-term vein bypass grafts in moderately hypercholesterolemic non-human primates. *Circulation* 1997;96:968–974.

18 Hill EG, Lundberg W, Titus JL. Experimental atherosclerosis in swine. A comparison of menhaden-oil supplements in tallow and coconut-oil diets. *Mayo Clin Proc* 1971;46:613–620.

19 Weiner BH, Ockene IS, Levine PH, et al. Inhibition of atherosclerosis by cod-liver oil in a hyperlipidemic swine model. *N Eng J Med* 1986;315:841–846.

20 Hartog JM, Lamers JM, Essed CE, et al. Does platelet aggregation play a role in the reduction in localized intimal proliferation in normolipemic pigs with fixed coronary artery stenosis fed dietary fish oil? *Arteriosclerosis* 1989;76:79–88.

21 Kim DN, Ho HT, Lawrence DA, et al. Modification of lipoprotein patterns and retardation of atherogenesis by a fish oil supplement to a hyperlipidemic diet for swine. *Atherosclerosis* 1989;76:35–54.

22 Sassen LM, Lamers JM, Sluiter W, et al. Development and regression of atherosclerosis in pigs. Effects of n-3 fatty acids, their incorporation into plasma and aortic plaque lipids, and granulocyte function. *Arterioscler Thromb* 1993;13:651–660.

23 Sassen LMA, Hartog JM, Lamers JMJ, et al. Mackerel oil and atherosclerosis in pigs. *Eur Heart J* 1989;10:838–846.

24 Barbeau ML, Klemp KF, Guyton JR, et al. Dietary fish oil. Influence on lesion regression in the porcine model of atherosclerosis. *Arterioscler Thromb Vasc Biol* 1997;17: 688–694.

25 Withman SC, Fish JR, Rand ML, et al. n-3 fatty acid incorporation into LDL particles renders them more susceptible to oxidation *in vitro* but not necessarily more atherogenic *in vivo*. *Arterioscler Thromb* 1994;14: 1170–1176.

26 Zhu BQ, Sievers RE, Isenberg WM, et al. Regression of atherosclerosis on cholesterol-fed rabbits: effects of fish oil and verapamil. *J Am Coll Cardiol* 1990;15:231–237.

27 Demiroglu C, Ozder A, Altug T, et al. Suppression of atherogenesis by n-3 fatty acids in the cholesterol-fed rabbit. *Angiology* 1991;42:323–330.

28 Chen M-F, Hsu H-C, Liau C-S, et al. The role of vitamin E on the anti-atherosclerotic effect of fish oil in diet induced hypercholesterolemic rabbits. *Prostag Other Lipid Mediat* 1999;57:99–111.

29 Thiery J, Seidel D. Fish oil feeding results in an enhancement of cholesterol-induced atherosclerosis. *Atherosclerosis* 1987;63:53–56.

30 Rogers KM, Adelstein R. MaxEPA fish oil enhances cholesterol-induced intimal foam cell formation in rabbits. *Am J Pathol* 1990;137:945–951.

31 Kristensen S, Roberts KM, Lawry J, et al. The effect of fish oil on atherogenesis and thrombopoiesis in rabbits on high cholesterol diet. *Artery* 1988;15: 250–258.

32 Campos C, Michalek VN, Matts JP, et al. Dietary marine oil supplements fail to affect cholesterol metabolism or inhibit atherosclerosis in rabbit with diet-induced hypercholesterolemia. *Surgery* 1989;106:177–184.

33 Chen M-F, Hsu H-C, Lee Y-T. Fish oil supplementation attenuates myointimal proliferation of the abdominal aorta after balloon injury in diet induced hypercholesterolemic rabbits. *Prostaglandins* 1995;49:295–310.

34 Faggin E, Puato M, Chiavegato A, et al. Fish oil supplementation prevents neointima formation in nonhypercholesterolemic balloon-injured rabbit carotid artery by reducing medial and adventitial cell activation. *Arterioscler Thromb Vasc Biol* 2000;20: 152–163.

35 Fincham JE, Gouws E, Woodroof CW, et al. Atherosclerosis: chronic effects of fish oil and a therapeutic diet in non-human primates. *Arterioscler Thromb* 1991; 11:719–732.

36 Rich S, Miller Jr JF, Charous S, et al. Development of atherosclerosis in genetically hyperlipidemic rabbits during chronic fish oil ingestion. *Arteriosclerosis* 1989;9:189–194.

37 Clubb FJ, Schmitz LM, Butler M, et al. Effect of dietary omega-3 fatty acids on serum lipids, platelets function and atherosclerosis in Watanabe heritable hyperlipidemic rabbits. *Arteriosclerosis* 1989;9:529–537.

38 Litchman AH, Clinton SK, Iiyama K, et al. Hyperlipidemia and atherosclerotic lesion development in LDL receptor-deficient mice fed defined semipurified diets with

and without cholate. *Arterioscler Thromb Vasc Biol* 1999;19.

39 Mortensen A, Hansen BF, Hansen JF, et al. Comparison of the effects of fish oil and olive oil on blood lipids and aortic atherosclerosis in Watanabe heritable hyperlipidaemic rabbits. *Br J Nutr* 1998;80:565–573.

40 Reiner G, Skamene E, DeSanctis J, et al. Dietary polyunsaturated fatty acids prevent the development of atherosclerotic lesion in mice. *Arterioscler Thromb* 1993;13:1515–1524.

41 Miles EA, Wallace FA, Calder PC. Dietary fish oil reduces intercellular adhesion molecule 1 and scavenger receptor expression on murine macrophages. *Atherosclerosis* 2000;152:43–50.

42 Breslow JL. Mouse models of atherosclerosis. *Science* 1996;272:685–688.

43 Ishibashi S, Brown MS, Goldstein JL, et al. Hypercholesterolemia in low-density lipoprotein receptor knock out mice and its reversal by adenovirus-mediated gene delivery. *J Clin Invest* 1993;92: 883–893.

44 Plump AS, Smith JD, Hayek T, et al. Severe hypercholesterolemia and atherosclerosis in apolipoprotein E-deficient mice created by homologous recombination in ES cells. *Cell* 1992;71:343–353.

45 Zhang SH, Reddick RL, Piedrahita JP, et al. Spontaneous, hypercholesterolemia and arterial lesion in mice lacking apolipoprotein E. *Science* 1992;258:468–471.

46 Tangirala RK, Rubin EM, Palinski W. Quantitation of atherosclerosis in murine models: correlation between lesions in the aortic origin and in the entire aorta, and differences in the extent of lesions between sexes in LDL receptor-deficient and apolipoprotein E-deficient mice. *J Lipid Res* 1995;36:2320–2328.

47 Calleja L, Paris MA, Paul A, et al. Low-cholesterol and high-fat diets reduce atherosclerotic lesion development in apoE-knockout mice. *Arterioscler Thromb Vasc Biol* 1999;19:2368–2375.

48 (a) Adan Y, Shibata K, Sato M, et al. Concentration of serum lipids and aortic lesion size in female and male apo E-deficient mice fed docosahexaenoic acid. *Biosci Biotechnol Biochem* 1999;63:309–313; (b) Zampolli A, Bysted A, Leth T, et al. Contrasting effect of fish oil supplementation on the development of atherosclerosis in murine models. *Atherosclerosis* 2006;184:78–85.

49 Daviglus ML, Stamler J, Orencia AJ, et al. Fish consumption and the 30-year risk of fatal myocardial infarction. *N Engl J Med* 1997;336:1046–1053.

50 Albert CM, Campos H, Stampfer MJ, et al. Blood levels of long-chain n-3 fatty acids and the risk of sudden death. *N Engl J Med* 2002;346:1113–1118.

51 Kris-Etherton P, Harris W, Appel L. Omega-3 fatty acids and cardiovascular disease. New recommendations from the American Heart Association. *Arterioscler Thromb Vasc Biol* 2003;23:151–152.

52 Middaugh J. Cardiovascular death among Alaskan natives 1980–1986. *Am J Public Health* 1990;80:282–285.

53 Newman W, Middaugh J, Propst M, et al. Atherosclerosis in Alaskan natives and non-natives. *Lancet* 1993;341:1056–1057.

54 Sacks FM, Stone PH, Gibson CM, et al. Controlled trial of fish oil for regression of human coronary atherosclerosis. HARP Research Group. *J Am Coll Cardiol* 1995;25.

55 von Shacky C, Angerer P, Kothny W, et al. The effect of dietary omega-3 fatty acids on coronary atherosclerosis. A randomized, double-blind, placebo-controlled trial. *Ann Intern Med* 1999;130:554–562.

56 Angerer P, Kothny W, Stork S, et al. Effect of dietary supplementation with omega-3 fatty acids on progression of atherosclerosis in carotid arteries. *Cardiovasc Res* 2002;54:183–190.

57 Angerer P, von Shacky C. n-3 polyunsaturated fatty acids and the cardiovascular system. *Curr Opin Lipidol* 2000;11:57–63.

58 Eritsland J, Arnesen H, Gronseth K, et al. Effect of supplementation with n-3 fatty acids on graft patency in patients undergoing coronary artery bypass operation. Result from the SHOT study. *Eur heart J* 1994; 15:29 [Abstract 351].

59 Slack J, Pinkerton C, Van Tassel J. Can oral fish oil supplement minimize re-stenosis after percutaneous transluminal angioplasty? *J Am Coll Cardiol* 1987;9:64A [Abstract].

60 Dehmer GJ, Popma JJ, van den Berg EK, et al. Reduction in the rate of early restenosis after coronary angioplasty by a diet supplemented with n-3 fatty acids. *N Engl J Med* 1988;241:733–740.

61 Grigg L, Kay T, Valentine P, et al. Determinants of restenosis and lack of effect of dietary supplementation with eicosapentaenoic acid on the incidence of coronary artery restenosis after angioplasty. *J Am Coll Cardiol* 1989;13:665–672.

62 Milner MR, Gallino RA, Leffingwell A, et al. Usefulness of fish oil supplements in preventing clinical evidence of restenosis after percutaneous transluminal coronary angioplasty. *Am J Cardiol* 1989;64:294–299.

63 Reis G, Boucher T, Sipperly ME, et al. Randomised trial of fish oil for prevention of restenosis after coronary angioplasty. *Lancet* 1989;11:177–181.

64 Nye E, Ilsley C, Ablett M, et al. Effect of eicosapentaenoic acid on restenosis rate, clinical course and blood lipids in patients after percutaneous transluminal coronary angioplasty. *Aust NZ J Med* 1990;20:549–552.

65 Bairati I, Roy L, Meyer F. Double-blind, randomized, controlled trial of fish oil supplements in prevention of

recurrence of stenosis after coronary angioplasty. *Circulation* 1992;85(Suppl I):950–956.

66 Kaul U, Saghvi S, Bahl V, et al. Fish oil supplements for prevention of restenosis after coronary angioplasty. *Int J Cardiol* 1992;35:87–93.

67 Franzen D, Schannwell M, Oette K, et al. A prospective, randomized, and double-blind trial on the effect of fish oil on the incidence of restenosis following PTCA. *Cathet Cardiovasc Diagn* 1993;28:301–310.

68 Bellamy C, Schofield P, Faragher E, et al. Can supplementation with omega-3 polyunsaturated fatty acids reduce coronary angioplasty restenosis rate? *Eur Heart J* 1992;3: 1626–1631.

69 Leaf A, Jorgensen M, Jacobs A, et al. Do fish oils prevent restenosis after coronary angioplasty? *Circulation* 1994;90(Suppl I):2248–2257.

70 Cairns J, Gill J, Morton B, et al. Fish oils and low-molecular-weight heparin for the reduction of restenosis after percutaneous transluminal coronary angioplasty. The EMPAR Study. *Circulation* 1996;94(Suppl I): 1553–1560.

71 (a) Maresta A, Balducelli M, Varani E, et al. Prevention of postcoronary angioplasty restenosis by omega-3 fatty acids: main results of the Esapent for Prevention of Restenosis ITalian Study (ESPRIT). *Am Heart J* 2002;143:E5; (b) Yokoyama M, Origasa H. Effects of eicosapentaenoic acid on cardiovascular events in Japanese patients with hypercholesterolemia: rationale, design, and baseline characteristics of the Japan EPA Lipid Intervention Study (JELIS). *Am Heart J* 2003;146:613–620; (c) Yokoyama M, for the Japan EPA Lipid Intervention Study (JELIS). Effects of eicosapentaenoic acid (EPA) on major cardiovascular events in hypercholesterolemic patients. *Circulation* 2005, American Heart Association Meeting, Dallas, TX, November 13–16, 2005 [Abstract].

72 De Caterina R. Endothelial dysfunctions: common denominators in vascular disease. *Curr Opin Lipidol* 2000;11:9–23.

73 Ross R. The pathogenesis of atherosclerosis: a perspective for the 1990s. *Nature* 1993;362:801–809.

74 De Caterina R, Libby P, Peng H-B, et al. Nitric oxide decreases cytokine-induced endothelial activation. *J Clin Invest* 1995;96:60–68.

75 Falk E, Shah PK, Fuster V. Coronary plaque disruption. *Circulation* 1995;92:657–671.

76 Leaf A, Weber PC. Cardiovascular effects of n-3 fatty acids. *N Eng J Med* 1988;318:549–557.

77 Harris WS. n-3 Fatty acids and serum lipoproteins: human studies. *Am J Clin Nutr* 1997;65:1645S–1654S.

78 Endres S, Ghorbani R, Kelley VE. The effect of dietary supplementation with n-3 polyunsaturated fatty acid on the synthesis of interleukin-1 and tumor necrosis factor by mononuclear cells. *N Eng J Med* 1989;320: 265–271.

79 Fox PL, DiCorleto PE. Fish oil inhibit endothelial cell production of platelet-derived growth factor-like protein. *Science* 1988;241:453–456.

80 Kaminski WE, Jendraschk E, Kiefl R, et al. Dietary omega-3 fatty acids lower levels of platelet-derived growth factor mRNA in human mononuclear cells. *Blood* 1993;81: 1871–1879.

81 Hansen JB, Olsen JO, Wilsgard L, et al. Effects of dietary supplementation with cod liver oil on monocyte thromboplastin synthesis, coagulation and fibrinolysis. *J Intern Med* 1989;225(Suppl):133–139.

82 Shimokawa H, Vanhoutte PM. Dietary omega-3 fatty acids and endothelium dependent relaxation in porcine coronary artery. *Am J Physiol* 1989;256: H968–H973.

83 Baumann K, Hessel F, Larass I, et al. Dietary omega-3, omega-6, and omega-9 unsaturated fatty acids and growth factor and cytokine gene expression in unstimulated and stimulated monocytes. A randomized volunteer study. *Arterioscler Thromb Vasc Biol* 1999;19: 59–66.

84 De Caterina R, Cybulsky M, Clinton S, et al. DHA inhibits cytokine-induced endothelial activation. *Proceedings of the Scientific Conference on Omega-3 Fatty Acids in Nutrition, Vascular Biology and Medicine*, Houston, Texas, April 1994:17–19.

85 De Caterina R, Cybulsky M, Clinton S, et al. Omega-3 fatty acids and endothelial leukocyte adhesion molecules. *Prostag Leukot Essent Fatty Acids* 1995;52: 191–195.

86 Weber C, Erl W, Pietsch A, et al. Docosahexaenoic acid selectively attenuates induction of vascular cell adhesion molecule-1 and subsequent monocytic cell adhesion to human endothelial cells stimulated by tumor necrosis factor-alpha. *Arterioscler Thromb Vasc Biol* 1995;15: 622–628.

87 Collins T. Endothelial nuclear factor-B and the initiation of the atherosclerotic lesion. *Lab Invest* 1993;68: 499–508.

88 Collins T, Read M, Neish A, et al. Transcriptional regulation of endothelial cell adhesion molecules: NF-B and cytokine-inducible enhancers. *FASEB J* 1995;9: 899–909.

89 De Caterina R, Bernini W, Carluccio M, et al. Structural requirements for inhibition of cytokine-induced endothelial activation by unsaturated fatty acids. *J Lipid Res* 1998;39:1062–1070.

90 Carluccio MA, Massaro M, Bonfrate M, et al. Oleic acid inhibits endothelial activation. A direct vascular antiatherogenic mechanism of a nutritional component of the Mediterranean diet. *Arterioscler Thromb Vasc Biol* 1999;19:220–228.

91 De Caterina R, Libby P, Peng HB et al. Nitric oxide decreases cytokine-induced endothelial activation. Nitric

oxide selectively reduces endothelial expression of adhesion molecules and proinflammatory cytokines. *J Clin Invest* 1995;96:60–68.

92 Dyerberg J, Bang H, Stofferson E, et al. Eicosapentaenoic acid and prevention of thrombosis and atherosclerosis. *Lancet* 1978;2:117–119.

93 De Caterina R, Massaro M. Omega-3 fatty acids and the regulation of expression of endothelial pro-atherogenic and pro-inflammatory genes. *J Membrane Biol* 2005;206: 103–116.

94 De Caterina R. *Attivazione Endoteliale e Aterogenesi.* Pisa: Primula, 2000.

CHAPTER 21

Treatment of endothelial dysfunction and atherosclerosis by cholesterol lowering

Masanori Aikawa, MD, PhD *& Peter Libby,* MD

Introduction

Accumulating evidence suggests that inflammation plays a pivotal role in the chronic processes of plaque progression and the onset of its acute complications such as myocardial infarction. Features common in other inflammatory diseases, e.g., endothelial cell (EC) activation, oxidative stress, and leukocyte invasion into the tissue, occur in atherosclerosis as well. Hypercholesterolemia, particularly elevated low-density lipoprotein (LDL) cholesterol, contributes importantly to risk of coronary thrombotic complications. In the last two decades, vascular biology provided an enormous amount of evidence linking elevated cholesterol, oxidative stress, and vascular inflammation. More recently, clinical and preclinical studies demonstrated that cholesterol lowering reduces risk of acute coronary complications in patients, in part by limiting inflammation of atherosclerotic plaques rather than simply reducing the lesion size. This chapter will review the role of hypercholesterolemia in vascular inflammation and EC dysfunction, and then discuss the evidence for mechanisms by which cholesterol lowering reduces acute coronary events.

Hypercholesterolemia as a major coronary risk factor

Hypercholesterolemia participates in the pathogenesis of vascular inflammation and atherosclerosis [1–6]. Particularly, clinical and epidemiologic studies have established that elevated plasma LDL particles increase the risk of acute coronary syndromes including acute myocardial infarction, unstable angina, and sudden cardiac death [7,8]. Since the early 20th century, animal studies have shown that hypercholesterolemia can cause atherosclerotic lesion formation [9–12]. Perplexing *in vitro* observations, however, have long suggested that native LDL itself does not convert macrophages into lipid-laden foam cells [13]. In the 1980s, the "oxidation hypothesis" finally resolved the missing link between LDL and atherosclerosis proposing that oxidized LDL (oxLDL) can exert pro-inflammatory and atherogenic actions [14–16]. Since then, vascular biology has provided much evidence that hypercholesterolemic induces oxidative stress, which leads to vascular inflammation and acute coronary complications [17].

Oxidative stress induces atherogenic molecules and suppresses anti-atherogenic molecules in EC

Where and how oxidation of LDL occurs *in vivo* remains speculative. However, accumulating evidence suggests that oxLDL exist in both human and experimental atherosclerotic plaques [14–16,18–20] (Figure 21.1(a), top panels). Excess infiltration of LDL into and retention within the arterial wall due to elevated plasma LDL levels likely accelerates this process. Atherosclerotic arteries intrinsically produce excess reactive oxygen species (ROS) such as

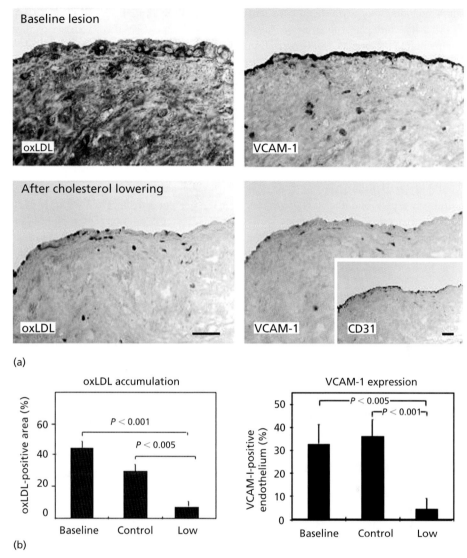

Figure 21.1 Lipid lowering reduced oxLDL accumulation and VCAM-1 expression in rabbit atherosclerotic plaques. (a) *Top panels*: oxLDL epitopes (MDA-lysine) accumulated in the aortic intima beneath VCAM-1-positive EC in hyper-cholesterolemic rabbits which consumed the atherogenic diet for 4 months (Baseline). *Bottom panels*: oxLDL epitopes (MDA-lysine) and VCAM-1 expression by EC were barely detectable in the intima of rabbit aorta after 16 months of lipid lowering, while CD31, an EC marker, indicated an intact monolayer. The lesions from Control animals that continued the atherogenic diet for 16 months continued to feature high levels of oxLDL and VCAM-1. Scale bar: 50 μM. Original magnification ×400. (b) Quantitative data for oxLDL and VCAM-1 from Baseline, Control and Treated Groups are reported as percent of immunopositive areas for oxLDL antibody and percent of CD31-positive endothelium also bearing VCAM-1, respectively, measured by computer-assisted color image analysis. Bars represent SEM. Reproduced from Ref. [20] with permission.

superoxide anion (O_2^-), hydrogen peroxide (H_2O_2), hypochlorous acid (HOCl), and peroxynitrite ($ONOO^-$), thus promoting further oxidative modification of LDL. oxLDL instigate an inflammatory response on arterial EC. A number of *in vitro* studies suggest that oxLDL and their derivatives increase the expression of cell adhesion molecules such as vascular cell adhesion molecule 1 (VCAM-1) and chemokines, including monocyte chemoattractant protein 1 (MCP-1), which play critical roles in leukocyte recruitment into the intima [21–23]. Activation of nuclear factor kappa B (NF-κB), a key transcription factor in inflammation, mediates EC production of VCAM-1 and MCP-1 in response to oxLDL [24]. In rabbits, hypercholesterolemia induces VCAM-1 expression in aortic EC [20,25] (Figure 21.1(a)). Nitric oxide (NO) exerts anti-atherogenic actions such as the inhibition of monocyte adhesion to EC or suppression of EC expression of VCAM-1 and MCP-1 [26–29]. Apparently normal EC constitutively express endothelial NO synthase (eNOS), which produces NO from L-arginine. However, inflammation impairs expression and/or bioavailability of eNOS in humans and experimental animals [20,30,31]. Oxidative stress decreases eNOS expression by cultured EC and also diminishes the bioavailability of NO [32].

The role of macrophages in acute thrombotic complications

During the 1980s, pathologic and angiographic studies challenged our classical view that acute myocardial infarctions usually occur within a coronary artery that has developed considerable luminal stenosis, as detected by angiography [33–35]. These studies provided new insight that rupture of the thin fibrous cap of coronary atherosclerotic plaques with preserved lumen often triggers acute fatal thrombosis [1,36]. Pathologic observations also taught us that vascular inflammation contributes critically to the onset of acute coronary events [17]. The so-called "vulnerable" atherosclerotic plaques prone to rupture and subsequent thrombus formation usually contain a prominent accumulation of macrophages, key mediators of inflammatory responses [1,37,38]. Lesional macrophages overexpress various proteinases, e.g., matrix metalloproteinases or MMP [1,39]. Collagenases of the MMP family found in human atherosclerotic plaques (MMP-1/collagenase-1, MMP-8/collagenase-2, and MMP-13/collagenase-3) cleave interstitial collagen [40–42]. Content of fibrillar collagen, particularly collagen type I, determines stability and durability of many tissues [43]. The so-called "vulnerable" plaques also have thin, collagen-poor fibrous caps overlying macrophage-rich cores. These characteristically

thin caps likely result from collagenolysis catalyzed by macrophage-derived collagenases of the MMP family. Mice bearing a genetically engineered collagen resistant to cleavage by the MMP-family collagenases develop atheroma with increased collagen content [44]. More recently, studies in MMP-13-deficient mice provided further evidence for the critical role of collagenase in collagen architecture [45]. Macrophages in atherosclerotic plaques also express tissue factor, a potent initiator of the blood coagulation cascade [46,47]. The fibrous cap usually separates thrombogenic macrophages from coagulation factors in the bloodstream. However, once disruption of the cap occurs, physical contact of the blood with tissue factor may accelerate thrombus formation at the site of rupture.

Macrophages also release ROS and may oxidatively modify lipids in atherosclerotic plaques. Macrophage-derived myeloperoxidase converts H_2O_2 into HOCl, a more cytotoxic ROS, and can promote lipid peroxidation [48]. Atherosclerotic plaques contain macrophages expressing myeloperoxidase, and HOCl-modified proteins with signs of physical disruption localize in human coronary plaques [49]. Clinical evidence also recognizes myeloperoxidase as an independent risk predictor of acute coronary events [50]. These clinical and experimental data suggest that macrophages contribute critically to oxidative stress in atherosclerotic plaques by producing myeloperoxidase, leading to the onset of acute coronary thrombosis.

The role of EC dysfunction in acute coronary syndromes

Activated EC may contribute to the formation of vulnerable plaques rich in proteolytically active and thrombogenic macrophages [51–54]. Monocytes in the circulating blood attach to adhesion molecules such as VCAM-1 on the endothelium and then enter the arterial wall by diapedesis between EC (Figure 21.2, top panel). MCP-1 may mediate much of this monocyte migration [55]. Studies in genetically altered mice have demonstrated *in vivo* a critical role of VCAM-1 and MCP-1 in the formation of macrophage-rich atherosclerotic plaques [56–58]. Recent studies suggest that lipoproteins containing apolipoprotein CIII (apoCIII) predict coronary risk [59]. apoCIII inhibits lipoprotein

Baseline lesion

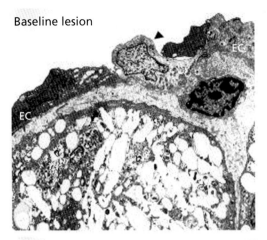

After cholesterol lowering

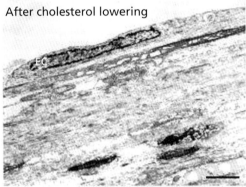

Figure 21.2 Ultrastructure of activated EC in rabbit atherosclerotic plaques and its normalization during cholesterol lowering. *Top panel*: Aortic EC of cholesterol-fed rabbits showed a cuboidal or rounded structure, typical of an "activated" phenotype. A monocytic cell (indicated by the arrowhead) appears to be entering the intima through the gap between EC. The circular cells containing abundant lipid particles in the subendothelial space of the aorta of the baseline lesion are probably macrophage-derived foam cells. *Bottom panel*: The aortic EC of treated animals had a more squamous morphology. The size, density, and amount of cytoplasmic organelles of EC of the plaque of treated animals are substantially smaller than those in the hypercholesterolemic animals. Accumulation of organized collagen fibrils was more prominent in the intima of the treated animals than in lesions of the high-cholesterol-fed rabbits. Original magnification: ×3000. Reproduced from Ref. [20] with permission.

catabolism in plasma. Our recent studies suggest that apoCIII promotes monocyte adhesion to activated EC, indicating a new mechanism for atherogenesis of dyslipidemia [60,61,61a].

NO inhibits monocyte–EC interaction [26–29]. Additionally, reduced production and bioavailability

of this athero-protective molecule in activated EC in atherosclerotic plaques should favor macrophage accumulation [20,30,31]. Decreased production of NO, well known as an endothelium-derived relaxing factor, reflects impaired endothelial functions beyond vasodilation [62]. Accumulating clinical evidence suggests a close association between endothelial dysfunction and future coronary events [63, 64]. Moreover, development of microvessels within the plaque may promote the formation of macrophage-rich vulnerable lesions by providing an extended surface area of activated EC [65–70].

In addition to its involvement in macrophage accumulation, EC activation may contribute more directly to the onset of acute coronary events. Although it occurs less commonly than rupture of the fibrous cap, superficial erosion of the plaque due to EC detachment plays an important role in the onset of acute thrombotic complications [71]. However, the molecular and cellular mechanisms of plaque erosion remain largely unknown. oxLDL induces EC expression of membrane type 1-MMP (MT1-MMP) that can activate MMP-2 [72]. Since MMP-2 cleaves type IV collagen, a major component of basement membrane beneath the endothelium, EC activation by oxidative stress may cause plaque erosion. More recently, we demonstrated that macrophage-derived myeloperoxidase, which potently induces lipid peroxidation, promotes EC apoptosis and tissue factor production *in vitro*, suggesting a role for vascular inflammation in plaque erosion and subsequent thrombosis [73].

In addition, activated EC may affect the fibrinolytic balance in the atherosclerotic plaques. While relatively normal EC express fibrinolytic molecules such as tissue-type plasminogen activator (tPA), activated EC increase the production of endogenous inhibitors of plasminogen activators (i.e., PAI-1) [74]. Such imbalance of fibrinolytic activity due to EC dysfunction likely stabilizes clots and favors the formation of a symptomatic or even fatal, occlusive thrombus.

Cholesterol lowering by HMG-CoA reductase inhibitors prevents acute coronary syndromes

During the 1990s, clinical studies established that cholesterol-lowering therapy by HMG-CoA reductase inhibitors (statins), a class of potent LDL-lowering drugs, substantially reduces the onset of acute coronary syndromes [1,75,76]. These trials demonstrated that the extent of cholesterol reduction positively correlates with risk reduction, further supporting the important causative role for elevated LDL in acute coronary events [8]. However, a number of angiographic trials revealed that benefits of statins for prevention of coronary events associated with little improvement in luminal stenoses [77]. This discrepancy introduced the concept that LDL lowering may modify the vulnerable plaque in a functional manner ("stabilization") rather than simply reduce lesion size ("regression") [36]. Many animal studies previously focused on plaque regression by cholesterol lowering [78,79]. However, more recent preclinical studies, including our own, explored evidence that supports the "plaque stabilization" hypothesis and sought mechanistic understanding of the clinical benefits of LDL lowering [1]. Clinical and preclinical studies also suggest various direct, or pleiotropic, effects of statins independent of LDL lowering [1,76,80].

Cholesterol lowering improves atheroma biology associated with plaque vulnerability and thrombogenicity

Throughout the 20th century, scientists accumulated increasing knowledge of hypercholesterolemic rabbits, whose arterial lesions mimic chronic atherosclerotic plaques in humans [9–12]. Rabbit aortic lesions created by combined mechanical injury and atherogenic diet contained several features typical of "vulnerable" plaques in humans: prominent macrophage accumulation, a thin and collagen-poor fibrous cap, expression of MMP and tissue factor and their inducers, CD40 ligand (or CD154) and CD40 [20,81–83]. Monitoring these factors during cholesterol withdrawal by diet alone in such atherosclerotic rabbits increased our understanding of the effects of cholesterol lowering itself, independent of any possible direct vascular effects of statins (Table 21.1) [20,81–83]. Dietary cholesterol lowering in rabbit atherosclerotic plaques reduced the accumulation of macrophages that express MMP including MMP-1/collagenase-1, and, in parallel, increased interstitial collagen content, a key determinant of

plaque stability [81]. A rabbit study by Kockx et al. and a clinical study by Crisby et al. reported similar findings of increased collagen in atherosclerotic plaques following cholesterol lowering [84,85]. These preclinical and clinical studies suggest that cholesterol lowering prevents acute coronary events in part by increasing the plaque's mechanical strength. Evidence that directly links collagenases of the MMP family and mechanical properties of arteries remains scant. However, our recent study on MMP-13-deficient mice demonstrated that genetic absence of this collagenolytic enzyme increased organization and alignment of fibrillar collagen in atherosclerotic plaques [45]. Cholesterol lowering also reduced the expression and activity of tissue factor and its inducers, CD154 and CD40, suggesting decreased thrombogenic potential, another major contributor to acute coronary events [82]. We furthermore reported that cholesterol lowering by statin treatment reduces the expression of MMP, tissue factor, and CD154 in Watanabe heritable hyperlipidemic rabbits [44,86]. Smooth muscle cells (SMC) undergo phenotypic modulation during the development of atherosclerosis [67]. SMC in the fibrous cap of rabbit atherosclerotic plaques also exhibited an immature phenotype compared with apparently normal medial SMC [83]. After dietary cholesterol lowering, however, the phenotype of SMC accumulated in the fibrous cap had a more mature phenotype and expressed less MMP and tissue factor compared with the baseline lesions of rabbit atherosclerosis [82,83].

Cholesterol lowering improves oxidative stress and EC dysfunction in atherosclerotic plaques

The series of rabbit studies mentioned above demonstrated the reduction of macrophage accumulation in rabbit lesions during dietary cholesterol lowering. However, the mechanisms by which cholesterol lowering diminished macrophages remained open. As discussed above, atherosclerotic arteries produce excess ROS and contain oxLDL. Such oxidative stress induces EC expression of VCAM-1 and MCP-1 and decreases eNOS expression, which favors macrophage infiltration in the atherosclerotic plaques. We therefore tested the

Table 21.1 Effects of cholesterol lowering on atherosclerotic plaques of hypercholesterolemic rabbits.

	Diet	Statins
LDL accumulation	Decreased	Decreased
ROS production (O_2^-)	Decreased	ND
oxLDL accumulation	Decreased	Decreased
Plasma autoantibody for oxLDL	Decreased	ND
EC functions		
VCAM-1	Decreased	ND
MCP-1	Decreased	ND
eNOS	Increased	ND
Microvessels	Decreased	ND
Macrophage accumulation	Decreased	Decreased
Macrophage proliferation	ND	Decreased
Macrophage apoptosis	ND	No change
MMP expression/activity	Decreased	Decreased
Collagen content	Increased	Increased*
Tissue factor expression/activity	Decreased	Decreased
PAI-1 expression	ND	Decreased
CD154 (CD40L) expression	Decreased	Decreased
PDGF-B expression	Decreased	ND
SMC maturity	Increased	ND
SM1 and SM2, a marker for mature SMCs	Increased	ND
SMemb, a nonmuscle or embryonic myosin	Decreased	ND

CD40L: CD40 Ligand; ND: not determined; and PDGF-B: platelet-derived growth factor B.

*No change with fluvastatin.

hypothesis that cholesterol lowering reduces oxidative stress and EC activation in the plaque (Table 21.1) [20]. Atherosclerotic aortas of cholesterol-fed rabbits elaborated high levels of ROS, including superoxide anion (O_2^-). However, cholesterol lowering by diet alone decreased ROS production to levels similar to those of normal aortas, concurring with previous work by Ohara et al. on an early stage of rabbit atherosclerosis [87]. Baseline lesions in hypercholesterolemic rabbits contained a prominent accumulation of oxLDL underlying activated EC that expressed VCAM-1 (Figure 21.1(a), top panels). In contrast, few if any EC in the plaque expressed eNOS. Dietary cholesterol lowering reduced oxLDL accumulation and VCAM-1 expression concomitantly, while lesions from control animals that continued the atherogenic diet maintained levels of both oxLDL and VCAM-1 (Figures 21.1(a), bottom panels, and (b)). Furthermore, plasma levels of autoantibodies against oxLDL epitopes

(MDA–LDL) decreased during cholesterol lowering. Dietary cholesterol lowering in these hypercholesterolemic rabbits increased eNOS expression substantially. After cholesterol lowering, aortic EC also exhibited a more normal ultrastructure compared with those of the atherosclerotic intima, which had features typical of activated EC (Figure 21.2, bottom panel). In aortic atherosclerotic plaques of cholesterol-fed rabbits, EC as well as SMCs and macrophages contained immunoreactive MCP-1 [20]. However, MCP-1 fell to barely detectable levels following cholesterol lowering. Collectively, these preclinical results suggest that statin treatment in hypercholesterolemic patients ameliorates oxidative stress and EC dysfunction by reducing LDL, a source of oxLDL, favoring feature of plaques associated with stability (Figure 21.3). Oxidized phospholipids (oxPL) are also pro-inflammatory. A recent study by Tsimikas et al., in collaboration with us, demonstrated that, in cholesterol-fed rabbits, the ratio of

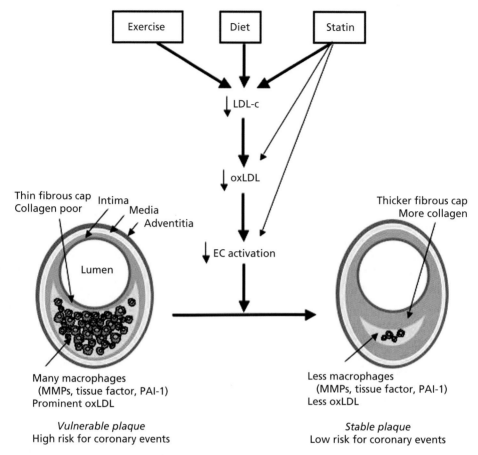

Figure 21.3 Potential mechanisms of atherosclerotic plaque stabilization by statin treatment. Decreased LDL levels by statin treatment should limit oxidative modification of LDL. Reduced oxLDL improves EC functions (e.g., reduced expression of VCAM-1), leading to diminished accumulation of proteolytic and prothrombotic macrophages in the plaque. Reduced oxidative stress also suppresses macrophage proliferation and activation. These changes may stabilize the plaque and prevent the onset of acute coronary syndromes. However, statins may also exert direct effects on oxidative modification of lipids, EC activation, and macrophage growth and activation. LDL-c: LDL-cholesterol.

oxPL and apOB-100 in plasma increased while oxPL accumulation decreases within the plaques. These results indicate that the plasma oxPL/apOB ratio may serve as a biomarker of lipid depletion from or regression of atherosclerotic plaques during cholesterol lowering [87a]. Additionally, *in vitro* evidence suggests that statins reduce macrophage uptake of oxLDL [88]. Despite the absence of consistent clinical evidence that associates statins with reduced LDL oxidation, more direct anti-oxidant properties of some statins or their metabolites might also mute vascular inflammation [89–93].

Cholesterol lowering vs direct effects of statins on EC dysfunction

A number of clinical studies suggest that LDL lowering by statins improves EC-dependent arterial relaxation. These benefits seem to involve at least two mechanisms: cholesterol lowering itself [94–96] and the direct vascular effects of statins [97–100]. Our rabbit study showed that dietary cholesterol reduction diminishes ROS production and oxLDL accumulation in lesions, which should by itself help restore normal EC functions [20]. The same study also showed increased EC expression of eNOS, an enzyme that generates NO. Thus, LDL lowering may itself improve EC-dependent vasorelaxation. On the other hand, considerable evidence indicates that statin treatment improves vasomotion independent of LDL lowering. Simvastatin preserved relaxation of coronary arteries of cholesterol-fed pigs in the absence of LDL reduction [97]. Laufs et al. demonstrated in a small human study that atorvastatin treatment (80 mg/day) improved endothelial function, as determined via forearm blood flow, within 24 h in normocholesterolemic subjects [99]. Changes in vascular functions in this study did not associate with changes in cholesterol levels, suggesting rapid effects of high-dose statin treatment on EC, independent of cholesterol reduction. Diabetic patients treated with cerivastatin for 3 days also showed improved EC-dependent dilation of brachial arteries [98]. Furthermore, a more recent clinical study demonstrated that a single dose (40 mg) of pravastatin, a hydrophilic statin, improved coronary EC function within 24 h [100]. EC vasodilator dysfunction correlates with risks for future coronary events [63,64]. Therefore, these reported rapid effects on EC functions provide mechanistic insight into the early benefits of acute statin treatment in the prevention of vascular events observed in some studies. However, the mechanisms by which statins, particularly hydrophilic statins that cannot penetrate easily into peripheral cells, produce such rapid vascular effects independent of LDL lowering remain obscure. Furthermore, little clinical evidence provides insight regarding statins' relative contribution of LDL-dependent and -independent mechanisms in the prevention of acute coronary events [101]. A recent meta-analysis suggested that statins' pleiotropic effects may not contribute additional risk reduction beyond LDL lowering [102].

Other preclinical studies support various cholesterol-independent effects of statins on EC functions [101]. This class of drugs suppresses cholesterol biosynthesis by inhibiting its rate-limiting enzyme, HMG-CoA reductase. Statins decrease not only cholesterol, but also isoprenoid intermediates including farnesylpyrophosphate and geranylgeranylpyrophosphate. These isoprenoids post-translationally modify proteins involved in cell functions, i.e., small G proteins Ras and Rho [103,104]. Simvastatin and atorvastatin increase eNOS expression and decrease endothelin-1 expression in EC by inhibiting Rho geranylgeranylation [105,106]. Atorvastatin also promotes NO production in EC by reducing caveolin-1 expression [107]. Kureishi et al. demonstrated that simvastatin induces phosphorylation of eNOS and increases NO production and survival of EC by activating the protein kinase Akt [108]. Yoshida et al. reported that cerivastatin suppresses monocyte–EC interaction under physiologic flow conditions *in vitro* by modulating of Rho activation [109]. Inhibition of the Rho-independent pathway and activation of Akt by statin treatment also reduce tissue factor expression in EC [110]. Masamura et al. further demonstrated that pitavastatin induces EC expression of thrombomodulin, an antithrombotic property of this cell type, via inhibition of the Rho family proteins [111]. *In vitro* studies including our own indicate that statin treatment reduced PAI-1 expression and increased tPA expression in EC, indicating an improvement of the fibrinolytic imbalance in the plaque [112,113].

More recent preclinical studies have explored effects of statins on angiogenesis both *in vitro* and *in vivo* [108,114–116]. However, considering the possible role of intraplaque microvessels in monocyte recruitment into the intima and in the formation of macrophage-rich plaques, the benefits of stimulation of angiogenesis by statins in coronary plaques in patients remain uncertain [65–70]. Lipid lowering by diet alone reduces the number of neovessels in rabbit atherosclerotic plaques, possibly favoring plaque stabilization (Figure 21.4) [1]. Other preclinical studies demonstrated cholesterol-independent effects of statins on other cell types related to vascular inflammation and atherogenesis, including activation and replication of macrophages [1,80, 86, 117–119]. Overall, these various effects on EC and macrophage functions illustrate mechanisms by which statins may exert anti-inflammatory and anti-atherothrombotic effects, although whether actions beyond cholesterol lowering contribute to clinical benefits remains unproven.

Conclusions and the future perspectives

Recent advances in clinical cardiology and vascular biology resolved several missing links between hypercholesterolemia and the onset of acute

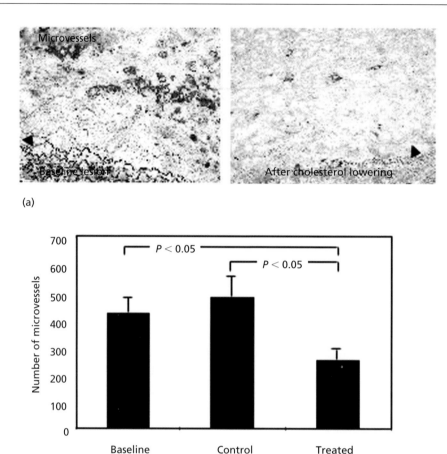

(a)

(b)

Figure 21.4 Cholesterol lowering reduced intraplaque microvessels. (a) Microvessels (lectin staining, BS-I) accumulated in the aortic intima of hypercholesterolemic rabbits after 4 months on a high-cholesterol diet (Baseline lesion). Sixteen month of dietary cholesterol lowering reduced microvessels in atherosclerotic plaques. The control animals that consumed the atherogenic diet for 16 more months contained many microvessels (data not shown). Original magnification ×400. (b) Quantitative data demonstrates the number of microvessels detected by BS-I staining in three experimental groups. Baseline indicates Baseline group; Control, high group; Treated, treated group. Bars represent SEM. Reproduced from Ref. [1] with permission.

coronary syndromes. Among them, in particular, oxidative stress and EC dysfunction play pivotal roles in hypercholesterolemia-induced vascular inflammation that triggers acute thrombotic complications. This chapter has highlighted the importance of cholesterol management in the prevention of thrombotic complications (Figure 21.3). We discussed unambiguous evidence that cholesterol lowering in rabbits by diet alone improves a number of features associated with inflammation, stability, and thrombogenicity of atherosclerotic plaques (Table 21.1). Although optimal LDL-cholesterol levels in humans remain unclear [120], recent

clinical evidence determined that intense lipid lowering provides greater benefit to patients at risk [8,121–126]. Indeed, the recently issued National Cholesterol Education Program (NCEP) update to the Adult Treatment Panel III (ATP III) guidelines proposes the option of lowered targets for blood concentrations of LDL-cholesterol ($<70 \, mg/dL$) for very high-risk individuals, e.g., existing coronary disease, diabetes, cigarette smoking, risk factors of metabolic syndrome, or history of a recent acute coronary event [127]. A recent clinical study on the effects of highly intense statin therapy used 40 mg/d rosuvastatin to achieve an average

LDL-cholesterol of 60.8 mg/dL and increased HDL-cholesterol by 14.7% and demonstrated significant plaque regression determined by intravascular ultrasound [127a].

The rapid clinical benefits of aggressive cholesterol lowering suggests direct effects of this class of drugs. Yet, establishing whether LDL-independent effects of statins provide additional benefits in the prevention of events in patients will require further studies [102]. Intensive life style changes remain an essential clinical approach to cardiovascular risk reduction. Exploration of new targets for anti-inflammatory therapies beyond LDL lowering, including inhibition of the renin–angiotensin–aldosterone system and activation of peroxisome proliferator-activated receptors (see Chapters 22 and 23), merits further investigation [128,129]. Treatment of atherosclerosis with drug combinations or with drugs containing multiple agents, including a less-than-maximal statin dose, e.g., co-therapy of a statin with a fibrate, cholesterol-absorption inhibitor, anti-hypertensive drug, or niacin, may become more common in the near future [130–136]. Furthermore, combining sensitive biomarkers that identify new risk factors beyond lipid profiles with novel imaging modalities that can detect luminal stenoses as well as the more "qualitative" features typical of vulnerable plaques [137] should provide better and more individualized approaches to the prevention of acute coronary syndromes.

Acknowledgment

This work was supported in part by grants from the National Institutes of Health, National Heart, Lung, and Blood Institute (P01-HL48743, Merit Award, and R01-HL80472 to Dr. Libby; SCOR P50HL56985 to Drs. Libby and Aikawa; and R01-HL66086 to Dr. Aikawa), Donald W. Reynolds Foundation and Leducq Foundation (to Dr. Libby), and the Japan Heart Foundation (to Dr. Aikawa). We acknowledge Ms. Karen E. Williams for her editorial assistance.

References

1 Aikawa M, Libby P. The vulnerable atherosclerotic plaque; pathogenesis and therapeutic approach. *Cardiovasc Pathol* 2004;13:125–138.

2 Ridker PM, Libby P. Risk factors for atherothrombotic disease. In: Zipes DP, Libby P, Bonow RO, Braunwald E, eds. *Braunwald's Heart Disease.* Philadelphia, PA: Elsevier Saunders; 2005:939–958.

3 Steinberg D. Thematic review series: the pathogenesis of atherosclerosis. An interpretive history of the cholesterol controversy: Part I. *J Lipid Res* 2004;45:1583–1593.

4 Steinberg D. Thematic review series: the pathogenesis of atherosclerosis. An interpretive history of the cholesterol controversy: Part II: The early evidence linking hypercholesterolemia to coronary disease in humans. *J Lipid Res* 2005;46:179–190.

5 LaRosa JC, Hunninghake D, Bush D, et al. The cholesterol facts. A summary of the evidence relating dietary fats, serum cholesterol, and coronary heart disease. A joint statement by the American Heart Association and the National Heart, Lung, and Blood Institute. The Task Force on Cholesterol Issues, American Heart Association. *Circulation* 1990; 81:1721–1733.

6 Yusuf S, Hawken S, Ounpuu S, et al. Effect of potentially modifiable risk factors associated with myocardial infarction in 52 countries (the INTERHEART study): case-control study. *Lancet* 2004; 364:937–952.

7 Libby P, Aikawa M, Schonbeck U. Cholesterol and atherosclerosis. *Biochim Biophys Acta* 2000;1529: 299–309.

8 Law MR, Wald NJ, Rudnicka AR. Quantifying effect of statins on low density lipoprotein cholesterol, ischaemic heart disease, and stroke: systematic review and meta-analysis. *BMJ* 2003;326:1423.

9 Anitschkow N, Chalatow S. On experimental cholesterin steatosis and its significance in the origin of some pathological processes (1913). *Reprinted in Arteriosclerosis* 1983;3:178–182.

10 Vesselinovitch D. Animal models and the study of atherosclerosis. *Arch Pathol Lab Med* 1988;112:1011–1017.

11 Armstrong ML, Heistad DD. Animal models of atherosclerosis. *Atherosclerosis* 1990;85:15–23.

12 Aikawa M, Fukumoto Y, Rabkin E, et al. Rabbit models of atherosclerosis. In: Daniel I. Simon, Rogers C, eds. *Vascular Disease and Injury: Preclinical Research.* Totowa, NJ: Humana Press; 2000:175–191.

13 Steinberg D. Thematic review series: the pathogenesis of atherosclerosis: an interpretive history of the cholesterol controversy: Part III: Mechanistically defining the role of hyperlipidemia. *J Lipid Res* 2005;46:2037–2051.

14 Steinberg D, Parthasarathy S, Carew TE, et al. Beyond cholesterol. Modifications of low-density lipoprotein that increase its atherogenicity. *N Engl J Med* 1989; 320:915–924.

15 Berliner JA, Navab M, Fogelman AM, et al. Atherosclerosis: basic mechanisms. Oxidation, inflammation, and genetics. *Circulation* 1995;91:2488–2496.

16 Tshimikas S, Glass CK, Steinberg D, et al. Lipoprotein oxidation, macrophages, immunity, and atherogenesis. In: Chein KR, ed. *Molecular Basis of Cardiovascular Disease.* Philadelphia, PA: Saunders; 2004:385–413.

17 Libby P. Inflammation in atherosclerosis. *Nature* 2002;420:868–874.

18 Haberland ME, Fong D, Cheng L. Malondialdehyde-altered protein occurs in atheroma of Watanabe heritable hyperlipidemic rabbits. *Science* 1988;241: 215–218.

19 Yla-Herttuala S, Palinski W, Rosenfeld ME, et al. Evidence for the presence of oxidatively modified low density lipoprotein in atherosclerotic lesions of rabbit and man. *J Clin Invest* 1989;84:1086–1095.

20 Aikawa M, Sugiyama S, Hill C, et al. Lipid lowering reduces oxidative stress and endothelial cell activation in rabbit atheroma. *Circulation* 2002;106:1390–1396.

21 Kume N, Cybulsky MI, Gimbrone MA Jr. Lysophosphatidylcholine, a component of atherogenic lipoproteins, induces mononuclear leukocyte adhesion molecules in cultured human and rabbit arterial endothelial cells. *J Clin Invest* 1992;90:1138–1144.

22 Khan BV, Parthasarathy SS, Alexander RW, et al. Modified low density lipoprotein and its constituents augment cytokine-activated vascular cell adhesion molecule-1 gene expression in human vascular endothelial cells. *J Clin Invest* 1995;95:1262–1270.

23 Cushing SD, Berliner JA, Valente AJ, et al. Minimally modified low density lipoprotein induces monocyte chemotactic protein 1 in human endothelial cells and smooth muscle cells. *Proc Natl Acad Sci USA* 1990;87:5134–5138.

24 Collins T, Cybulsky MI. NF-kappa B: pivotal mediator or innocent bystander in atherogenesis? *J Clin Invest* 2001;107:255–264.

25 Li H, Cybulsky MI, Gimbrone MA Jr, et al. An atherogenic diet rapidly induces VCAM-1, a cytokine-regulatable mononuclear leukocyte adhesion molecule, in rabbit aortic endothelium. *Arterioscler Thromb* 1993; 13:197–204.

26 Tsao PS, McEvoy LM, Drexler H, et al. Enhanced endothelial adhesiveness in hypercholesterolemia is attenuated by L-arginine. *Circulation* 1994;89:2176–2182.

27 De Caterina R, Libby P, Peng HB, et al. Nitric oxide decreases cytokine-induced endothelial activation. Nitric oxide selectively reduces endothelial expression of adhesion molecules and proinflammatory cytokines. *J Clin Invest* 1995;96:60–68.

28 Khan BV, Harrison DG, Olbrych MT, et al. Nitric oxide regulates vascular cell adhesion molecule 1 gene expression and redox-sensitive transcriptional events in human vascular endothelial cells. *Proc Natl Acad Sci USA* 1996;93:9114–9119.

29 Tsao PS, Wang B, Buitrago R, et al. Nitric oxide regulates monocyte chemotactic protein-1. *Circulation* 1997;96: 934–940.

30 Oemar BS, Tschudi MR, Godoy N, et al. Reduced endothelial nitric oxide synthase expression and production in human atherosclerosis. *Circulation* 1998;97: 2494–2498.

31 Huang AL, Vita JA. Effects of systemic inflammation on endothelium-dependent vasodilation. *Trends Cardiovasc Med* 2006;16:15–20.

32 Liao JK, Shin WS, Lee WY, et al. Oxidized low-density lipoprotein decreases the expression of endothelial nitric oxide synthase. *J Biol Chem* 1995; 270:319–324.

33 Davies MJ, Thomas AC. Plaque fissuring – the cause of acute myocardial infarction, sudden ischaemic death, and crescendo angina. *Br Heart J* 1985;53:363–373.

34 Ambrose JA, Tannenbaum MA, Alexopoulos D, et al. Angiographic progression of coronary artery disease and the development of myocardial infarction. *J Am Coll Cardiol* 1988;12:56–62.

35 Hackett D, Davies G, Maseri A. Pre-existing coronary stenoses in patients with first myocardial infarction are not necessarily severe. *Eur Heart J* 1988;9: 1317–1323.

36 Libby P. Molecular bases of the acute coronary syndromes. *Circulation* 1995;91:2844–2850.

37 van der Wal AC, Becker AE, van der Loos CM, et al. Site of intimal rupture or erosion of thrombosed coronary atherosclerotic plaques is characterized by an inflammatory process irrespective of the dominant plaque morphology. *Circulation* 1994;89:36–44.

38 Moreno PR, Bernardi VH, Lopez-Cuellar J, et al. Macrophage infiltration predicts restenosis after coronary intervention in patients with unstable angina. *Circulation* 1996;94:3098–3102.

39 Visse R, Nagase H. Matrix metalloproteinases and tissue inhibitors of metalloproteinases: structure, function, and biochemistry. *Circ Res* 2003;92:827–839.

40 Galis ZS, Sukhova GK, Lark MW, et al. Increased expression of matrix metalloproteinases and matrix degrading activity in vulnerable regions of human atherosclerotic plaques. *J Clin Invest* 1994;94:2493–2503.

41 Sukhova G, Schoenbeck U, Rabkin E, et al. Evidence of increased collagenolysis by interstitial collagenases-1 and -3 in vulnerable human atheromatous plaques. *Circulation* 1999;99: 2503–2509.

42 Herman MP, Sukhova GK, Libby P, et al. Expression of neutrophil collagenase (matrix metalloproteinase-8) in human atheroma: a novel collagenolytic pathway suggested by transcriptional profiling. *Circulation* 2001; 104:1899–1904.

43 Lee RT, Libby P. The unstable atheroma. *Arterioscler Thromb Vasc Biol* 1997;17:1859–1867.

44 Fukumoto Y, Deguchi JO, Libby P, et al. Genetically determined resistance to collagenase action augments interstitial collagen accumulation in atherosclerotic plaques. *Circulation* 2004;110: 1953–1959.

45 Deguchi J, Aikawa E, Libby P, et al. Matrix metallopro-teinase-13/collagenase-3 deletion promotes collagen accu-mulation and organization in mouse atherosclerotic plaques. *Circulation* 2005;112:2708–2715.

46 Wilcox JN, Smith KM, Schwartz SM, et al. Localization of tissue factor in the normal vessel wall and in the atheroscle-rotic plaque. *Proc Natl Acad Sci USA* 1989; 86:2839–2843.

47 Libby P, Mach F, Schoenbeck U, et al. Regulation of the thrombotic potential of atheroma. *Thromb Haemost* 1999;82:736–741.

48 Heinecke JW. Oxidative stress: new approaches to diag-nosis and prognosis in atherosclerosis. *Am J Cardiol* 2003;91:12A–16A.

49 Sugiyama S, Okada Y, Sukhova GK, et al. Macrophage myeloperoxidase regulation by granulocyte macrophage colony-stimulating factor in human atherosclerosis and implications in acute coronary syndromes. *Am J Pathol* 2001;158:879–891.

50 Baldus S, Heeschen C, Meinertz T, et al. Myeloperoxidase serum levels predict risk in patients with acute coronary syndromes. *Circulation* 2003;108:1440–1445.

51 Poole JCF, Florey HW. Changes in the endothelium of the aorta and the behavior of macrophages in experimen-tal atheroma of rabbits. *J Path Bact* 1958;75:245–253.

52 Faggiotto A, Ross R, Harker L. Studies of hypercholes-terolemia in the nonhuman primate: Part I: Changes that lead to fatty streak formation. *Arteriosclerosis* 1984;4: 323–340.

53 Cotran RS, Briscoe DM. Endothelial cells in inflammation. In: Kelly W, Harris E, Ruddy S, Sledge C, eds. *Textbook of Rheumatology.* Philadelphia, PA: WB Saunders Publishing Co.; 1997:183–198.

54 Gimbrone MA, Topper JN. Biology of the vessel wall: endothelium. In: Chein KR, ed. *Molecular Basis of Cardiovascular Disease.* Philadelphia, PA: WB Saunders; 1999:331–348.

55 Rollins BJ. Chemokines. *Blood* 1997;90:909–928.

56 Cybulsky MI, Iiyama K, Li H, et al. A major role for VCAM-1, but not ICAM-1, in early atherosclerosis. *J Clin Invest* 2001;107:1255–1262.

57 Gu L, Okada Y, Clinton SK, et al. Absence of monocyte chemoattractant protein-1 reduces atherosclerosis in low density lipoprotein receptor-deficient mice. *Mol Cell* 1998;2: 275–281.

58 Boring L, Gosling J, Cleary M, et al. Decreased lesion for-mation in CCR2−/− mice reveals a role for chemokines in the initiation of atherosclerosis. *Nature* 1998;394: 894–897.

59 Sacks FM, Alaupovic P, Moye LA, et al. VLDL, apolipoproteins B, CIII, and E, and risk of recurrent coronary events in the Cholesterol and Recurrent Events (CARE) trial. *Circulation* 2000;102:1886–1892.

60 Kawakami A, Aikawa M, Libby P, et al. Apolipoprotein CIII in apoB lipoproteins enhances the adhesion of

human monocytic cells to endothelial cells. *Circulation* 2006;113:691–700.

61 Kawakami A, Aikawa M, Alcaide P, et al. Apolipoprotein CIII induces expression of vascular cell adhesion mole-cule-1 in vascular endothelial cells and increases adhe-sion of monocytic cells. *Circulation* 2006;114:681–687.

61a Kawakami A, Aikawa M, Nitta N, et al. Apolipoprotein CIII-induced cell adhesion to endothelial cells involves pertussis toxin-sensitive G-protein kinase Ca-mediated nuclear factor-κB activation. *Arteriolscler Thromb Vasc Biol* (in Press).

62 Davignon J, Ganz P. Role of endothelial dysfunction in atherosclerosis. *Circulation* 2004;109:III27–III32.

63 Suwaidi JA, Hamasaki S, Higano ST, et al. Long-term fol-low-up of patients with mild coronary artery disease and endothelial dysfunction. *Circulation* 2000;101:948–954.

64 Halcox JP, Schenke WH, Zalos G, et al. Prognostic value of coronary vascular endothelial dysfunction. *Circulation* 2002;106:653–658.

65 O'Brien KD, Allen MD, McDonald TO, et al. Vascular cell adhesion molecule-1 is expressed in human coro-nary atherosclerotic plaques. Implications for the mode of progression of advanced coronary atherosclerosis. *J Clin Invest* 1993;92:945–951.

66 Brogi E, Winkles JA, Underwood R, et al. Distinct pat-terns of expression of fibroblast growth factors and their receptors in human atheroma and nonatherosclerotic arteries. Association of acidic FGF with plaque microvessels and macrophages. *J Clin Invest* 1993; 92:2408–2418.

67 Aikawa M, Sivam PN, Kuro-o M, et al. Human smooth muscle myosin heavy chain isoforms as molecular markers for vascular development and atherosclerosis. *Circ Res* 1993;73: 1000–1012.

68 O'Brien ER, Garvin MR, Dev R, et al. Angiogenesis in human coronary atherosclerotic plaques. *Am J Pathol* 1994;145: 883–894.

69 Moulton KS, Heller E, Konerding MA, et al. Angiogenesis inhibitors endostatin or TNP-470 reduce intimal neovas-cularization and plaque growth in apolipoprotein E-deficient mice. *Circulation* 1999;99: 1726–1732.

70 Celletti FL, Waugh JM, Amabile PG, et al. Vascular endothelial growth factor enhances atherosclerotic plaque progression. *Nat Med* 2001;7:425–429.

71 Farb A, Burke AP, Tang AL, et al. Coronary plaque erosion without rupture into a lipid core. A frequent cause of coronary thrombosis in sudden coronary death. *Circulation* 1996; 93: 1354–1363.

72 Rajavashisth TB, Liao JK, Galis ZS, et al. Inflammatory cytokines and oxidized low density lipoproteins increase endothelial cell expression of membrane type 1-matrix metalloproteinase. *J Biol Chem* 1999;274:11924–11929.

73 Sugiyama S, Kugiyama K, Aikawa M, et al. Hypochlorous acid, a macrophage product, induces

endothelial apoptosis and tissue factor expression. Involvement of myeloperoxidase-mediated oxidant in plaque erosion and thrombogenesis. *Arterioscler Thromb Vasc Biol* 2004:1309–1314.

74 Schneiderman J, Sawdey MS, Keeton MR, et al. Increased type 1 plasminogen activator inhibitor gene expression in atherosclerotic human arteries. *Proc Natl Acad Sci USA* 1992;89:6998–7002.

75 Gotto AM, Farmer JA. Lipid-lowering trials. In: Braunwald E, Zipes DP, Libby P, eds. *Heart Disease: A Text Book of Cardiovascular Medicine*. Philadelphia, PA: WB Saunders; 2001:126–146.

76 Libby P, Aikawa M. Stabilization of atherosclerotic plaques: new mechanisms and clinical targets. *Nature Med* 2002;8:1257–1262.

77 Vaughan CJ, Gotto Jr AM, Basson CT. The evolving role of statins in the management of atherosclerosis. *J Am Coll Cardiol* 2000;35:1–10.

78 Small DM. George Lyman Duff memorial lecture. Progression and regression of atherosclerotic lesions. Insights from lipid physical biochemistry. *Arteriosclerosis* 1988;8:103–129.

79 Wissler RW, Vesselinovitch D. Can atherosclerotic plaques regress? Anatomic and biochemical evidence from nonhuman animal models. *Am J Cardiol* 1990;65: 33F–40F.

80 Davignon J. Beneficial cardiovascular pleiotropic effects of statins. *Circulation* 2004;109:III39–III43.

81 Aikawa M, Rabkin E, Okada Y, et al. Lipid lowering by diet reduces matrix metalloproteinase activity and increases collagen content of rabbit atheroma: a potential mechanism of lesion stabilization. *Circulation* 1998;97:2433–2444.

82 Aikawa M, Voglic SJ, Sugiyama S, et al. Dietary lipid lowering reduces tissue factor expression in rabbit atheroma. *Circulation* 1999; 100:1215–1222.

83 Aikawa M, Rabkin E, Voglic SJ, et al. Lipid lowering promotes accumulation of mature smooth muscle cells expressing smooth muscle myosin heavy chain isoforms in rabbit atheroma. *Circ Res* 1998;83:1015–1026.

84 Kockx MM, De Meyer GR, Buyssens N, et al. Cell composition, replication, and apoptosis in atherosclerotic plaques after 6 months of cholesterol withdrawal. *Circ Res* 1998;83:378–387.

85 Crisby M, Nordin-Fredriksson G, Shah PK, et al. Pravastatin treatment increases collagen content and decreases lipid content, inflammation, metalloproteinases, and cell death in human carotid plaques: implications for plaque stabilization. *Circulation* 2001;103: 926–933.

86 Aikawa M, Rabkin E, Sugiyama S, et al. An HMG-CoA reductase inhibitor, cerivastatin, suppresses growth of macrophages expressing matrix metalloproteinases and tissue factor *in vivo* and *in vitro*. *Circulation* 2001; 103:276–283.

87 Ohara Y, Peterson TE, Sayegh HS, et al. Dietary correction of hypercholesterolemia in the rabbit normalizes endothelial superoxide anion production. *Circulation* 1995;92: 898–903.

87a Tsimikas S, Aikawa M, Miller FJ, et al. Increased plasma oxidized phospholipid: apolipoprotein B-100 ratio with concomitant depletion of oxidized phospholipids from atherosclerotic lesions following dietary lipid lowering: a potential biomarker of early atherosclerosis regression. *Arteriolscler Thromb Vasc Biol* (in Press)

88 Fuhrman B, Koren L, Volkova N, et al. Atorvastatin therapy in hypercholesterolemic patients suppresses cellular uptake of oxidized-LDL by differentiating monocytes. *Atherosclerosis* 2002;164: 179–185.

89 Giroux LM, Davignon J, Naruszewicz M. Simvastatin inhibits the oxidation of low-density lipoproteins by activated human monocyte-derived macrophages. *Biochim Biophys Acta* 1993;1165:335–338.

90 Leonhardt W, Kurktschiev T, Meissner D, et al. Effects of fluvastatin therapy on lipids, antioxidants, oxidation of low density lipoproteins and trace metals. *Eur J Clin Pharmacol* 1997;53:65–69.

91 Aviram M, Fuhrman B. LDL oxidation by arterial wall macrophages depends on the oxidative status in the lipoprotein and in the cells: role of prooxidants vs. antioxidants. *Mol Cell Biochem* 1998;188:149–159.

92 Franzoni F, Quinones-Galvan A, Regoli F, et al. A comparative study of the *in vitro* antioxidant activity of statins. *Int J Cardiol* 2003;90:317–321.

93 Shishehbor MH, Brennan ML, Aviles RJ, et al. Statins promote potent systemic antioxidant effects through specific inflammatory pathways. *Circulation* 2003;108: 426–431.

94 Egashira K, Hirooka Y, Kai H, et al. Reduction in serum cholesterol with pravastatin improves endothelium-dependent coronary vasomotion in patients with hypercholesterolemia. *Circulation* 1994;89:2519–2524.

95 Treasure CB, Klein JL, Weintraub WS, et al. Beneficial effects of cholesterol-lowering therapy on the coronary endothelium in patients with coronary artery disease. *N Engl J Med* 1995;332:481–487.

96 Anderson TJ, Meredith IT, Yeung AC, et al. The effect of cholesterol-lowering and antioxidant therapy on endothelium-dependent coronary vasomotion. *N Engl J Med* 1995;332:488–493.

97 Wilson SH, Simari RD, Best PJ, et al. Simvastatin preserves coronary endothelial function in hypercholesterolemia in the absence of lipid lowering. *Arterioscler Thromb Vasc Biol* 2001;21:122–128.

98 Tsunekawa T, Hayashi T, Kano H, et al. Cerivastatin, a hydroxymethylglutaryl coenzyme a reductase inhibitor, improves endothelial function in elderly diabetic patients within 3 days. *Circulation* 2001;104: 376 379.

99 Laufs U, Wassmann S, Hilgers S, et al. Rapid effects on vascular function after initiation and withdrawal of atorvastatin in healthy, normocholesterolemic men. *Am J Cardiol* 2001;88: 1306–1307.

100 Wassmann S, Faul A, Hennen B, et al. Rapid effect of 3-hydroxy-3-methylglutaryl coenzyme a reductase inhibition on coronary endothelial function. *Circ Res* 2003;93:e98–e103.

101 Aikawa M. Effects of statin therapy on vascular dysfunction. *Coron Artery Dis* 2004;15:227–233.

102 Robinson JG, Smith B, Maheshwari N, et al. Peliotropic effects of statins: benefits beyond cholesterol reduction? *J Am Coll Cardiol* 2005;46:1855–1862.

103 Goldstein JL, Brown MS. Regulation of the mevalonate pathway. *Nature* 1990;343:425–430.

104 Liao JK. Isoprenoids as mediators of the biological effects of statins. *J Clin Invest* 2002;110:285–288.

105 Laufs U, Liao JK. Post-transcriptional regulation of endothelial nitric oxide synthase mRNA stability by Rho GTPase. *J Biol Chem* 1998;273:24266–24271.

106 Hernandez-Perera O, Perez-Sala D, Soria E, et al. Involvement of Rho GTPases in the transcriptional inhibition of preproendothelin-1 gene expression by simvastatin in vascular endothelial cells. *Circ Res* 2000;87:616–622.

107 Feron O, Dessy C, Desager JP, et al. Hydroxy-methylglutaryl-coenzyme A reductase inhibition promotes endothelial nitric oxide synthase activation through a decrease in caveolin abundance. *Circulation* 2001; 103:113–118.

108 Kureishi Y, Luo Z, Shiojima I, et al. The HMG-CoA reductase inhibitor simvastatin activates the protein kinase Akt and promotes angiogenesis in normocholesterolemic animals. *Nat Med* 2000;6:1004–1010.

109 Yoshida M, Sawada T, Ishii H, et al. HMG-CoA reductase inhibitor modulates monocyte– endothelial cell interaction under physiological flow conditions *in vitro*: involvement of Rho GTPase-dependent mechanism. *Arterioscler Thromb Vasc Biol* 2001;21: 1165–1171.

110 Eto M, Kozai T, Cosentino F, et al. Statin prevents tissue factor expression in human endothelial cells: role of Rho/Rho-kinase and Akt pathways. *Circulation* 2002; 105:1756–1759.

111 Masamura K, Oida K, Kanehara H, et al. Pitavastatin-induced thrombomodulin expression by endothelial cells acts via inhibition of small G proteins of the Rho family. *Arterioscler Thromb Vasc Biol* 2003;23:512–517.

112 Essig M, Nguyen G, Prie D, et al. Friedlander G. 3-Hydroxy-3-methylglutaryl coenzyme A reductase inhibitors increase fibrinolytic activity in rat aortic endothelial cells. Role of geranylgeranylation and Rho proteins. *Circ Res* 1998;83:683–690.

113 Bourcier T, Libby P. HMG CoA reductase inhibitors reduce plasminogen activator inhibitor-1 expression by

human vascular smooth muscle and endothelial cells. *Arterioscler Thromb Vasc Biol* 2000;20:556–562.

114 Weis M, Heeschen C, Glassford AJ, et al. Statins have biphasic effects on angiogenesis. *Circulation* 2002;105: 739–745.

115 Urbich C, Dernbach E, Zeiher AM, et al. Double-edged role of statins in angiogenesis signaling. *Circ Res* 2002;90:737–744.

116 Walter DH, Rittig K, Bahlmann FH, et al. Statin therapy accelerates reendothelialization: a novel effect involving mobilization and incorporation of bone marrow-derived endothelial progenitor cells. *Circulation* 2002;105: 3017–3024.

117 Sakai M, Kobori S, Matsumura T, et al. HMG-CoA reductase inhibitors suppress macrophage growth induced by oxidized low density lipoprotein. *Atherosclerosis* 1997;133:51–59.

118 Colli S, Eligini S, Lalli M, et al. Vastatins inhibit tissue factor in cultured human macrophages. A novel mechanism of protection against atherothrombosis. *Arterioscler Thromb Vasc Biol* 1997;17:265–272.

119 Bellosta S, Via D, Canavesi M, et al. HMG-CoA reductase inhibitors reduce MMP-9 secretion by macrophages. *Arterioscler Thromb Vasc Biol* 1998;18:1671–1678.

120 O'Keefe Jr JH, Cordain L, Harris WH, et al. Optimal low-density lipoprotein is 50 to 70 mg/dl: lower is better and physiologically normal. *J Am Coll Cardiol* 2004;43:2142–2146.

121 Group HPSC. MRC/BHF Heart Protection Study of cholesterol lowering with simvastatin in 20,536 high-risk individuals: a randomised placebo-controlled trial. *Lancet* 2002;360:7–22.

122 Kinlay S, Timms T, Clark M, et al. Comparison of effect of intensive lipid lowering with atorvastatin to less intensive lowering with lovastatin on C-reactive protein in patients with stable angina pectoris and inducible myocardial ischemia. *Am J Cardiol* 2002;89: 1205–1207.

123 van Wissen S, Trip MD, Smilde TJ, et al. Differential hs-CRP reduction in patients with familial hypercholesterolemia treated with aggressive or conventional statin therapy. *Atherosclerosis* 2002;165:361–366.

124 Taylor AJ, Kent SM, Flaherty PJ, et al. ARBITER: Arterial Biology for the Investigation of the Treatment Effects of Reducing Cholesterol: a randomized trial comparing the effects of atorvastatin and pravastatin on carotid intima medial thickness. *Circulation* 2002;106: 2055–2060.

125 Cannon CP, Braunwald E, McCabe CH, et al. Intensive versus moderate lipid lowering with statins after acute coronary syndromes. *N Engl J Med* 2004;350: 1495–1504.

126 Nissen SE, Tuzcu EM, Schoenhagen P, et al. Effect of intensive compared with moderate lipid-lowering

therapy on progression of coronary atherosclerosis: a randomized controlled trial. *JAMA* 2004;291: 1071–1080.

127   Grundy SM, Cleeman JI, Merz CN, et al. Implications of recent clinical trials for the National Cholesterol Education Program Adult Treatment Panel III guidelines. *Circulation* 2004; 110:227–239.

127a Nissen SE, Nicholls SJ, Sipahi I, et al. Effect of very high-intensity statin therapy on regression of coronary atherosclerosis: the ASTEROID trial. *JAMA* 2006;295: 1556–1565.

128   Weiss D, Sorescu D, Taylor WR. Angiotensin II and atherosclerosis. *Am J Cardiol* 2001;87:25C–32C.

129   Ziouzenkova O, Perrey S, Marx N, et al. Peroxisome proliferator-activated receptors. *Curr Atheroscler Rep* 2002;4:59–64.

130   Farnier M, Salko T, Isaacsohn JL, et al. Effects of baseline level of triglycerides on changes in lipid levels from combined fluvastatin + fibrate (bezafibrate, fenofibrate, or gemfibrozil). *Am J Cardiol* 2003;92: 794–797.

131   Ballantyne CM, Houri J, Notarbartolo A, et al. Effect of ezetimibe coadministered with atorvastatin in 628 patients with primary hypercholesterolemia: a prospective, randomized, double-blind trial. *Circulation* 2003;107:2409–2415.

132   Kastelein J. What future for combination therapies? *Int J Clin Pract Suppl* 2003:45–50.

133   Wald NJ, Law MR. A strategy to reduce cardiovascular disease by more than 80%. *BMJ* 2003;326:1419.

134   Nickenig G. Should angiotensin II receptor blockers and statins be combined? *Circulation* 2004;110: 1013–1020.

135   Davidson MH, Ballantyne CM, Kerzner B, et al. Efficacy and safety of ezetimibe coadministered with statins: randomised, placebo-controlled, blinded experience in 2382 patients with primary hypercholesterolemia. *Int J Clin Pract* 2004;58:746–755.

136   Kosoglou T, Statkevich P, Yang B, et al. Pharmacodynamic interaction between ezetimibe and rosuvastatin. *Curr Med Res Opin* 2004;20:1185–1195.

137   Deguchi J, Aikawa M, Tung CH, et al. Inflammation in atherosclerosis: visualizing matrix metalloproteinase action in macrophages *in vivo*. *Circulation* 2006;114: 55–62.

CHAPTER 22

Antioxidants and endothelial protection

Domenico Praticò, MD

Introduction

Long considered merely a semi-permeable membrane, the endothelium in the last 20 years has gained recognition as a complex organ system that controls vascular homeostasis by integrating signals between the vascular wall and the vessel lumen. Today it is widely accepted that the endothelium plays important roles in maintaining normal vascular tone and blood fluidity, reducing platelet activity and leukocyte adhesion, and limiting vascular inflammatory reactions [1]. Under normal conditions, the endothelium regulates vascular homeostasis by elaborating a variety of factors such as nitric oxide (NO), prostacyclin, and endothelin. However, in particular situations the endothelium can also modify its phenotype, thus facilitating vasoconstriction, inflammation, and thrombotic events. Such abnormal responses occur in the absence of any morphological change of the vessel and manifest in conditions such as hypercholesterolemia, hypertension, and diabetes mellitus [2]. Increasing evidence suggests that such functional changes (endothelial dysfunctions, ED) foreshadow atherosclerosis and predict future vascular events [3]. The etiology of these altered endothelial functions is multifactorial, and underlying mechanisms are complex and incompletely elucidated. Among these factors, altered receptor signaling due to membrane changes, alterations of endothelial nitric oxide synthase (eNOS) expression and activity, decreased availability of tetrahydrobiopterin, and increased generation of superoxide radicals have all been considered responsible for these alterations [4]. However, the mechanism most frequently implicated in the pathogenesis of ED relate to increased production of reactive oxygen species (ROS). ROS deplete the bioavailability of NO and exacerbate local oxidative stress by reacting directly with NO to form peroxynitrite, which in turn further sustains oxidative injury to the endothelium [5]. If the hypothesis that an imbalance between ROS formation and the endothelial capacity to dispose of ROS plays a causative role in these altered endothelial functions, molecules capable of scavenging ROS might reverse or prevent them. Thus, any pharmacological intervention with exogenous antioxidants should protect vascular endothelium specifically via a ROS-scavenging activity and the restoration of NO bioavailability. This chapter will therefore focus on the role of exogenous antioxidants in the protection of normal endothelial functions.

Antioxidants and ED

The term ED has been used very broadly to describe several pathological conditions, such as altered anti-coagulant properties of the endothelium or dysregulation of vascular remodeling (see Chapter 1). Currently, however, in its clinical acception, ED commonly refers to reduced endothelium-dependent vasodilatory capacity of the coronary and peripheral circulation to acetylcholine. Since this type of vasorelaxation associates with endothelial cell production of NO, which acts in turn on smooth muscle cells, we typically attribute ED to decreased production and/or increased catabolism of endothelium-derived NO. Accumulating evidence suggests that increased oxidative stress can account for a significant portion of this phenomenon. Increased production of ROS not efficiently destroyed by endogenous antioxidant systems could deplete local NO production or its bioavailability by reacting and scavenging NO itself to form peroxynitrite. Several potential enzymatic sources of ROS in vascular cells can be responsible for the reduction of NO bioavailability, particularly xantine oxidase, NADH/NADPH oxidase, lipooxygenases, and cyclooxygenases [6]. Additionally, ROS may participate in ED by regulating the expression levels of eNOS. The integrity of eNOS protein expression and the preservation of its enzymatic activity are essential to maintaining availability of continuous and adequate NO to the endothelium. Surprisingly, however, *in vitro* data show that ROS cause increased levels of eNOS protein, generally considered a secondary reaction to local NO deficiency [7].

Animal studies

Mugge et al. first reported ROS-impaired endothelial function *in vivo* in atherosclerotic rabbits, and restoration of impaired endothelium-dependent vasorelaxation in cholesterol-fed-rabbits by the administration of polyethylene glycol conjugated superoxide dismutase (SOD) [8]. Another group showed that dietary treatment with the lipid-soluble antioxidants vitamin E, and β-carotene preserves endothelium-dependent vasorelaxation in cholesterol-fed-rabbits [9]. Although directly associated with the accumulation of these vitamins in vascular tissue, such improvements were unrelated to any alteration in lipoproteins, and were independent of the extent of atherosclerosis [9]. Protection of endothelium-dependent relaxation by vitamin E has been observed in pathophysiological states associated with increased oxidative stress. Thus, chronic vitamin E supplementation has been reported to be protective in diabetic rats as well as hypercholesterolemic rabbits [10,11]. Recent reports suggest that long-term dietary supplementation with vitamin E associates with improved endothelial vasodilatory function in heart failure [12]. Another study examined the effect of dietary supplements with vitamin A, vitamin E, and selenium in rats consuming a high-fat diet for 6 months [13]. In such conditions, treatment with dietary antioxidants increased antioxidant tissue levels and

preserved endothelium-dependent vasorelaxation, even in the absence of significant changes in lipid levels. In hypercholesterolemic pigs, the combined administration of vitamin E and vitamin C reduced vascular inflammation, normalized NO bioactivity, and preserved coronary endothelial function [14]. Moreover, the long-term administration of vitamin C had beneficial effect on ED in vascular beds of apolipoprotein E-deficient mice by increasing vascular tetrahydrobiopterin levels and nitric oxide synthase (NOS) activity [14,15]. Chronic administration of vitamin C or glutathione prevented microvascular dysfunction secondary to experimental endothelial injury in pigs [16].

Finally, the hydroxymethylglutaryl coenzyme A (HMGCoA) reductase inhibitors simvastatin and pravastatin protect the endothelium [17,18], an effect independent of the lipid-lowering activity of these drugs and more likely secondary to antioxidant mechanisms (i.e., reduction of low-density lipoproteins (LDL) oxidation, increased SOD, and gluthatione peroxidase activities).

Human studies

Increasingly, human studies in peripheral as well as in coronary vessels have investigated the effects of antioxidants on ED; most have shown positive results. Vitamin C improved ED in chronic smokers, subjects with type 1 and type 2 diabetes mellitus, hypercholesterolemia, essential and reno-vascular hypertension, chronic heart failure, and in healthy subjects as well [19–27]. However, only a few of these studies investigated the effectiveness of vitamin C, at the dosage administered, in reducing any biomarker of oxidative stress. Therefore, it is difficult to fully support an antioxidant mechanism of action for these vitamins in these studies.

Vitamin E treatment improved ED and decreased levels of thiobarbituric acid-reactive substances (TBARS) in patients with vasospastic angina pectoris [28]. The long-term supplementation of vitamin E also ameliorated ED in hypercholesterolemic smokers, and decreased auto-antibody levels against oxidized LDL (oxLDL) [29]. Finally, vitamin E preserved intact endothelial vasomotor function in patients with coronary atherosclerosis [30] and after methionine loading [31]. More recently, HMGCoA reductase inhibitors reversed ED by increasing

Table 22.1 *In vivo* effects of antioxidants on various vascular functions.

Function	Human studies	References	Animal studies	References
ED	Positive	[19–33]	Positive	[8–18]
Leukocyte–endothelium interactions	Positive	[50–52,56,57]	Positive	[46,55]
Thrombosis/fibrinolysis	Positive	[68–71]	Positive	[63–65]

Data from human and animal studies.

eNOS levels and decreasing oxidative stress in the absence of lipid lowering [32,33].

Despite conflicting data from clinical trials of antioxidants in cardiovascular diseases [34], findings on the therapeutic benefit of antioxidants in protecting from ED are surprisingly consistent. Thus, both animal and clinical studies indicate that increased ROS formation and subsequent oxidative stress associate with impaired vasodilation that occurs in response to the production of endothelial NO. Reduced NO bioavailability, at least partially attributable to concomitant ROS production, contributes significantly to these effects, and supplementation with exogenous antioxidants normalizes altered vascular responses (Table 22.1).

Antioxidants and leukocyte–endothelium interactions

In addition to altered endothelium-dependent vasodilation, ROS have also been studied in relation to leukocyte–endothelial interactions. Leukocytes can be source of ROS, and their activation and migration from the circulation to areas of vascular damage may play a significant role in the pathogenesis of altered endothelial function [35,36]. Several inflammatory cytokines can initiate leukocyte adhesion and penetration into the arterial intima, mediated by membrane adhesion molecules expressed on leukocytes and their respective vascular ligands. Among them, vascular cell adhesion molecule-1 (VCAM-1) and intercellular adhesion molecule-1 (ICAM-1) are particularly important (see Chapter 2). Normal vascular endothelial cells generally express very low levels of VCAM-1 and ICAM-1, which increase in the atherosclerotic endothelium. Although the nature of factors responsible for switching a normal quiescent endothelial cell to one that avidly recruits leukocytes remains

incompletely elucidated, oxidative stress likely participates in this mechanism. Interestingly, the isoprostane (iP) $F_{2\alpha}$-III, a stable end product of lipid peroxidation produced *in vivo* under conditions of oxidative stress, induces rapidly and selectively increased neutrophil adhesiveness [37]. Further, exposure to high glucose concentrations *in vitro* leads to increased levels of some adhesion molecules on the endothelial cells via an antioxidant-sensitive mechanism [38]. On the other hand, antioxidants can modulate the increased expression of key adhesion molecules on monocyte–macrophages and neutrophils that occurs shortly after exposure to cytokines or lipid oxidation products [39–42].

Several studies have shown that enrichment with vitamin E decreases adhesiveness of monocytes and neutrophils *in vitro* and *in vivo*, secondary to decreased adhesion molecule expression [43–45]. The overexpression of Cu, Zn SOD, and catalase reduced the expression of cell-adhesion molecules, and inhibited the adherence of leukocytes to endothelial cell more efficiently than the overexpression of SOD or catalase alone [46]. Long-term supplementation with vitamin C reduced leukocyte adhesion in the central microcirculation of diabetic rats [47,48]. Smoking, a major risk factor in atherogenesis, induces ROS formation *in vivo*. Cigarette smoke elicits leukocyte adhesion to the endothelium in animal models; this enhanced adherence of monocytes to endothelial cells is considered an initial event in the pathogenesis of cigarette smoke-related ED [49]. Additionally, pretreatment with SOD or vitamin C, but not vitamin E, inhibits smoke-induced leukocyte adhesion to the endothelium [49,50]. Further, oral supplementation with vitamin C for 10 days reversed the increased monocyte adhesion to human endothelial cells *ex vivo* in smokers to levels found in non-smokers [50]. In addition, vitamin E supplementation decreased circulating levels of ICAM-1 and NO metabolites in hypercholesterolemic patients as well as in healthy subjects [51,52].

Leukocyte–endothelium interactions also participate importantly in ischemia–reperfusion injury, generally thought to be caused by endothelial damage secondary to leukocyte-derived ROS formation [53,54]. In this setting, pre-treatment with antioxidants (vitamin C or vitamin E) protects against ischemia–reperfusion injury [55,56]. Finally, a recent double-blind prospective study demonstrated that antioxidant supplements retard the progression of cardiac transplant-associated arteriosclerosis [57].

Regulated interactions between leukocytes and the endothelial cell membranes are key events in preserving a normal vascular homeostasis. In oxidative stress, the normally quiescent endothelium becomes active and begins to attract and recruit leukocytes, an important and necessary initial event in the pathogenesis of the atherosclerotic response of the endothelium. Exogenous antioxidants consistently reverse this pathological situation *in vitro* and *in vivo* (Table 22.1).

Antioxidants and endothelial cell thrombotic and fibrinolytic properties

Endothelial cells provide a number of components important to thrombosis and fibrinolysis, which confer another extremely important property to the endothelium: the maintenance of a delicate balance between pro- and anti-thrombotic events. Physiologically, endothelial cells possess excess plasminogen activators, thrombomodulin, and prostacyclin, which all protect against anti-fibrinolytic, procoagulant, and platelet-activating states. However, the endothelium can change its phenotype and manifest opposing activities when exposed to different stimuli. Several *in vitro* studies have indeed demonstrated that minimally oxLDL, but not native LDL, increase tissue factor (TF) expression by endothelial cells, an action prevented by antioxidants [58,59]. OxLDL also induce thrombomodulin mRNA, thrombomodulin antigen and activity, reduce tissue plasminogen activator (tPA), and increase the release of plasminogen activator-inhibitor-1 (PAI-1) from human endothelial cells [60,61]. Transition metals such as copper and iron,

known to initiate ROS formation and lipid peroxidation, increase the expression levels (mRNA and protein) as well as activity of TF, effects all completely reversed by antioxidants such as vitamin E and butylated hydroxytoluene [62]. In addition, a seleno-organic antioxidant, ebselen, has been shown to be beneficial after experimental embolic stroke in rabbits by enhancing the neuroprotective activity of low-dose tPA [63]. The same compound was also effective in delaying microvascular thrombus formation in rat microvessel preparations [64]. Both α- and γ-tocopherol decreased platelet aggregation and delay intra-arterial thrombus formation in an experimental model of thrombosis [65].

Clinical studies have demonstrated that subjects with hyperlipidemia, a condition associated with oxidative stress, have a significant reduction in the free form of TF pathway inhibitor, while the form of TF pathway inhibitor associated with LDL increases [66]. High levels of cholesterol also associate with prolonged euglobulin lysis, suggesting an altered balance between pro- and anti-fibrinolytic factors, secondary to altered levels and the ratio between tPA and PAI-1, which both originate at least in part in the endothelium [67]. Additionally, protein S and von Willebrand factor levels were higher in subjects with coronary heart disease compared with healthy controls [67]. Interestingly, another study reported that plasma protein oxidation markers in healthy subjects correlate directly with procoagulant markers, and vitamin E treatment restores the equilibrium between pro- and anti-coagulant pathways [68]. A hemostatic imbalance, characterized by clotting activation, is evident in some patients with liver failure, secondary to an accelerated thrombin generation rate *in vivo*. In this clinical setting, the administration of vitamin E for 4 weeks significantly decreases TF antigen and prothrombin fragment 1 + 2, and associates with a reduction in systemic oxidative stress [69]. Finally, vitamin C levels correlate inversely with several hemostatic factors, and the administration of vitamin C improved fibrinolysis [70,71], although other studies did not confirm these data [72].

Most data accumulated thus far therefore suggest an association between ROS formation, oxidative stress, and altered endothelial hemostatic balance, *in vitro* and in animal models (Table 22.1). However, current evidence insufficiently supports the hypothesis that antioxidants can reverse this situation *in vivo*.

Antioxidants and endothelial cell apoptosis

Several experiments using different types of endothelial cells have shown clearly that the endothelium can undergo apoptosis under oxidative stress and in the presence of oxidized lipids, and that vitamin C and vitamin E can prevent these events [73,74]. However, how these observations relate to the *in vivo* situation is still not completely clear.

The antioxidant paradox

As mentioned earlier, many of the altered endothelial functions described in this chapter are considered precursors of vascular atherosclerosis, and antioxidants have a beneficial effect on them. This observation would support the hypothesis that these compounds should also protect from atherogenesis. While the vast majority of animal studies showed that administration of antioxidants did in fact ameliorate the disease process in experimental models of atherogenesis, the outcomes of clinical trials have been disappointing [34,75]. The results of large prospective, controlled clinical trials assessing the efficacy of antioxidant supplementation (mostly with vitamin E) in preventing cardiovascular disease are somewhat controversial. Two trials (CHAOS and SPACE) found vitamin E to be efficacious, but seven others (ATBC, GISSI, PPP, SECURE, HOPE, HPS, and VEAPS) failed to show any benefit [76]. The reasons for this discrepancy are not clear, but factors such as the selection of patients with different levels of oxidative stress, and doses of antioxidants may have influenced the results. These studies used a wide range of vitamin E from 55 to 800 IU/day. In none of them measures of oxidative stress were included to assess its levels and the ability of the antioxidants to lower it. However, it is also possible that in these trials the therapy was initiated too far down the natural history of the disease to have an effect.

Conclusion

Antioxidants may regulate and protect some aspects of endothelial functions through mechanisms unrelated to antioxidant activity. For example, vitamin E can modulate prostaglandin biosynthesis [77], alter the activation of protein kinase C [78], or increase guanyl cyclase expression [12]. Thus, antioxidant therapy and agents designed to scavenge ROS potentially act both through a pure antioxidant mechanism and through other mechanisms [79–84] (Table 22.2). Current data preclude full support of the hypothesis that antioxidants discussed here act through a pure antioxidant mechanism.

However, substantial evidence suggests that many endothelial functions are sensitive to ROS and subsequent oxidative stress. Studies accumulated over the past decade have shown positively that exogenous antioxidants can normalize endothelium-dependent vasodilatory responses in healthy subjects and also in several conditions at risk for atherosclerosis. This is also the case for altered endothelium–leukocyte interactions, where antioxidants limit leukocyte recruitment and migration to the intima. Much less is known about the participation of antioxidants in protecting the endothelium from an imbalance between pro- and antithrombotic stimuli, or cell apoptosis. Further *in vitro* studies and clinical trials are required to elucidate these issues and thus achieve a better understanding of the mechanisms of altered endothelial functions, as well as new and more specific therapies to prevent or reverse them.

Table 22.2 Genes modulated by vitamin E with possible involvement in endothelial homeostasis.

Gene	Function	Effect	References
SR-AI/II, SR-BI, CD36	Uptake of oxLDL	Inhibition	[79–82]
IL-1β, IL-4, TGF-β	Chemotaxis, inflammation	Inhibition	[79]
ICAM-1, E- and L-selectin	Rolling, adhesion to endothelial cells	Inhibition	[79,83]
α-Tropomyosin	Vascular smooth cells proliferation	Inhibition	[79,84]

References

1 Gimbrone Jr MA. Vascular endothelium: an integrator of pathophysiologic stimuli in atherosclerosis. *Am J Cardiol* 1995;75:67B–70B.

2 Drexler H. Endothelial dysfunction: clinical implications. *Prog Cardiovasc Dis* 1997;39:287–324.

3 Halcox JP, Schenke WH, Zalos G, et al. Prognostic value of coronary vascular endothelial dysfunction. *Circulation* 2002;106:653–658.

4 Gokce N, Keaney JF, Vita JA. Endotheliopathies: clinical manifestations of endothelial dysfunction. In: Loscalzo J, Scafer A, eds. *Thrombosis and Hemorrhage.* Baltimore: Williams and Wilkins; 1998:901–924.

5 Cai H, Harrison DG. Endothelial dysfunction in cardiovascular diseases: the role of oxidant stress. *Circ Res* 2000;87:840–844.

6 Harrison DG. Endothelial function and oxidant stress. *Clin Cardiol* 1997;20 (Suppl II):11–17.

7 Drummond GR, Cai H, Davis ME, et al. Transcriptional and posttranscriptional regulation of endothelial nitric oxide synthase expression by hydrogen peroxide. *Circ Res* 2000;86:347–354.

8 Mugge A, Elwell JH, Peterson TE, et al. Chronic treatment with polyethylene-glycolated superoxide dismutase partially restores endothelium-dependent vascular relaxations in cholesterol-fed rabbits. *Circ Res* 1991;69:1293–1300.

9 Keaney Jr JF, Gaziano JM, Xu A, et al. Dietary antioxidants preserve endothelium-dependent vessel relaxation in cholesterol-fed rabbits. *Proc Natl Acad Sci USA* 1993;90:11880–11884.

10 Stewart-Lee AL, Forster LA, Nourooz-Zadeh J, et al. Vitamin E protects against impairment of endothelium-mediated relaxations in cholesterol-fed rabbits. *Arterioscl Thromb* 1994;14:494–499.

11 Keegan A, Walbank H, Cotter MA, et al. Chronic vitamin E treatment prevents defective endothelium-dependent relaxation in diabetic rat aorta. *Diabetologia* 1995;38:1475–1478.

12 Bauersachs J, Fleming I, Fraccarollo D, et al. Prevention of endothelial dysfunction in heart failure by vitamin E: attenuation of vascular superoxide anion formation and increase in soluble guanylyl cyclase expression. *Cardiovasc Res* 2001;51:344–350.

13 Sato J, O'Brien T, Katusic ZS, et al. Dietary antioxidants preserve endothelium dependent vasorelaxation in overfed rats. *Atherosclerosis* 2002;161:327–333.

14 d'Uscio LV, Milstien S, Richardson D, et al. Long-term vitamin C treatment increases vascular tetrahydrobiopterin levels and nitric oxide synthase activity. *Circ Res* 2003;92:88–95.

15 Matsumoto T, d'Uscio LV, Eguchi D, et al. Protective effect of chronic vitamin C treatment on endothelial function of apolipoprotein E-deficient mouse carotid artery. *J Pharmacol Exper Ther* 2003;306:103–108.

16 Aikawa K, Saitoh SI, Muto M, et al. Effects of antioxidants on coronary microvascular spasm induced by epicardial artery endothelial injury in pigs. *Coron Artery Dis* 2004;15:21–30.

17 Rodriguez-Porcel M, Lerman LO, Holmes Jr DR, et al. Chronic antioxidant supplementation attenuates nuclear factor-kappa B activation and preserves endothelial function in hypercholesterolemic pigs. *Cardiovasc Res* 2002;53:1010–1018.

18 Carneado J, Alvarez de Sotomayor M, Perez-Guerrero C, et al. Simvastatin improves endothelial function in spontaneously hypertensive rats through a superoxide dismutase mediated antioxidant effect. *J Hypertens* 2002;20:429–437.

19 Heitzer T, Just H, Munzel T. Antioxidant vitamin C improves endothelial dysfunction in chronic smokers. *Circulation* 1996;94:6–9.

20 Ting HH, Timimi FK, Boles KS, et al. Vitamin C improves endothelium-dependent vasodilation in patients with non-insulin-dependent diabetes mellitus. *J Clin Invest* 1996;97:22–28.

21 Timimi FK, Ting HH, Haley EA, et al. Vitamin C improves endothelium-dependent vasodilation in patients with insulin-dependent diabetes mellitus. *J Am Coll Cardiol* 1998;31:552–557.

22 Ting HH, Timimi FK, Haley EA, et al. Vitamin C improves endothelium-dependent vasodilation in forearm resistance vessels of humans with hypercholesterolemia. *Circulation* 1997;95:2617–2622.

23 Taddei S, Virdis A, Ghiadoni L, et al. Vitamin C improves endothelium-dependent vasodilation by restoring nitric oxide activity in essential hypertension. *Circulation* 1998;97:2222–2229.

24 Higashi Y, Sasaki S, Nakagawa K, et al. Endothelial function and oxidative stress in renovascular hypertension. *N Engl J Med* 2002;346:1954–1962.

25 Hornig B, Arakawa N, Kohler C, et al. Vitamin C improves endothelial function of conduit arteries in patients with chronic heart failure. *Circulation* 1998;97:363–368.

26 Mak S, Egri Z, Tanna G, et al. Vitamin C prevents hyperoxia-mediated vasoconstriction and impairment of endothelium-dependent vasodilation. *Am J Physiol Heart Circ Physiol* 2002;282:H2414–H2421.

27 Hirooka Y, Eshima K, Setoguchi S, et al. Vitamin C improves attenuated angiotensin-II-induced endothelium-dependent vasodilation in human forearm vessels. *Hypertens Res* 2003;26:953–959.

28 Motoyama T, Kawano H, Kugiyama K, et al. Vitamin E administration improves impairment of endothelium-dependent vasodilation in patients with coronary spastic angina. *J Am Coll Cardiol* 1998;32:1672–1679.

29 Heitzer T, Yla Herttuala S, Wild E, et al. Effect of vitamin E on endothelial vasodilator function in patients with hypercholesterolemia, chronic smoking or both. *J Am Coll Cardiol* 1999;33:499–505.

30 Kinlay S, Fang JC, Hikita H, et al. Plasma alpha-tocopherol and coronary endothelium-dependent vasodilator function. *Circulation* 1999;100:219–221.

31 Raghuveer G, Sinkey CA, Chenard C, et al. Effect of vitamin E on resistance vessel endothelial dysfunction induced by methionine. *Am J Cardiol* 2001;88:285–290.

32 Wilson SH, Simari RD, Best PJ, et al. Simvastatin preserves coronary endothelial function in hypercholesterolemia in the absence of lipid lowering. *Arterioscl Thromb Vasc Biol* 2001;21:122–128.

33 Tsunekawa T, Hayashi T, Kano H, et al. Cerivastatin, a hydroxymethylglutaryl coenzyme a reductase inhibitor, improves endothelial function in elderly diabetic patients within 3 days. *Circulation* 2001;104:376–379.

34 Pratico D. Vitamin E: murine studies versus clinical trials. *Ital Heart J* 2001;2:878–881.

35 Ellis GR, Anderson RA, Lang D, et al. Neutrophil superoxide anion–generating capacity, endothelial function and oxidative stress in chronic heart failure: effects of short- and long-term vitamin C therapy. *J Am Coll Cardiol* 2000;36:1474–1482.

36 Lopez BL, Christopher TA, Yue TL, et al. Carvedilol, a new beta-adrenoreceptor blocker antihypertensive drug, protects against free-radical-induced endothelial dysfunction. *Pharmacology* 1995;51:165–173.

37 Fontana L, Giagulli C, Minuz P, et al. 8-iso-PGF2 alpha induces beta2-integrin-mediated rapid adhesion of human polymorphonuclear neutrophils: a link between oxidative stress and ischemia/reperfusion injury. *Arterioscl Thromb Vasc Biol* 2001;21:55–60.

38 Kado S, Wakatsuki T, Yamamoto M, et al. Expression of intercellular adhesion molecule-1 induced by high glucose concentrations in human aortic endothelial cells. *Life Sci* 2001;68:727–737.

39 Lehr HA, Krober M, Hubner C, et al. Stimulation of leukocyte/endothelium interaction by oxidized low-density lipoprotein in hairless mice. Involvement of CD11b/CD18 adhesion receptor complex. *Lab Invest* 1993;68:388–395.

40 Jialal I, Devaraj S, Kaul N. The effect of alpha-tocopherol on monocyte proatherogenic activity. *J Nutr* 2001;131:389S–394S.

41 Blouin E, Halbwachs-Mecarelli L, Rieu P. Redox regulation of beta2-integrin CD11b/CD18 activation. *Eur J Immunol* 1999;29:3419–3431.

42 Yoshikawa T, Yoshida N, Manabe H, et al. Alpha-tocopherol protects against expression of adhesion molecules on neutrophils and endothelial cells. *Biofactors* 1998;7:15–19.

43 Islam KN, Devaraj S, Jialal I. Alpha-tocopherol enrichment of monocytes decreases agonist-induced adhesion

to human endothelial cells. *Circulation* 1998;98:2255–2261.

44 Martin A, Foxall T, Blumberg JB, et al. Vitamin E inhibits low-density lipoprotein-induced adhesion of monocytes to human aortic endothelial cells *in vitro*. *Arterioscl Thromb Vasc Biol* 1997;17:429–436.

45 Steiner M, Li W, Ciaramella JM, et al. Dl-alpha-tocopherol, a potent inhibitor of phorbol ester induced shape change of erythro- and megakaryoblastic leukemia cells. *J Cell Physiol* 1997;172:351–360.

46 Yang H, Shi M, Richardson A, et al. Attenuation of leukocyte-endothelium interaction by antioxidant enzymes. *Free Radical Biol Med* 2003;35:266–276.

47 Jariyapongskul A, Patumraj S, Yamaguchi S, et al. The effect of long-term supplementation of vitamin C on leukocyte adhesion to the cerebral endothelium in STZ-induced diabetic rats. *Clin Hemoreol Microcirc* 2002;27:67–76.

48 Zanardo RC, Costa Cruz JW, Oliveira MA, et al. Ascorbic acid supplementation restores defective leukocyte–endothelial interaction in alloxan-diabetic rats. *Diabetes Metab Res Rev* 2003;19:60–68.

49 Lehr HA, Kress E, Menger MD, et al. Cigarette smoke elicits leukocyte adhesion to endothelium in hamsters: inhibition by CuZn-SOD. *Free Radical Biol Med* 1993;14:573–581.

50 Weber C, Erl W, Weber K, et al. Increased adhesiveness of isolated monocytes to endothelium is prevented by vitamin C intake in smokers. *Circulation* 1996;93:1488–1492.

51 Desideri G, Marinucci MC, Tomassoni G, et al. Vitamin E supplementation reduces plasma vascular cell adhesion molecule-1 and von Willebrand factor levels and increases nitric oxide concentrations in hypercholesterolemic patients. *J Clin Endocrinol Metab* 2002;87:2940–2945.

52 van Dam B, van Hinsbergh VW, Stehouwer CD, et al. Vitamin E inhibits lipid peroxidation-induced adhesion molecule expression in endothelial cells and decreases soluble cell adhesion molecules in healthy subjects. *Cardiovasc Res* 2003;57:563–571.

53 Kurose I, Wolf RE, Grisham MB, et al. Hypercholesterolemia enhances oxidant production in mesenteric venules exposed to ischemia/reperfusion. *Arterioscl Thromb Vasc Biol* 1998;18:1583–1588.

54 Panes J, Kurose I, Rodriguez-Vaca D, et al. Diabetes exacerbates inflammatory responses to ischemia–reperfusion. *Circulation* 1996;93:161–167.

55 Lafont AM, Chai YC, Cornhill JF, et al. Effect of alpha-tocopherol on restenosis after angioplasty in a model of experimental atherosclerosis. *J Clin Invest* 1995;95:1018–1025.

56 Tardif JC, Cote G, Lesperance J, et al. Probucol and multivitamins in the prevention of restenosis after coronary

angioplasty. Multivitamins and probucol study group. *N Engl J Med* 1997;337:365–372.

57 Fang JC, Kinlay S, Beltrame J, et al. Effect of vitamins C and E on progression of transplant-associated arteriosclerosis: a randomised trial. *Lancet* 2002;359:1108–1113.

58 Fei H, Berliner JA, Parhami F, et al. Regulation of endothelial cell tissue factor expression by minimally oxidized LDL and lipopolysaccharide. *Arterioscl Thromb* 1993;13:1711–1717.

59 Drake TA, Hannani K, Fei HH, et al. Minimally oxidized low-density lipoprotein induces tissue factor expression in cultured human endothelial cells. *Am J Pathol* 1991;138:601–607.

60 Ishii H, Kizaki K, Horie S, et al. Oxidized low density lipoprotein reduces thrombomodulin transcription in cultured human endothelial cells through degradation of the lipoprotein in lysosomes. *J Biol Chem* 1996;271:8458–8465.

61 Grafe M, Auch-Schwelk W, Hertel H, et al. Human cardiac microvascular and macrovascular endothelial cells respond differently to oxidatively modified LDL. *Atherosclerosis* 1998;137:87–95.

62 Crutchley DJ, Que BG. Copper-induced tissue factor expression in human monocytic THP-1 cells and its inhibition by antioxidants. *Circulation* 1995;92:238–243.

63 Lapchak PA, Zivin JA. Ebselen, a seleno-organic antioxidant, is neuroprotective after embolic strokes in rabbits. Synergism with low-dose tissue plasminogen activator. *Stroke* 2003;34:2013–2018.

64 Lindenblatt N, Schareck W, Belusa L, et al. Anti-oxidant ebselen delays microvascular thrombus formation in the rat cremaster muscle by inhibiting platelet P-selectin expression. *Thromb Haemost* 2003;90:882–892.

65 Saldeen T, Li D, Metha JL. Differential effects of alpha- and gamma-tocopherol on low-density lipoprotein oxidation, superoxide activity, platelet aggregation and arterial thrombogenesis. *J Am Coll Cardiol* 1999;34:1208–1215.

66 Kokawa T, Enjyoji K, Kumeda K, et al. Measurement of the free form of TFPI antigen in hyperlipidemia. Relationship between free and endothelial cell-associated forms of TFPI. *Arterioscl Thromb Vasc Biol* 1996;16:802–808.

67 Dart AM, Cooper B, Kay SB, et al. Relationships between protein C, protein S, von willebrand factor and euglobulin lysis time and cardiovascular risk factors in subjects with and without coronary heart disease. *Atherosclerosis* 1998;140:55–64.

68 De Cristofaro CR, Rocca B, Marchioli R, et al. Plasma protein oxidation is associated with an increase of procoagulant markers causing an imbalance between pro- and anticoagulant pathways in healthy subjects. *Thromb Haemost* 2002;87:58–67.

69 Ferro D, Basili S, Pratico D, et al. Vitamin E reduces monocyte tissue factor expression in cirrhotic patients. *Blood* 1999;93:2945–2950.

70 Khaw KT, Woodhouse P. Interrelation of vitamin C, infection, haemostatic factors, and cardiovascular disease. *Br Med J* 1995;310:1559–1563.

71 Bordia AK. The effect of vitamin C on blood lipids, fibrinolytic activity and platelet adhesiveness in patients with coronary artery disease. *Atherosclerosis* 1980;35:181–187.

72 Tofler GH, Stec JJ, Stubbe I, et al. The effect of vitamin C supplementation on coagulability and lipid levels in healthy male subjects. *Thromb Res* 2000;100:35–41.

73 Chen TH, Tseng HP, Yang JY, et al. Effect of antioxidant in endothelial cells exposed to oxidized low-density lipoproteins. *Life Sci* 1998;62:PL277–PL282.

74 Dimmeler S, Haendeler J, Galle J, et al. Oxidized low-density lipoprotein induces apoptosis of human endothelial cells by activation of cpp32-like proteases. A mechanistic clue to the "response to injury" hypothesis. *Circulation* 1997;95:1760–1763.

75 Kritharides L, Stocker R. The use of antioxidant supplements in coronary artery disease. *Atherosclerosis* 2002;164:211–219.

76 Pratico D. Antioxidants and endothelium protection. *Atherosclerosis* 2006;181:215–224.

77 Kunisaki M, Umeda F, Inoguchi T, et al. Vitamin E restores reduced prostacyclin synthesis in aortic endothelial cells cultured with a high concentration of glucose. *Metabolism* 1992;41:613–621.

78 Keaney JF Jr, Guo Y, Cunningham D, et al. Vascular incorporation of alpha-tocopherol prevents endothelial dysfunction due to oxidized LDL by inhibiting protein kinase C stimulation. *J Clin Invest* 1996;98:386–394.

79 Azzi A, Gysin R, Kempna P, et al. Regulation of gene and protein expression by vitamin E. *Free Radical Res* 2002;36:30–35.

80 Ricciarelli R, Zingg JM, Azzi A. Vitamin E reduces the uptake of oxidized LDL by inhibiting CD36 scavenger receptor expression in cultured human aortic smooth muscle cells. *Circulation* 2000;102:82–87.

81 Teupser D, Thiery J, Seidel D. Alpha-tocopherol down-regulates scavenger receptor activity in macrophages. *Atherosclerosis* 1999;144:109–115.

82 Devaraj S, Hugou I, Jialal I. Alpha-tocopherol decreases CD36 expression in human monocyte-derived macrophages. *J Lipid Res* 2001;42:521–527.

83 Yoshida N, Manabe H, Terasawa Y, et al. Inhibitory effects of vitamin E on endothelial-dependent adhesive interactions with leukocytes induced by oxidized low density lipoprotein. *Biofactors* 2000;13:279–288.

84 Aratri E, Spycher SE, Breyer I, et al. Modulation of alpha-tropomyosin expression by alpha-tocopherol in rat vascular smooth muscle cells. *FEBS Lett* 1999;447:91–94.

CHAPTER 23

Angiotensin-converting enzyme inhibitors and angiotensin II type 1 receptor blockers to reverse endothelial dysfunction

G.B. John Mancini, MD, FRCP(C), FACC *&*
Sammy Y. Chan, MD, FRCP(C)

The purpose of this chapter is to summarize current information on the effect of sustained treatment with angiotensin-converting enzyme (ACE) inhibitors as a means of preserving and enhancing endothelial function. Emerging evidence pertaining to angiotensin II type 1 receptor blockers (AT1RB's, sartans) will also be summarized. The importance of these approaches to therapy is underscored by studies indicating the prognostic importance of endothelial dysfunction measurements. Such studies are also summarized in this context.

By far the commonest methods utilized in clinical investigations to assess endothelial function rely on endothelium-dependent vasodilatory function of either the conduit arteries (e.g., dilation of proximal coronary arteries, or of the brachial artery) or the resistance vessels (e.g., changes of coronary or forearm blood flow). A distinction must be made between interventions that either stimulate the production of nitric oxide (NO) through NO synthase (NOS) (e.g., stimulation through shear stress, acetylcholine etc.), inhibit the basal/tonic release of NO by inhibition of NOS (e.g., the infusion of L-NG-monomethylarginine (L-NMMA)), provide precursors of NO (e.g., the administration of L-arginine), or serve to enhance the bioavailability of NO by inhibiting premature oxidative destruction (e.g., the use of antioxidants, or inhibitors of NADP/NADPH generation of superoxide and other

reactive oxygen species by blockade of angiotensin II effects). These effects are generally contrasted to the vascular response to a non-endothelium-dependent dilator such as nitrates (e.g., nitrate-mediated dilation or NMD). Through complex interactions outlined in prior chapters, these pathways are also linked to prothrombotic/pro-adhesive properties of the endothelium, as well as to barrier functions for macromolecules both in the systemic vasculature or in specific vascular beds (e.g., the glomerular/mesangial complex in the kidney). Importantly, drug-induced changes in these endothelial mechanisms can be measured relatively quickly (from minutes to months), in contrast to NO-mediated effects on smooth muscle cell growth and remodeling, which may take years before they are measurable in clinical studies (e.g., gluteal biopsy retrieval of arterial resistance vessels, angiographic or ultrasound progression/regression studies).

Important mechanisms of action of ACE inhibitors and sartan's on the endothelium

Figure 23.1 provides an intentionally oversimplified framework for the interpretation of the ACE inhibitor and sartan studies summarized in this chapter. Each of the pathways depicted may be the dominant determinant or the least important

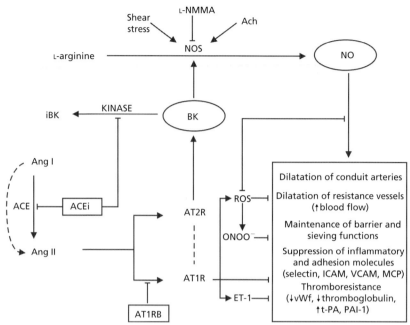

Figure 23.1 A simplified overview is here provided of the pathways investigated in the studies reviewed in this chapter. NOS converts L-arginine to NO in the basal state and also in response to stimuli such as shear stress, acetylcholine and bradykinin (BK). NO released by the intact endothelium then induces dilation of large vessels (measured as a diameter change) or resistance vessels (measured as a change in blood flow). This pathway can be blocked with L-NMMA. Angiotensin-converting enzyme inhibitors (ACEI) block the degradation of BK, which in turn can stimulate NOS to produce NO. BK also stimulates the elaboration of other vasodilatory compounds such as prostacyclin and endothelium-derived hyperpolarizing factor. ACEI inhibit conversion of angiotensin I (Ang I) to angiotensin II (Ang II), but do not block conversion through alternate pathways (dotted arrow, e.g., the chymase pathway). Thus, the degree of angiotensin II type 1 (AT1) and type 2 (AT2) stimulation allowed by such agents may be variable. AT1-mediated actions are effectively blocked by the AT1RB's, sartans while allowing the purported vasculoprotective effects mediated through AT2 to persist. The dashed line between AT1 and AT2 indicates increasing evidence to suggest the existence of a "crosstalk" between these two receptor types. There is also evidence to suggest that the vasodilatory effects mediated through the AT-2 receptor are BK/NO dependent. Reactive oxygen species (ROS) and endothelin-1 (ET-1) generation can occur through multiple mechanisms, and Ang II is a prominent facilitator of these processes. Ang II and ET-1 constrict vessels and antagonize the effects of NO. ROS degrade NO and decrease its bioavailability. Moreover, ONOO⁻ and other peroxynitrites, formed through the degradation of NO and its interaction with ROS may directly and adversely affect endothelial function.

determinant of improved endothelial dysfunction. In the context of a discussion of ACE inhibitors and sartans, it is important to point out that by blocking the degradation of bradykinin, ACE inhibitors potentiate the ability of bradykinin to stimulate the release of tissue-type plasminogen activator (t-PA) from the endothelium, an effect not seen with the sartans [1,2]. Even so, clinical studies generally do not allow distinction along these lines and many measure only one facet of endothelial function (e.g., vasodilatory properties are measured, but adhesive properties or fibrinolytic properties are not, or vice versa). Therefore our goal is merely to provide a summary of the mechanistic studies indicating that these classes of drugs have important effects on all of these important pathways of endothelial function, yielding net improvement in many aspects of endothelial integrity and vascular health. Due to the burgeoning literature in this area, we have limited our review to those studies that have the greatest relevance to the typical, clinical utilization of these drugs as oral agents used chronically. We have specifically focused our attention on patients with hypertension, coronary disease, diabetes, or congestive heart failure.

Endothelial function is of prognostic importance

An increasing body of literature suggests that endothelial function is of prognostic importance in patients with coronary artery disease, hypertension, peripheral vascular disease, and congestive heart failure [3–14]. Several such studies imply that changes in endothelial function induced by treatment may also be of prognostic importance [13,14]. For example, we followed 152 subjects with known coronary artery disease enrolled in an intensive risk factor modification rehabilitation program. Endothelial function was assessed with brachial artery flow-mediated dilation (FMD), and the atherosclerotic burden was estimated by carotid ultrasound [13]. Over a follow-up period of 34 months, 22 vascular events occurred. Multivariate analysis showed that brachial artery FMD/NMD ratio and carotid plaque area were independent predictors of adverse outcome. These two parameters interacted. Subjects with a high atherosclerotic burden had higher risk of events. In these subjects, a superior FMD/NMD ratio was associated with a better outcome. Subjects with a low atherosclerotic burden had a lower risk of adverse events. In this group, there was no difference in outcome between subjects with high or low FMD/NMD ratios. Moreover, deterioration of endothelial function during follow-up, in spite of aggressive risk factor treatment, was also predictive of adverse cardiac events.

The prognostic importance of endothelial dysfunction and change during treatment is also suggested by the study of Modena et al., who investigated 400 postmenopausal females with hypertension [14]. Endothelial function was assessed with brachial artery FMD before and after 6 months of anti-hypertensive therapy. Two hundred and fifty subjects showed an improvement in endothelial function (FMD > 10% compared with baseline) and 150 showed persistent impaired endothelial function. There was no difference in the blood pressure attained in the two groups. Over a mean follow-up period of 67 months, there were 32 events in subjects with persistent endothelial dysfunction, but only 14 events in subjects with improved endothelial function. This study illustrated the reversibility of endothelial function after adequate anti-hypertensive treatment, and that improvement

in prognosis was dependent on the enhancement in endothelial function. This study also demonstrated that endothelial function may be a better therapeutic target than mere blood pressure reduction.

A number of studies have shown a prognostic role of serum or plasma levels of soluble adhesion molecules (see also Chapter 18). Hwang et al. studied three groups of subjects from the Atherosclerosis Risk in Communities Study [15]. Two hundred and four developed incident coronary heart disease (CHD) events during the follow-up. Two hundred and seventy-two had evidence of carotid atherosclerosis. Three hundred and sixteen subjects served as controls. Serum soluble (s)ICAM 1 were higher in subjects with CHD and carotid atherosclerosis than controls. Subjects in the highest quartile of sICAM-1 had a 5.5 times risk of developing CHD than subjects in the lowest quartile after adjusting for established cardiac risk factors. Ridker et al. analyzed data from a 9-year follow-up of the Physicians' Health Study [16]. Using a nested-case–control design, they found an 80% relative increase in the risk of myocardial infarction (MI) in subjects in the highest quartile of sICAM-1. There were no significant changes in risk after adjustments for lipids, smoking, or C-reactive protein. In contrast, there was no relation between serum sVCAM-1 levels and subsequent MI in the same subjects. Malik et al. analyzed data from the British Regional Heart Study [17]. They found an increased odds ratio of 1.68 (95% CI 1.32–2.14) in a comparison of subjects in the top tertile of sICAM-1 with the bottom tertile. The odds decreased to 1.11 (95% CI 0.75–1.64) after adjustments for classical risk factors and socio-economic indicators.

Soluble adhesion molecules have also been evaluated for prognosis in subjects with coronary artery disease (see also Chapter 18). Blankenberg et al. assessed the usefulness of sICAM-1 and sVCAM-1 in association with classical risk factors and high-sensitivity C-reactive protein (hsCRP) in 1240 subjects [18]. Serum sVCAM-1 levels correlated with hsCRP. Median levels of sVCAM-1 and sICAM-1 were higher in subjects who subsequently died of cardiovascular causes. In multivariate Cox regression analysis, both sVCAM-1 and sICAM-1 remained significant predictors of subsequent cardiovascular death even after adjustments for classical risk factors, extent of coronary disease, extent of

MI, statin therapy, and intervention procedure. After further adjustment for ejection fraction, sVCAM-1 remained an independent predictor. Interestingly, sVCAM-1 was the strongest predictor of all variables tested. In the multivariate model, sVCAM-1 was the only variable that emerged. The prognostic value of sVCAM-1 was also independent of hsCRP.

ACE inhibitors in hypertensive patients

The role of ACE inhibitors in improving endothelial function has been studied most extensively within the area of hypertension [19]. Some studies are negative, but all of these negative studies involved a period of treatment of 12 months or less, and some were based on assessment of the response of resistance vessel endothelial dysfunction [20–23]. It is conceivable that this vascular bed is more resistant to the benefit of ACE inhibitors because a 2-year study by Schiffrin and Deng indicated a mild improvement in the vasodilatory properties of resistance vessels harvested from patients subjected to gluteal biopsy after long-term therapy with cilazapril [24]. In contrast, an assessment at 1 year in this same group showed no such improvement, in spite of evidence for improved arteriolar structure based on a reduced and normalized media-to-lumen ratio [21]. In contrast to resistance vessel function, two groups reported reversal of conduit artery dysfunction after active therapy for only 3–8 months [25–27].

A subgroup of studies comparing ACE inhibitors with other effective anti-hypertensive drugs is also interesting [21,24,28–35]. The commonest comparator is the drug class of calcium channel blockers. Several very small studies suggest that the two classes of agent are comparable in their effects on the endothelium and that this benefit parallels the comparability of blood pressure lowering [28,32,35]. However, a large observational study that included 175 patients receiving a calcium channel blocker and a smaller, prospective, randomized study using similar methodology show clearly an ineffectiveness of the calcium channel blocker class when compared with ACE inhibitors [33,34]. Finally, Ghiadoni et al. compared nifedipine gastrointestinal therapeutic system (GITS), amlodipine, atenolol, nebivolol, telmisartan and perindopril and found that only perindopril augmented FMD after 6 months of treatment even though this agent reduced oxidative stress and increased plasma antioxidant capacity to the same extent as telmisartan, nifedipine and amlodipine [36]. Thus, the most consistent finding within the hypertension literature is that the calcium channel blockers do not improve endothelial function and that, among many options, ACE inhibitors most reliably lead to improvement in endothelial vasodilatory function.

Limited information is available about the effects of ACE inhibitors on soluble adhesion molecules. Ferri et al., however, did show that enalapril treatment for 3 months induced reductions in sICAM-1, sVCAM-1 and sE-selectin [37].

Sartans in hypertension

Schiffrin et al. examined 19 untreated subjects with mild, essential hypertension, who were randomly assigned to either losartan or atenolol in a double-blind fashion [38]. Dosages were not reported, but equivalent blood pressure control was achieved by both agents. Resistance arteries dissected from gluteal fat biopsies were harvested before and after treatment, and studied *in vitro*. Endothelium-dependent relaxation induced by acetylcholine was improved in the losartan group but not in the atenolol group, after 1 year of therapy (Figure 23.2). Moreover, the ratio of the media width to the lumen diameter was diminished (improved) only in the patients treated with losartan. When patients were switched from chronic atenolol therapy to irbesartan for 1 year, benefits in resistance vessel endothelial dysfunction and media-to-lumen ratio were detected [39]. Von zur Huhlen et al., using forearm venous plethysmography, were also able to demonstrate the efficacy of irbesartan for resistance vessel endothelial function after only 3 months of treatment [40]. In this study, however, the benefits of irbesartan were not distinct from those of atenolol.

Ghiadoni et al. assessed resistance vessel function, based on maximal forearm blood flow with the use of forearm plethysmography, in a cohort of 15 hypertensive patients and 15 controls [41]. They evaluated not only the effects of acetylcholine stimulation of NOS, but also the inhibition of it with L-NMMA. Endothelin-A/-B receptor blockade was also evaluated. Candesartan (8–16 mg daily) for

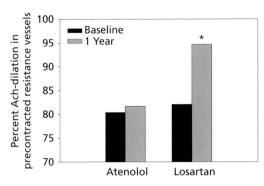

Figure 23.2 Resistance vessels obtained from gluteal biopsies were examined before and after a year of treatment with either atenolol or losartan. The losartan treatment led to an improvement in endothelium-dependent relaxation induced by acetylcholine (Ach). (Figure drawn from data presented in Ref. [38]).

2 and 12 months was evaluated. Candesartan significantly enhanced vasoconstriction to L-NMMA after 2 and 12 months, meaning that candesartan improved the tonic release of NOS-generated NO. Endothelin-A/-B blockade induced less vasodilation at 2 months and almost no vasodilation after 12 months. The latter was paralleled by a fall in endothelin-1 levels in response to the candesartan, indicative of a decrease in angiotensin II-mediated release of endothelin-1 from activated endothelial cells. Finally, stimulated release of NO in response to acetylcholine was improved, but only after 12 months, and not at the 2-month assessment.

Deng et al. used a unique echocardiographic protocol to assess the dilatory response of the left main coronary artery to cold pressor testing [42]. A dysfunctional, constrictor response at baseline was dramatically improved after 3 months of treatment with losartan.

Raham et al. utilized eprosartan for 1 month in hypertensive patients, and demonstrated a reduction in sVCAM-1, monocyte chemotactic protein 1 (MCP-1), superoxide anion, and low-density lipoprotein (LDL) oxidation [43].

Several studies contrast the effects of sartans on endothelial function with those of alternative anti-hypertensive agents, showing disparate results [36,44–47]. However, an important study by Rizzoni et al. in hypertensive patients with type 2 diabetes mellitus showed that both candesartan (8–16 mg/day) and enalapril (10–20 mg/day) for 1 year induced

favorable remodeling of small resistance arteries obtained by gluteal biopsy and equal improvements in endothelium-dependent vasodilation [47].

ACE inhibitors in diabetic patients

Three studies reported a benefit on resistance vessel endothelial function in either type 1 or type 2 diabetic patients [48–50]. However negative findings in type 1 diabetic patients were reported by Mullen [51] and McFarlane et al. [52]. Both studies assessed brachial (conduit) artery dilation. In contrast, Arcaro and associates demonstrated that ACE inhibitors could improve femoral (conduit) artery dilation after only 1 week of treatment in type 1 diabetic patients with microalbuminuria [53].

Another paper suggests that patients with type 1 diabetes have degrees of endothelial dysfunction similar to patients with hypercholesterolemia or patients who smoke, but only the latter two groups respond to L-arginine, with an improvement in FMD of the brachial artery [54]. This contrasts sharply with the study by Giugliano and associates, who demonstrated an improvement in blood flow to the leg with L-arginine infusion after perindopril treatment in type 2 diabetic patients. These patients, however, were also mildly hypertensive [49].

Although there may be differences in the response to therapy between type 1 and type 2 diabetic patients, the small, short-term trials by O'Driscoll and colleagues do not support such a distinction [48,50]. Enalapril improved resistance vessel endothelial dysfunction in both types of diabetes. Borcea and associates enrolled both type 1 and type 2 patients in their open-label, prospective study [55]. They did not disaggregate the two populations, because baseline soluble thrombomodulin levels were equal in both types. There were more type 2 diabetic patients in the ramipril-treated group than in the control group. These investigators determined that ramipril was the only major predictor of improved soluble thrombomodulin levels, but they did not include the type of diabetes in their multiple regression model. Therefore this study does not shed light on whether one group or the other responds more readily to ACE inhibitors.

In two studies assessing barrier function, the results were concordant in indicating that ACE inhibitors can improve it [56,57]. The reduction in proteinuria seen in diabetic patients under treatment cannot be explained solely by changes in blood pressure and intraglomerular pressures. Evidence suggests that other effects bearing directly on the mesangial and endothelial cells and their ability to serve a barrier function play a significant role. Morelli and colleagues undertook an investigation of the dextran barrier function test in patients with type 1 diabetes mellitus who had diabetic nephropathy with proteinuria [56]. The dextran barrier test would allow the examination of the sieving behavior of the glomeruli of proteinuric diabetic patients toward uncharged and non-reabsorbable dextrans having a broad size distribution. The sieving behavior of the glomeruli can be considered to represent a function that is at least partly dependent on endothelial integrity and function, and maintains the physiological properties of normal mesangial cells and the basement membrane. It has been suggested that ACE inhibitors may reduce mesangial contraction and increase the surface area of glomerular filtration, improve the metabolism of mesangial cells, or decrease permeability. Some of these effects are thought to be due to NO or bradykinin, or both, and may, therefore, be induced by ACE inhibitors. Indeed, in the study by Morelli et al., a 90-day course of enalapril resulted in greater barrier function. This was selective for the larger particles, and could not be accounted for solely by anticipated changes in glomerular pressure. Thus, a direct effect of ACE inhibitors on "pore" size, as mediated by the mesangial (endothelial) cell barrier was evident [56]. In a related study, Nielsen and colleagues examined type 2 diabetic patients with diabetic nephropathy and hypertension [57]. They contrasted the effects of lisinopril and atenolol by monitoring the transcapillary escape rate of albumin as an index of total body endothelial barrier function. The transcapillary escape rate of albumin was diminished by ACE inhibitors, but not by beta-blocking agents. It is of interest that levels of von Willebrand Factor (vWF) failed to change. Perhaps vWF is a less-sensitive index of endothelial integrity or activation.

Finally, Gasic et al. showed that sVCAM-1 (but not sICAM, sE-selectin, plasminogen activator inhibitor 1 (PAI-1) or t-PA) was favorably altered by a 3-month course of fosinopril in type 2 diabetic patients with microalbuminuria [58]. As already

indicated above, Borcea and associates demonstrated a decrease in plasma soluble thrombomodulin after 1.5 years of therapy with ramipril [55].

Thus, in diabetic patients, there is some inconsistency in the demonstration of benefits of ACE inhibitors on vasodilatory function. In general, benefits are readily seen in patients with microalbuminuria. However, because therapy with ACE inhibitors is already indicated in diabetic patients with microalbuminuria or with hypertension, new studies should include cohorts with uncomplicated diabetes, similar to those studied by Mullen and colleagues, to clarify the existence of vasodilatory effects.

Sartans and diabetic endothelial dysfunction

Investigators at the University of Western Australia have published a series of papers on the effects of losartan (50 mg daily for 4 weeks) in both type 1 and type 2 diabetic patients [59–61]. In the first study, 11 subjects with type 1 diabetes and without evidence of significant concomitant problems (i.e., smoking, renal impairment/proteinuria, significant microalbuminuria or retinopathy, hepatic impairment, gout/hyperuricemia, more than mild hypercholesterolemia or hypertension) were randomized to receive either losartan or placebo, in a double-blind, placebo-controlled cross-over protocol. Resistance vessel endothelial dysfunction was assessed using forearm plethysmography and intrabrachial artery infusions of acetylcholine and sodium nitroprusside. Losartan failed to improve the blood flow response to acetylcholine. This result was surprising in view of the group's prior success in treating resistance vessel endothelial dysfunction in type 1 diabetic patients using enalapril [48]. However, the authors conjecture was that this particular group of type 1 diabetic patients had virtually normal endothelial function at baseline. It is not clear, therefore, whether the results are due to the inefficacy of losartan or to the possibility that resistance vessel endothelial dysfunction was simply not present in these patients.

The same investigators used the same approach to assess the endothelium-dependent response of resistance vessels to losartan 50 mg daily for 4 weeks in nine subjects with type 2 diabetes [60]. In this study, a beneficial effect was noted on acetylcholine-induced forearm blood flow changes. Losartan, however, did not improve the tonic release of NO as assessed by the inhibition of basal NOS activity with L-NMMA infusion (Figure 23.3). Finally, they assessed conduit vessel, brachial artery FMD in 12, uncomplicated type 2 diabetic subjects and showed a beneficial effect [61]. This short-term benefit (obtained with 1 month of treatment) was not confirmed by the longer term (6 month) study of Tan et al. [62] There were, however, major differences between the two patient populations investigated in these two studies. While Tan et al. studied patients with significant microalbuminuria [62], Cheetham et al. excluded such patients [61]. Also, both endothelium- dependent and -independent vasodilation were diminished at baseline in Tan's study [62]. Both these issues suggest that the endothelium was more severely compromised in Tan's study. Of even greater interest is that Tan et al. showed that microalbuminuria was ameliorated in spite of the lack of changes in conduit vessel endothelial function [62]. Thus, the specific effect of sartans in type 2 diabetic patients in improving conduit vessel endothelial dysfunction is unclear at the moment, and the single study showing an improvement in resistance vessel function requires confirmation.

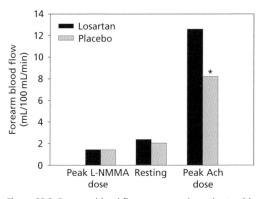

Figure 23.3 Forearm blood flow responses in patients with type 2 diabetes mellitus are shown in response to L-NMMA and acetylcholine (Ach). Losartan induced a statistically significant (*) increase in endothelium-dependent forearm blood flow stimulated by Ach. Tonic NOS effects, however, were not altered, as evidenced by the lack of differential effects of L-NMMA between the placebo- and losartan-treated patients. (Figure drawn from data presented in Ref. [60]).

ACE inhibitors in patients with coronary artery disease

Several studies are of relevance to patients with coronary artery disease [63–71]. Three of the studies pertain to stable patients with a recent MI, and the remainder to stable patients with coronary artery disease. All studies reported positive results, and suggested that ACE inhibitors improve endothelium-mediated conduit function and endothelium-mediated fibrinolytic function after relatively brief courses of therapy (1–6 months). The studies by Vaughan and colleagues and Oshima and associates, involving patients recruited very soon after infarction, are concordant with respect to a beneficial role of ACE inhibitors in normalizing endothelium-mediated fibrinolytic function [65,66]. Indeed, improvement of the fibrinolytic state can also be shown in non-coronary patients treated with ACE inhibitors [2,72]. Thus, ACE inhibitors improve endothelium-mediated processes affecting conduit artery vasodilatory properties and the systemic fibrinolytic status, and this effect may be related to a bradykinin effect [1,2,72]. A Doppler sub-study by Schlaifer and colleagues suggests that amelioration may also extend to endothelium-dependent resistance vessel vasodilatory function [73]. Another post-hoc analysis by this group showed that smokers in particular derive benefit from treatment with ACE inhibitors [74]. This is consistent with the results seen in smokers without other diseases [75].

The trial by Koh and associates is of particular interest because, in addition to measuring conduit artery dilation, they also measured indices of LDL oxidation, inflammation (soluble(s) E-selectin, sICAM-1, sVCAM-1, interleukin-6), and fibrinolysis (PAI-1, D-dimer) [67]. None of the blood parameters were significantly altered. Additionally, a decrease in total serum nitrate/nitrite concentration was shown. This was interpreted as indicating reduced synthesis of NO by constitutive NOS as a result of reduced degradation of NO through angiotensin II-dependent superoxide production. This purported antioxidant effect, however, was insufficient to lower serum levels of oxidized LDL. Overall, this study suggests that flow-mediated responses are the easiest and earliest to change in response to treatment with ACE inhibitors.

Several trials are of special interest due to the inclusion of sartans and other vasoactive agents [68,70,76]. These studies are discussed more fully below.

Zhou and coworkers undertook a unique study in a small group of patients treated with ACE inhibitors while awaiting elective bypass surgery [71]. Portions of the internal mammary artery were harvested at the time of surgery and analyzed for the expression of NOS. Compared with patients not receiving ACE inhibitors, a striking increase in eNOS and iNOS expression were seen in both the endothelial cells and the smooth muscle cells. This occurred in conjunction with a decrease in the vascular expression of ACE and an upregulation of the AT1R. Although circulating and vascular levels of angiotensin II were diminished, the upregulation of AT1R raises the question of whether sartans might be better than ACE inhibitors in sustaining improved endothelial function or whether they should be added to the therapy of patients already taking ACE inhibitors.

Lee and associates showed that ACE inhibitors can improve forearm resistance vessel endothelial function in patients with hypercholesterolemia characterized by average LDL in the range of 4.5 mmol/L in spite of lipid-lowering therapy [77]. Levels this high in patients with coronary artery disease are inappropriate, and lipid lowering is an effective means of improving endothelial dysfunction. The study by Esper et al. indicates that the beneficial effects of lipid lowering and ACE inhibitors on endothelial dysfunction are additive [69].

Sartans and coronary artery disease

Anderson and colleagues were the first to assess the comparative roles of daily doses of quinapril (20 mg), enalapril (10 mg), losartan (50 mg), and amlodipine (5 mg) on brachial artery FMD in patients with coronary artery disease [68]. In a partial-block, cross-over design trial, patients were randomized to one of four different sequences for assessing the effects of three of the four agents. The treatment periods were 8 weeks in duration, followed by a 2-week washout before another agent was assessed. Losartan induced an improvement in FMD second in magnitude only to that of quinapril. But only quinapril treatment induced a statistically significant

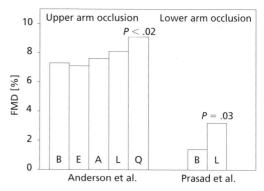

Figure 23.4 FMD is compared at baseline (B) and after 8 weeks of treatment with enalapril (E), amlodipine (A), losartan (L), and quinapril (Q). Anderson and coworkers used upper arm occlusion to induce FMD, and concluded that only quinapril induced a significant improvement in FMD. In contrast, Prasad and coworkers used lower arm occlusion and concluded that L effectively improved FMD. The two methods of assessing FMD may account for the differences in magnitude of the FMD measurements. (Figure drawn from data presented in Refs. [68,78]).

improvement in FMD compared with baseline values (Figure 23.4).

These negative results using losartan stand in contrast to a report from Prasad et al. who also examined brachial FMD in coronary patients [78]. The cohort of patients treated chronically consisted of 31 patients given losartan for 8 weeks. The majority (24/31 patients) received 50 mg/day and the remainder only 25 mg. Even so, the overall results showed an improvement in endothelial dysfunction induced by losartan over the course of 8 weeks (Figure 23.4).

Hornig et al. showed that high-dose losartan (50 mg, twice daily, $n = 17$) given for 4 weeks, instead of 8 as in the studies reported above, induced an improvement in endothelial dysfunction equivalent to ramipril (10 mg daily, $n = 18$) (Figure 23.5) [70]. Improvements were seen both in resistance (radial artery flow) and in conduit vessel function (radial artery dilation). The authors were able to relate these benefits to a reduction in oxidative stress within the arterial wall, mediated in part by an increase in endothelial cell superoxide dismutase [70].

Navalkar et al. demonstrated a reduction in superoxide anion, consistent with the findings of Hornig et al. [70,79]. Moreover, these authors showed that

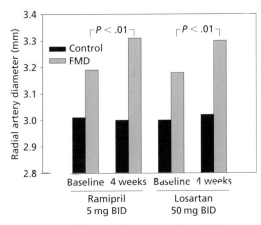

Figure 23.5 Radial artery diameters are shown in the control state and after FMD. High doses of ramipril and losartan led to equally effective increases in FMD after 4 weeks of treatment. (Figure drawn from data presented in Ref. [70]).

irbesartan also reduced sVCAM-1. Prasad et al. used relatively low doses of losartan and did not see a change in endothelial soluble adhesion molecules [80]. However, his group did find that the leukocyte adhesion molecule L-selectin was improved even by this dose of losartan. L-selectin is expressed on the leukocyte and is responsible for the initial attachment of leukocytes to the endothelium. It is rapidly shed after leukocyte activation, and its expression appears to be decreased in inflammatory states. Trevelyan et al. examined the role of both enalapril (10 mg twice daily) and losartan (50 mg daily) in coronary patients awaiting bypass surgery [76]. They showed equal benefits of the two agents on FMD, but the responses were modulated by the underlying ACE genotype. Patients with the ACE II genotype had lower FMD at baseline but improved more readily that those with the DI or the DD genotype. In a small study of patients with coronary disease, Preumont et al. assessed FMD of the brachial artery and changes in myocardial blood flow during cold pressor testing and positron emission tomography imaging [81]. Candesartan was administered chronically at a dose of 8–16 mg daily. Although there was no overall change in brachial FMD, there was an improvement in myocardial perfusion, and this improvement was correlated to changes in FMD. This suggests that the coronary microvasculature was more sensitive to vascular benefit than implied

by the measure of endothelial function in the brachial artery. Thus, these studies suggest that low doses of sartans may have a specific and favorable effect of diminishing leukocyte adhesive properties, that higher doses also diminish adhesive properties of the endothelium itself and that the dilatory effects may be modulated by patients' characteristics such as the ACE genotype.

ACE inhibitors in patients with congestive heart failure

In spite of the undisputed role of ACE inhibitors in the therapy of congestive heart failure, there are very few studies that examine improvements in endothelial function as a mechanism of the benefit. Moreover, the results have been highly heterogeneous, and the studies included very few patients [82–86]. The study by Bridges and associates, based on t-PA and PAI-1 measurements, was negative [82]. The short-term observations of Drexler and associates showed concordant trends in symptomatology, resistance vessel endothelial function, and soluble adhesion molecule levels, but in only eight symptomatic responders out of a total of 13 patients studied [83]. The remaining five had abnormalities that were not improved by ACE inhibitors. The study by Stephens and colleagues showed a slight worsening of *ex vivo* endothelium-dependent relaxation of small resistance vessels in patients treated for 6–43 months with ACE inhibitors [84]. These patients had had New York Heart Association class II–III ischemic heart failure, occurring within 3–10 days of infarction. This finding remains unexplained and is completely incongruous with all available information. Perhaps the main lesson of this chapter is that the cohort of patients really had no demonstrable endothelial dysfunction, even in the placebo-treated patients. Gibbs et al. examined hemorheological, endothelial, and platelet functions in patients with chronic heart failure and in sinus rhythm [85]. In ACE inhibitor-naïve patients, the addition of up to 20 mg daily of lisinopril caused a significant fall in von Willebrand Factor (vWF) and fibrinogen within 3–6 months. Such effects were not seen in a separate group treated with beta-blockers. Jorde and coworkers assessed the controversial issue of tissue affinity as a distinguishing feature among ACE inhibitors [86]. Thirty patients were studied in a randomized, double-blind trial of the low tissue affinity ACE inhibitor enalapril or the high tissue affinity ACE inhibitor trandolapril. There were no differences between these agents with respect to suppression of the renin–angiotensin system, or endothelial function. Indeed, neither treatment materially improved endothelial function. Accordingly, endothelial dysfunction in resistance vessels is not uniformly present in patients with heart failure, especially the milder forms. In patients in whom endothelial dysfunction exists, Drexler and associates showed that this may improve in response to ACE inhibitors, but the likelihood was only 62% (8 of 13) [83]. These observations in very small numbers of patients need to be expanded through larger, more detailed investigations. Because ACE inhibitors are indicated in patients with heart failure, a major question to answer is whether those with or without endothelial dysfunction (in conduit or resistance arteries, or both) have a different outcome and whether measurements of endothelial function in response to the drug might determine those patients who might benefit from more aggressive treatment.

Sartans in patients with congestive heart failure

Only one study utilizing chronic, oral sartans was identified. Ellis and coworkers added candesartan (8–16 mg daily) for 1 month to the treatment of patients with heart failure who were already on stable doses of ACE inhibitors [87]. In addition to measures of brachial artery FMD, they measured numerous parameters pertaining to oxidative stress and exercise performance. None of these indexes were improved by the addition of candesartan.

Conclusions

Endothelial dysfunction is a multifaceted and fundamental process underlying a myriad of disease states associated with significant cardiovascular morbidity and mortality. The concept has emerged from the basic science laboratories and brought to the bedside, being now measurable in patients through non-invasive methods and various serum markers. Far from being a mere curiosity, evidence has emerged to indicate that the status of endothelial function of the

vascular wall is of prognostic importance and may, in time, become a therapeutic target in disease management. ACE inhibitors and sartans affect many of the key pathways that determine the status of endothelial function. Further work is however required to more completely understand the role of these agents in the complex vasculopathy of diabetic patients and in patients with diverse forms or severities of congestive heart failure. The available evidence in patients with hypertension and coronary artery disease, however, indicates that these agents, particularly ACE inhibitors, have vasculoprotective effects that are not solely a function of blood pressure lowering. Such data therefore suggest that improvement in endothelial dysfunction is very likely to be one of the major underlying mechanisms that explains the success of these agents in some recently completed outcome trials, including the initial landmark HOPE and LIFE trials [88,89]. Endothelial dysfunction is an early marker of vascular disease, it is of prognostic importance and appears to modify the impact of underlying structural vascular disease. This chapter has summarized therapeutic options for treatment of endothelial dysfunction in a limited number of disease states. The exploration of other disease states with demonstrable endothelial dysfunction and the assessment of potential therapy with ACE inhibitors and sartans should also be a fruitful area of research.

References

1 Vaughan DE, Lazos SA, Tong K. Angiotensin II regulates the expression of plasminogen activator inhibitor-1 in cultured endothelial cells: a potential link between the renin–angiotensin system and thrombosis. *J Clin Invest* 1995;95:995–1001.

2 Brown NJ, Gainer JM, Stein CM, et al. Bradykinin stimulates tissue plasminogen activator release in human vasculature. *Hypertension* 1999;33:1431–1435.

3 Mancini GBJ. Vascular structure versus function: is endothelial dysfunction of independent prognostic importance or not? *J Am Coll Cardiol* 2004;43:624–628.

4 Cohn JN, Quyyumi A, Hollenberg NK, et al. Surrogate markers for cardiovascular disease: functional markers. *Circulation* 2004;109(Suppl IV):IV-31–IV-46.

5 Katz SD, Katarzyna H, Hriljac I, et al. Vascular endothelial dysfunction and mortality risk in patients with chronic heart failure. *Circulation* 2005;111:310–314.

6 Takase B, Hamabe A, Satomura K, et al. Comparable prognostic value of vasodilator response to acetylcholine in brachial and coronary arteries for predicting long-term

cardiovascular events in suspected coronary artery disease. *Circ J* 2006;70:49–56.

7 Suwaidi J, Hamasaki S, Higano ST, et al. Long term follow-up of patients with mild coronary artery disease and endothelial dysfunction. *Circulation* 2000;101: 948–954.

8 Schachinger V, Britten MB, Zeiher AM. Prognostic impact of coronary vasodilator dysfunction on adverse long-term outcome of coronary heart disease. *Circulation* 2000; 101:1899–1906.

9 Neunteufl T, Heher S, Katzenschlager R, et al. Late prognostic value of flow-mediated dilation in the brachial artery of patients with chest pain. *Am J Cardiol* 2000; 86:207–210.

10 Heitzer T, Schlinzig T, Krohn K, et al. Endothelial dysfunction, oxidative stress, and risk of cardiovascular events in patients with coronary artery disease. *Circulation* 2001; 104:2673–2678.

11 Perticone F, Ceravolo R, Pujia A, et al. Prognostic significance of endothelial dysfunction in hypertensive patients. *Circulation* 2001;104:191–196.

12 Halcox JP, Schenke WH, Zalos G, et al. Prognostic value of coronary vascular endothelial dysfunction. *Circulation* 2002;106:653–658.

13 Chan SY, Mancini GBJ, Burns S, et al. Normal endothelial function attenuates the risks associated with high plaque burden. *Circulation* 2001;104:II-486.

14 Modena MG, Bonetti L, Coppi F, et al. Prognostic role of reversible endothelial dysfunction in hypertensive postmenopausal women. *J Am Coll Cardiol* 2002; 40:505–510.

15 Hwang SJ, Ballantyne CM, Sharrett AR, et al. Circulating adhesion molecules VCAM-1, ICAM-1, and E-selectin in carotid atherosclerosis and incident coronary heart disease cases: the Atherosclerosis Risk In Communities (ARIC) study. *Circulation* 1997;96:4219–4225.

16 Ridker PM, Hennekens CH, Roitman-Johnson B, et al. Concentration of soluble intercellular adhesion molecule 1 and risks of future myocardial infarction in apparently healthy men. *Lancet* 1998;351:88–92.

17 Malik I, Danesh J, Whincup P, et al. Soluble adhesion molecules and prediction of coronary heart disease: a prospective study and meta-analysis. *Lancet* 2001;358: 971–976.

18 Blankenberg S, Rupprecht HJ, Bickel C, et al. Circulating cell adhesion molecules and death in patients with coronary artery disease. *Circulation* 2001;104:1336–1342.

19 Mancini GBJ. Long-term use of angiotensin-converting enzyme inhibitors to modify endothelial dysfunction: a review of clinical investigations. *Clin Invest Med* 2000;23:144–161.

20 Creager MA, Roddy MA. Effect of captopril and enalapril on endothelial function in hypertensive patients. *Hypertension* 1994;24:499–505.

21 Schiffrin EL, Deng LY, Larochelle P. Effects of a b-blocker or a converting enzyme inhibitor on resistance arteries in essential hypertension. *Hypertension* 1994;23:83–91.

22 Kiowski W, Linder L, Nuesch R, et al. Effects of cilazapril on vascular structure and function in essential hypertension. *Hypertension* 1996;27(3 Pt 1):371–376.

23 Riondino S, Pignatelli P, Pulcinelli FM, et al. Platelet function in hypertensive older patients is controlled by lowering blood pressure. *J Am Geriatr Soc* 1999;47: 943–947.

24 Schiffrin EL, Deng LY. Comparison of effects of angiotensin I-converting enzyme inhibition and b-blockade for 2 years on function of small arteries from hypertensive patients. *Hypertension* 1995;25:699–703.

25 Asmar RG, Pannier B, Santoni JP, et al. Reversion of cardiac hypertrophy and reduced arterial compliance after converting enzyme inhibition in essential hypertension. *Circulation* 1988;78:941–950.

26 Asmar RG, Journo HJ, Lacolley PJ, et al. Treatment for one year with perindopril: effect on cardiac mass and arterial compliance in essential hypertension. *J Hypertens* 1988;6:S33–S39.

27 Tomiyama H, Kimura Y, Mitsuhashi H, et al. Relationship between endothelial function and fibrinolysis in early hypertension. *Hypertension* 1998;31:321–327.

28 Lyons D, Webster J, Benjamin N. The effect of antihypertensive therapy on responsiveness to local intra-arterial NG-monomethyl-L-arginine in patients with essential hypertension. *J Hypertens* 1994;12:1047–1052.

29 Mimran A, Ribstein J, DuCailar G. Contrasting effect of antihypertensive treatment on the renal response to L-arginine. *Hypertension* 1995;26:937–941.

30 Iwatsubo, H, Nagano M, Sakai T, et al. Converting enzyme inhibitor improves forearm reactive hyperemia in essential hypertension. *Hypertension* 1997;29:286–290.

31 Higashi Y, Oshima T, Sasaki S, et al. Angiotensin-converting enzyme inhibition, but not calcium antagonism, improves a response of the renal vasculature to L-arginine in patients with essential hypertension. *Hypertension* 1998;32:16–24.

32 Takase H, Sugiyama M, Nakazawa A, et al. Long-term effect of antihypertensive therapy with calcium antagonist or angiotensin converting enzyme inhibitor on serum nitrite/nitrate levels in human essential hypertension. *Drug Res* 2000;50:530–534.

33 Higashi Y, Sasaki S, Nakagawa K, et al. A comparison of angiotensin-converting enzyme inhibitors, calcium antagonists, beta-blockers and diuretic agents on reactive hyperemia inpatients with essential hypertension: a multicenter study. *J Am Coll Cardiol* 2000;35:284–289.

34 Higashi Y, Saski S, Nakagawa K, et al. Effect of the angiotensin-converting enzyme inhibitor imidapril on reactive hyperemia in patients with essential hypertension: relationship between treatment periods and resistance

artery endothelial function. *J Am Coll Cardiol* 2001;37: 863–870.

35 On YK, Kim CH, Oh BH, et al. Effects of angiotensin converting enzyme inhibitor and calcium antagonist on endothelial function in patients with essential hypertension. *Hypertens Res* 2002;25:365–371.

36 Ghiadoni L, Magagna A, Versari D, et al. Different effect of antihypertensive drugs on conduit artery endothelial function. *Hypertension* 2003;41:1281–1286.

37 Ferri C, Desideri G, Baldoncini R, et al. Early activation of vascular endothelium in non-obese, nondiabetic essential hypertensive patients with multiple metabolic abnormalities. *Diabetes* 1998;47:660–667.

38 Schiffrin EL, Park JB, Intengan HD, et al. Correction of arterial structure and endothelial dysfunction in human essential hypertension by the angiotensin receptor antagonist losartan. *Circulation* 2000;101:1653–1659.

39 Schiffrin EL, Park JB, Pu Q. Effect of crossing over hypertensive patients from a beta-blocker to an angiotensin receptor antagonist on resistance artery structure and on endothelial function. *J Hypertens* 2002;20:71–78.

40 Von zur Huhlen B, Kahan T, Hagg A, et al. Treatment with irbesartan or atenolol improves endothelial function in essential hypertension. *J Hypertens* 2001;19: 1813–1818.

41 Ghiadoni L, Virdis A, Magagna A, et al. Effect of the angiotensin II type 1 receptor blocker candesartan on endothelial function in patients with essential hypertension. *Hypertension* 2000;35:501–506.

42 Deng Y-B, Wang D-W, Li C-L, et al. Effects of the angiotensin receptor antagonist losartan on the response of the left main coronary artery to cold pressor test in patients with essential hypertension as assessed by echocardiography. *Can J Cardiol* 2002;18:389–396.

43 Raham ST, Bauten WB, Khan QA, et al. Effects of eprosartan versus hydrochlorothiazide on markers of vascular oxidation and inflammation and blood pressure (renin–angiotensin system antagonists, oxidation, and inflammation). *Am J Cardiol* 2002;89:686–690.

44 Chung NA, Beevers G, Lip GYH. Effects of losartan versus hydrochlorothiazide on indices of endothelial damage/dysfunction, angiogenesis and tissue factor in essential hypertension. *Blood Pressure* 2004;13:183–189.

45 Leu HB, Charng MJ, Ding PYA. A double blind randomized trial to compare the effects of eprosartan and enalapril on blood pressure, platelets, and endothelium function in patients with essential hypertension. *Jpn Heart J* 2004;45:623–635.

46 Tomiyama H, Motobe K, Zaydun G, et al. Insulin sensitivity and endothelial function in hypertension. *Am J Hypertens* 2005;18:178–182.

47 Rizzoni D, Porteri E, De Ciuceis C, et al. Effect of treatment with candesartan or enalapril on subcutaneous

small artery structure in hypertensive patients with noninsulin-dependent diabetes mellitus. *Hypertension* 2005; 45(Pt 2):659–665.

48 O'Driscoll G, Green D, Rankin J, et al. Improvement in endothelial function by angiotensin-converting enzyme inhibition in insulin-dependent diabetes mellitus. *J Clin Invest* 1997;100:678–684.

49 Giugliano D, Marfella R, Acampora R, et al. Effects of perindopril and carvedilol on endothelium-dependent vascular functions in patients with diabetes and hypertension. *Diabetes Care* 1998;21:631–636.

50 O'Driscoll G, Green D, Maiorana A, et al. Improvement in endothelial function by angiotensin-converting enzyme inhibition in non-insulin-dependent diabetes mellitus. *J Am Coll Cardiol* 1999;33:1506–1511.

51 Mullen MJ, Clarkson P, Donald AE, et al. Effect of enalapril on endothelial function in young insulin-dependent diabetic patients: a randomized, double-blind study. *J Am Coll Cardiol* 1998;31:1330–1335.

52 McFarlane R, McCredie RJ, Bonney MA, et al. Angiotensin converting enzyme inhibition and arterial endothelial function in adults with type 1 diabetes mellitus. *Diabetic Med* 1999;16:62–66.

53 Arcaro G, Zenere BM, Saggiani F, et al. ACE inhibitors improve endothelial function in type 1 diabetic patients with normal arterial pressure and microalbuminuria. *Diabetes Care* 1999;22:1536–1542.

54 Thorne S, Mullen MJ, Clarkson P, et al. Early endothelial dysfunction in adults at risk from atherosclerosis: different responses to L-arginine. *J Am Coll Cardiol* 1998;32: 110–116.

55 Borcea V, Morcos M, Isermann B, et al. Influence of ramipril on the course of plasma thrombomodulin in patients with diabetes mellitus. *Vasa* 1999;28:172–180.

56 Morelli E, Loon N, Meyer T, et al. Effects of converting-enzyme inhibition on barrier function in diabetic glomerulopathy. *Diabetes* 1990;39:76–82.

57 Nielsen FS, Rossing P, Gall MA, et al. Lisinopril improves endothelial dysfunction in hypertensive NIDDM subjects with diabetic nephropathy. *Scand J Clin Lab Invest* 1997;57:427–434.

58 Gasic S, Wagner OF, Fasching P, et al. Fosinopril decreases levels of soluble vascular cell adhesion molecule-1 in borderline hypertensive type II diabetic patients with microalbuminuria. *Am J Hypertens* 1999;12:217–222.

59 Munro N, Riche N, McIntosh C, et al. Losartan, an angiotensin type 1 receptor inhibitor, and endothelial vasodilator function in type 1 diabetes mellitus. *Diabetic Med* 2000;17:550–560.

60 Cheetham C, Collis J, O'Driscoll G, et al. Losartan, an angiotensin type 1 receptor antagonist, improves endothelial function in non-insulin-dependent diabetes. *J Am Coll Cardiol* 2000;36:1461–1466.

61 Cheetham C, O'Driscoll G, Stanton K, et al. Losartan, an angiotensin type 1 receptor antagonist, improves conduit vessel endothelial function in type II diabetes. *Clin Sci* 2001;100:13–17.

62 Tan KCB, Chow W-S, Ai VHG, et al. Effects of angiotensin II receptor antagonist on endothelial vasomotor function and urinary albumin excretion in type 2 diabetic patients with microalbuminuria. *Diabetes Metab Res Rev* 2002;18:71–76.

63 Wright RA, Flapan AD, Alberti KG, et al. Effects of captopril therapy on endogenous fibrinolysis in men with recent, uncomplicated myocardial infarction. *J Am Coll Cardiol* 1994;24:67–73.

64 Mancini GB, Henry GC, Macaya C, et al. Angiotensin-converting enzyme inhibition with quinapril improves endothelial vasomotor dysfunction in patients with coronary artery disease. *Circulation* 1996;94:258–265.

65 Vaughan DE, Rouleau JL, Ridker PM, et al. Effects of ramipril on plasma fibrinolytic balance in patients with acute anterior myocardial infarction. *Circulation* 1997;96: 442–447.

66 Oshima S, Ogawa H, Mizuno Y, et al. The effects of the angiotensin-converting enzyme inhibitor imidapril on plasma plasminogen activator inhibitor activity in patients with acute myocardial infarction. *Am Heart J* 1997;134: 961–966.

67 Koh KK, Bui MN, Hathaway L, et al. Mechanism by which quinapril improves vascular function in coronary artery disease. *Am J Cardiol* 1999;83:327–331.

68 Anderson TJ, Elstein E, Haber H, et al. Comparative study of ACE-inhibition, angiotensin II antagonism, and calcium channel blockade on flow-mediated vasodilation in patients with coronary disease (BANFF study). *J Am Coll Cardiol* 2000;35:60–66.

69 Esper RJ, Machado R, Vilarino J, et al. Endothelium-dependent responses in patients with hypercholesterolemic coronary artery disease under the effects of simvastatin and enalapril, either separately or combined. *Am Heart J* 2000;140:684–689.

70 Hornig B, Landmesser U, Kohler C, et al. Comparative effect of ACE inhibition and angiotensin II type 1 receptor antagonism on bioavailability of nitric oxide in patients with coronary artery disease. *Circulation* 2001;103: 799–805.

71 Zhou JL, Mendelsohn FAO, Ohishi M. Perindopril alters vascular angiotensin-converting enzyme, AT1 receptor, and nitric oxide synthase expression in patients with coronary heart disease. *Hypertension* 2002;39:634–638.

72 Brown NJ, Agirbasli MA, Williams GH, et al. Effect of activation and inhibition of the renin–angiotensin system on plasma PAI-1. *Hypertension* 1998;32:965–971.

73 Schlaifer JD, Wargovich TJ, O'Neill B, et al. Effects of quinapril on coronary blood flow in coronary artery disease patients with endothelial dysfunction. *Am J Cardiol* 1997;80:1594–1597.

74 Schlaifer JD, Mancini GB, O'Neill BJ, et al. Influence of smoking status on angiotensin-converting enzyme inhibition-related improvement in coronary endothelial function. *Cardiovasc Drugs Ther* 1999;13:201–209.

75 Butler R, Morris AD, Struthers AD. Lisinopril improves endothelial function in chronic cigarette smokers. *Clin Sci* 2001;101:53–58.

76 Trevelyan J, Needham EWA, Morris A, et al. Comparison of the effect of enalapril and losartan in conjunction with surgical coronary revascularisation versus revascularisation alone on systemic endothelial function. *Heart* 2005;91:1053–1057.

77 Lee AF, Dick JB, Bonnor CE, et al. Lisinopril improves arterial function in hyperlipidemia. *Clin Sci* 1999;96: 441–448.

78 Prasad A, Tupas-Habib T, Schenke BS, et al. Acute and chronic angiotensin-1 receptor antagonism reverses endothelial dysfunction in atherosclerosis. *Circulation* 2000;101:2349–2354.

79 Navalkar S, Parthasarathy S, Santanam N, et al. Irbesartan, an angiotensin type 1 receptor inhibitor, regulates markers of inflammation in patients with premature atherosclerosis. *J Am Coll Cardiol* 2001;37:440–444.

80 Prasad A, Kon K, Schenke WH, et al. Role of angiotensin II type 1 receptor in the regulation of cellular adhesion molecules in atherosclerosis. *Am Heart J* 2001;142: 248–253.

81 Preumont N, Unger P, Goldman S, et al. Effect of long-term angiotensin II type 1 receptor antagonism on peripheral and coronary vasomotion. *Cardiovasc Drug Ther* 2004;18:197–202.

82 Bridges AB, McLaren M, Belch JJ. A comparative study of captopril and enalapril on endothelial cell function in congestive heart failure patients. *Angiology* 1995;46: 811–817.

83 Drexler H, Kurz S, Jeserich M, et al. Effect of chronic angiotensin-converting enzyme inhibition on endothelial function in patients with chronic heart failure. *Am J Cardiol* 1995;76:13E–18E.

84 Stephens N, Drinkhill MJ, Hall AS, et al. Structure and in vitro function of human subcutaneous small arteries in mild heart failure. *Am J Physiol* 1998;274:C1298–C1305.

85 Gibbs CR, Blann AD, Watson RDS, et al. Abnormalities of hemorheological, endothelial, and platelet function in patients with chronic heart failure in sinus rhythm: effects of angiotensin-converting enzyme inhibitor and beta-blocker therapy. *Circulation* 2001;103:1746–1751.

86 Jorde UP, Vittorio TJ, Dimayuga CA, et al. Comparison of suppression of the circulating and vascular renin–angiotensin system by enalapril versus trandolapril in chronic heart failure. *Am J Cardiol* 2004;94:1501–1505.

87 Ellis GR, Nightingale AK, Blackman DJ, et al. Addition of candesartan to angiotensin converting enzyme inhibitor therapy in patients with chronic heart failure does not reduce levels of oxidative stress. *Eur J Heart Fail* 2002;4:193–199.

88 The Heart Outcomes Evaluation Study Investigators. Effects of an angiotensin-converting enzyme inhibitor, ramipril, on cardiovascular events in high-risk patients. *N Engl J Med* 2000;342:145–153.

89 Dahlof B, Devereux RB, Kjeldsen SE, et al. Cardiovascular morbidity and mortality in the losartan intervention for endpoint reduction in hypertension study (LIFE): a randomized trial against atenolol. *Lancet* 2002;359:995–1003.

CHAPTER 24

PPARs in atherosclerosis

Ouliana Ziouzenkova, PhD, *Nikolaus Marx,* MD,
Peter Libby, MD, *& Jorge Plutzky,* MD

PPARs: ligand-activated transcriptions implicated in metabolism, inflammation, and atherosclerosis

More than a decade of extensive work has established a central role for peroxisome proliferator-activated receptors (PPARs) in the transcriptional regulation of key metabolic pathways [1]. More recently, considerable attention has focused on the possible role of PPARs in atherosclerosis and inflammation [2]. Several factors contribute to this burgeoning interest. We currently know that all three PPAR isoforms are expressed in all major vascular and inflammatory cells, with gene targets relevant to atherosclerosis and inflammation. Synthetic PPAR agonists are used clinically to treat type 2 diabetes mellitus (T2DM) and dyslipidemia, making their vascular effects immediately applicable to common clinical scenarios. Furthermore, current experience with PPAR agonists establishes precedent, rationale, and even the need for later generation PPAR activators that remain under wide pursuit. Epidemiologic evidence documenting the expanding, intertwined problems of diabetes/insulin resistance, obesity, dyslipidemia, and atherosclerosis also indicate the need for additional therapeutic interventions. Finally, the nature of PPAR-activating drugs as transcriptional modulators illustrates how the alteration of gene expression might be used as a therapeutic approach [3]. We review here basic science insight into PPARs, and then focus on evidence for the participation of PPAR-α and PPAR-γ in inflammation and atherosclerosis. Despite rapidly emerging new insight into PPAR-δ, [4] we defer detailed

discussion of this data due to the lack of a PPAR-δ agonist in current clinical use.

PPARs: basic mechanisms

Like other members of the steroid nuclear receptor family, PPAR proteins contain five major domains, including a ligand-binding (LBD) and a DNA-binding domain (DBD) [1]. The interaction between a given PPAR-LBD and its specific cognate ligand(s) – either synthetic or naturally occurring – leads to receptor activation. Thus, one major component of PPAR specificity depends on the chemical structure of the ligand and its binding to the ligand pocket [5]. Such specificity may determine not only the selectivity toward PPAR subtypes, but also particular PPAR isotype responses. For example, troglitazone, a partial agonist, and rosiglitazone, a full agonist, may generate different metabolic effects among synthetic PPAR-γ agonists, a possibility that has supported the notion that selective PPAR modulators (SPARMS) may exist, much like selective estrogen-like molecules (selective estrogen receptor modulators (SERMs)). While circulating hormones activate estrogen, corticosteroid, and thyroid receptors, PPARs and other related receptors, e.g., pregnane X receptors (PXRs) and retinoid X receptors (RXRs), respond to a large variety of dietary lipids, vitamins, and/or xenobiotics. The conformational state of PPARs change in response to ligand binding, fostering to the formation of a transcriptional complex that includes a PPAR heterodimeric nuclear receptor partner, the retinoid X receptor (RXR), activated by its own presumed ligand, 9-*cis*-retinoic acid [6]. This activated transcription complex also involves small accessory molecules, either released (co-repressors) or recruited (co-activators) [7]. These coordinated events result in the binding of the PPAR:RXR complex to PPAR response elements (PPRE) in the promoter region of specific target genes and induce the expression of these target genes. In addition, PPAR activation can inhibit the expression of other target genes through so-called trans-repression, a process that remains incompletely understood.

PPARs include three known isoforms: PPAR-α, PPAR-δ (also known as PPAR-β), and PPAR-γ [1]. Multiple levels of control account for the specific roles ascribed to PPAR-α, -γ, and -δ, including the nature of the ligand, the LBD sequence, the DBD sequence, and the PPREs, as well as differing patterns of expression for each isoform.

PPAR-α: a central mediator of fatty acid metabolism

PPAR-α was first identified through the observation that certain industrial compounds, including fibric acids, increased the size and number of peroxisomes, sub-cellular organelles, in rodents [1,8]. Ultimately this was found to be the result of nuclear receptor activation; importantly, less PPAR-α expression and negligible peroxisomal proliferation has been found in humans [9]. In addition to identifying fibric acid derivatives like gemfibrozil, fenofibrate, and clofibrate as PPAR-α ligands, several landmark studies reported that certain fatty acids (FA), especially long-chain FA, could also bind to PPAR-α, although that occurred only *in vitro* and at high concentrations [10,11]. Extensive work by many groups ultimately defined PPAR-α as a key regulator of FA metabolism. PPAR-α target genes include enzymes of FA beta-oxidation, a highly efficient energy-generating process [12]. Consistent with this, PPAR-α is expressed abundantly in high-energy-utilization tissues, such as the heart and the skeletal muscle, as well as the liver [13]. Its hepatic expression links to its key role in lipoprotein metabolism. PPAR-α target genes include apolipoprotein A1 (ApoA1), lipoprotein lipase (LPL), the endogenous inhibitor of LPL ApoCIII, FA transporters, and the ATP-binding cassette transporter A1 (ABCA1), a transporter involved in cholesterol efflux [14,15]. Thus, this constellation of target genes reveals the critical role of PPAR-α in regulating triglyceride (TG) uptake in the periphery, the processing, and composition of lipoproteins in the liver, and the proportion of triglyceride-rich lipoproteins (TRL) and HDL in blood.

Gonzalez and colleagues provided major insight into the role of PPAR-α by generating PPAR-α-deficient mice [16] that lack peroxisomal response to peroxisome proliferators, a fundamental proof of concept. The critical role of PPAR-α in lipid metabolism and energy balance under stress conditions is evident from the acute lipid accumulation in the liver during starvation or high-fat diet. Under basal conditions, PPAR-α-deficient mice have modestly lower HDL, perhaps resulting from increased catabolism. Mice lacking PPAR-α also demonstrate low energy production, with resulting impairment of physical activity and thermogenesis. Interestingly, humans with the V162 allele mutation, which results in impaired activation of ligand-mediated PPAR-α, show associated hyperapolipoprotein B dyslipidemia [17,18].

Further insight into PPAR-α action in humans derives from clinical trials with PPAR-α-activating drugs, namely fibrates [15]. Not surprisingly, given the *in vitro* and animal data cited above, fibrates are used to lower TG and raise HDL levels [19]. Angiographic studies reveal that gemfibrozil and fenofibrate can reduce coronary artery stenoses [20]. The Veterans Administration HDL Intervention Trial (VA-HIT) demonstrated, in a cohort of patients with low high-density lipoproteins (HDL) (32 mg/dL), modestly increased TG (160 mg/dL), and average-to-low-density lipoproteins (LDL) levels (104 mg/dL), that primary cardiovascular endpoints decrease significantly following treatment with the fibrate gemfibrozil compared with placebo [21]. Such baseline lipid parameters are quite typical for patients with diabetes mellitus; indeed, some 25% of VA-HIT subjects had diabetes, and approximately 50% had underlying insulin resistance. In VA-HIT, HDL levels increased only modestly (~32 to ~35 mg/dL) while *post hoc* analyses argued that TG lowering (30%) did not explain the clinical benefit, leaving the mechanism(s) underlying the trial's positive results unclear. One alternate hypothesis would be that the outcomes may have derived from the direct activation by fibrates of PPAR-α in vascular and inflammatory cells [22].

Many studies have established PPAR-α expression in all the major cells of the vasculature and also in the invading inflammatory cells that characterize atherosclerosis, including endothelial cells (EC), vascular smooth muscle cells (VSMC), monocytes–macrophages, and T lymphocytes. In these various cellular settings, PPAR-α agonists have been shown to repress key pro-inflammatory and pro-atherosclerotic target genes. For example, in VSMC PPAR-α ligands decrease the critical upstream responses of the inflammatory regulator interleukin-6 (IL-6) as well as of cyclooxygenase-2 (COX-2) [23]. In monocyte–macrophages, PPAR-α activation decreases the expression of tissue factor, a major contributor to plaque atherogenicity [24,25]. Moreover, PPAR-α ligands potently repress the expression of proximal pro-inflammatory cytokines such as tumor necrosis factor alpha (TNF-α) and IL-1 in T lymphocytes [26].

In EC, PPAR-α ligands limit cytokine-induced expression of vascular cell-adhesion molecule-1 (VCAM-1) [27], a key step in atherogenesis as well as atherosclerosis (Figure 24.1). PPAR-α activation

may also contribute to the clinical cardiovascular benefits garnered from fish-enriched diets and fish oil [28,29]. For example, oxidized eicosapentaenoic acid, a major component of fish oil, activates PPAR-α and represses adhesion molecule expression [29]. Indeed, oxEPA repressed adhesion molecule expression and decreased leukocyte adhesion in vivo in wild-type but not PPAR-α-deficient mice. This finding is consonant with several others that have found more potent PPAR activation by oxidized – as opposed to native – forms of certain molecules [30–32]. Such data, as well as studies in EC isolated from PPAR-α-deficient mice, provide genetic evidence that anti-inflammatory, anti-atherosclerotic responses occur through PPAR-α itself, as opposed to mechanisms triggered by PPAR-α activation indirectly.

The search for an underlying mechanism for regulating adhesion molecule expression through PPAR-α reveals likely transcriptional interaction between PPAR-α and the central inflammatory regulators nuclear factor kappa B (NF-κB) and activator protein-1 (AP-1) [27]. PPAR modulation

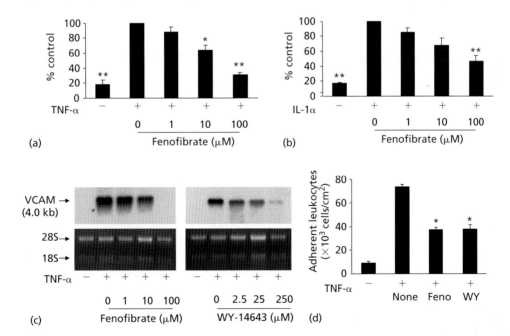

Figure 24.1 PPAR-α agonists decrease endothelial inflammatory responses. Treatment of human EC with the indicated concentrations of PPAR-α agonists fenofibrate or WY-14643 decreases TNF-α-induced (a) and IL-1α-induced (b) VCAM-1 levels, as shown by flow-cytometric analysis. (c) As expected for the effects of a transcription factor, VCAM-1 mRNA is also repressed. (d) Functional assays of leukocyte adhesion demonstrate similar decreases in adhesion.

of NF-κB and AP-1 represents a common mechanism of trans-repressive effects [5,33]. PPAR-α can interact physically with the p65 subunit of NF-κB and also increase the expression of inhibitory I-κB alpha. In addition, many other pro-inflammatory target genes also appear repressed by PPAR-α through NF-κB-mediated mechanisms. In fact, NF-κB activation may increase basally in association with aging in PPAR-α-deficient mice [34–36]. PPAR-α-mediated inhibition of NF-κB activation also may occur through the inhibition of oxidative pathways. PPAR-α activates the expression of two antioxidative enzymes, catalase and superoxide dismutase, thereby decreasing free-radical formation intra- and possibly extracellularly [34–36]. Additionally, recent reports suggest that PPAR-α activation may limit oxidation through ApoA1 induction [37]. In humans, fenofibrate data also support a possible PPAR-α anti-inflammatory effect, as suggested by decreased inflammatory markers for coronary heart disease, e.g., C-reactive protein and fibrinogen [23].

The prior positive data for gemfibrozil in VA-HIT reviewed earlier, combined with the extensive recent data for PPAR-α activation as limiting inflammation and atherosclerosis, suggested that fenofibrate, as a more potent PPAR-α activator than gemfibrozil, might be particularly effective in decreasing cardiovascular events. As such, the results of the FIELD study, which tested the effects of fenofibrate on cardiovascular events in patients with diabetes in either the presence or absence of cardiovascular disease, were highly anticipated [38]. Unfortunately FIELD subjects on fenofibrate had no improvement in outcomes as compared to those who received placebo [38]. Various explanations have been offered for these somewhat surprising results, including a modest increase in HDL (2%) and a significant "drop-in" rate of statin usage that occurred disproportionately in the placebo as compared to the fenofibrate arm. Statin use would have been expected to decrease risk within this group, as suggested by post hoc analyses. Statistically significant improvements in secondary endpoints in response to fenofibrate included decreased cardiovascular events among those with no prior history of coronary artery disease (CAD) and also a surprising decrease in microvascular disease. The fenofibrate may have had some untoward effect on cardiovascular disease

that offset benefits that might have otherwise been seen. Although not statistically significant, an increase in cardiovascular mortality was found in FIELD in response to fenofibrate. Such data could be consistent with some lines of evidence that have implicated PPAR-α in hypertension and cardiomyopathy, at least in mice [39–41].

The FIELD results underscore the importance of separating clinical responses to synthetic PPAR-α agonists from the role of PPAR-α itself *in vivo*, where extensive data identifies this nuclear receptor as an important regulator of fundamental cellular and systemic processes under physiologic conditions. Extrapolation of some of the *in vitro* and *in vivo* effects of synthetic PPAR-α agonists might suggest that endogenous PPAR-α activation could represent a mechanism protecting against dyslipidemia, inflammation, and atherosclerosis. Relatively little had been known previously about natural PPAR ligands or their mechanism of generation. The first reported natural PPAR ligands, based largely on *in vitro* assays, were certain long-chain FA [10,11]. In these landmark studies, saturated FA was shown to activate PPAR-α, with less effect on PPAR-δ, while polyunsaturated FA (PUFA) activated all PPAR isoforms. These broad isoform-independent effects toward all PPAR isoforms left issues of selective PPAR activation unresolved, while also offering no link to lipid metabolism pathways. Additionally, such findings were sometimes inconsistent with separate *in vivo* data. For example, saturated and monounsaturated FAs fail to reproduce the lipid-lowering and anti-inflammatory effects seen with synthetic PPAR-α ligands. Moreover, the lipid-lowering effect of PUFA persists in PPAR-α-deficient mice. Recent work demonstrates that activation of selective PPAR through TRL lipolysis may offer some resolution for this apparent paradox [42,43]. LBD and direct ligand displacement studies demonstrate that LPL, the predominant enzyme in TRL catabolism, acts on circulating lipoproteins to release PPAR ligands [44] (Figure 24.2). These LPL-mediated responses reveal selectivity for PPAR isotypes (PPAR-α ≫ PPAR-δ > PPAR-γ), lipoprotein substrate (VLDL ≫ LDL > HDL), and among lipases, evident with some but not other FA-releasing enzymes. LPL action liberates FA from their esterified state within lipoproteins and induces classic PPAR-α responses, including PPAR-α target

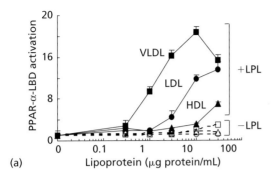
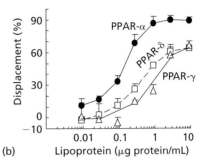

Figure 24.2 LPL-mediated generation of PPAR ligands demonstrates selectivity for VLDL as a substrate and PPAR-α as the targeted PPAR [37]. (a) PPAR-α LBD/GAL4 assays were performed across a concentration gradient of common circulating lipoproteins, revealing preferential activation by LPL treatment of VLDL. Subsequent studies showed this response to depend on intact LPL catalytic activity. (b) The ability of LPL-treated VLDL to directly displace the binding of known high potency PPAR radioligands to expressed PPAR proteins is a rigorous test of ligand activity. Such studies reveal results similar to those of ligand-binding assays, namely preferential PPAR-α activation by LPL-treated VLDL at the lipoprotein concentrations shown.

expression and peroxisomal proliferation (in mice and murine-derived cells). Such effects include increased LPL expression, suggesting that a positive feedback loop may be at work since LPL itself is PPAR regulated. Interestingly, like synthetic PPAR-α agonists, LPL-treated VLDL represses VCAM-1 expression, suggesting a novel anti-inflammatory role for intact TG-metabolism through LPL. In delineating an endogenous mechanism for PPAR-α ligand generation, these data may offer a connection between dietary responses and PPAR activation, and also suggest that the known association of LPL dysfunction and atherosclerosis may occur in part through a failure to generate PPAR-α ligands. Concurrent work also suggested that LPL might act on very low-density lipoproteins (VLDL) in macrophages to preferentially activate PPAR-δ in macrophages [45], raising the possibility of cell-specific effects. Recent data have extended this lipolytic model of PPAR activation to other lipoprotein substrates and other lipases, including endothelial lipase [46,47].

The proposed production of natural PPAR ligands through lipoxygenase pathways represents a pathway that likely operates under pro-inflammatory conditions to limit inflammatory responses. The 15- or 5-lipoxygenase leads to 15-HETE and leukotriene B4 formation, which activates PPAR-α and helps terminate the inflammatory response [48]. Oxidized linoleic acid, i.e., 9- or 13-HODE, which forms during non-specific or lipoxygenase-mediated oxidation, may be a natural ligand for both PPAR-α and PPAR-γ [30,49]. Again, in distinction to LPL pathways active under physiologic conditions, HODEs likely form in pathologic settings of oxidative stress. All of these catabolites may form in atheroma; but their relevance to systemic PPAR activation *in vivo* is unclear.

Although most of the PPAR-α literature supports its putative anti-inflammatory, anti-atherosclerotic effects, this is not uniformly the case. PPAR-α agonists have been reported to induce the chemokine monocyte chemoattractant protein-1 (MCP-1) in wild-type but not in PPAR-α-deficient mice [50]. In contrast, MCP-1 levels appear stable in patients receiving PPAR-α activators, possibly reflecting species or experimental differences. Notably, ApoE-deficient mice also lacking PPAR-α had more atherosclerosis, contrary to the decrease expected if PPAR-α were anti-atherosclerotic [39]. The explanations for these findings remain unclear but, as noted earlier, could conceivably contribute to the somewhat disappointing FIELD results. Variations among species may contribute to such disparity, as could the specific models employed. Importantly, PPAR-α agonists decreased atherosclerosis in ApoE-deficient mice expressing human ApoA1 [51], consistent with most prior studies. Early reports also suggest that treatment with PPAR-α agonists decreases atherosclerosis in mouse models.

PPAR-γ: key mediator of adipogenesis, lipid metabolism, and glucose control

PPAR-γ was initially identified as a member of a transcriptional complex that controls the expression of a fat-specific target gene [52]. Serendipitous chemical screening led to the identification of thiazolidinediones (TZDs) as insulin-sensitizing antidiabetic agents and the subsequent realization that such effects occurred due to TZD binding to PPAR-γ [53]. Members of the TZD class identified thus far include rosiglitazone, pioglitazone, ciglitazone, and troglitazone; all increase insulin sensitivity. Consistent with the model of ligand/receptor interaction described earlier, the synthetic ligand's structure determines much of its functional profile. Notably, structural variability may be an issue especially for PPAR-γ, due to its particularly large LBD, even as compared with other nuclear receptors [1]. A linear relationship exists between the avidity of PPAR-γ-binding and insulin sensitization responses. Troglitazone, the structure of which includes not only a TZD but also an alpha-tocopherol (Vitamin E) moiety, may have partial PPAR agonist properties. This unique structure contributed to occasional and apparently rare irreversible liver damage, leading to its removal from the market. Currently used TZDs do not have this side effect. Rosiglitazone (Avandia) is a full PPAR-γ agonist, consistent with its efficacy at lower doses. Some PPAR-α binding, at least *in vitro*, has been reported for pioglitazone (Actos). In one head-to-head trial, pioglitazone has been shown to lower TG to a greater extent than rosiglitazone although the clinical significance of this is not clear. Both rosiglitazone and pioglitazone significantly increase HDL to levels that rival those seen with drugs used specifically for that purpose, e.g., gemfibrozil, supporting the prospect of cardiovascular benefit via TZD therapy.

TZDs could theoretically limit atherosclerosis through two distinct pathways. Certainly, the greater insulin sensitivity, lower glucose levels, and improved lipid profiles produced by TZD therapy may indirectly ameliorate atherosclerosis or its complications. Alternatively, the demonstration by many groups of PPAR-γ expression throughout the vasculature, e.g., inflammatory cells such as monocytes–macrophages and T lymphocytes, as well as in

human atherosclerosis itself (Figure 24.3) raises the possibility that PPAR-γ activation might directly affect atherosclerosis [55,56]. The list of PPAR-γ-regulated targets relevant to vascular biology and atherosclerosis continues to expand rapidly, and now includes the trans-repression of cytokines in macrophages and T lymphocytes, chemokines and chemokine receptors, and matrix metalloproteinases (MMPs), matrix-degrading enzymes strongly implicated in plaque rupture. PPAR-γ activation also decreases VSMC cell cycling and proliferation, which may result from changes in transcription factor EGR-1 [56]. Further, PPAR-γ ligands induce the promoter for PPAR-γ itself, indicating relevant feedback mechanisms that participate in determining responses. Interestingly, some studies suggest that the anti-inflammatory effects of PPAR-γ agonists may persist in PPAR-γ-deficient murine macrophages, although variables including animal model, the concentration and nature of agonists, and the experimental system may have contributed to the results [57].

Similar to PPAR-α, reports of untoward effects through PPAR-γ also exist. For example, PPAR-γ mediates the induction of the FA transporter, CD-36, which facilitates uptake of oxidized LPL in monocytes [58]. Although initial reports suggesting this response could promote foam cell formation, subsequent work has argued against a critical role for CD-36 in macrophage development [59], supported by decreased mouse atherosclerosis in response to PPAR-γ agonists (see below). CD-36 induction in other tissues may be protective, providing a "sink" for lipoproteins in less pathologic locales, or PPAR-γ activation may induce offsetting cholesterol efflux through induction of ABCA1 [59–61]. These effects would be consistent with anti-inflammatory responses of PPAR-γ agonists in atherosclerosis. Direct effects of PPAR-γ agonists on the myocardium have also been raised, although with variable results.

Mouse models of atherosclerosis support an antiatherosclerotic effect through PPAR-γ activation (see above). At least four different reports have found significant decreases in atherosclerotic lesions in response to PPAR-γ ligands, including various TZDs administered to ApoE- and LDL receptor-deficiency models. Although one early report found responses restricted to male mice [62], subsequent studies in other models have reported benefits in

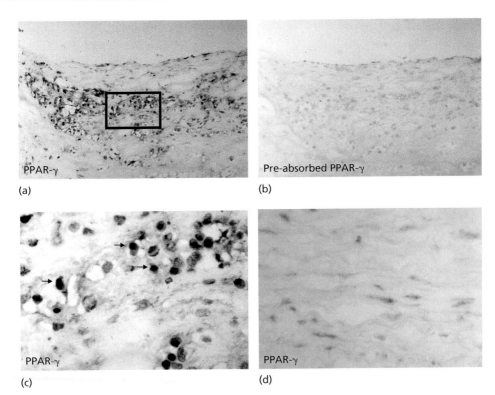

Figure 24.3 PPAR-γ is expressed in human atherosclerotic lesions. (a) Low power view of sections from human carotid lesions reveals immunoreactive PPAR-γ in the shoulder region of the lipid core (LC), a location enriched in macrophages. (b) No immunoreactive PPAR-γ is detected in parallel sections of **A** stained with pre-absorbed PPAR-γ antibodies, suggesting PPAR-γ specificity. (c) High power view of the area indicated by the square in **A**, shows PPAR-γ staining restricted to the nuclei of these macrophages, as would be expected for a PPAR. (d) In non-atherosclerotic arteries (*n* = 5), little PPAR-γ staining could be detected, except for mild staining in occasional VSMC (*N* = 12, similar results) [54].

both genders [57]. Interestingly, in these studies CD-36 induction has been seen despite decreased atherosclerosis, although with absent PPAR-γ-mediated repression of VCAM or MCP-1 [63]. An abundance of other pro-inflammatory and pro-atherosclerotic targets may also contribute to the benefits seen [64].

The explosion of data suggesting anti-atherosclerotic and anti-inflammatory benefits for PPAR-γ agonists has generated considerable interest in whether similar responses occur in humans. Early surrogate cardiovascular studies supported the concept that PPAR-γ agonists might limit inflammation and atherosclerosis. PPAR-γ agonist treatment with both troglitazone [65] and pioglitazone [66] decreased carotid artery intima–media thickness. These changes, seen as early as 3 months, suggest not only the usual decrease in atherosclerotic

progression but also actual regression, creating some skepticism regarding the results. TZD agonists may decrease in-stent restenosis, a process driven largely by VSMC proliferation, matrix remodeling, and inflammation, all known PPAR-γ-regulated responses [67–69]. Recent studies reporting that PPAR-γ agonists decreased serum levels of MMP-9, as well as the anti-inflammatory marker C-reactive protein, strongly implicated as a predictor of atherosclerosis [70,71], have been particularly encouraging (Figure 24.4). Additionally, TZDs improve endothelial function [72].

The potential effects of PPAR-γ agonists on the coagulation system remain unresolved. PPAR-γ agonists clearly decrease serum plasminogen activator inhibitor-1 (PAI-1) levels in patients with polycystic ovarian syndrome (PCOS), a well-recognized insulin-resistance state, possibly resulting from

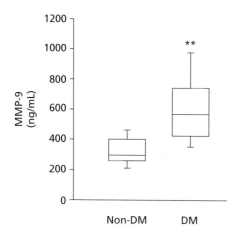

Figure 24.4 The PPAR-γ-agonist rosiglitazone (4 mg/day) decreases serum circulating MMP-9 levels in a group of patients with T2DM and CAD as compared to placebo. Data are presented as 25th percentile, median, and 75th percentile. *$P < 0.05$ compared with baseline. ($N = 21$ patients with angiographically proven CAD). Similar results have been seen by others [59].

various clinical effects, such as improved insulin sensitivity, lower TG, or improved glucose levels [73]. Putative natural ligands such as 15d-PGJ2 increase PAI-1 promoter responses [74], while various effects have been seen with synthetic PPAR-γ ligands, including responses independent of PPAR-γ [75,76]. Various factors, e.g., experimental systems or differing cell types, might contribute to these differences. All results with 15d-PGJ2 may stem from its PPAR-γ-independent effects on I-κB kinase. EC apoptosis has also been reported with 15d-PGJ2 [77].

In advanced atheroma, synthetic PPAR-γ ligands have been reported to decrease neovascularization, a process thought essential for lesion development [78]. PPAR-γ ligands prevent EC migration induced by leptin, and abrogate microtubuli formation in response to basic fibroblast growth factor (b-FGF) and vascular endothelial growth factor (VEGF) as well as mitogenic stimuli. Such PPAR-γ-meditated inhibition of angiogenesis may result from changes in a host of targets including MMP-9, IL-8, PLA2, and PAI-2. In addition, the EC response to PGJ2 can result in apoptosis, although this apparently does not occur with the synthetic agonists.

This fairly large database for PPAR-γ agonists in limiting atherosclerosis provided a rationale for large-scale cardiovascular trials with TZDs, several of which are now underway and the first of which has been reported. The PROactive study tested the effects of pioglitazone versus active anti-diabetic therapy in a group of patients with fairly advanced cardiovascular disease. In this study, pioglitazone failed to decrease a combined cardiovascular endpoint, including coronary and peripheral artery revascularization [79]. Interestingly, a secondary endpoint, identified prior to unblinding of the data and consisting of the more clinically relevant and objective endpoints of stroke, myocardial infarction (MI) and cardiovascular death, was different between groups, with a 13% decrease seen with pioglitazone ($P < 0.05$). An increase in edema, as previously noted to be associated with TZD use, was found, although these events were not well adjudicated [80]. Additional data from future TZD studies may help address these issues.

Independent of these trials, other studies continue to support cardiovascular benefits from TZDs. In the PIUS trial, pioglitazone treatment over 6 months decreased neointimal volume as measured by intracoronary ultrasound in a group of non-diabetic patients [81]. In the PIONEER trial, the effects of pioglitazone were compared to glimepiride under titration conditions geared toward matching hemoglobin A1C levels in both arms [82]. In spite of similar levels of glucose control, those who received the TZDs had significantly greater decreases in inflammatory markers as compared to glimepiride treatment. Particularly intriguing was the observation that these anti-inflammatory effects were evident even among TZD-treated patients who failed to lower their hemoglobin A1C levels. These results suggest that the anti-inflammatory effects of TZDs may be distinct from its insulin-sensitizing glucose effects. Together, these studies continue to support the notion that PPAR-γ agonists may have benefits on atherosclerosis and indicate the need for studies that add to the PROactive results.

One separate effect of PPAR-γ agonists may be in delaying or perhaps even preventing the development of diabetes. Indeed, troglitazone decreased the conversion to new diabetes among women with a prior history of gestational diabetes [83], a clinical condition with an exceptionally high conversion rate to T2DM. The treated group, which had >50%

reduction in the development of T2DM compared with placebo, continued to show a significant difference in diabetes rates for 8 months off therapy, arguing against a simple "masking effect" due to treating undiagnosed diabetes and raising instead the prospect of a fundamental change in the disease process. Intriguingly, data in animal models suggests that TZDs may lead to beta cell preservation [84]; additional data in this regard should be available soon. Metformin, ACE-inhibitors, and regular modest exercise have also been shown to decrease the conversion to new T2DM [85,86]. The possibility of delaying or preventing diabetes in "pre-diabetic" conditions could have major implications for the incidence of atherosclerosis in this high-risk population, although this has not yet been established.

A separate line of evidence for PPAR involvement in metabolism and vascular disease includes experiments of nature in which mutations have altered PPAR function. More data have emerged for PPAR-γ in this regard. O'Rahilly and colleagues reported a dominant-negative PPAR-γ mutation with altered LBD [87]. In the identified kindred, subjects had severe insulin resistance as well as hypertension, and subsequent data suggested a form of lipodystrophy. Other PPAR-γ mutations have been seen with similar phenotypes [88]. The cardiovascular status of such individuals remains unelucidated. Additionally, Pro-Ala 12, a single-nucleotide polymorphism (SNP) for PPAR-γ, has been reported in several small cohorts [89]. Despite some variability in initial studies, combination of the data in a meta-analysis and an investigation in a larger cohort revealed that the Pro-Ala 12 mutation likely associates with decreased incidence of T2DM [89]. Recently, we found a lower incidence of MI associated with this SNP [90]. This mutation is particularly intriguing since in-vitro studies with this variant suggest it is a mutation with "loss-of-function" for PPAR-γ [91], leaving investigators to ponder how lower PPAR-γ function can be reconciled with a lower incidence of T2DM. It remains possible that these in-vitro data do not reflect in vivo PPAR activity in the presence of this variant, although similar discrepancies exist throughout the PPAR literature. For example, some data argue for metabolic benefits through PPAR-γ antagonism or partial PPAR-γ agonists, as opposed to full agonists [92,93].

Likewise, PPAR-γ heterozygous-deficient mice have less, not more diabetes [94,95]. A better understanding of the receptor and its biology may help resolve these interesting issues.

PPAR-γ agonists may have some untoward effects in cardiovascular patients. For example, an apparent paradox may exist in TZDs increasing insulin sensitivity and lowering markers of inflammation while also inducing a modest weight gain [70,96]. Some of this weight gain may result from fluid retention. Indeed, a second concern involves the precipitation of congestive heart failure with TZDs, a clinical response that more likely occurs in conjunction with insulin administration [97]. Numerous studies are underway to examine whether this is indeed congestive heart failure or simply right-sided failure with pedal edema. TZDs do have vasodilatory effects, similar to other pedal edema-inducing agents like nifedipine. Several hypotheses may explain the benefits seen despite weight gain, including: a shift in fat from visceral stores, where it may have more untoward effects, to a subcutaneous location; a qualitative change in the fat itself, with the induction of younger, smaller, and more responsive adipocytes; or changes in gene expression and protein levels in fat, e.g., increased amounts of adiponectin, which may have anti-inflammatory, anti-diabetic effects [98].

Integrating PPAR biology into vascular biology: an evolving perspective

The potential role of PPARs is an exciting arena that will continue to evolve rapidly along parallel tracks of basic science and clinical investigation, bolstered by the combination of many unanswered questions, the clinical use of currently approved PPAR agonists in high-risk conditions like T2DM and dyslipidemia, and the ongoing development of new PPAR agonists. These new PPAR agonists include higher potency PPAR ligands, non-TZD PPAR-γ agonists, and compounds capable of activating both PPAR-α and PPAR-γ. This latter possibility, already under study in clinical trials, holds out the promise of agents that would improve dyslipidemia and decrease insulin resistance. It remains to be seen whether such an approach offers benefits that exceed the use of separate PPAR-α and -γ ligands. Additionally, such work will likely pave routes for the development of agonists for the increasing list of other nuclear receptors currently implicated in lipid metabolism and atherosclerosis, including PPAR-δ, liver X receptor (LXR), RXR, farnesoid X receptor (FXR), and PXR. For now, several short-term issues exist on the horizon regarding PPAR-α and PPAR-γ. Do these agents decrease atherosclerosis, or, more importantly, clinical cardiovascular events in a clinically significant manner and with an acceptable level of safety and tolerability? Is inflammation a legitimate PPAR-regulated target, and if so, does the PPAR-mediated decrease in inflammation stem from improved metabolism or direct regulation of specific inflammatory target genes? What is the dose–response relationship for these PPAR-mediated responses? To what extent do cardiovascular and inflammatory effects of PPAR agonists occur through the PPAR itself? All these questions are in the process of being answered. Indeed, the obvious importance in asking and answering these questions serves to underscore the evident but still evolving role of PPARs as regulators and possible therapeutic targets in atherosclerosis and vascular biology.

References

1 Willson TM, Brown PJ, Sternbach DD, et al. The PPARs: from orphan receptors to drug discovery. *J Med Chem* 2000;43:527–550.

2 Marx N, Libby P, Plutzky J. Peroxisome proliferator-activated receptors (PPARs) and their role in the vessel wall: possible mediators of cardiovascular risk? *J Cardiovasc Risk* 2001;8:203–210.

3 Plutzky J. PPARs as therapeutic targets: reverse cardiology? *Science* 2003;302:406–407.

4 Michalik L, Desvergne B, Wahli W. Peroxisome proliferator-activated receptors beta/delta: emerging roles for a previously neglected third family member. *Curr Opin Lipidol* 2003;14:129–135.

5 Berger J, Moller DE. The mechanisms of action of PPARs. *Annu Rev Med* 2002;53:409–435.

6 Mangelsdorf DJ, Evans RM. The RXR heterodimers and orphan receptors. *Cell* 1995;83:841–850.

7 Westin S, Kurokawa R, Nolte RT, et al. Interactions controlling the assembly of nuclear-receptor heterodimers and co-activators. *Nature* 1998;395: 199–202.

8 Pineda Torra I, Gervois P, Staels B. Peroxisome proliferator-activated receptor alpha in metabolic disease, inflammation, atherosclerosis and aging. *Curr Opin Lipidol* 1999; 10:151–159.

9 Holden PR, Tugwood JD. Peroxisome proliferator-activated receptor alpha: role in rodent liver cancer and species differences. *J Mol Endocrinol* 1999;22:1–8.

10 Kliewer SA, Sundseth SS, Jones SA, et al. Fatty acids and eicosanoids regulate gene expression through direct interactions with peroxisome proliferator-activated receptors alpha and gamma. *Proc Natl Acad Sci USA* 1997;94: 4318–4323.

11 Forman BM, Chen J, Evans RM. Hypolipidemic drugs, polyunsaturated fatty acids, and eicosanoids are ligands for peroxisome proliferator-activated receptors alpha and delta. *Proc Natl Acad Sci USA* 1997;94:4312–4317.

12 Reddy JK, Hashimoto T. Peroxisomal beta-oxidation and peroxisome proliferator-activated receptor alpha: an adaptive metabolic system. *Annu Rev Nutr* 2001;21: 193–230.

13 Barger PM, Kelly DP. PPAR signaling in the control of cardiac energy metabolism. *Trends Cardiovasc Med* 2000; 10:238–245.

14 Kelly DP. The pleiotropic nature of the vascular PPAR gene regulatory pathway. *Circ Res* 2001;89:935–937.

15 Duez H, Fruchart JC, Staels B. PPARS in inflammation, atherosclerosis and thrombosis. *J Cardiovasc Risk* 2001;8: 187–194.

16 Lee SS, Pineau T, Drago J, et al. Targeted disruption of the alpha isoform of the peroxisome proliferator-activated receptor gene in mice results in abolishment of the pleiotropic effects of peroxisome proliferators. *Mol Cell Biol* 1995;15:3012–3022.

17 Flavell DM, Pineda Torra I, Jamshidi Y, et al. Variation in the PPARalpha gene is associated with altered function *in vitro* and plasma lipid concentrations in Type II diabetic subjects. *Diabetologia* 2000;43:673–680.

18 Tai ES, Demissie S, Cupples LA, et al. Association between the PPARA L162V polymorphism and plasma lipid levels: the Framingham Offspring Study. *Arterioscler Thromb Vasc Biol* 2002;22:805–810.

19 Auwerx J, Schoonjans K, Fruchart JC, et al. Transcriptional control of triglyceride metabolism: fibrates and fatty acids change the expression of the LPL and apo C-III genes by activating the nuclear receptor PPAR. *Atherosclerosis* 1996;124(Suppl):S29–S37.

20 Hahmann HW, Bunte T, Hellwig N, et al. Progression and regression of minor coronary arterial narrowings by quantitative angiography after fenofibrate therapy. *Am J Cardiol* 1991;67:957–961.

21 Rubins HB, Robins SJ, Collins D, et al. Gemfibrozil for the secondary prevention of coronary heart disease in men with low levels of high-density lipoprotein cholesterol. Veterans Affairs High-Density Lipoprotein Cholesterol Intervention Trial Study Group. *N Engl J Med* 1999;341: 410–418.

22 Ziouzenkova O, Perrey S, Marx N, et al. Peroxisome proliferator-activated receptors in the vasculature. *Curr Atheroscler Rep* 2002;4:59–64.

23 Staels B, Koenig W, Habib A, et al. Activation of human aortic smooth-muscle cells is inhibited by PPARalpha but not by PPARgamma activators. *Nature* 1998;393: 790–793.

24 Marx N, Mackman N, Schonbeck U, et al. PPARalpha activators inhibit tissue factor expression and activity in human monocytes. *Circulation* 2001;103:213–219.

25 Neve BP, Corseaux D, Chinetti G, et al. PPARalpha agonists inhibit tissue factor expression in human monocytes and macrophages. *Circulation* 2001;103:207–212.

26 Marx N, Kehrle B, Kohlhammer K, et al. PPAR activators as antiinflammatory mediators in human T lymphocytes: implications for atherosclerosis and transplantation associated arteriosclerosis. *Circ Res* 2002;90:703–710.

27 Marx N, Sukhova GK, Collins T, et al. PPARalpha activators inhibit cytokine-induced vascular cell adhesion molecule-1 expression in human endothelial cells. *Circulation* 1999;99:3125–3131.

28 Neschen S, Moore I, Regittnig W, et al. Contrasting effects of fish oil and safflower oil on hepatic peroxisomal and tissue lipid content. *Am J Physiol Endocrinol Metab* 2002; 282:E395–E401.

29 Sethi S, Ziouzenkova O, Ni H, et al. Oxidized omega-3 fatty acids in fish oil inhibit leukocyte-endothelial interactions through activation of PPAR alpha. *Blood* 2002; 100:1340–1346.

30 Nagy L, Tontonoz P, Alvarez JG, et al. Oxidized LDL regulates macrophage gene expression through ligand activation of PPARgamma. *Cell* 1998;93: 229–240.

31 Delerive P, Furman C, Teissier E, et al. Oxidized phospholipids activate PPARalpha in a phospholipase A2-dependent manner. *FEBS Lett* 2000; 471:34–38.

32 Davies SS, Pontsler AV, Marathe GK, et al. Oxidized alkyl phospholipids are specific, high affinity peroxisome proliferator-activated receptor gamma ligands and agonists. *J Biol Chem* 2001;276:16015–16023.

33 Plutzky J. Peroxisome proliferator-activated receptors in endothelial cell biology. *Curr Opin Lipidol* 2001;12: 511–518.

34 Poynter ME, Daynes RA. Peroxisome proliferator-activated receptor alpha activation modulates cellular redox status, represses nuclear factor-kappaB signaling, and reduces inflammatory cytokine production in aging. *J Biol Chem* 1998;273:32833–32841.

35 Inoue I, Noji S, Awata T, et al. Bezafibrate has an antioxidant effect: peroxisome proliferator-activated receptor alpha is associated with Cu2+, Zn2+-superoxide dismutase in the liver. *Life Sci* 1998;63:135–144.

36 Yoo HY, Chang MS, Rho HM. Induction of the rat Cu/Zn superoxide dismutase gene through the peroxisome proliferator-responsive element by arachidonic acid [In Process Citation]. *Gene* 1999;234:87–91.

37 Nofer JR, Kehrel B, Fobker M, et al. HDL and arteriosclerosis: beyond reverse cholesterol transport. *Atherosclerosis* 2002;161:1–16.

38 Keech A, Simes RJ, Barter P, et al. Effects of long-term fenofibrate therapy on cardiovascular events in 9795 people with type 2 diabetes mellitus (the FIELD study): randomised controlled trial. *Lancet* 2005;366:1849–1861.

39 Tordjman K, Bernal-Mizrachi C, Zemany L, et al. PPARalpha deficiency reduces insulin resistance and atherosclerosis in apoE-null mice. *J Clin Invest* 2001;107: 1025–1034.

40 Bernal-Mizrachi C, Weng S, Feng C, et al. Dexamethasone induction of hypertension and diabetes is PPAR-alpha dependent in LDL receptor-null mice. *Nat Med* 2003; 9;1069–1075.

41 Finck BN, Bernal-Mizrachi C, Han DH, et al. A potential link between muscle peroxisome proliferator-activated receptor-alpha signaling and obesity-related diabetes. *Cell Metab* 2005;1:133–144.

42 Chawla A, Schwarz EJ, Dimaculangan DD, et al. Peroxisome proliferator-activated receptor (PPAR) gamma: adipose-predominant expression and induction early in adipocyte differentiation. *Endocrinology* 1994; 135:798–800.

43 Ziouzenkova O, Gieseg SP, Ramos P, et al. Factors affecting resistance of low density lipoproteins to oxidation. *Lipids* 1996;31(Suppl):S71–S76.

44 Ziouzenkova O, Perrey S, Asatryan L, et al. Lipolysis of triglyceride-rich lipoproteins generates PPAR ligands: Evidence for an antiinflammatory role for lipoprotein lipase. *Proc Natl Acad Sci USA* 2003;5:2730–2735.

45 Chawla A, Lee CH, Barak Y, et al. PPARdelta is a very low-density lipoprotein sensor in macrophages. *Proc Natl Acad Sci USA* 2003;100:1268–1273.

46 Ziouzenkova O, Asatryan L, Sahady D, et al. Dual roles for lipolysis and oxidation in peroxisome proliferation-activator receptor responses to electronegative low density lipoprotein. *J Biol Chem* 2003;278:39874–39881.

47 Ahmed W, Ziouzenkova O, Orasanu G, et al. Hydrolysis of HDL Generates PPAR-alpha Activation: A Candidate Mechanism for HDL's Anti-Inflammatory Effects. *Circ Res* 2006;98(4):490–498.

48 Devchand PR, Keller H, Peters JM, et al. The PPARalpha-leukotriene B4 pathway to inflammation control [see comments]. *Nature* 1996;384: 39–43.

49 Huang JT, Welch JS, Ricote M, et al. Interleukin-4-dependent production of PPAR-gamma ligands in macrophages by 12/15-lipoxygenase. *Nature* 1999;400: 378–382.

50 Lee H, Shi W, Tontonoz P, et al. Role for peroxisome proliferator-activated receptor alpha in oxidized phospholipid-induced synthesis of monocyte chemotactic protein-1 and interleukin-8 by endothelial cells. *Circ Res* 2000;87:516–521.

51 Duez H, Chao YS, Hernandez M, et al. Reduction of atherosclerosis by the PPARalpha agonist fenofibrate in mice. *J Biol Chem* 2002;107:1.

52 Tontonoz P, Graves RA, Budavari AI, et al. Adipocyte-specific transcription factor ARF6 is a heterodimeric complex of two nuclear hormone receptors, PPAR gamma and RXR alpha. *Nucleic Acids Res* 1994; 22:5628–5634.

53 Willson TM, Lehmann JM, Kliewer SA. Discovery of ligands for the nuclear peroxisome proliferator-activated receptors. *Ann NY Acad Sci* 1996;804:276–283.

54 Marx N, Sukhova G, Murphy C, et al. Macrophages in human atheroma contain PPARgamma: differentiation-dependent peroxisomal proliferator-activated receptor gamma(PPARgamma) expression and reduction of MMP-9 activity through PPARgamma activation in mononuclear phagocytes *in vitro*. *Am J Pathol* 1998;153: 17–23.

55 Bishop-Bailey D. Peroxisome proliferator-activated receptors in the cardiovascular system. *Br J Pharmacol* 2000; 129:823–834.

56 Wakino S, Law RE, Hsueh WA. Vascular protective effects by activation of nuclear receptor PPARgamma. *J Diabetes Complicat* 2002;16:46–49.

57 Hsueh WA, Bruemmer D. Peroxisome proliferator-activated receptor gamma: implications for cardiovascular disease. *Hypertension* 2004;43:297–305.

58 Tontonoz P, Nagy L, Alvarez JG, et al. PPARgamma promotes monocyte/macrophage differentiation and uptake of oxidized LDL. *Cell* 1998;93: 241–252.

59 Moore KJ, Rosen ED, Fitzgerald ML, et al. The role of PPAR-gamma in macrophage differentiation and cholesterol uptake. *Nat Med* 2001;7:41–47.

60 Chinetti G, Lestavel S, Bocher V, et al. PPAR-alpha and PPAR-gamma activators induce cholesterol removal from human macrophage foam cells through stimulation of the ABCA1 pathway. *Nat Med* 2001;7:53–58.

61 Chawla A, Boisvert WA, Lee CH, et al. A PPAR gamma-LXR-ABCA1 pathway in macrophages is involved in cholesterol efflux and atherogenesis. *Mol Cell* 2001;7: 161–171.

62 Li AC, Brown KK, Silvestre MJ, et al. Peroxisome proliferator-activated receptor gamma ligands inhibit development of atherosclerosis in LDL receptor-deficient mice. *J Clin Invest* 2000;106: 523–531.

63 Li XX, Liao WS. Expression of rat serum amyloid A1 gene involves both C/EBP-like and NF kappa B-like transcription factors. *J Biol Chem* 1991;266:15192–15201.

64 Staels B, Vu Dac N, Kosykh VA, et al. Fibrates downregulate apolipoprotein C-III expression independent of induction of peroxisomal acyl coenzyme A oxidase. A potential mechanism for the hypolipidemic action of fibrates. *J Clin Invest* 1995;95:705–712.

65 Minamikawa J, Tanaka S, Yamauchi M, et al. Potent inhibitory effect of troglitazone on carotid arterial wall thickness in type 2 diabetes. *J Clin Endocrinol Metab* 1998;83:1818–1820.

66 Koshiyama H, Shimono D, Kuwamura N, et al. Rapid communication: inhibitory effect of pioglitazone on carotid arterial wall thickness in type 2 diabetes. *J Clin Endocrinol Metab* 2001;86:3452.

67 Marx N, Schonbeck U, Lazar MA, et al. Peroxisome proliferator-activated receptor gamma activators inhibit gene expression and migration in human vascular smooth muscle cells. *Circ Res* 1998;83:1097–1103.

68 Law RE, Goetze S, Xi XP, et al. Expression and function of PPARgamma in rat and human vascular smooth muscle cells. *Circulation* 2000;101(11):1311–1318.

69 De Dios ST, Bruemmer D, Dilley RJ, et al. Inhibitory Activity of Clinical Thiazolidinedione Peroxisome Proliferator Activating Receptor-{gamma} Ligands Toward Internal Mammary Artery, Radial Artery, and Saphenous Vein Smooth Muscle Cell Proliferation. *Circulation* 2003;107(20):2548–2550.

70 Haffner SM, Greenberg AS, Weston WM, et al. Effect of rosiglitazone treatment on nontraditional markers of cardiovascular disease in patients with type 2 diabetes mellitus. *Circulation* 2002; 106:679–684.

71 Marx N, Froehlich J, Siam L, et al. Antidiabetic PPAR gamma-activator rosiglitazone reduces MMP-9 serum levels in type 2 diabetic patients with coronary artery disease. *Arterioscler Thromb Vasc Biol* 2003;23: 283–288.

72 Campia U, Matuskey LA, Panza JA. Peroxisome proliferator-activated receptor-gamma activation with pioglitazone improves endothelium-dependent dilation in nondiabetic patients with major cardiovascular risk factors. *Circulation* 2006;113:867–875.

73 Ehrmann DA, Schneider DJ, Sobel BE, et al. Troglitazone improves defects in insulin action, insulin secretion, ovarian steroidogenesis, and fibrinolysis in women with polycystic ovary syndrome. *J Clin Endocrinol Metab* 1997;82:2108–2116.

74 Marx N, Bourcier T, Sukhova GK, et al. PPARgamma activation in human endothelial cells increases plasminogen activator inhibitor type-1 expression: PPARgamma as a potential mediator in vascular disease. *Arterioscler Thromb Vasc Biol* 1999;19:546–551.

75 Kato T, Sawamura Y, Tada M, et al. p55 and p75 tumor necrosis factor receptor expression on human glioblastoma cells. *Neurol Med Chir (Tokyo)* 1995;35:567–574.

76 Liu HB, Hu YS, Medcalf RL, et al. Thiazolidinediones inhibit TNFalpha induction of PAI-1 independent of PPARgamma activation. *Biochem Biophys Res Commun* 2005;334:30–37.

77 Bishop-Bailey D, Hla T. Endothelial cell apoptosis induced by the peroxisome proliferator-activated receptor (PPAR) ligand 15-deoxy-Delta12, 14-prostaglandin J2. *J Biol Chem* 1999;274:17042–17048.

78 Margeli A, Kouraklis G, Theocharis S. Peroxisome proliferator activated receptor-gamma (PPAR-gamma)

ligands and angiogenesis. *Angiogenesis* 2003;6: 165–169.

79 Dormandy JA, Charbonnel B, Eckland DJ, et al. Secondary prevention of macrovascular events in patients with type 2 diabetes in the PROactive Study (PROspective pioglitAzone Clinical Trial In macroVascular Events): a randomised controlled trial. *Lancet* 2005;366:1279–1289.

80 Yki-Jarvinen H. The PROactive study: some answers, many questions. *Lancet* 2005;366:1241–1242.

81 Marx N, Wohrle J, Nusser T, et al. Pioglitazone reduces neointima volume after coronary stent implantation: a randomized, placebo-controlled, double-blind trial in nondiabetic patients. *Circulation* 2005;112:2792–2798.

82 Pfutzner A, Marx N, Lubben G, et al. Improvement of cardiovascular risk markers by pioglitazone is independent from glycemic control: results from the pioneer study. *J Am Coll Cardiol* 2005;45:1925–1931.

83 Buchanan TA, Xiang AH, Peters RK, et al. Preservation of pancreatic beta-cell function and prevention of type 2 diabetes by pharmacological treatment of insulin resistance in high-risk hispanic women. *Diabetes* 2002;51: 2796–2803.

84 Finegood DT, McArthur MD, Kojwang D, et al. Beta-cell mass dynamics in Zucker diabetic fatty rats. Rosiglitazone prevents the rise in net cell death. *Diabetes* 2001;50: 1021–1029.

85 Effects of ramipril on cardiovascular and microvascular outcomes in people with diabetes mellitus: results of the HOPE study and MICRO-HOPE substudy. Heart Outcomes Prevention Evaluation Study Investigators. *Lancet* 2000;355:253–259.

86 Knowler WC, Barrett-Connor E, Fowler SE, et al. Reduction in the incidence of type 2 diabetes with lifestyle intervention or metformin. *N Engl J Med* 2002;346:393–403.

87 Barroso I, Gurnell M, Crowley VE, et al. Dominant negative mutations in human PPARgamma associated with severe insulin resistance, diabetes mellitus and hypertension [see comments]. *Nature* 1999;402:880–883.

88 Garg A. Acquired and inherited lipodystrophies. *N Engl J Med* 2004;350:1220–1234.

89 Altshuler D, Hirschhorn JN, Klannemark M, et al. The common PPARgamma Pro12Ala polymorphism is associated with decreased risk of type 2 diabetes. *Nat Genet* 2000;26:76–80.taf/dynapage.taf?file=/ncb/genetics/v26/n1/full/ng0900_76.html taf/dynapage.taf?file=/ncb/genetics/v26/n1/abs/ng0900_76.html

90 Ridker PM, Cook NR, Cheng S, et al. Alanine for proline substitution in the peroxisome proliferator-activated receptor Gamma-2 (PPARG2) gene and the risk of incident myocardial infarction. *Arterioscler Thromb Vasc Biol* 2003;23: 859–863.

91 Deeb SS, Fajas L, Nemoto M, et al. A Pro12Ala substitution in PPARgamma2 associated with decreased receptor activity, lower body mass index and improved insulin sensitivity. *Nat Genet* 1998;20:284–287.

92 Rieusset J, Touri F, Michalik L, et al. A new selective peroxisome proliferator-activated receptor gamma antagonist with antiobesity and antidiabetic activity. *Mol Endocrinol* 2002;16: 2628–2644.

93 Camp HS, Li O, Wise SC, et al. Differential activation of peroxisome proliferator-activated receptor-gamma by troglitazone and rosiglitazone. *Diabetes* 2000;49: 539–547.

94 Miles PD, Barak Y, He W, et al. Improved insulin-sensitivity in mice heterozygous for PPAR-gamma deficiency. *J Clin Invest* 2000;105:287–292.

95 Yamauchi T, Waki H, Kamon J, et al. Inhibition of RXR and PPARgamma ameliorates diet-induced obesity and type 2 diabetes. *J Clin Invest* 2001;108:1001–1013.

96 Larsen TM, Toubro S, Astrup A. PPARgamma agonists in the treatment of type II diabetes: is increased fatness commensurate with long-term efficacy? *Int J Obes Relat Metab Disord* 2003;27:147–161.

97 Tang WH, Francis GS, Hoogwerf BJ, et al. Fluid retention after initiation of thiazolidinedione therapy in diabetic patients with established chronic heart failure. *J Am Coll Cardiol* 2003;41:1394–1398.

98 Pajvani UB, Scherer PE. Adiponectin: systemic contributor to insulin sensitivity. *Curr Diab Rep* 2003;3:207–213.

CHAPTER 25

Stem cells in atherosclerosis and atherosclerosis-related vascular disorders

Yong-Jian Geng, MD, PhD *& Rosalinda Madonna,* MD, PhD

Introduction

Life expectancy and atherosclerosis

Toward the end of the 20th century, life expectancy in the Western hemisphere reached an average of 76 years (male, 73 years; female, 79 years) [1], and most health improvements likely resulted from a significant decline ($\approx 50\%$) in the annual death rate for atherosclerosis-related cardiovascular disease. Decreased cardiovascular mortality appears more prominent among young- and middle-aged patients with coronary heart disease. According to data from the Atherosclerosis Risk in Communities Study [2], this favorable trend is the result of improved treatment of acute disease as well as secondary prevention [3]. Additionally, other social and medical achievements, including improved living conditions, decline of a variety of infectious diseases, and advances in diagnostic techniques and therapies, contribute greatly to improved human longevity.

Despite the reduction in cardiovascular death rates, however, cardiovascular disease remains the leading cause of death [4]. One-third of men and one-tenth of women in the United States currently develop major cardiovascular disease before the age of 60 years [5]. Current projections from the World Health Organization indicate coronary heart disease and stroke will still hold the first and fourth places for overall death and disability, respectively, in the year 2020 despite continued steady progress in treatment [6].

For many years, scientists and physicians have devoted great efforts delineating the etiology and pathophysiology behind atherosclerosis, and developing new medicines or therapies to prevent or treat atherosclerotic lesion development. However, the pathogenesis of this disease remains largely unknown, and atherosclerosis-associated heart attack and stroke persist as the top killers of humans. The histopathological alterations of atherosclerosis occur in the arterial intima, resulting in a fibromuscular hyperplasia associated with variable degrees of lipids, inflammatory cell infiltration, and connective tissue formation as well as calcification. As the disease progresses, arterial tissue may undergo encroachment on the lumen or aneurismal dilation [7]. Although the arterial intima is the major site of atherosclerotic lesion development, particularly in the early stages of atherogenesis, the arterial media may display abnormalities including medial cell death, and calcification, as well as the phenotypic switch of smooth muscle cells (SMC) from contractile to synthetic phenotype. Among the most characteristic and microscopically visible alterations in vascular cell morphology is the formation and accumulation of lipid-laden foam cells, which likely occurs from macrophages and, to a lesser extent, SMC transformation.

Proposed by Ross and colleagues [9], the "response-to-injury" hypothesis represents the classical paradigm of atherogenesis. A variety of pro-atherogenic factors such as hypercholesterolemia, hypertension, diabetes, obesity, smoking, and aging can damage the vessel wall and provoke a cellular repair response to tissue injury. Traditional view holds that, in response to injury, adjacent endothelial cells (ECs) expand and replace damaged EC, while SMC in the medial layers migrate into the intima and thereafter start proliferation. However, compelling evidence from recent stem cell studies now challenges the traditional view about EC replacement and SMC proliferation during the development of atherosclerosis. Through stem cell research, investigators are now been beginning to understand the complexity of vascular cellular response to injury.

Rapid progress in the nascent field of stem cell biology and regenerative medicine has recently attracted great attention from both the lay press and biomedical professionals. Recent studies on cardiovascular stem cells reveal new mechanisms underlying the development of coronary heart disease [8]. In the heart suffering from atherosclerotic coronary disease, chronic ischemia causes degeneration and progressive loss of cardiovascular cells, and ultimately triggers myocardial dysfunction or heart failure. Various types of stem cells from embryonic and adult tissues can potentially regenerate functional cardiovascular cells in the heart undergoing ischemic injury. However, native or exogenous stem cells in ischemic hearts are exposed to various pro-apoptotic or cytotoxic factors. Furthermore, certain numbers of cells newly produced during repopulation and differentiation may die by apoptosis during cardiovascular tissue remodeling and morphogenesis. Genetically programmed to apoptosis, embryonic and adult stem cells may have different life spans. Endogenous and environmental factors, including inflammatory cytokines, growth factors, surface receptors, proteolytic enzymes, mitochondrial respiration, nuclear proteins, telomerase activity, hypoxia-responding proteins, and stem-cell–host-cell interaction, play important roles in the regulation of stem cells. Clarification of the molecular mechanisms may aid our understanding and design of stem cell therapies. Recent research has focused largely on the role played by external stem cells in the repair of the injured blood vessels and the maintenance of the integrity of the blood vessel wall, and also on the pathogenesis of atherosclerosis. Hence, a new paradigm of atherogenesis is emerging as scientists unveil abnormalities of vascular stem cells during intimal hyperplasia and vascular tissue remodeling. This chapter will review the putative mechanisms for stem cell participation in vascular repair during atherosclerotic lesion formation and the aging process of the arterial wall. Further, we will outline potential pathogenic and therapeutic implications for stem cell biology and technology in atherosclerotic vascular disease.

Definition of stem cells

Regardless of their sources, stem cells are defined by their indefinite capability of self-renewal (proliferation) and unlimited potential to generate specialized tissue cells (differentiation). Currently, scientists are working on two major types of stem cells, embryonic and adult, which share three characteristic properties:

1 *Stem cells are premature, undifferentiated, or unspecialized.* Stem cells lack a tissue-specific structure that allows performance of specialized functions. For example, a stem cell cannot work with its neighbors to pump blood through the body (like a heart muscle cell); cannot carry molecules of oxygen through the bloodstream (like a red blood cell); and cannot fire electrochemical signals to other cells that allow the body to move or speak (like a nerve cell). However, unspecialized stem cells can generate specialized cells, including heart muscle cells, blood cells, or nerve cells.

2 *Stem cells can divide and renew themselves for long periods.* Unlike muscle cells, red blood cells, or nerve cells – which normally do not replicate themselves – stem cells may replicate, or proliferate, many times. An initial population of stem cells that proliferates for many months in the laboratory can yield millions of cells. If the resulting cells remain unspecialized, like the parent stem cells, they likely are capable of long-term self-renewal.

3 Stem cells can respond to exogenous or endogenous signals by generating specialized cell types. When unspecialized stem cells develop into specialized cells, the process is called *differentiation*. Signals both inside and outside cells that trigger stem cell differentiation remain incompletely identified. The internal signals controlled by a number of cell genes, which intersperse across long strands of DNA, carry coded instructions for all cell structures and functions. External signals for cell differentiation include

chemicals secreted by other cells, physical contact with neighboring cells, and certain molecules in the microenvironment.

Different terms currently describe the stemness, or pluripotency, of stem cells, and their capacity for long-term survival, growth, and differentiation. Depending on their maturity or potential to generate specialized cell types, a given type of stem cell might be denoted as *totipotent, pluripotent, multipotent, oligopotent,* and *unipotent.* By analyzing the behavior of the cells in the intact organism (*in vivo*), under specific laboratory conditions (*in vitro*), or after transplantation *in vivo,* investigators have established and characterized stem cell lines for decades. For example, the fertilized egg is defined to be *totipotent.* The proxy *toti,* derived from the Latin word *totus,* means "entire." Totipotent stem cells or fertilized eggs potentially can generate all the cells and tissues that form an embryo and support embryonic development *in utero.* The fertilized egg divides and differentiates until it produces a mature organism. Most scientists use the term pluripotent to describe stem cells that can generate cells derived

from all three embryonic germ layers: *mesoderm, endoderm,* and *ectoderm.* All of the many different kinds of specialized cells in the body derive from one of these germ layers (Figure 25.1). "Pluri," which derives from the Latin *plures,* means several or many. Thus, pluripotent cells potentially can generate any type of cell, a property observed in the natural course of embryonic development and under certain laboratory conditions. Thus far, only embryonic stem cells, derived from the inner mass of blastocyst (Figure 25.1), can produce all the three layers of cell types. Embryonic stem cells have been used for a long time for cardiovascular medical research.

Compared with embryonic stem cells, adult stem cells have limited potency of differentiation. They are often committed to one or few types of cells in a given tissue. *Unipotent* stem cells, a term usually applied to cells in an adult organism, are capable of differentiating along only one lineage. "Uni" derives from the Latin word *unus,* or one. Usually, a certain number of *adult stem cells* reside in many differentiated, undamaged tissues. In terms of stemness, they are typically defined as multipotent,

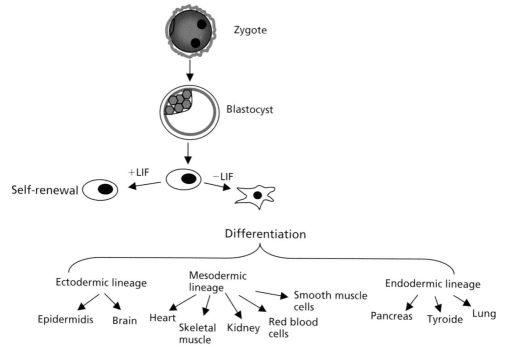

Figure 25.1 Schematic representation of embryonic stem (ES) cell origin from embryos prior to gastrulation and its alternative fates in the presence or absence of leukemia inhibitory factor (LIF). In the absence of LIF, ES cells may initiate differentiation and produce derivatives of all three primary germ layers: ectoderm, mesoderm, and endoderm.

oligopotent, or unipotent stem cells, and they generate only a dozen (multipotent), several (oligopotent), or only one (unipotent) cell types under normal conditions. This process would allow a steady state of self-renewal for the tissue.

Regenerative medicine requires delivery of stem cells into diseased tissues or organs. Many issues require attention prior to the initiation of stem cell transplantation, i.e., source, quality and quantity, biosafety, and availability of stem cells. Embryonic stem cells, the most potent, hold great promise for the development of cellular therapy, but several critical issues in ethics, potential contamination, and immunocompatibility should be considered before a cellular therapy is initiated. Hence, most of embryonic stem cell transplantation remains in the laboratory.

In contrast, adult stem cells offer immediate opportunities for regenerative medicine. Although less potent than embryonic stem cells, adult stem cells from bone marrow and other tissues can differentiate into cardiovascular cells in laboratory animals; in some cases, they have been used clinically for patients with atherosclerotic coronary diseases. On the other hand, recent advances in stem cell vascular biology have deepened our understanding of the molecular and cellular basis of vascular adult stem cell growth and differentiation as well as the potential for using stem cells to treat various diseases, including heart disease. In this chapter, we will focus on several fundamental issues in adult vascular stem cell biology in atherosclerosis.

Stem cells in atherogenesis

Smooth muscle and endothelium are two essential structures for the architecture of the blood vessels. Vascular stem cells, a group of multipotent heterogeneous stem cells, largely fall into two subgroups: endothelial and SMC progenitors (Figure 25.2). EC progenitors develop closely from CD34+ bone marrow stem cells, in particular those committed to the monomyeloid cell lineage, whereas SMC progenitors may belong or originate together in mesenchymal stem cells, which are negative for CD34. Atherosclerosis may damage the arterial wall and impair the capacity of both vascular stem cell types to regenerate neovascular tissue, or may trigger

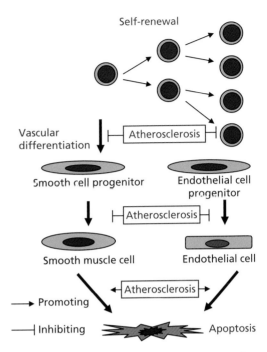

Figure 25.2 Schematic presentation of vascular stem cell growth and differentiation, and the impact of atherosclerosis on these biological processes.

abnormal proliferation or death by apoptosis under different pathological conditions (Figure 25.2).

Stem cell motivation in response to vascular injury in atherosclerosis

Recent studies have documented the role for stem cells in the pathogenesis of atherosclerosis (Table 25.1). The classic "response-to-injury" theory [9] postulates that atherogenesis represents a non-specific response to endothelial damage, which occurs in various forms – mechanical, hemodynamic, immunological, toxic, or metabolic, such as that caused by homocysteine and modified low-density lipoprotein (LDL). Regardless of the nature of insult, i.e. chemical or physical, structural or functional, injury to the arterial wall results in alteration of EC function and the ultimate loss of the anti-thrombogenic properties of the endothelium. The atherosclerotic arterial wall shows augmented adherence of platelets and inflammatory cell infiltration. Exposure to subendothelial connective tissue and tissue factor in plaques activates platelets and promotes platelet aggregation and thrombus formation.

Table 25.1 Stem cells used for atherosclerosis research.

Origin	Type	Model	Reference
Embryos	ESC	*In vitro* gene profiling	[53]
Embryos	ESC	Transgenic atherosclerosis	[54]
Blood	EPC	Angiogenesis in atherosclerosis	[55]
BM	SMPC	Graft atherosclerosis	[56]
Blood	EPC/SMPC	Aging and atherosclerosis	[57]

BM: bone marrow; ESC: embryonic stem cells; SPC: smooth muscle progenitor cells.

Meanwhile, various inflammatory cytokines and growth factors such as platelet-derived growth factor (PDGF) are released from the injured arterial wall, which in turn stimulates migration of SMC normally resident in the arterial tunica media into the intima, where they proliferate, produce extracellular matrix, and, together with blood-borne leukocytes, constitute the major cellular components of the intimal lesions, i.e., atherosclerotic plaques. SMC hyperplasia induced by vessel injury also occurs in other pathological conditions such as post-angioplasty restenosis, in-stent stenosis, and transplant arteriopathy [10].

Although the kinetics of post-atherosclerotic arterial repair and remodeling has been well documented through last decades, the origin of the cells that participate in this repair process is less clear [11]. In the response-to-injury theory, neointimal SMC in vascular lesions likely originate locally from SMC of the medial layer [12]. However, more recent data suggest other sources of vascular cells, such as those circulating or resident in tissues. Vascular cells may also derive from other types of tissue cells through the process of *transdifferentiation*. Adult, undifferentiated stem cells are frequently released from the stem cell reservoirs in the body, most actively in the bone marrow. Indeed, the attachment of circulating mononuclear cells to the luminal side of the injured artery occurs prior to the development of neointimal hyperplasia exclusively due to SMC proliferation [13]. In addition, neointimal tissue may develop in the absence of medial cells, based on a model of medial SMC deprivation by severe injury [14]. Moreover, other studies [15,16] have reported that blocking chemokines or adhesion molecules, which play a crucial role in recruiting blood cells but have no effect on the migration and proliferation of differentiated SMC,

might prevent SMC hyperplasia. Finally, neointimal SMC are distinct from medial SMC in phenotype and pattern of gene expression [17].

Stem cells and hyperplasia in atherosclerotic lesions

Contrary to the conventional assumption that local parenchymal cells repair damaged tissues, a great wealth of evidence indicates that somatic stem cells might mobilize to remote organs, differentiate into the required cell lineages, and participate in organ repair and regeneration [18–20]. Vascular stem cells may contribute to vascular repair and pathological remodeling in models of post-angioplasty restenosis, transplant-associated arteriosclerosis, and hyperlipidemia-induced atherosclerosis. Studies from Asahara and colleagues in 1997 reported circulating CD34+ mononuclear cells from human peripheral blood capable of differentiating into EC *in vitro*, and also incorporating at sites of angiogenesis *in vivo* [18]. In contrast, peripheral blood mononuclear cells seeded on collagen nets in the presence of PDGF-BB transform into smooth muscle-like cells that express α-smooth muscle actin, myosin heavy chain, calponin, and several integrins [21]. Such findings indicate a common vascular progenitor cell that can differentiate into either endothelial or SMC or both in the presence of lineage-specific stimuli such as vascular endothelial growth factor (VEGF) and PDGF-BB. The cytoplasticity of adult stem cells challenges the traditional view that vascular progenitor cells are confined to limited vascular tissue and to bone marrow or peripheral circulation. Current evidence suggests that vascular progenitor cells distribute widely throughout peripheral tissues including, but not limited to, the vessel wall, which can be activated in response to injury. Furthermore, *in vivo* studies support the concept that mature endothelium itself may generate SMC in the arteries through transdifferentiation. Vascular cell plasticity refers to the ability of a mature cell to acquire some or all of the characteristics of another mature cell. Two research teams recently demonstrated that adult EC transdifferentiate into SMC in a TGF-β dependent manner [22,23]. However, only a small percentage (0.01–0.03%) of EC has been shown capable of differentiation or transdifferentiation.

Origin of SMC in transplant arteriosclerosis

Transplant vasculopathy, characterized by concentric myointimal proliferation in the arteries of the graft, resembles atherosclerosis. The thickened neointima of graft arteries consists of proliferating vascular SMC, and contributes to progressive occlusion of the artery, leading to downstream ischemic tissue damage and fibrosis [24,25]. Saiura et al. [26] have studied the role of bone-marrow-derived stem cells in graft vasculopathy through heterotypic cardiac transplantation between wild-type mice and ROSA26 mice, which express *LacZ* ubiquitously. Immunohistochemical staining with X-gal revealed that the majority of the neointima in the allograft vessels was composed of recipient cells expressing LacZ. Immunofluorescence studies revealed that *LacZ+* cells in the neointima expressed various markers for SMC, including myosin heavy chain, calponin, h-caldesmon, and α-smooth muscle actin [14]. Conversely, *LacZ−* neointima developed on the *LacZ+* coronary arteries following transplantation of *LacZ+* hearts into wild-type mice. Such results indicate that the majority of neointimal cells derived from recipient cells, but not from the medial cells of donor origin (Table 25.2).

Sata et al. also identified the source of recipient cells in the atherosclerotic allograft [14]. In their studies, they transplanted bone marrow stem cells from *LacZ* mice to wild-type mice and, after 4–8 weeks, transplanted wild-type hearts into bone-marrow-transplanted wild-type mice. Four weeks after cardiac transplantation, most neointimal cells were LacZ+ and accumulated on the luminal side of the graft coronary arteries. Furthermore, some of the LacZ+ cells in graft vasculopathy revealed α-smooth muscle actin expression. These results indicate that recipient bone marrow cells can circulate through the body and localize in atherosclerotic lesions, where they contribute to vascular remodeling and neointima formation, generating both EC and SMC (Table 25.2).

Table 25.2 Origin of neointimal cells during atherogenesis.

Species	Organ	Cell type	Cell source	Final event	Reference
Human	Aorta, heart	SMC	Cytokine and PDGF released from injured arterial wall	Migration of SMC into the intima, proliferation, and matrix secretion	[9]
Human	Aorta	Mononuclear cells	Peripheral blood	Transdifferentiation into neointimal smooth muscle-like cells	[21]
Human, in vitro analysis	Aorta	ECs	Arterial wall	Transdifferentiation into neointimal smooth muscle-like cells	[22,23]
Human mouse	Aorta, heart	Stem/progenitor cells	Bone marrow	Differentiation into neointimal smooth muscle-like cells	[14,26,27, 29,34]
Mouse	Aorta	Stem/progenitor cells	Periadventitial tissues (such as adipose tissue)	Differentiation into neointimal smooth muscle-like cells	[29,30,69]
Human		Stem/progenitor cells	Peripheral blood	Differentiation into neointimal smooth muscle-like cells	[32,33]

Several groups have addressed the issue of bone marrow involvement in the process of neointimal development and SMC hyperplasia. Shimizu and colleagues used a mouse aortic allotransplant model [27,70]. In the model of bone-marrow-chimeric LacZ-transgenic mice, Li et al. determined that approximately 11% of neointimal SMC originated in bone marrow [28]. Following vein grafting in LacZ-transgenic normal and bone-marrow-chimeric mice, Hu et al. concluded that approximately 40% of neointimal SMC were recipient derived, whereas 60% remained donor original [29,69]. They also showed that large numbers of vascular cell progenitors localized in the adventitia may contribute to proliferation and accumulation of intimal vascular cells in a similar model [30]. However some controversial reports do not favor the notion that SMC originate from bone marrow. A study on bone-marrow-chimeric rats [31] showed that host-derived EC in advanced neointimal lesions of aortic allograft were primarily not bone marrow derived (Table 25.2).

Taken together, although bone marrow can contribute to the SMC population found in neointimal lesions, non-bone-marrow resources can provide precursor cells to transplant-related atherosclerotic lesions (Figure 25.3). Recent studies show that human peripheral blood contains circulating SMC precursors, suggesting a possible alternative explanation to bone marrow as the origin of vascular progenitor cells. Furthermore, Simper et al. [21] showed that human mononuclear blood cells in culture can generate SMC in the presence of PDGF. Adipose tissue may contain precursors that might enter the vessel wall from the adventitia through *vasa vasorum*. Additionally, circulating SMC precursors or progenitors might also originate from other sources, such as transdifferentiation of EC [32] or non-bone-marrow-derived fibroblast-like cells residing in the peripheral blood [33]. In any case, it is possible that SMC precursors recruited from a variety of resources participate in vascular tissue repair or remodeling (Figure 25.4). When vessel damage occurs, medial SMC can migrate into the intima, where they serve as a new source of neointimal SMC. More severe and prolonged vascular damage might signal the need of SMC growth from adjacent vessels. Severe and time-restricted vessel damage will lead to recruitment from non-bone-marrow sources, whereas similar

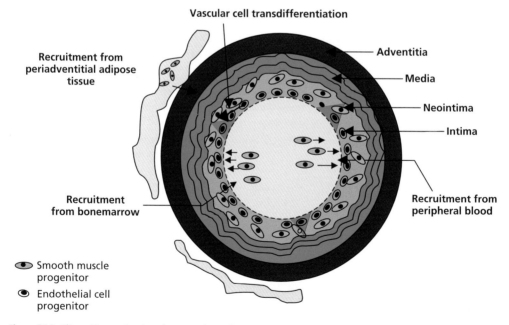

Figure 25.3 Alternative mechanisms for transplant atherosclerosis development. Neointima originates from vascular precursor cells recruited from various sources, including bone marrow, blood, and periadventitial tissues that contain adipose tissue. Transdifferentiation of ECs into neointimal SMC provides an additional mechanism for neointimal formation.

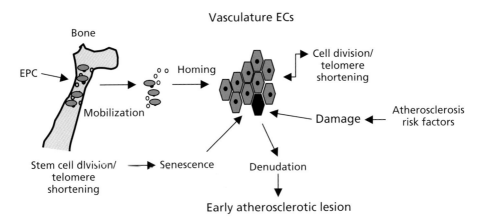

Figure 25.4 Schematic overview of the role of EC division, progenitor cell homing, and telomere shortening in atherosclerosis. Upon EC damage, neighboring cells divide, and EPCs home into the endothelium to fill up the discontinuities. Stem cells in bone marrow divide to maintain a constant concentration of EPC. EC and stem cells division lead to telomere shortening. Excessive telomere erosion induces the exhaustion of endothelial repair processes, with EC denudation and formation of early atherosclerotic lesion.

damage over a prolonged period of time will probably need additional SMC precursors from the bone marrow.

Origin of vascular cells in vascular remodeling and hyperlipidemia

The origin of SMC in atherosclerotic lesions remains undetermined. Recent work by Sata and colleagues [14] points to the contribution of bone-marrow-derived stem cells to the pathogenesis of lesion formation after mechanical vascular injury as well as atherosclerotic plaque formation after hyperlipidemia. In this study, bone marrow of wild-type mice was replaced with that of LacZ mice. Four to eight weeks after bone marrow transplantation, a large wire inserted into the femoral artery of mice led to endothelial denudation and apoptosis of SMC. X-gal staining revealed LacZ+ cells attached to the luminal side of the injured vessels, whereas immunofluorescent staining for SMC and endothelial markers showed that some of bone-marrow-derived LacZ cells in the neointimal lesions expressed SMC α-actin or CD31. Such results indicate that bone marrow cells generate vascular cells, thereby contributing to arterial remodeling after mechanical injury.

Bone marrow transplantation from green fluorescent protein positive (GFP+) mice and LacZ+ mice to 8-week-old apolipoprotein E-deficient (apoE −/−) mice fed a Western-type diet for 8 weeks showed GFP+ or *LacZ*+ cells in atherosclerotic lesions [14]. Immunofluorescence studies revealed that GFP-positive cells accumulating in atherosclerotic plaques developed differentiation markers for smooth muscle in the aorta of bone-marrow-transplanted mice. For instance, most of the GFP+ cells expressed markers for SMC α-actin, indicating that bone marrow cells generate SMC-like cells observed in hyperlipidemia-induced atherosclerotic plaques. Further analysis of bone marrow cells that potentially can generate vascular cells suggests that SMC may derive from a hematopoietic stem cell (HSC) enriched fraction positive for c-kit and Sca-1 but negative for Lin. Evidence in support of this hypothesis has been provided by Sata and colleagues [14]. In this study, the HSC-enriched fraction (c-kit+, Sca-1+, Lin−) isolated from the bone marrow of LacZ mice was injected into lethally irradiated wild-type mice. At 4 weeks from irradiation, the femoral arteries of recipient mice were injured mechanically. At 4 weeks from the injury, arteries showed hyperplasia in the neointima, in which LucZ + cells expressing α-SMA were identified. These findings indicate that the c-Kit+, Sca-1+ Lin− fraction of bone marrow cells potentially can differentiate into either SMC or EC, thereby contributing to vascular remodeling (Table 25.2).

Endothelial repair

Impaired endothelial function is commonly believed to result from arterial injury due to acute or chronic exposure to cardiovascular risk factors such as smoking, a hypercaloric diet, elevated cholesterol, a sedentary life-style, diabetes, and high blood pressure. Therefore, several emerging lines of evidence suggest that impaired vascular repair reflects this ongoing injury, and disequilibrium between the magnitude of vascular injury and capacity of repair can lead to atherosclerosis. Although some morphological studies indicate that stem cells contribute to the regeneration of the arterial wall with atherosclerosis and mechanical injury, little is known about the role of stem cells in functional recovery. Because a functionally defective artery might be more vulnerable to pro-atherogenic injury, full installation of endothelial and SMC function is vital for a fully functioning arterial wall. Angioplasty through a balloon catheter has been used routinely to treat patients with coronary or other vascular diseases caused by atherosclerosis. Here it is highly likely that EC progenitors normally repair mechanically damaged EC.

Vascular stem cells in aging arteries

The impact of aging on vascular cell progenitors. The production of vasoactive molecules, cytokines, and growth factors during atherogenesis triggers not only a paracrine effect on the adjacent arterial wall, but also an endocrine signal perceived by responsive remote tissues [34]. Local migration and proliferation of EC adjacent to the site of injury reflects the response of the vessel wall to the injury. Therefore, in virtue of endocrine function acquired by damaged tissues of the vessel wall, peripheral tissues such as bone marrow initiate a repair process through the mobilization of vascular progenitor cells and their incorporation into the sites of injury [18,34–37]. It is important in vascular repair to identify particular cell populations from bone marrow. Intermediate vascular progenitor cells (CD31+/CD45−) and more primitive stem cells (CD34+/VEGFR2+), which comprise the total population of endothelial progenitor cells (EPCs) and share DiI-acLDL uptake, explain the atheroprotective property of bone marrow. Using apoE-deficient mice (i.e., mice specifically bred to develop severe atherosclerosis and high

cholesterol levels [68]), Rauscher and colleagues investigated the effects of injected bone marrow cells and their distributions in the disease process, and monitored the distribution and engraftment of bone-marrow-derived vascular progenitor cells into sites of atherosclerosis [34,71]. Investigators intravenously injected bone marrow cells from normal mice (10^6 cells every 2 weeks) into atherosclerosis-prone, apoE-deficient mice over a 14-week period, starting at 3 weeks of age. As a control, an equal number of atherosclerosis-prone mice were left untreated or sham treated. Results showed an accumulation of progenitors along the arterial surface, particularly along the proximal, thoracic, and abdominal aorta, where atherosclerotic lesions are most pronounced. Such accumulation was not observed in animals that did not receive bone marrow cells or those at low risk of developing atherosclerosis. A majority of the engrafted marrow cells differentiated into EC. These results demonstrate that bone marrow cells are capable of homing in the atherosclerosis-prone regions of the aorta and also participate in the repair process. In particular, EPCs can provide a pool of cells that could form a cellular patch at the site of injured vessel wall.

Atherogenesis requires an imbalance between injury and repair, and bone-marrow-derived vascular progenitor cells may participate Thus, understanding the triggers and mechanisms leading to an altered repair capacity of marrow cells is important. Rauscher et al. first observed that progenitor cells originating from the bone marrow become incompetent with aging – the most powerful risk factor for atherosclerosis – and in the presence of other risk factors. In such conditions, the cells lose their capacity to repair the arterial wall, which then becomes dysfunctional and develops atherosclerotic lesions [34]. These authors treated apoE-deficient mice with intravenous injections of cells obtained from the marrow of either young (3–4 weeks of age, before any atherosclerotic lesion could be detected) or old (6 months) apoE-deficient mice. Whereas the young apoE-deficient bone marrow cells maintained a repair capacity not detectably different from that of wild-type marrow cells, the beneficial effect of old apoE-deficient bone marrow cells disappeared. Analysis for specific cell populations in the bone marrow of young and old wild-type apoE-deficient mice indicated that EPCs tend to disappear in the marrow of old apoE-deficient mice. Such results indicate that aging, combined with ongoing injury such as hyperlipidemia, causes increased susceptibility to atherosclerosis through the progressive exhaustion of bone-marrow-derived progenitor cells, in particular EPC, with capacity for repair of the damaged arterial wall.

Cardiovascular risk factors, vascular repair, and vascular progenitor cells are strongly linked in humans as well. Statin therapy increases the levels of circulating EPCs [38–40]. Recent studies from Tepper and colleagues showed that EPC from patients with type 2 diabetes exhibit impaired proliferation, adhesion, and incorporation into vascular structures, thus accounting for the impaired neo-vascularization observed in such individuals [41]. Furthermore, circulating EPC from high-risk subjects (with diabetes, hypertension, elevated serum cholesterol levels, and aging) are less numerous and also become senescent more rapidly compared with low-risk subjects [42]. Similarly, previous studies have noted qualitative differences between EPC from patients with symptomatic coronary artery disease and those from control subjects [40]. Low levels of circulating EPC in patients with increasing cardiovascular risk could result from several mechanisms. By modulating the levels of oxidative stress, nitric oxide activity, or other endothelial physiological processes, risk factors might directly influence the mobilization or half-life of EPC. Alternatively, continuous endothelial damage or dysfunction may lead to depletion or exhaustion of a finite supply of EPC.

Animal studies have documented a link between loss of repair and early phases of atherogenesis, such as vascular inflammation. Because inflammatory markers, such as C-reactive protein (CRP) and interleukin-6 (IL-6), an interleukin that regulates production of CRP by the liver, identify patients at risk for cardiovascular events [43], Rauscher and colleagues, by studying IL-6 levels in the apoE-deficient mice model of atherosclerosis, tested the hypothesis that the inflammatory process is linked to a deficient repair process of the arterial wall due to bone marrow senescence [34]. Indeed, IL-6 levels increased in wild-type mice on regular chow and in apoE-deficient mice on a high-fat diet. In these mice, increased IL-6 paralleled the changes in total cholesterol observed, and substantially decreased after the administration of bone marrow

cells. Interestingly, while marrow cells obtained from wild-type mice on a regular chow brought IL-6 levels to near background, marrow cells from apoE-deficient mice on a high-fat diet were significantly less able to reduce IL-6. These data support the hypothesis that inflammatory molecules increase beyond the capacity of the organism to downregulate them in the absence of production of repair cells by the bone marrow (e.g., an aging marrow in the presence of risk factors), thus overcoming a negative feedback loop that begins with the production and release of vascular progenitor cells able to repair the damaged arterial wall. Therefore, inflammatory molecules begin to recruit inflammatory cells, such as activated macrophages, that potentially can increase the injury to the artery (positive feedback loop).

Mechanisms for vascular cell progenitor survival and stemness maintenance

Vascular stem cells play a key role in the maintenance of endothelial monolayer integrity by replacing apoptotic or damaged EC and SMC. However, it is important to understand the capability of vascular stem cells to survive in atherosclerotic lesions, where pro-inflammatory and pro-apoptotic factors accumulate. Atherosclerosis may be viewed as a long-term battle between death and division of vascular cells surrounding or within the lesions. Also, the balance between recruitment and deletion of vascular cell stem cells from the bone marrow or other sources constantly changes. Recent studies have shown that changes in the number of surviving circulating EC progenitors are important markers of the risk for coronary disease. A large number of high-quality stem cells is essential for a healthy arterial wall [44].

How can we evaluate the quality of stem cells? Each cell division leads to telomere shortening, and eventually to cellular senescence once the shortening telomere length reaches a critical threshold. Telomerase is a ribonucleoprotein complex that contains RNA-dependent DNA polymerase (reverse transcriptase) activity with its RNA component (complementary to the telomeric single-stranded overhang) as a template to synthesize the TTAGGG repeats directly onto telomeric ends [45]. Telomerase catalyzes the addition of oligonucleotide (TTAGGG) repeats onto the repetitive DNA structure, telomeres, at the ends of linear chromosomes [45]. Telomerase-catalyzed DNA addition prevents telomere shortening and stabilizes chromosomes [46]. Extension of the 3′ DNA template permits additional replication of the 5′ end of the lagging strand, thus compensating for telomere shortening that occur in its absence. Although telomerase exists abundantly in embryonic stem cells and adult germline cells, it is almost undetectable in mature somatic cells except for actively proliferating cells of renewal tissues [47]. The telomerase-mediated maintenance of telomere length contributes to the pluripotency, or "stemness," of cellular lineage differentiation in mammalian tissues.

In vivo, telomeres shorten more rapidly in EC located at regions susceptible to atherosclerosis, such as the arterial sites exposed to the high shear stress and turbulent blood flow [48–50], and exposure to atherosclerotic risk factors that lead to oxidative stress modulate telomere shortening [51]. For instance, exposure of cultured EC to homocysteine-induced oxidative stress significantly accelerates the rate of EC senescence and telomere length shortening [52]. Okuda et al. reported a higher rate of age-dependent telomere attrition in both the intima and the media of the distal vs proximal human abdominal aorta [49], and also determined a negative correlation between telomere length and atherosclerotic grade, suggesting that telomere attrition contributes to age-dependent endothelial dysfunction [49]. EC with senescence-associated phenotypes localize in human atherosclerotic lesions [53]; and overexpression of a dominant-negative mutant of telomerase reverse transcriptase (TERT) induces this phenotype in cultured human aortic EC [53]. Average telomere length in leukocytes of patients with coronary artery disease is significantly shorter compared with controls with normal angiograms after adjustment for age and sex [54]. In another study comparing 203 cases of premature myocardial infarction and 180 age and sex-adjusted controls, mean telomere length of patients was significantly shorter than that of controls [55]. These studies might suggest that telomere attrition might be a primary abnormality that renders the organism more susceptible to cardiovascular risk factors. However, the rate of

telomere shortening augments in most somatic cells with increasing cell divisions [45,48]. Therefore the data just mentioned do not necessary support the hypothesis that telomere shortening is a primary abnormality in atherosclerosis. Indeed, reduced leukocyte telomere length occurs in patients with cardiovascular disease possibly, and likely, as a mere consequence of increased cell turnover induced by the chronic inflammatory response underlying atherogenesis. Nevertheless, Poch et al. [56] provided other exciting data assessing the impact of telomere attrition on atherogenesis induced by dietary cholesterol in apoE-deficient mice, a well-established model of experimental atherosclerosis [57]. They found that late-generation mice doubly deficient in apoE and TERT had shorter telomeres and were better protected from atherosclerosis compared with apoE-null mice with an intact TERT gene. In this study, the beneficial effect of short telomeres seems to correlate with impaired proliferative capacity of lymphocytes and macrophages [56]. These conflicting findings might be reconciled if one can assume that accumulation of cellular damage imposed by prolonged exposure to cardiovascular risk factors ultimately prevails over protective mechanisms, including telomore shortening.

Therapeutic implications of vascular progenitor cells

In consideration of the classical dogma that atherosclerosis develops as an abnormality of tissue response to vascular damage, many past and current treatments aim to eliminating risk factors and prevent further vascular injury [12,58–61]. The novel model of vascular injury and repair in atherosclerosis points to deficiency in vascular repair secondary to the obsolescence of somatic stem cells in bone marrow and other tissues, including the arterial wall itself. Such abnormality of vascular stem cells in tissue regeneration and repair critically determines disease initiation and progression [34,41,42]. This defect may inspire an alternative approach aiming at slowing progression and promoting repression of atherosclerosis. This new therapeutic approach is based on either restoring the capacity of bone marrow to produce vascular repair EPCs or administering exogenous EPCs to stabilize patients with a markedly impaired arterial repair process. Outsourcing of progenitor cells has been reported in children with Hurler syndrome, a lysosomal storage disorder first discovered in 1919, characterized by the accumulation of acid mucopolysaccharides in the central nervous system and peripheral tissues [62,63]. These patients develop premature and accelerated atherosclerosis that leads to myocardial infarction and heart failure at ages of 10–20 years. In Hurler syndrome, the development of atherosclerotic lesions occurs due to mucopolysaccharide-mediated insult to the vascular wall. Administration of umbilical blood stem cells from normal children to the diseased children with Hurler syndrome has been reported to completely normalize the physical appearance and mental levels of the patients, with substantially remitting signs of overt coronary artery disease [63]. Successful stem cell treatment in this unique atherosclerosis-prone genetic disorder opens great potential for the use of stem cells to develop anti-atherosclerosis therapies. However one has to caution on the fact that, in certain stages of atherogenesis or in complications of atherosclerosis, controlling stem cell overgrowth may also be important, considering the fact that stem cells from the bone marrow may contribute to intimal hyperplasia and neointima formation [14,26–29,31]. In this regard, systemic or local (e.g., drug eluting stents) strategies may inhibit smooth muscle progenitor cells in vascular lesions.

Our recent work has shown that transendocardial injections of autologous mononuclear bone marrow cells in patients with end-stage ischemic heart disease could safely promote neovascularization and improve perfusion and myocardial contractility [64]. The relative safety of intramyocardial injections of bone-marrow-derived stem cells in humans with severe heart failure points to the potential for using stem cells to improve myocardial blood flow with associated enhancement of regional and global left ventricular function [65]. We demonstrated, in experimental animals with chronic heart failure, that transplanted mesenchymal stem cells from autologous bone marrow tissue can enhance circulation by generating neovascular tissue and improving collateral blood supply [65]. Using an *in vitro* system, we very recently

demonstrated that treatment with a cholesterol-lowering drug may attenuate expression of inducible nitric oxide synthase, a key enzyme responsible for inflammation and regulation of cell apoptosis [66].

Conclusions

Stem cells are characterized by their capability of unlimited self-renewal and potential of differentiation into specialized tissue cells. Recent studies have provided both *in vitro* and *in vivo* evidence that abnormality of stem cells occurs and contributes to tissue response and remodeling in the arterial wall with atherosclerosis. Vascular stem cells are progenitors of endothelial and SMC. Although less potent than embryonic stem cells in terms of the potential of growth and cell lineage differentiation, vascular stem cells actively participate in arterial tissue repair and regeneration in atherosclerosis. Studies with embryonic stem cells can help characterizing the cellular and molecular pathways that regulate vascularization and angiogenesis [66,67]. In adults, many tissues, including bone marrow, blood, and connective tissue such as the adipose tissue, contain vascular stem cells. Atherogenic stimulation triggers a response to injury in a way that leads to mobilization of stem cells. Abnormal activation, proliferation, and death of stem cells may serve as the cellular basis for the development of atherosclerotic lesions in the arteries. Stem cells also provide potential opportunities to repair damaged blood vessels and treat or prevent atherosclerosis. In order to develop therapeutic strategies for atherosclerosis and its complication, we must understand the phenotype and differentiation profiles of bone-marrow- or other tissue-derived vascular progenitor cells.

Acknowledgments

This work is supported by grants awarded to Dr. Yong-Jian Geng from the National Institutes of Health, the Texas Higher Educational Coordination Board, and the Department of Defense T5 program.

References

1 *Der Fischer Weltalmanach 1996.* Frankfurt: *Fischer Taschenbuch* Verlag.

2 Lenfant C. Heart research: celebration and renewal. *Circulation* 1997;96:3822–3823.

3 Rosamond WD, Chambless LE, Folsom AR, et al. Trends in the incidence of myocardial infarction and in mortality due to coronary heart disease. *N Engl J Med* 1998;339: 1987–1994.

4 National Center of Health Statistics. *United States, 1990.* Washington, DC: US Government Printing Office; 1991.

5 Statistics NCoH. *Mortality*, Part A. Washington, DC: Statistics NCoH; 1991.

6 Murray JL, Lopez AD. Global burden disease study. *Lancet* 1997;349:1269–1276.

7 Gertz D, Kurgan A, Eisenberg D. Aneurysm of the rabbit common carotid artery induced by periarterial application of calcium chloride in vivo. *J Clin Invest* 1988; 81:649–656.

8 Geng YJ. Molecular mechanisms for cardiovascular stem cell apoptosis and growth in the hearts with atherosclerotic coronary disease and ischemic heart failure. *Ann NY Acad Sci* 2003;1010:687–697.

9 Ross R. *The Pathogenesis of Atherosclerosis*. Philadelphia, PA: Lippincott-Raven; 1996.

10 Moore S. Pathogenesis of atherosclerosis. *Metabolism* 1985;34(Suppl 1):13–16.

11 Schwartz SM, De Blods D, O' Brien ER. The intimal soil for atherosclerosis and restenosis. *Circ Res* 1995;77: 445–465.

12 Ross R. Atherosclerosis: an inflammatory disease. *N Engl J Med* 1999;340:115–126.

13 Feldman LJ, Mazighi M, Scheuble A. Differential expression of matrix metalloproteinases after stent implantation and balloon angioplasty in the hypercholesterolemic rabbit. *Circulation* 2001;103:3117–3122.

14 Sata M, Saiura A, Kumisato A. Hematopoietic stem cells differentiate into vascular cells that participate in the pathogenesis of atherosclerosis. *Nat Med* 2002; 8:403–409.

15 Furukawa Y, Matsumori A, Ohashi N. Anti-monocyte chemoattractant protein-1/monocyte chemotactic and activating factor antibody inhibits neointimal hyperplasia in injured rat carotid arteries. *Circ Res* 1999;84: 306–314.

16 Hayashi S, Watanabe N, Nakazawa K. Roles of P-selectin in inflammation, neointimal formation, and vascular remodelling in balloon-injured rat carotid arteries. *Circulation* 2000;102:1710–1717.

17 Zohlnofer D, Klein CA, Richter T. Gene expression profiling of human stent-induced neointima by cDNA array analysis of microscopic specimens retrieved by helix cutter atherectomy: detection of FK506-binding protein 12 upregulation. *Circulation* 2001; 103:1396–1402.

18 Asahara T, Murohara T, Sullivan A. Isolation of putative progenitor endothelial cells for angiogenesis. *Science* 1997;275:964–967.

19 McKay R. Stem cells: hype and hope. *Nature* 2000; 406:361–364.

20 Orlic D, Kajstura J, Chimenti S. Mobilized bone marrow cells repair the infarcted heart, improving function and survival. *Proc Natl Acad Sci USA* 2001;98: 10344–10349.

21 Simper D, Stadboerger PG, Panetta CJ. Smooth muscle progenitor cells in human blood. *Circulation* 2002;106: 1199–1204.

22 Frid MG, Kale VA, Stenmark KR. Mature vascular endothelium can give rise to smooth muscle cells via endothelial mesenchymal differentiation: *in vitro* analysis. *Circ Res* 2002;90:1189–1196.

23 Ishisaki A, Hayashi S, Li A-J, et al. Human umbilical vein endothelium-derived cells retain potential to differentiate into smooth muscle like cells. *J Biol Chem* 2003;278: 1303–1309.

24 Orosz CG, Pelletier RP. Chronic remodelling pathology in grafts. *Curr Opin Immunol* 1997;9:676–680.

25 Billingham ME. Cardiac transplant atherosclerosis. *Transplant Proc* 1987;19:19–25.

26 Saiura A, Sata M, Hirata Y. Circulating smooth muscle progenitor cells contribute to atherosclerosis. *Nat Med* 2001;7:382–383.

27 Shimizu K, Sugiyama S, Aikawa M, et al. Host bone-marrow cells are a source of donor intimal smooth muscle-like cells in murine aortic transplant arteriopathy. *Nat Med* 2001;7:738–741.

28 Li J, Han X, Jiang J, et al. Vascular smooth muscle cells of recipient origin mediate intimal expansion after aortic allotransplantation in mice. *Am J Pathol* 2001;158: 1943–1947.

29 Hu Y, Mayr M, Metzler B, et al. Both donor and recipient origins of smooth muscle cells in vein graft atherosclerotic lesions. *Circ Res* 2002;91:e13–e20.

30 Hu Y, Zhang Z, Torsney E, et al. Abundant progenitor cells in the adventitia contribute to atherosclerosis of vein grafts in ApoE-deficient mice. *J Clin Invest* 2004; 113:1258–1265.

31 Hillebrands JL, Klatter FA, van Dijk WD, et al. The bone marrow does not contribute substantially to host-derived endothelial cells replacement in transplant arteriosclerosis. *Nat Med* 2002;8:2–3.

32 Gittenberger-de Groot AC, DeRuiter MC, Berwerff M, et al. Smooth muscle cell origin and its relation to heterogeneity in development and disease. *Arterioscler Thromb Vasc Biol* 1999;19:1589–1594.

33 Bucala R, Spiegel LA, Chesney J, et al. Circulating fibrocytes define a new leukocyte subpopulation that mediates tissue repair. *Mol Med* 1994;1:71–81.

34 Rauscher FM, Goldschmidt-Clermont PJ, Davis BH. Aging, progenitor cells exhaustion and atherosclerosis. *Circulation* 2003;108:457–463.

35 Rafii S. Circulating endothelial precursors: mystery, reality and promise. *J Clin Invest* 2000;105:17–19.

36 Patterson C. The Ponzo effect: endothelial progenitor cells appear on the horizon. *Circulation* 2003;107: 2995–2997.

37 Hristov M, Erl W, Weber PC. Endothelial progenitor cells: mobilization, differentiation and homing. *Arterioscler Thromb Vasc Biol* 2003;23:1185–1189.

38 Llevadot J, Murasawa S, Kureishi Y. HMG-CoA reductase inhibitor mobilizes bone marrow-derived endothelial progenitor cells. *J Clin Invest* 2001;108:399–405.

39 Dimmeler S, Aicher A, Vasa M. HMG-CoA reductase inhibitors (statins) increase endothelial progenitor cells via the PI3-kinase/Akt pathway. *J Clin Invest* 2001;108: 391–397.

40 Vasa M, Fichtlscherer S, Adler K. Increase in circulating endothelial progenitor cells by statin therapy in patients with stable coronary artery disease. *Circulation* 2001;103: 2885–2890.

41 Tepper OM, Galiano RD, Capla JM, et al. Human endothelial progenitor cells from type II diabetics exhibit impaired proliferation, adhesion and incorporation into vascular structures. *Circulation* 2002;106:2781–2786.

42 Hill JM, Zalos G, Halcox JPJ, et al. Circulating endothelial progenitor cells, vascular function and cardiovascular risk. *N Engl J Med* 2003;348:593–600.

43 Ridker PM. Clinical application of C-reactive protein for cardiovascular disease detection and prevention. *Circulation* 2003;107:363–369.

44 Hill JM, Zalos G, Halcox JPJ, et al. Circulating endothelial progenitor cells, vascular function and cardiovascular risk. *N Engl J Med* 2003;348:593–600.

45 Harley CB, Villeponteau B. Telomeres and telomerase in aging and cancer. *Curr Opin Genet Dev* 1995;5: 249–255.

46 Cech TR, Lingner J. Telomerase and the chromosome end replication problem. *Ciba Found Symp* 1997;211: 20–28.

47 Odorico JS, Kaufman DS, Thomson JA. Multilineage differentiation from human embryonic stem cell lines. *Stem Cells* 2001;19:193–204.

48 Chang E, Harley CB. Telomere length and replicative aging in human vascular tissues *Proc Natl Acad Sci USA* 1995;92:11190–11194.

49 Okuda K, Khan MY, Skurnick J, et al. Telomere attrition of the human abdominal aorta: relationships with age and atherosclerosis. *Atherosclerosis* 2000;152:391–398.

50 Davies PF, Remuzzi A, Gordon EJ, et al. Turbulent fluid shear stress induces vascular endothelial cell turnover *in vitro*. *Proc Natl Acad Sci USA* 1986;83:2114–2117.

51 Von Zglinicki T. Oxidative stress shortens telomeres. *Trend Biochem Sci* 2002;27:339–344.

52 Xu D, Neville R, Finkel T. Homocysteine accelerates endothelial cell senescence. *FEBS Lett* 2000;470: 20–24.

53 Minamino T, Miyauchi H, Yoshida T, et al. Endothelial cell senescence in human atherosclerosis: role of telomere in endothelial dysfunction. *Circulation* 2002;105: 1541–1544.

54 Samani NJ, Boultby R, Butler R, et al. Telomere shortening in atherosclerosis. *Lancet* 2001;358:472–473.

55 Brouilette S, Singh RK, Thompson JR, et al. White cell telomere length and risk of premature myocardial infarction. *Arterioscler Thromb Vasc Biol* 2003;23:842–846.

56 Poch E, Carbonell P, Franco S, et al. Short telomeres protect from diet-induced atherosclerosis in apolipoprotein E-null mice. *FASEB J* 2004;18:418–420.

57 Breslow JL. Mouse models of atherosclerosis. *Science* 1996;272:685–688.

58 Lusis AJ. Atherosclerosis. *Nature* 2000;407:233–241.

59 Boisvert WA, Spangenberg J, Curtiss LK. Treatment of severe hypercholesterolemia in apolipoprotein E-deficient mice by bonemarrow transplantation. *J Clin Invest* 1995;96:1118–1124.

60 Linton MF, Atkinson JB, Fazio S. Prevention of atherosclerosis in apolipoprotein E-deficient mice by bone marrow transplantation. *Science* 1995;267:1034–1037.

61 Hurler G. Uber einen typ multiper Abartungen, vorwiegend am Skelettsystem. *Zeitschrift Kinderheilkd* 1919; 24:220–234.

62 Dorfman A, Matalon R. The Hurler and Hunter syndromes. *Am J Pathol* 1969;47:691–707.

63 Peters C, Balthazor M, Shapiro EG. Outcome of unrelated donor bone marrow transplantation in 40 children with Hurler syndrome. *Blood* 1996;87:4894–4892.

64 Perin EC, Dohmann HF, Borojevic R, et al. Transendocardial, autologous bone marrow cell transplantation for severe, chronic ischemic heart failure. *Circulation* 2003;107:2294–2302.

65 Silva GV, Litovsky S, Assad JA, et al. Mesenchymal stem cells differentiate into an endothelial phenotype, enhance vascular density, and improve heart function in a canine chronic ischemia model. *Circulation* 2005;111: 150–156.

66 Madonna R, Di Napoli P, Massaro M, et al. Simvastatin attenuates expression of cytokine-inducible nitric oxide synthase in embryonic cardiac myoblasts. *J Biol Chem* 2005;280(14):13503–13511.

67 Lindmark H, Rosengren B, Hurt-Camejo E, et al. Gene expression profiling shows that macrophages derived from mouse embryonic stem cells is an improved in vitro model for studies of vascular disease. *Exp Cell Res* 2004; 300:335–344.

68 Breslow JL. Transgenic mouse models of lipoprotein metabolism and atherosclerosis. *Proc Natl Acad Sci USA* 1993;90:8314–8318.

69 Xu Q, Zhang Z, Davison F, et al. Circulating progenitor cells regenerate endothelium of vein graft atherosclerosis, which is diminished in ApoE-deficient mice. *Circ Res* 2003;93:e76–e86.

70 Shimizu K, Mitchell RN. Stem cell origins of intimal cells in graft arterial disease. *Curr Atheroscler Rep* 2003; 5:230–237.

71 Rauscher FM, Goldschmidt-Clermont PJ, Davis BH, et al. Aging, progenitor cell exhaustion, and atherosclerosis. *Circulation* 2003;108:457–463.

CHAPTER 26

Endothelium-targeted gene and cell-based therapy for cardiovascular disease

Luis G. Melo, PhD, *Alok S. Pachori,* PhD, *Deling Kong,* PhD,
Massimiliano Gnecchi, PhD *& Victor J. Dzau,* MD

Long perceived as a mere selective permeability barrier directing the movement of water and solutes across the blood vessel wall, the vascular endothelium has emerged in the last two decades as a very complex organ involved in the regulation of all aspects of vascular function and homeostasis [1]. Due to its strategic localization, the endothelium functions as an interface that senses hemodynamic and hormonal changes and elaborates a wide variety of vasomodulatory substances that can initiate compensatory adjustment in vascular tone to normalize blood flow and pressure [2]. The endothelium also produces and releases a variety of anti-inflammatory, antithrombotic and cytostatic substances that protect the vessel wall against inflammatory cell adhesion, thrombus formation, atherosclerosis, and vascular cell proliferation [3]. Under normal physiological conditions, the endothelium maintains vascular homeostasis by establishing a balance between the production of vasodilatory, vasoconstrictive, and adhesion molecules [4]. Disruption of this balance by pathological conditions such as oxidative stress, hyperlipidemia, and inflammation results in endothelial dysfunction due to reduced availability of vasodilatory and growth-inhibiting moieties such as nitric oxide (NO) and prostacyclin (PGI_2) and concomitant increases in vasoconstrictive and growth-promoting substances such as endothelin-1, angiotensin II, and thromboxanes. This imbalance, which results in increased vascular reactivity, inflammatory cell and platelet adhesion, and proliferation of the medial smooth muscle cells, typically precedes the development of vascular disease [4].

Since the endothelium plays a pivotal role in the pathogenesis of vascular and myocardial dysfunction, it is an attractive therapeutic target for treatment of vascular disease. Genetic modulation of endothelial phenotype may offer new opportunities to modify the course of common cardiovascular diseases such myocardial infarction (MI), hypertension, atherosclerosis, thrombosis, and graft failure. Furthermore, the recent identification of putative endothelial progenitor cells (EPC) in peripheral blood may permit the design of cell-based strategies for the rescue of ischemic tissue and the repair and bioengineering of damaged vessels and prosthetic grafts [5]. Several experimental endothelium-targeted gene and cell-based therapeutic strategies have evolved in the last few years. Although the majority of these novel therapies have been tested only in animal models of cardiovascular disease, some have or currently are undergoing early phase clinical evaluation to determine their feasibility safety and efficacy [6,7] Successful transition from the pre-clinical stage to therapeutic applications will depend on the availability of safe and efficacious vectors and tools for delivery of the therapeutic genetic material. Recent improvements in vector platforms and delivery tools [8–11] already may have partially filled the prerequisite for enhanced safety and efficacy of gene transfer protocols that could eventually help pave the way to clinical application of these novel therapeutic modalities.

This chapter reviews the major advances in gene- and cell-based therapies for cardiovascular diseases, and particularly emphasizes strategies for modulating endothelial function. We will highlight the major breakthroughs and potential obstacles that may be encountered during the transition from pre-clinical evaluation to clinical application. We end with a perspective on the future developments opportunities in this fledgling field.

Strategies for genetic manipulation of the vessel wall

Augmentation of gene function

The archetypical somatic gene therapy strategy for cardiovascular disease involves exogenous transfer and overexpression of a gene whose endogenous activity may be attenuated due to mutation or disease, or otherwise normal but insufficient to counteract the pathological process. The goal of such therapy is to augment the function of the deficient or undercompensating gene in order to restore normal function or reverse disease progression. In this setting, a vector system capable of expressing the therapeutic protein delivers a full length or partial cDNA encoding the deficient gene (Figure 26.1). The therapeutic gene may encode an intracellular protein, in which case the therapeutic effect is predominantly autocrine, or, alternatively, the therapeutic protein may be secreted by the targeted cells and exert physiological effects in a paracrine or endocrine fashion. Such "gain-of-function" gene transfer strategies have been tested in diverse experimental models of cardiovascular disease such as myocardial ischemia, restenosis, hypertension, and atherosclerosis, for review see Refs. [12,13].

Inhibition of gene function

In some situations, the silencing (loss-of-function) of genes involved in the pathogenesis of cardiovascular disease may be desirable. Treatment with short single-stranded antisense oligodeoxynucleotides, ribozymes and more recently, using RNA interference technology can achieve acute inhibition of transcription and translation [14–17] (Figure 26.1). These molecules inhibit the synthesis of proteins by hybridizing the target mRNA in a sequence-specific complementary fashion. Double-stranded "decoy" oligonucleotides bearing DNA-consensus-binding sequences (*cis*-elements) also inhibit the transactivating activity of target transcription factors (TF), for review see Ref. [18] (Figure 26.1). The decoy is usually delivered in molar excess, effectively sequestering the target TF and rendering it incapable of binding to the promoter region of the target gene. In some instances, short-term inhibition of a pathogenic gene may sufficiently prevent disease development. Because the target TF may control several genes and several TF may influence the target gene, a major limitation of this strategy involves potential absence of specificity. Recently developed nucleic acid [19] and peptide [20] aptamers can inhibit protein function without altering the genetic complement of the host. The use of aptamers in cardiovascular therapeutics remains unevaluated.

Tools for genetic manipulation of the vessel wall

A major hindrance to the development of effective gene therapies for vascular disease has been the unavailability of efficient tools for genetic manipulation of the vessel wall. Although a variety of vectors, delivery tools, and strategies have evolved over the years [21,22], none of the vectors and delivery platforms currently in use displays all of the desired features of the ideal delivery system, i.e., safety, versatility, specificity, and efficiency of gene delivery. The majority of vectors used in vascular gene transfer lack tissue specificity, incurring in the risk of systemic biodistribution and ectopic transgene expression. With few exceptions, transgene expression is unregulated and driven by strong constitutive viral promoters [21]. Furthermore, transgene expression by most of the current vectors is transient, rendering them unsuitable for gene transfer in chronic vascular disease. Various modifications to these vectors have attempted to enhance the efficiency of vascular uptake [22,23], and several recently developed targeting systems improve specificity of transgene delivery and expression [24,25]. A number of catheter types are now available for both intravascular and periadventitial gene delivery *in vivo* and *ex vivo* [24]. Cell-based strategies using genetically engineered vascular smooth muscle and

(A) Gene transfer

(B) Gene blockade

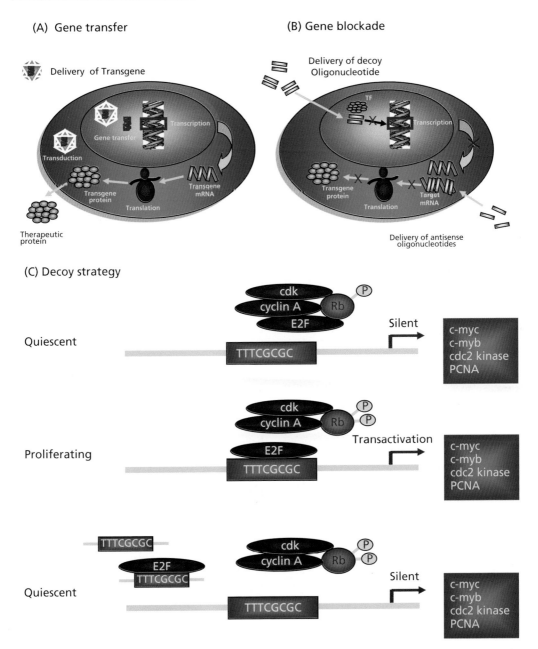

Figure 26.1 Strategies for genetic manipulation in the cardiovascular system. (A) Gene transfer involves the delivery of one or several exogenous genes (transgenes) by a vector capable of expressing the therapeutic protein in the host cells. The overall goal is to increase the activity of a gene(s) (gain-of-function) whose endogenous function may be deficient or attenuated and cause disease. (B) Gene blockade involves inhibition of genes whose overactivity may lead to disease. Two strategies are commonly used to inhibit gene activity at the transcriptional or translational level. Short single-stranded deoxyoligonucleotides complementary to the target gene mRNA (antisense oligonucleotides) are delivered to the target cells or tissue by transfection or with the aid of a vector. The antisense deoxyoligonucleotide binds to the target mRNA transcript and prevents it from being translated. (C) The decoy strategy employs double-stranded deoxyoligonucleotides containing the consensus-binding sequences (decoy oligonucleotides) for transcriptional factors involved in the activation of pathogenic genes. Transfection of a molar excess of the decoy oligonucleotide prevents the binding and transactivation of the genes regulated by the target transcriptional factor. Less commonly, short segments of RNA with enzymatic activity (ribozymes) are used to degrade target mRNA transcripts.

endothelial cells also accomplish gene transfer to injured vessels [26,27]. Despite significant advances, however, the efficiency of gene transfer to intact and injured vessels remains suboptimal in most conditions.

Vectors for gene transfer to the vasculature

As a general rule, the type of vector used for delivery of the therapeutic gene, the route of delivery, the permissiveness of the target cells to the vector [28], and to a lesser extent, the dosage and volume of delivery of the genetic material all influence the efficiency of gene transfer [29]. The principal characteristics of the vectors currently used for gene transfer are summarized in Table 26.1. Several non-viral, viral, and cell-based vectors used in vascular gene transfer have achieved variable degrees of success [21,30]. Non-viral vectors, including naked plasmids, cationic liposomes and hybrid formulations, synthetic peptides, and several physical methods, for review see Ref. [31] usually yield low vascular gene transfer efficiency due to lack of genomic integration and rapid degradation of the vector. Nevertheless, there have been examples of naked plasmid-mediated gene transfer to the vasculature that have led to a sustained therapeutic effect [32], and some protocols using naked plasmid DNA have entered into clinical trials [33]. Although naked DNA is simple and safe, the low efficiency of gene transfer and transient gene expression limits the use of this method. Encapsulating plasmid in neutral liposomes fused to the viral coat of the Sendai virus (hemagglutaning virus of Japan, HVJ) [34] or conjugating it to cationic liposomes can improve plasmid gene transfer [35], but transgene expression remains highly transient because lysosomal enzymes rapidly degrade the complexes. Application of non-distending pressure in an enclosed environment has been used to deliver oligonucleotides *ex vivo* to the heart [36] and vein grafts [37], highlighting a potential application of this technique for genetic engineering of blood vessels and other organs in preparation for transplantation. Recently, we reported that applying ultrasound at the time of gene delivery significantly enhances vascular transgene uptake [38], suggesting potential adjunctive use in vascular gene transfer protocols. A promising new delivery technology uses synthetic peptide carriers containing a nuclear localization signal to facilitate nuclear uptake of the target cDNA [39]. These peptide-DNA heteroplexes are recognized by intracellular receptor proteins and imported into the nucleus, where the target cDNA is transcribed.

Because recombinant viruses, i.e., replication-deficient viral particles that retain their ability to penetrate target cells and deliver genetic material with higher efficiency than non-viral vectors [21,40], generally yield higher gene transfer efficiencies than non-viral methods, they have become the preferred vectors for vascular gene transfer [21]. Furthermore, some viral vectors can integrate the host genome, leading to sustained expression of the therapeutic gene [22]. Prolonged transgene expression may be desirable for gene transfer in chronic vascular diseases such as myocardial ischemia, atherosclerosis, and hypertension. Unfortunately, the host may trigger a robust immune reaction in response to viral proteins synthesized by the vector, possibly reducing gene transfer efficiency and the sustainability of transgene expression [41]. Moreover, although the viral vectors used in gene therapy are replication deficient these vectors may revert to replication proficiency, thus raising safety concerns about biological hazards such as oncogenesis and insertional mutagenesis (Table 26.1) [21].

A variety of viral vectors have been used over the years [21,40]. Adenoviruses of serotype 2 or 5, the most widely used, for review see Ref. [21,40] can transduce both dividing and terminally differentiated vascular cell types and can accommodate large (up to $\cong 7.5$ kb) DNA inserts [40]. Adenoviruses transduce endothelial cells with >90% efficiency in intact vessels, but transduce medial smooth muscle with only ~10% efficiency after intraluminal delivery [42]. Modifications of the vector backbone, e.g., incorporating motifs that recognize matrix metalloproteinases, improve the efficiency and specificity of vascular adenoviral uptake [43]. The problems most commonly encountered with the use of adenoviruses include cytotoxicity associated with induction of the immune response, rapid loss of transgene expression due to episomal localization of the viral genomes, and widespread systemic biodistribution after vascular delivery [40,44]. Additionally, local adenoviral delivery may increase expression of adhesion molecules in the vessel wall and lead to neointima deposition [45,46]. A new generation of "gutted" adenoviral

Table 26.1 Vectors used for transfer and manipulation of genetic material in cardiovascular tissues.

Vector	Chromosomal integration	Transfer efficiency in vivo	Onset of transgene expression	Sustainability of therapeutic effect	Level of expression	Target cells	Host immune response	Potential risks	References
Non-viral									
Cationic liposomes	No	+	Rapid	Short	+	Quiescent and dividing	+	Cytotoxicity	[30,31]
HVJ-liposomes	No	+++	Rapid	Short	++	Quiescent and dividing	+	Cytotoxicity	[34,162]
Naked plasmid	No	+	Moderate	Short	+	Quiescent and dividing	+	Cytotoxicity	[31,32]
Viral									
Retrovirus	Yes	++	Rapid	Life-long	++	Dividing	+	Cytotoxicity oncogenesis	[21,40,52]
Lentivirus	Yes	+++	Rapid	Life-long	+++	Quiescent and dividing	+	Cytotoxicity viral mutation	[21,40,53]
Adenovirus	No	+++++	Rapid	Moderate	++++	Quiescent and dividing	++++	Cytotoxicity viral mutation	[21,40,43,44,47]
Adeno-associated virus	Yes	+++	Slow	Life-long	+++	Quiescent and dividing	+	Oncogenesis viral mutation	[48,49,51]
Herpes Simplex virus	No	+++	Moderate	Long	+++	Quiescent and dividing	+++	Cytotoxicity viral mutation	[21,40,54]
Alphavirus	No	++	Very rapid	Short	+++	Quiescent and dividing	+++	Cytotoxicity viral mutation	[21,40,55]
Cell-based									
Autologous endothelial cells	vd	vd	vd	vd	vd	Dividing	0	None	[57,58]
Endothelial progenitor cells	vd	vd	vd	vd	vd	Dividing	0	None	[5,59]
Vascular smooth muscle cells	vd	vd	vd	vd	vd	Dividing	0	None	[60]

vd: vector-dependent.

vectors attenuates host inflammatory response by removing all adenoviral coding sequences [47].

Due to its low immunogenicity and ability to stably transduce terminally differentiated cells with high efficiency, adeno-associated virus (AAV) has emerged as the vector of choice in several gene-therapy applications [48]. The vector transduces endothelial and vascular smooth muscle cells (VSMC) in culture and *in vivo* with moderate efficiency [49,50]. The major limitation of the vector involves its inability to accommodate large DNA inserts (transgene size is restricted to 4 kb or less); [48] however, a recent strategy involves trans-splicing between two separate AAV vectors to deliver genes >4 kb [51]. Similar to adenovirus, biodistribution and ectopic transgene expression can also occur after local AAV delivery [48].

Initially used for *in vivo* arterial gene transfer, RNA-based retroviral vectors have not found widespread application in *in vivo* vascular gene transfer protocols for several biological and technical reasons [52]. Most currently used retroviral vectors derive from Moloney murine leukemia virus (MLV). More recently, vectors derived from murine stem cell virus (MSCV) efficiently transduce EPC. These single-stranded vectors integrate randomly into the host genome, leading to the possibility of stable long-term transgene expression [52]. However, retroviral integration requires cell division, rendering these vectors inefficient transducers of quiescent vascular cells. Furthermore, retrovirally delivered transgenes are prone to transcription silencing, which may significantly shorten the duration of transgene expression, and the random integration of the viral DNA into the host genome poses a possible risk of oncogenesis [52].

Other viral vector systems currently used for gene transfer, such as lentivirus, Herpes Simplex viruses (HSV), and alphaviruses, have had limited application in vascular gene transfer [21,40]. Lentiviruses can infect both dividing and quiescent cells [53]. The vector transduces human umbilical vein endothelial cells in culture with high efficiency [53]. However, the efficiency of these vectors for *in vivo* vascular gene transfer remains unevaluated. HSV-based vectors can accommodate very large DNA fragments, and have advantages for transferring very large or multiple genes [54]. The positive strand RNA alphaviruses based on the Semliki Forest (SFV) and Sendibis virus can express transgenes within 24 hours

of transduction with minimal cytotoxicity, suggesting their potential application for acute gene manipulation of the vessel wall [55].

Several vascular cell types have also been employed as vectors for delivery of genetic material to tissues, for review see Ref. [56]. Genetically modified autologous and heterologous endothelial cells overexpressing therapeutic genes can seed injured blood vessels, prosthetic grafts, and vascular stents [57,58] in order to repair damaged endothelium. EPC originating from adult bone marrow have been isolated recently from peripheral blood [5]. These EPC can be expanded *ex vivo* to yield sufficient numbers for therapeutic application, and can be genetically engineered with viral vectors capable of expressing therapeutic genes [59]. The use of autologous EPC circumvents the host immune response induced by heterologous cells. VSMC can deliver genes to the vessel wall systemically [60], but the therapeutic value of this approach remains unproven.

Routes and devices for gene transfer to the vessel wall

The anatomical localization of the vascular endothelium renders it easily accessible for gene transfer by intraluminal delivery, and since the elastic lamina is impermeable to most vectors, relatively endothelial-specific transgene delivery can, in principle, be achieved via this route. However, only a few studies have considered endothelial-specific expression of therapeutic genes, due partly to vector inefficiency and partly to the preponderance of studies on models of vascular injury characterized by endothelial denudation. For review see Ref. [61,62]. For the same reason, the relative imperviousness of the internal elastic lamina renders luminal gene transfer to the media difficult in intact vessels, requiring high concentration of vector delivered at high pressure [62]. However, intimal damage caused by balloon injury facilitates gene transfer to the media, suggesting that this could be used to deliver antiproliferative and antithrombotic genes for the inihibition of neointima hyperplasia and atherosclerosis after angioplasty [62]. Delivering the vector directly to the site in large arteries, or percutaneously using special catheters can achieve site-specific adventitial gene transfer, for review see Ref. [63].

Delivery of genetic material to the vascular wall has been achieved using a variety of methods [61,63].

However, vector delivery to the vascular wall poses significant technical challenges due to the barrier properties of the vessel wall and the branching pattern of the arterial beds. The simplest approach for local delivery involves the surgical isolation of the target arterial segment between two ligatures and infusion of the vector. This invasive "dwell" method requires prolonged incubation periods, during which the segment is rendered ischemic. Several modified double-balloon catheters, hydrogel coated-porous and channeled balloon catheters have been used for percutaneous gene delivery of the vectors locally to the vessel wall [63]. However, gene transfer to the vessel wall using such catheters usually requires pressure or mechanical facilitation to aid passive diffusion of the vector into the vessel wall [63], and balloon inflation may cause trauma to the vessel wall [61,63]. Furthermore, vector uptake usually requires prolonged incubation times that may cause tissue ischemia, and the risk of systemic distribution of the vector cannot be prevented, for review see Ref. [63]. The Dispatch™ catheter is a sophisticated autoperfusion catheter variant of the balloon catheter that allows local delivery at multiple infusion sites without impairing distal perfusion of the arterial bed [64]. This catheter has been used for gene delivery to the endothelium and the media with moderate efficiency in normal and atherosclerotic vessels [64]. A novel approach for vascular gene transfer employs coated stents seeded with endothelial cells or viral vectors [63,65]. The feasibility of this approach has been demonstrated [66,67], suggesting that it may yield therapeutic potential in vascular gene transfer.

Targets for endothelial gene and cell-based therapy

Endothelial cell-specific targeting
Endothelial cell-specific transgene expression has been achieved by incorporating a variety of promoters in the gene transfer vectors [68] or by enhancing the tropism of the vectors for the endothelium [69]. Minimal promoters derived from the pro-angiogenic factor angiopoietin Tie II receptor exhibit specificity and high level of basal transgene expression in endothelial cells [70]. Other promoters reported to direct endothelial-specific gene expression include those derived from Flt-1 (VEGFR-1) [68], von Willebrand factor [71], thrombomodulin [72],

E-selectin [73] and intercellular adhesion molecule-2 (ICAM-2) [74]. Flt-1 promoter-driven vectors have yielded transgene expression efficiencies comparable to cytomegalovirus (CMV) promoter-driven vectors in cultured human umbilical vein endothelial cells, and demonstrate endothelial cell-specific expression after *ex vivo* transduction of intact human vein or following systemic administration [71]. Several modifications to vector backbones also have increased the tropism of viral vectors for the endothelium. Replacement of the native enhancer sequences in murine leukemia virus (MLV) retrovirus (RV) with regulatory sequences of the preproendothelin-1 promoter results in endothelial-specific expression of reporter gene [75], while replacement of the adenovirus type 5 fiber by the endothelium-binding peptide SIGYPLP [76] leads to selective endothelial transgene expression.

The potential benefits of endothelium-specific transgene expression are obvious. First, since endothelial dysfunction plays a central role in a majority of cardiovascular diseases [4], genetic manipulations aimed at improving endothelial function should yield therapeutic benefits. Secondly, the targeted delivery and expression of therapeutic transgene to the endothelium averts potential cytotoxic effects associated with indiscriminate expression of the therapeutic protein, thereby enhancing the specificity and safety of the therapeutic strategy. The combination of physiologically regulated enhancer element(s) and tissue-specific promoter in a single vector may provide the optimal strategy for achieving maximal therapeutic efficiency with minimal side effects. The efficacy of such a combinatorial approach already has been partially validated. Transient transfection of endothelial cells derived from endothelioma with retroviral vectors incorporating hypoxia responsive elements and endothelial-specific enhancer sequences derived from the flk-1 promoter confers endothelial-specific expression of a luciferase reporter gene, which was induced several fold by exposure to hypoxia [77]. This strategy permits both spatial and temporal control of transgene expression, such that the therapeutic protein is produced where and when needed.

Therapeutic targets
Endothelial dysfunction is the most pervasive harbinger of cardiovascular disease [3,4] and plays a central role in the pathogenesis of all major

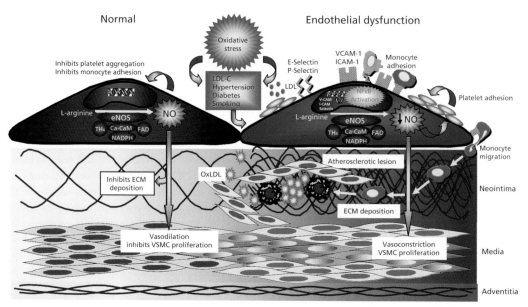

Figure 26.2 Pathophysiology of endothelial dysfunction. (a) In normal conditions, the endothelial cell plays a pivotal role in maintaining vessel wall homeostasis by producing a vasoactive anti-inflammatory, antithrombotic and cytostatic factors that help maintain vessel tone and protect the vessel wall against inflammatory cell and platelet adhesion, thrombus formation and vascular cell proliferation. NO released from the terminal guanidino group of L-arginine by eNOS plays a crucial role in maintenance of endothelial cell homeostasis. (b) Endothelial dysfunction ensues when endothelial homeostasis is disturbed by pathological stresses such as oxidative stress, hyperlipidemia, hypertension and diabetes. NO production is impaired and the balance between vasodilatory and vasoconstrictive moieties is disrupted leading to increased vessel tone. The endothelial cell becomes "activated" and synthesizes cell surface adhesion molecules such as selectins and integrins, which increase leukocyte and platelet adhesion and thrombus formation. The loss of growth-inhibiting mediators from the endothelium triggers the activation and migration of VSMC into the intimal space where they proliferate to form the neointima. In time the infiltration of inflammatory cells into the intimal space and accumulation of oxidized LDL results in the formation of the atherosclerotic lesion.

cardiovascular diseases including atherosclerosis, hypertension, diabetes, and coronary artery disease (CAD) and associated MI [4]. The alteration in endothelial function is characterized by impaired vessel relaxation and increased adhesiveness and platelet adherence [3,4], predisposing the vessel wall to vasoconstriction, inflammatory cell infiltration, plaque deposition, and thrombus formation (Figure 26.2) [4]. Many of the risk factors for cardiovascular disease associate with increased oxidative stress, indicating that alterations in redox state play a major role in endothelial dysfunction [78]. Reactive oxygen species (ROS) accelerate the catabolism of NO and activate TF such as nuclear factor kappa B (NF-κB), which upregulate the transcription of several inflammatory genes, chemokines, and adhesion molecules [78]. NO exerts multiple effects in the vessel wall including vasodilation, inhibition of vascular smooth muscle proliferation, and migration and downregulation of inflammatory and adhesion molecules [79]. Thus, NO participates crucially in the maintenance of vessel wall homeostasis, and decreased NO bioactivity provides a link between oxidative stress, endothelial dysfunction, and the pathogenesis of cardiovascular disease (Figure 26.2). Hence, therapeutic strategies aimed at reducing oxidative stress likely should increase NO bioavailability and help reverse endothelial dysfunction and the progression of cardiovascular diseases.

A number of genes could offer potential targets for genetic modulation of endothelial function. Endothelium-targeted overexpression of antithrombotic and antioxidant proteins, and/or the inhibition of pro-inflammatory and cell adhesion molecules may have therapeutic value as strategies to reduce thrombosis and inflammation of the vessel wall in atherosclerosis, whereas strategies for plaque stabilization and inhibition of platelet adhesion may be of benefit in reducing the occurrence of acute coronary events and MI, for review see Ref. [80–82]. Additionally, inhibition of endothelial cell activation and suppression of pro-inflammatory pathways and adhesion molecule activity may be useful in treatment of acute MI and as immunosuppressive therapy in transplantation [83–85]. Endothelial-targeted overexpression of vasodilatory substances such as NO or inhibition of vasoconstrictive peptides such as angiotensin II and endothelin may be effective antihypertensive strategies [86,87], whereas strategies aimed at modulating the activity of cell proliferation-regulating genes in the vessel wall may be useful in the treatment of vascular proliferative disease [88,89]. Targeted delivery of proangiogenic factors such as vascular endothelial growth factor (VEGF) and fibroblast growth factor (FGF) may be useful in the treatment of myocardial and peripheral ischemia [90–92]. The recent identification of putative EPC in peripheral blood [5] and the ability to expand and genetically engineer these cells [93] may allow the design of novel cell-based strategies for rescue and repair of ischemic tissue and damaged vessels as well as the bioengineering of vein and prosthetic grafts to render them resistant to atherosclerosis [5].

Gene therapy for hypertension, atherosclerosis and vascular proliferative disease

Hypertension and dyslipidemia are primary risk factors for peripheral and CAD. Such diseases often coexist under a common denominator of endothelial dysfunction [4,94]. Heightened vascular tone, hypercholesterolemia, inflammation, and VSMC proliferation and migration are prominent features of hypertension and atherosclerosis. VSMC proliferation into the intimal space is a major cause of post-angioplasty and in-stent restenosis, vein graft bypass failure, and transplant vasculopathy [95,96]. Accordingly, several experimental gene therapy strategies aimed at reducing vascular tone, plasma cholesterol levels, and vessel wall proliferation have been developed as potential treatments for these diseases [88,97,98]. While most of these experimental therapies have not been designed to specifically target the endothelium, a significant

component of their therapeutic effect can be attributed to improved endothelial function.

Gene therapy for hypertension

Two gene therapy strategies for hypertension have been tested in animal models. One strategy involves the inhibition of pressor pathways using antisense oligonucleotides against components of the renin–angiotensin system (RAS) [99–101] or the β-adrenergic signaling pathway (Table 26.2) [102]. Using AAV for intravenous delivery of angiotensinogen antisense cDNA, Tang et al. [99] showed a dose-dependent decrease in arterial blood pressure in adult spontaneously hypertensive rats (SHR) in association with reduced angiotensinogen levels, whereas the onset of hypertension was delayed up to 6 months in SHR after a single intracardiac injection of angiotensinogen antisense cDNA to newborn SHR rats [100]. Other components of the RAS signaling system including antisense inhibition of angiotensin I converting enzyme (ACE) [103] and AT_1 receptor have yielded comparable results [104,105]. Antisense inhibition of $β_1$-adrenergic receptor has achieved effective blood pressure reduction as well [102], suggesting that this strategy could be used as an alternative to pharmacological β-blockade.

The other gene therapy strategy for hypertension is based on the overexpression of vasodilatory genes such as nitric oxide synthase (NOS), atrial peptides and kinins (Table 26.2) [106–109]. Intravenous delivery of a plasmid encoding human endothelial NOS under the CMV promoter led to a sustained hypotensive effect in SHR rats that paralleled increased urinary cGMP and nitrite/nitrate levels [106]. Others have shown that systemic delivery of atrial natriuretic factor [107] kallikrein [108], or adrenomedullin [109] genes with a constitutively active adenoviral vector decreases blood pressure and attenuates renal and myocardial damage in salt-fed Dahl salt-sensitive and DOCA-salt rats. Overexpression of antioxidant genes such as heme oxygenase-1 (HO-1) [110] and extracellular superoxide dismutase (ecSOD) [111] have also been reported to reduce arterial pressure in hypertensive animals, indicating that oxidative stress contributes significantly to hypertension.

To date, the use of antihypertensive gene therapy has not been tested in human trials despite its simplicity and compelling pre-clinical evidence about

Table 26.2 Targets for gene-based therapy for hypertension, atherosclerosis and vascular proliferative disease.

Strategy	Therapeutic target	Genetic manipulation	Vector	Application	References
Blood pressure	*Vasodilation*				
	Kallikrein, eNOS, ANP, CNP, HO-1, ecSOD	Overexpression	AD, AAV	Hypertension, HF	[106–111]
	Vasoconstriction				
	ACE, AGT, AT_1	Inhibition	AAV-AS-ODN	Hypertension, HF	[99–105]
Atherosclerosis	*Plaque stabilization (CAD)*				
	CD40	Overexpression	ADV, α-virus, AAV(?)	CAD	[82]
	Cholesterol homeostasis				
	LDL-R, lipoprotein lipase, hepatic lipase, apoE, VLDL-R, SR-B1, apoA1	Overexpression	ADV	FH, CAD, PAD	[114–122]
	Thromboprotection				
	PAI-1, plasminogen activator, tissue factor, MCP-1	Inhibition	AS-ODN	CAD, MI, PAD	[113,123,124]
	t-PA, hirudin, urokinase	Overexpression	ADV, AAV, RV	CAD, MI, PAD	[124,127]
	Tissue factor pathway inhibitor				[129]
	Thrombomodulin, COX-1				[26,131]
	PGI_2 synthase				[130]
	eNOS, iNOS, HO-1, SOD				[132–138,140]
Vascular cell proliferation	*Cell-cycle proteins*				
	p16, p21, p27, p53, Rb	Overexpression	Plasmid, ADV, HVJ	Neointima hyperplasia	[155–159]
	Cdc2, cdk2, c-myb, c-myc, PCNA	Inhibition	AS-ODN,	Neointima hyperplasia	[146,147,153,154]
	E2F	Inhibition	Decoy-ODN	Neointima hyperplasia	[148–151]
	Cytotoxic/suicide genes				
	Thymidine kinase	Overexpression	ADV	Neointima hyperplasia	[145]
	Antiproliferative genes				
	eNOS, iNOS, ecSOD, HO-1	Overexpression	ADV, AAV	Neointima hyperplasia Graft atherosclerosis	[132,162–165]
	TF, cytokines, apoptotic and signaling molecules				
	NF-κB, BcL-X$_L$	Inhibition	Decoy-ODN, AS-ODN	Neointima hyperplasia	[88,143,160]
	Fas ligand, Gax, GATA-6β-interferon, VEGF	Overexpression	ADV	Neointima hyperplasia	[88,143]

ADV: adenovirus; AS-ODN: antisense oligodeoxynucleotide; HF: heart failure; PAI-1: plasminogen activator inhibitor-1; COX-1: cyclooxygenase-1; ANP: atrial natriuretic peptide; CNP: C-type natriuretic peptide; AGT: angiotensinogen. For other abbreviations refer to text.

its safety and efficacy. Enthusiasm for these novel approaches is tempered by the efficacy of current drug therapies. Nevertheless, the prospect of achieving long-term control of blood pressure by gene therapy in hypertensive patients could potentially overcome the problem of non-compliance frequently encountered in patients on antihypertensive medication.

Gene therapy for atherosclerosis and thrombosis

Plaque rupture and subsequent thrombosis and occlusion are the major causes of acute coronary episodes that result in MI and sudden cardiac death [112]. Gene therapy aimed at reducing cholesterol level and/or at increasing thromboresistance and tensile strength within the plaque may offer a novel and potentially effective alternative option to achieve long-term plaque stabilization and prevent the occurrence of acute coronary events (Table 26.2) [113].

Due to their monogenic etiology and refractoriness to drug treatment, the effect of lipid-lowering gene therapy has been evaluated mainly in inherited disorders of lipid metabolism such as familial hypercholesterolemia (FH) and apoE deficiency. Initial attempts to correct FH involved transplantation of autologous hepatocytes stably transduced *ex vivo* with a retroviral vector constitutively expressing the low-density lipoprotein (LDL) receptor in heritable hyperlipidemic Watanabe rabbits [114]. This initial study showed decreased plasma cholesterol levels (30–50%) for up to 6 months. The success of this animal study led to a small clinical trial, but the outcome was less impressive, showing a reduction of 6–23% in plasma LDL levels in 3 out of 5-treated patients [115], with a relatively short duration, possibly attributable to retroviral gene silencing. Other potential targets for correcting genetic hyperlipidemia include replacement of lipoprotein lipase and hepatic lipase genes [116,117], apoE [118], VLDL receptor [119], and scavenger receptor-B1 (SR-B1) (Table 26.2) [120].

Novel lipid lowering and plaque-stabilizing strategies are emerging [121]. For example, overexpression of apoprotein apoA1 in mice by intravenous adenoviral gene delivery increases serum HDL levels [122]. Blockade of monocyte infiltration and activation in the arterial wall by inhibiting monocyte chemoattractant protein-1 (MCP-1)

receptor activation retarded the onset of atheroma and limited progression and destabilization of established atherosclerotic lesions in apoE mice [123]. Overexpression of antithrombotic genes at sites in the vessel wall at risk of thrombosis may provide a feasible protective strategy for vulnerable plaque and prevention of acute coronary events, and delivery of anticoagulant, antifibrinolytic, and antiplatelet genes, such as thrombomodulin, for review see Ref. [124–126] tissue-specific plasminogen activator (t-PA) and urokinase type plasminogen activator (u-PA) [127], hirudin [128], tissue factor pathway inhibitor [129], prostacyclin synthase [130], and cyclooxygenase I [131], to the injured vessel wall reduces the incidence of thrombosis (Table 26.2).

Another important target for vascular protection is NOS, for review see Ref. [132,133]. Endothelium-derived NO exerts a plethora of vasculoprotective actions, including vasorelaxation, inhibition of VSMC proliferation and migration, inhibition of platelet activation and adhesion, and reduction of inflammation [79]. NOS gene transfer provides a mechanism to increase NO bioactivity and enhance the antiatherogenic properties of the vessel wall. Indeed, delivery of inducible nitric oxide synthase (iNOS) [134] by adenovirus abrogates aortic allograft atherosclerosis in rats, and neuronal nitric oxide synthase (nNOS) gene transfer reduces inflammatory cell infiltration and lipid deposition, and enhances vasomotor function in carotid arteries of cholesterol-fed rabbits [135]. The endothelial nitric oxide synthase (eNOS) isoform yielded similar results. Liposome-mediated delivery of eNOS reduced endothelial cell activation and leukocyte infiltration in transplanted rabbit hearts [136], and adenoviral eNOS gene transfer restored endothelial function in the aorta from angiotensin II-treated animals in association with reduced superoxide production [137]. Additionally, gene transfer of cytoprotective genes such as HO-1 and SOD exerts vasculoprotective effects. Adenovirus-mediated delivery of HO-1 attenuated the development of aortic lesions in apoE-deficient mice, and in parallel decreased iron deposition [138], likely due to the anti-inflammatory and antioxidant properties of HO-1 [139], whereas adenoviral delivery of manganese SOD improved vascular function in pre-atherosclerotic carotid arteries from hypercholesterolemic rabbits [140].

Gene therapy for vascular proliferative disease

Revascularization procedures using percutaneous transluminal angioplasty (PTCA), stenting, or coronary artery bypass grafting (CABG) are common treatment options for CAD. Every year more than 1.5 million revascularization procedures are performed worldwide [95,141]. Still, despite significant improvements in pharmacological therapies and the introduction of cytostatic drug-eluting stents [142], the failure rate of these procedures remains high due to restenosis and atherosclerosis, and often makes repeated interventions required. The ability to deliver antiproliferative and antithrombotic genes and to inhibit pro-proliferative genes in the vessel wall offers the opportunity to genetically engineer native vessels or grafts, rendering them resistant to atherosclerosis and neointimal hyperplasia (Table 26.2), for review see Ref. [143]. Using adenovirus to deliver thrombomodulin to jugular vein segments *ex vivo* prior to interpositional grafting in rabbits, Kim et al. [144] reported that genetic engineering of the graft led to thromboresistance and graft survival, whereas adenoviral delivery of tissue factor pathway inhibitor [128] or the suicide gene thymidine kinase [145] to balloon-injured atherosclerotic rabbit carotid arteries inhibits thrombus formation and reduces neointimal proliferation, demonstrating the potential of thrombolytic and cytotoxic gene therapy to inhibit restenosis.

Cytostatic gene therapy has yielded promising results in the treatment of vasculoproliferative disease (Table 26.2). The basic tenet of this strategy involves the inhibition of key proteins regulating cell-cycle progression [146]. Treatment of jugular veins *in vivo* with HVJ-liposome complexes containing an antisense oligonucleotide against cell-cycle regulators proliferating cell nuclear antigen (PCNA) and cdc2 kinase inhibited atherosclerosis and neointimal hyperplasia after carotid artery interpositional grafting in rabbits maintained on a high cholesterol diet [147]. We showed that treatment of vein grafts prior to implantation with a decoy deoxyoligonucleotide bearing the consensus-binding sequence of E2F-1, a transcriptional factor involved in cell-cycle progression, resulted in prolonged resistance to neointimal hyperplasia and improved graft patency of the graft after transplantation [148]. These findings led to a

phase I prospective, randomized double-blind trial of human saphenous vein graft treatment with E2F decoy (PREVENT-1) [149]. Using non-distending pressure to deliver the E2F decoy oligonucleotide *ex vivo* prior to arterial interpositional grafting in this safety and feasibility trial, the authors reported that E2F decoy treatment was safe and prevented graft atherosclerosis concomitant with inhibition of cell cycle progression. A Phase II trial designed to evaluate the effect of E2F decoy treatment on CABG failure recently confirmed these results Grube et al. American Heart Association meeting, November 2001, for commentary see Ref. [150]. Interestingly, we recently reported that the E2F decoy selectively targets VSMC proliferation without affecting the endothelial cell proliferative burst essential for healing after vein grafting [151]. We believe that this sparing effect on the endothelium contributes to the enhanced endothelial function previously reported by us in vein grafts treated with cell cycle regulatory proteins [152].

Other cytostatic strategies have yielded variable degrees of success in experimental models of restenosis. Treatment with antisense oligonucleotides against cell-cycle regulatory genes cdk2 kinase [153] and the proto-oncogenes c-myb [154] and c-myc [155], and overexpression of p21 [156] and p27 [157] cyclin-dependent kinase inhibitors, non-phosphorylatable retinoblastoma gene product [158], and p53 [159] all inhibit neointimal hyperplasia in animal models of arterial injury, as was the inhibition of intracellular signaling mediators of mitogen-dependent kinases, NF-κB, Bcl-x_L and growth factors, or overexpression of Fas ligand, gax and GATA-6 TF and cytokines such as β-interferon and VEGF (Table 26.2) for review see Ref. [88,143,160]. The application of VEGF gene transfer may be particularly useful in re-establishing vascular wall homeostasis after injury because of the ability of this endothelium-specific cytokine to promote re-endothelialization of the denuded arterial wall [161].

Delivery of antiproliferative genes such as those coding for the NOS offer another approach to achieve inhibition of neointima hyperplasia (Table 26.2). All three isoforms of NOS exert vasculoprotective and antiproliferative effects after gene transfer for review see Ref. [132]. The efficacy of endothelial and iNOS gene transfer in reducing neointimal thickening in balloon-injured vessels [162,163] resulted in at least one Phase I clinical trial (REGENT-I)AHA annual meeting, Nov 2001 to evaluate the ability of catheter-based iNOS gene delivery to prevent restenosis of coronary arteries treated by PTCA. Local delivery of antioxidant enzymes such as HO-1 [164] and ecSOD [165] by adenovirus inhibits neointimal hyperplasia in various animal models of restenosis, possibly due to reduction in inflammation and oxidative stress during the early phase of vascular injury, and the subsequent inhibition of vascular smooth muscle proliferation.

Despite these promising preclinical data, the use of gene therapy in treatment of vasculoproliferative disease still must overcome various feasibility, safety, and efficacy issues, and improvements in vector and delivery technologies are warranted. The complexity of the pathological processes leading to restenosis suggests that effective and sustained therapeutic benefit may require genetic manipulation of multiple targets. Because endothelial damage at the time of intervention plays a pivotal role in the subsequent development of restenosis and graft atherosclerosis, strategies to accelerate endothelial recovery should be considered as well [95,96,143]. Two potential strategies to achieve rapid endothelial recovery may involve the transplantation of genetically engineered autologous endothelial cells that could confer enhanced thromboresistance to damaged vessels or vascular grafts, or the mobilization of endogenous endothelial cells to the sites of injury. Several preliminary studies have already demonstrated the feasibility of these approaches [59,166,167], and future clinical trials should determine their therapeutic value in humans.

Gene therapy for myocardial ischemic disease

Myocardial ischemia secondary to CAD is a predominant cause of premature death in the industrialized world [168,169]. Acute episodes of myocardial ischemia are almost invariably symptomatic of CAD [82,168,169]. Depending on the severity of vessel occlusion, an acute coronary event may lead to MI and irreversible tissue damage resulting in sudden death [170]. Chronic myocardial ischemia leads to progressive impairment of cardiac function that may culminate in heart failure [170], a syndrome characterized by hemodynamic insufficiency and the inability of the heart to sustain metabolic requirements for normal activity [171]. Oxidative stress [78,172] and endothelial dysfunction [173,174] play pivotal roles in the pathogenesis of myocardial ischemia and infarction secondary to CAD. Increased levels of ROS cause endothelial dysfunction by reducing NO bioavailability [78] and by inducing endothelial activation of pro-inflammatory TF such as NF-κB and Egr-1, which stimulate the transcription of cytokines, chemokines, and adhesion molecules, thus impairing vessel relaxation, enhancing endothelial adhesion of platelets and leukocytes, and rendering the vessel prone to thrombosis [173,174] and occlusion.

While current "rescue" therapies for MI using primary percutaneous coronary interventions (PCI), fibrinolytic, and anti-platelet agents [170,175] effectively ameliorate the acute symptoms of the disease and reduce peri-MI death, reperfusion introduces a separate set of cellular stresses, brought about by oxidative stress, endothelial cell activation, and inflammation, that can exacerbate the damage initiated during ischemia [176,177]. Ironically, the improved survival of MI patients treated with thrombolytic therapies has led to a drastic increase in the number of patients who suffer from chronic heart disease [170]. The socio-economic impact of this problem calls for a fundamental paradigm shift in the therapeutic approach to the management of heart disease, requiring a change of focus from rescue to prevention and protection. The availability of sensitive risk assessment technologies [178], together with the identification of several potential therapeutic targets [179] and the availability of cardiotropic vectors such as AAV that are capable of long-term and stable protein expression with a single administration of therapeutic genes [180] may offer an opportunity for the design of gene-based therapies for both protection and rescue of the myocardium from ischemia and failure.

Gene therapy for protection from ischemia-induced myocardial injury

The development of gene therapies for acute MI has been difficult because the time required for transcription and translation of therapeutic genes with the current generation of vectors exceeds the window for successful intervention. For this reason, gene transfer of anticoagulant genes is not as feasible as primary thrombolytic therapy for acute MI, i.e., the time required for production of the therapeutic protein falls outside the time window for successful intervention after coronary thrombosis. However, antithrombotic gene therapy could have a role as an adjuvant to primary thrombolytic therapy to prevent the recurrence of thrombosis in the affected vessel, or during routine revascularization procedures such as CABG, stenting, or prosthetic graft implantation.

An alternative gene therapy for myocardial protection involves "preventing" ischemia/reperfusion (I/R) injury by transferring cytoprotective genes into the myocardium of high-risk patients using a gene delivery method that could confer long-term therapeutic gene expression (Table 26.3). This novel concept of "preventive" gene therapy would protect the heart from future I/R injury, thereby minimizing the need for acute intervention [181]. Given the role of oxidative stress in CAD and I/R injury, gene therapy strategies aimed at increasing endogenous antioxidant reserves should, in principle, provide a useful strategy for prevention/protection in patients at risk of acute MI. This strategy would potentiate the native protective response of the myocardium, rendering it resistant to future ischemic insults [172,176,177].

We have evaluated the feasibility of antioxidant enzyme gene transfer as a long-term first line of defense against I/R-induced oxidative injury, using an rAAV vector for intramyocardial delivery of HO-1 gene in a rat model of myocardial I/R injury [181]. Our findings showed that HO-1 gene delivery to the left ventricular risk area several weeks in advance of MI reduced infarct size by approximately 80%, in association with decreases in oxidative stress, inflammation, and interstitial fibrosis. Consistent with the histopathology, echocardiographic assessment showed post-infarction recovery of left ventricular function in the HO-1-treated animals, whereas the untreated control animals presented evidence of ventricular enlargement and depressed ventricular function. Gene transfer of ecSOD, a secreted metalloenzyme that plays an essential role in the maintenance of redox homeostasis by dismutating the oxygen free radical superoxide, yielded comparable findings [182–184]. We showed improved long-term survival after acute MI in ecSOD-treated animals relative to the untreated animals in parallel with smaller

infarcts and decreased myocardial inflammation [182]. Overexpression of other major antioxidant enzyme systems, such as Cu/Zn SOD [185] catalase [186] and glutathione peroxidase achieved efficient protection from I/R injury [187]. Thus, these findings suggest that AAV-mediated delivery of antioxidant genes may offer a viable therapeutic option for long-term myocardial protection from I/R injury in patients with CAD. Other genes that exert cardioprotective effects include stress-induced heat shock proteins such as HSP 70 [188] and HSP 27 [189], survival genes Bcl-2, Akt [190,191], and immunosuppressive cytokines [192] adenosine A_1 and A_3 receptors [193], kallikrein [194], caspase inhibitor [195], and hepatocyte growth factor (HGF) (Table 26.3) [196].

The inhibition of pro-inflammatory genes involved in the pathogenesis of I/R injury offers another option for cardioprotection (Table 26.3). Morishita et al. [197] showed that pretreatment with a decoy oligonucleotide capable of inhibiting the trans-activating activity of the pro-inflammatory TF NF-κB reduces myocardial infarct after coronary artery ligation in rats. Although the rapid *in vivo* degradation of oligonucleotides precludes their use in long-term myocardial protection, they may be useful in the treatment of acute myocardial ischemia and in cardiac transplantation by serving as a tool for inhibiting pro-oxidant, pro-inflammatory, and immunomodulatory genes activated by ischemia and reperfusion [198]. For example, treatment with antisense oligonucleotide directed against ICAM-1 prolonged cardiac allograft tolerance and long-term survival when administered *ex vivo* prior to transplantation into the host [199]. Thus, oligonucleotide-mediated inhibition of anti-inflammatory genes and adhesion molecules could be used to suppress the acute inflammatory response in donor organs in advance of transplantation to minimize reperfusion-induced injury.

The suitability of these experimental therapies for myocardial protection in humans remains unestablished, and further work is required to elucidate the mechanism by which exogenous gene delivery of antioxidant enzymes confers myocardial protection from ischemic injury. Conceivably, the increase in basal pro-oxidant scavenging activity imparted by constitutive overexpression of antioxidant enzymes may confer cytoprotection by

Table 26.3 Targets for gene-based therapy for myocardial protection and rescue from ischemia-induced injury.

Strategy	Therapeutic target	Genetic manipulation	Vector	Application	References
Protection/Prevention Myocardial ischemia	*Antioxidant genes*				
	HO-1, SOD, catalase, GPx	Overexpression	ADV, AAV, LV, α-virus	CAD, ACS, I/R injury	[181–187]
	Heat shock proteins				
	HSP 70, HSP 90, HSP 27	Overexpression	ADV, AAV, LV, α-virus	CAD, ACS, I/R injury	[188,189]
	Survival genes				
	Bcl-2, Akt, HGF	Overexpression	ADV, AAV, LV, α-virus	CAD, ACS, I/R, HF	[190–191,196]
	Inflammatory cytokines, adhesion molecules and TF				
	ICAM, VCAM, TNF-α	Inhibition	AS-ODN	MI, I/R injury, graft etherosclerosis, transplantation	[192]
	NF-κB		Decoy ODN ADV-AS-ODN, RV-AS-ODN		[197–199]
	Pro-apoptotic genes				
	Bad, caspase inhibitorp53, Fas ligand	Inhibition	AS-ODN Decoy ODN, ADV-AS-ODN	I/R injury, HF	[195]
	Coronary vessel tone				
	eNOS, adenosine (P1, P3) receptors	Overexpression	RV, ADV, AAV(?)	CAD, I/R injury, HF	[132,193]
Rescue Myocardial ischemia	*Pro-angiogenic factors*				
	VEGF$_{121, 165}$, FGF-1, 2,4, 5, HGF, Ang-1, MCP-1, G-CSF, PDGF-BB, IGF-1,2 HIF-1α/VP16, egr-1, Prox-1	Overexpression	Plasmid ADV, AAV, LV(?)	CAD, MI, HF	[200–204, 206–212, 218,219]

ACS: acute coronary syndromes; ADV: adenovirus; Ang-1: angiopoietin-1; AS-ODN: antisense oligonucleotide; egr-1: early growth response factor-1; GPx: glutathione peroxidase; HF: heart failure; HIF: hypoxia inducible factor; HSP: heat shock protein; IGF: insulin-like growth factor; LV: lentivirus; VCAM: vascular cell adhesion molecule. For other abbreviations refer to text.

preconditioning the myocardium to future I/R episodes. Nevertheless, these pre-clinical studies provide compelling evidence that antioxidant gene therapy may provide a viable strategy for protection from ischemic myocardial injury.

Gene therapy for rescue from ischemic heart disease

Gene therapy strategies for rescuing ischemic myocardium may be attainable in certain situations, for review see Ref. [90,200]. Therapeutic angiogenesis by delivery of genes coding pro-angiogenic growth factors promoted neovascularization and functional recovery of ischemic myocardium in several animal models and in humans with CAD (Table 26.3) [32,91,92,201–205]. This strategy offers a potentially efficacious method for the treatment of CAD in patients for whom percutaneous angioplasty or surgical revascularization has been excluded. Proof of principle has been demonstrated in several animal models of hindlimb and myocardial ischemia by gene transfer of VEGF [203,204,206], FGF [92,207,208], and HGF [202,209,210]. In all cases, improvement in tissue perfusion was accompanied by morphological and angiographic evidence of new vessel formation, thus establishing a relationship between improved tissue viability and neovascularization. For example, Mack et al. [201] showed that intramyocardial delivery of $VEGF_{121}$ to pigs by adenovirus improved regional myocardial perfusion and left ventricular function in response to stress in an aneroid constrictor model of chronic myocardial ischemia. Using intracoronary injection of an adenovirus vector encoding human FGF-5, Giordano et al. [92] also showed significantly improved blood flow and reduced stress-induced functional abnormalities (in association with an increase in capillary to fiber ratios) as early as 2 weeks after aneroid placement around the proximal left circumflex coronary artery in pigs.

Several Phase I, II, and III clinical trials of Angiogenic GENe Therapy (AGENT) have been carried out with patients suffering from myocardial and limb ischemia (Table 26.4) [203, 204,211–213, for review see Ref. 200,214]. Although these safety trials comprised small non-randomized patient samples, they demonstrate the potential of AGENT for treatment of ischemic heart disease. In a Phase I study in five male patients aged 53–71 years of age with

angiographic evidence of CAD that did not respond to conventional anti-anginal therapy, Losordo et al. [33] reported that direct intramyocardial delivery of naked plasmid encoding $VEGF_{165}$ into the ischemic myocardium resulted in significantly reduced anginal symptoms and modestly improved left ventricular function concomitant with reduced ischemia and improved Rentrop score. Using adenovirus for intramyocardial delivery of $VEGF_{121}$ into an area of reversible ischemia in the left ventricle as sole or adjunct therapy in patients undergoing conventional CABG, Rosengart et al. [203] showed improvements in regional ventricular function and wall motion in the region of vector administration in both groups of patients. Vale and colleagues [211] undertook a randomized, single-blinded placebo-controlled phase I trial in patients with chronic myocardial ischemia using catheter-based delivery of naked $VEGF_{165}$ assisted by electromechanical NOGA mapping of the left ventricle. The results of this study indicated significant reductions in weekly anginal attacks for as long as 1 year after gene delivery in the treated patients, in contrast to the patients receiving placebo. The reduction in anginal episodes was accompanied by improved myocardial perfusion, as evidenced by SPECT-sestamibi perfusion scanning and electromechanical mapping. Recently Grines and colleagues [212] completed the AGENT double-blinded, randomized, placebo-controlled trial using dose-escalating adenovirus-mediated intracoronary delivery of FGF-4 in patients with angina, in order to evaluate the safety an efficacy of this protocol in reducing ischemic symptoms. The authors reported increased exercise tolerance and improved stress echocardiograms at 4 and 12 weeks after gene transfer in the patients who received FGF-4 gene therapy compared to the patients receiving placebo. Unfortunately the long-term outcome beyond 12 weeks has not been reported.

The relative success of these initial small-scale trials warrant larger and more adequately controlled larger multicenter trials. Several issues relating to feasibility, safety, and sustainability require further investigation before therapeutic angiogenesis may be envisaged as a viable therapeutic option for treatment of heart and peripheral ischemic disease. The issue of safety of the approach requires systematic evaluation. This is particularly relevant in the light of recent evidence that transplantation of myoblasts

Table 26.4 Clinical trials using gene therapy for therapeutic angiogenesis in myocardial and peripheral ischemia.

Trial name/authors	Trial phase	Therapeutic agent	Vector and route of administration	Therapeutic target	Follow up	Therapeutic outcome
Losordo et al. *Circulation* 1998;98:2800	I	VEGF$_{165}$	plasmid, intramyocardial	CAD not amenable to revascularization	10 weeks	↑ SPECT-sestamibi, ↑ Rentrop score, ↓ NTG use
Losordo et al. *Circulation* 2002;105:2012	I/II	VEGF$_{165}$	plasmid, transendocardial with NOGA catheter	CAD not amenable to revascularization	12 weeks	↑ CCS angina class, ↑ exercise duration, ↑ Seattle angina questionnaire
Vale et al. *Circulation* 2001;103:2138	I	VEGF$_{165}$	plasmid, transendocardial with NOGA catheter	CAD not amenable to revascularization	1 year	↑ SPECT-sestamibi, ↑ Rentrop score, ↓ NTG use, ↓ weekly angina attacks
Symes et al. *Ann Thorac Surg* 1999;68:830	I	VEGF$_{165}$	plasmid, Intramyocardial	CAD not amenable to revascularization with Type III, IV angina	3 months	↑ SPECT-sestamibi, no rest ischemic pain, ↓ NTG use
Rosengart et al. *Circulation* 1999;100:468	I	VEGF$_{121}$	adenovirus, intramyocardial	CAD not amenable to revascularization	1 month	↑ SPECT-sestamibi, ↑ CCS angina class ↑ treadmill exercise
Hedman et al. KAT trial *Circulation* 2003;107:2635	I	VEGF$_{121}$	adenovirus, intracoronary	CAD at time of PTCA	6 months	↓ coronary restenosis, ↑ myocardial perfusion
Henry et al. VIVA trial *Circulation* 2003;107:1359	I	hrVEGF$_{165}$ protein	intracoronary with intravenous suppl.	CAD not amenable to revascularization	2 months	No change in ETT, ↓ angina episodes
Grines et al. AGENT trial *Circulation* 2002;105:1291	I/II	FGF-4	adenovirus, intracoronary	Class II or III angina, >1 vessel patent	1–3 months	↑ ETT, improved stress ECG
Simons et al. FIRST trial *Circulation* 2002;105:788	I/II	FGF-2	intracoronary bolus	Class II or III angina	90 and 180 days	↑ ETT, ↓ angina episodes at 90 days no differences at 180 days
Laham et al. *J Am Coll Cardiol* 2000;36:2132	I	FGF-2	intracoronary infusion	CAD not amenable to revascularization	1–6 months	↑ ETT, ↑ wall thickness and perfusion by MRI, improved quality of life
Unger et al. *Am J Cardiol* 2000;85:1414	I	FGF-2	intracoronary bolus	CAD with stable angina	1 month	↑ diameter of epicardial arteries

(continued)

Table 26.4 Continued

Trial name/authors	Trial phase	Therapeutic agent	Vector and route of administration	Therapeutic target	Follow up	Therapeutic outcome
Kleiman et al. J Am Coll Cardiol 2000;36:310	I	FGF-2	intracoronary infusion	CAD not amenable to revascularization	6 months	No differences between placebo and treatment groups
Schumacher et al. Circulation 1998;97:645	I	FGF-1	intramyocardial	Three vessel disease and distal LAD disease	12 weeks to 3 years	↑ angiogenesis distal to LAD, ↑ SPECT-sestamibi, ↓ NTG use
Seiler et al. Circulation 2001;104:1994	I	GM-CSF	intracoronary subcutaneous	CAD not amenable to revascularization	2 weeks	↑ coronary flow index, ↓ ECG abnormalities during balloon inflation
Baumgartner et al. Circulation 1998;97:1114	I	VEGF$_{165}$	plasmid, intramuscular	critical limb ischemia	2–11 months	↑ ankle-brachial index, ↑ exercise time, ↑ neovascularization, limb salvage
Makinen et al. Mol Ther 2002;6:127	I	VEGF$_{165}$	adenovirus, intraluminal after PTA	critical lim ischemia and infrainguinal occlusion	3 months	↑ neovascularization, ↑ ankle-brachial index
Isner et al. Lancet 1996;348:370	I	VEGF$_{165}$	plasmid, intraluminal	critical limb-ischemia	3 months	↑ neovascularization and Doppler flow,
Lederman et al. TRAFFIC trial Lancet 2002;359:2053	I	FGF-2	intraluminal	critical limb ischemia with intermittent claudication	3 months	↑ ETT

CAD: coronary artery disease; ETT: exercise tolerance time; LAD: left anterior descending coronary artery; NTG: nitroglycerin; PTA: percutaneous transluminal angioplasty.

constitutively expressing VEGF under a retroviral promoter into mouse hearts led to intramural angiomas followed by heart failure and death [215, for commentary see 216]. This observation underscores the necessity for regulated expression of pro-angiogenic factors. Such a strategy may require the incorporation of promoter sequences such as hypoxia-sensitive responsive elements capable of rendering expression of the therapeutic transgene subservient to the pathophysiological changes in myocardial oxygen tension. This concept has recently been validated by Su et al. [217] who demonstrated stimulation of VEGF expression by hypoxia in ischemic myocardium using an AAV vector encoding VEGF under transcriptional control by the erythropoietin hypoxia responsive element. Another approach to achieve regulated therapeutic angiogenesis uses engineered TF capable of activating endogenous VEGF expression as a strategy to induce VEGF expression in pathophysiological conditions [218,219]. These novel strategies may allow endogenous regulation of angiogenesis so that the magnitude of neovascularization is graded to the severity of the ischemic insult. Further work is also necessary in order to determine the safest and most efficacious route and method of gene delivery, in order to avert potentially hazardous side effects such as neovascularization of occult neoplasms or peripheral vascular effects that may result in edema and hypotension. In this context, the optimal strategy may require targeted tissue delivery by incorporation of cell-specific promoters for the expression of the transgene exclusively at the target sites and co-expression of an angiogenic factor capable of inducing lymph vessel angiogenesis. Regarding long-term therapeutic sustainability, researchers must establish whether a single administration of the therapeutic gene can achieve the desired long-term therapeutic effect, or whether multiple treatments may be required. Unless the new capillaries are accompanied by arterialization and furnished with blood supply, VEGF-induced neovessels tend to regress soon after termination of the transgene expression, indicating the necessity for carefully designed therapeutic angiogenesis protocols and optimized for dose and duration of angiogenic transgene expression [200]. The optimal gene therapy for therapeutic angiogenesis likely may require co-transfer of both angiogenic cytokines and growth factors, e.g., platelet-derived growth factor

(PDGF), that can recruit the cellular elements, e.g., pericytes, required for support and stabilization of the new vessels [200].

Endothelial cell-based therapy for myocardial and vascular disease

Recent isolation of blood-borne EPC has given rise to an exciting new field [5]. These cells can be expanded and genetically modified [59,93] *ex vivo* with relative ease, offering opportunities to design autologous cell-based therapies for neovascularization of ischemic tissues or repair of damaged vessels [220,221] and also for tissue engineering [222]. Cells mobilized from bone marrow in response to a variety of signals home preferentially to sites of injury such as infarcted myocardium and denuded blood vessels, where they may contribute to local tissue repair and regeneration [220,223, for review see Ref. 224]. Furthermore, the levels of circulating EPC increase in patients with MI [225], suggesting that these cells may play an essential role in neovascularization of the myocardium in response to ischemia. The therapeutic potential of EPC in tissue salvage and regeneration has been demonstrated in various animals models of myocardial and vascular injury [166,220,221,226,227, for review see Ref. 228], and transplantation of autologous EPC has been used in treatment of patients with MI [229]. The mobilization of EPC with bone marrow-mobilizing cytokines such as VEGF and granulocyte colony stimulating factor (G-CSF) offers a promising new strategy for potentiation of the endogenous repair mechanisms shown to accelerate angiogenesis of ischemic tissues [59,166,227,230,231] and re-endothelialization of damaged vessels and prosthetic grafts [167,221]. The recent discovery that HMG-CoA inhibitors (statins) can mobilize EPC to sites of injury [232–235] suggests that EPC may mediate the therapeutic benefit of these cholesterol-lowering drugs, at least in part.

Endothelial progenitor cells

Several studies have reported the identification and isolation of EPC from adult peripheral blood [5,236, for review see Ref. 224] The cells likely originate from a common hemangioblast precursor in the bone marrow [5,237] and express endothelial lineage markers such as CD34, Flk-1, VE-cadherin,

PECAM-1 (CD31), von Willebrand factor, eNOS, and E-Selectin [5,166,227,237,238 for review see Ref. 224]. Compared to native endothelial cells, EPC have high proliferative potential [5] and under specific growth conditions can differentiate into mature endothelial cells that can be expanded in culture to yield sufficient numbers for therapeutic applications [49,93,166,220,226,227, for review see Ref. 228]. Loss of hematopoietic stem cell marker CD133 expression usually coincides with EPC differentiation into cells with phenotypic and functional characteristics of endothelial cells. For review see Ref. [224]. The relative abundance of EPC in basal conditions is low [5,57], but the number of circulating cells increases several fold after exogenous stimulation with cytokines such as VEGF, granulocyte-colony stimulating factor (G-CSF), stem cell factor (SCF), and stromal cell-derived factor-1 (SDF-1) [59,166,227,230,231,239, for review see Ref. 224,228]. The mechanisms governing the mobilization, homing, and differentiation of EPC *in vivo* remain largely unknown. Several groups have reported that the cells are recruited predominantly to sites of injury, such as ischemic myocardium and damaged blood vessels [166,225,227, for review see Ref. 224], suggesting that signals emanating from the injury site may play a principal role in the mobilization, homing, and differentiation processes. Several cytokines, chemokines, adhesion molecules, and extracellular matrix proteins are locally released in response to injury. These agents may act in concert in mediating these processes. For example, ischemic tissues release increased levels of VEGF, G-CSF, SCF-1, and SDF-1, which stimulate hematopoietic cell mobilization from the bone marrow [240–242, for review see Ref. 243]. Furthermore, EPC express VEGF and SDF-1 receptors [224], and the respective ligands stimulate EPC mobilization and migration [224], suggesting that they may participate centrally in these processes. At the site of injury, the production of adhesion molecules may provide a microenvironment for implantation and subsequent proliferation and differentiation of the EPC.

Endothelial cell therapy for myocardial and peripheral ischemic disease

An alternative option for therapeutic angiogenesis involves the use of EPC as angiogenic substrate. Two strategies have achieved cell-based neovascularization of ischemic tissues. The most common approach involves the isolation of the mononuclear cell fraction ("buffy coat") from bone marrow (BM-MNC) or peripheral blood (PB-MNC) by density centrifugation (Figure 26.3). The mononuclear fraction may then be injected whole, submitted to further selection, or cultured and expanded *ex vivo* under selective growth conditions favouring endothelial cell differentiation to obtain sufficient number of cells for therapeutic application [5,57]. The cells are then used for transplantation without any further manipulation, or they may be genetically modified with vectors expressing therapeutic genes [59,244] and then delivered to the target area, where they may implant and promote new vessel growth in response to specific cues emanating from the ischemic area (Figure 26.3) for review see Ref. [228,245]. This approach has been tested and evaluated in several animal models of myocardial [166,220,223,246–250] and limb ischemia [59,93,226,251] and recently has been employed in several recent small-scale clinic studies in patients with MI [229,252–255] and unoperable peripheral limb ischemia [256] (Table 26.5). For example, transplantation of autologous CD31[+] EPC from peripheral blood induced new vessel formation and improved left ventricular perfusion and function in pig hearts rendered ischemic by placing an aneroid constrictor in the circumflex coronary artery [246]. Likewise, implantation of whole [220] or CD34[+]-selected [246] human PB-MNC into nude rats immediately after acute MI led to revascularization of the infarcted myocardium, resulting in reduced interstitial fibrosis and improved left ventricular function. Favorable results have also been reported with BM-MNC. Transendocardial delivery of autologous BM-MNC to hibernating myocardium in swine led to significantly increased basal systolic function in parallel with increases in collateral vessel formation and blood flow [247, 248,250]. Similarly, intravenous delivery of human CD34[+] BM-MNC to nude rats with MI led to neovascularization of the infarcted myocardium, resulting in reduced apoptosis of myocytes in the peri-infarct region, decreased interstitial fibrosis, and sustained improvement in left ventricular function [166], and implantation of bone marrow-derived Lin-c-kit[+] [257] cells into the infarct border or coronary infusion of side-population (SP) [259] from LacZ transgenic mice into lethally irradiated donors exposed to I/R injury led to dramatic recuperation of the infarcted myocardium and

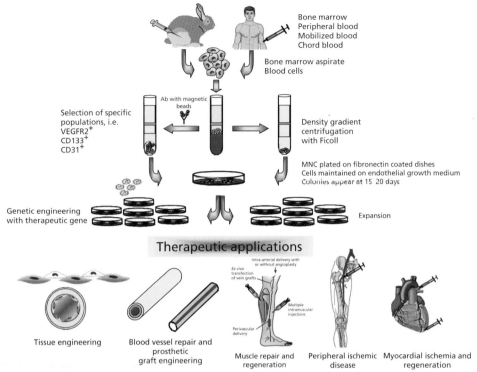

Figure 26.3 Isolation, cultivation and genetic engineering of EPC for therapeutic application. EPC can be isolated from the BM-MNC, peripheral blood or umbilical chord blood with or without further selection and purification. The mononuclear cells are expanded *ex vivo* under endothelial-specific growth conditions and may be genetically modified to overexpress one or several therapeutic genes. The differentiated cells are then used in transplantation protocols for rescue and repair of damaged tissues such as infarcted myocardium, ischemic limb or injured muscle. The cells may also be used for endothelialization of damaged blood vessels and vascular prosthetic grafts and in tissue engineering.

improved ventricular function in association with new vessel formation.

The success of these pre-clinical studies led to several recent small-scale feasibility and safety studies to evaluate the use of bone marrow cell transplantation in treatment of MI and ischemic heart disease (Table 26.5) [229,252–255]. In a recent small-scale phase I clinical trial, Stamm and colleagues [229] injected autologous AC133+ bone marrow cells into the infarct border during CABG in 6 patients with earlier acute transmural MI. The authors reported improved perfusion of the infarcted area and significant enhancement of global left ventricular function 3–9 months after surgery. The transplantation protocol appears safe and did not cause adverse cardiac effects. Strauer et al. [252] reported that intracoronary delivery of unfractionated autologous mononuclear bone marrow cells 6 days after infarction led to reduced infarct size and improved ventricular function and chamber geometry 10 weeks after transplantation. Intracoronary infusion of either BM-MNC or PB-MNC 4 days after infarction to a randomized group of 20 patients with reperfused acute MI led equally to significant improvements in global left ventricle ejection fraction and wall motion in the infarct zone as well as reduced end-systolic dimensions at 4 months follow-up, in association with increased coronary flow reserve in the infarct artery and myocardial viability in the infarct zone [253]. No adverse effects occurred with the transplantation protocol, and the authors suggested that autologous progenitor cell may provide a feasible strategy for preventing post-infarction ventricular remodeling and failure. Two other groups reported recently that transendocardial delivery of autologous BM-MNC using NOGA mapping led to significant improvements in left ventricular perfusion and performance, and reduced incidence of ischemic

Table 26.5 Pre-clinical and clinical cell-based therapy for therapeutic angiogenesis.

Target	Donor	Recipient	Type and source of cells	Method of delivery	Therapeutic effects	References
Myocardium						
Myocardial ischemia	Swine	Autologous	CD31$^+$, peripheral blood	Transendocardial with NOGA mapping	↑ Rentrop score, ↑ EF, ↑ capillary density	[246]
	Swine	Autologous	MNC, bone marrow	Transendocardial	↑ capillary density, ↑ collateral flow, ↑ myocardial contractility	[250]
Hibernating myocardium	Swine	Autologous	MNC, peripheral blood MNC, bone marrow	Transendocardial	↑ EF, ↑ capillary density, ↑ flow ↑ EF, ↑ collateral flow	[247,248]
Myocardial ischemia	Rat	Autologous	MNC, bone marrow	Intramyocardial	↑ capillary density	[249]
Myocardial infarction	Human	Nude rat	CD34$^+$, peripheral blood MNC, peripheral blood	Intramyocardial intravenous	↑ EF, ↑ capillary density, ↓ fibrosis ↑ EF, ↑ capillary density, ↓ fibrosis	[220,246]
	Human	Nude rat	CD34$^+$, bone marrow	Tail vein injection	↑ EF, ↑ capillary density, ↓ fibrosis, ↑ apoptosis, ↓ infarct size	[227]
	GFP-mouse	Syngenic mouse	Lin-c-kit$^+$, bone marrow	Peri-infarct region	↑ LVDP, ↑ capillary density, ↓ infarct	[257]
	Mouse	Autologous	Bone marrow mobilization	Homing	↑ EF, ↑ capillary density, ↓ remodeling	[258]
	Rosa-mouse	Syngenic	SP cells, bone marrow	periinfarct region	↑ capillary density, ↓ infarct	[259]
	Human	Autologous	CD133$^+$, bone marrow	Infarct border	↑ EF, ↑ collateral flow (SPECT)	[229]
	Human	Autologous	MNC, bone marrow MNC, peripheral blood	Intracoronary balloon catheter	↓ infarct size, ↑ wall motion, ↑ contractility, ↑ myocardial perfusion	[252,253]
Myocardial ischemia (Unstable angina)	Human	Autologous	MNC, bone marrow	Transendocardial with NOGA mapping	↓ anginal episodes, ↑ wall thickening, ↑ wall motion, ↑ EF	[254,255]
Ischemic limb disease						
Hindlimb ischemia	Rat	Autologous	MNC, bone marrow	Intramuscular injection in gastrocnemius	↑ capillary density, ↑ blood flow, ↑ AVDO$_2$, ↑ exercise capacity	[226]
	Rabbit	Autologous	MNC, bone marrow	Intramuscular injection in thigh	↑ capillary density, ↑ blood flow	[223]
	Human	Athymic mice	MNC, peripheral blood	Intracardiac injection	↑ capillary density, ↑ blood flow	[93]
	Human	Athymic mice	MNC, peripheral blood overexpressing VEGF	Tail vein injection	↓ autoamputation, ↑ capillary density, ↑ blood flow	[59]
	Human	Nude rat	MNC, peripheral blood MNC, chord blood	Intramuscular injection in thigh	↑ capillary density, ↑ blood flow	[251,260]
	Human	Autologous	MNC, bone marrow	Intramuscular injection in Gastrocnemius	↑ ankle-brachial index, ↑ pain-free walking, ↑ transcutaneous PO$_2$	[256]

AVDO$_2$: arteriovenous oxygen difference; EF: ejection fraction; MNC: mononuclear cells; PO$_2$: partial pressure of oxygen.

episodes in patients with end-stage ischemic heart disease [254] or stable angina [255], suggesting that BM-MNC transplantation may be useful as a strategy to improve myocardial function in patients with severe ischemic heart disease.

Progenitor cells also have potential therapeutic value in treatment of critical limb ischemia (Table 26.5) [59,93,223,226,230,251,256]. Local intramuscular delivery of autologous BM-MN restored blood flow and exercise capacity in rat ischemic limb, in association with new vessel formation in the ischemic muscle [226]. Similarly, administration of human BM-MNC or PB-MNC to nude rats [251,260] or athymic mice [59,93] induced angiogenesis in the ischemic limb, leading to improved perfusion and reduced incidence of autoamputation. Interestingly, the transplanted PB-MNC in one study [251] did not incorporate into the new capillaries, but contributed to new vessel formation by secreting pro-angiogenic cytokines. Recently, autologous BM-MNC were injected in the gastrocnemius muscle of patients with unilateral or bilateral leg ischemia due to severe peripheral artery disease [256]. Four weeks after cell-transplantation, ankle–brachial indexes significantly improved in legs treated with BM-MNC but not in cells treated with saline. Rest pain and pain-free walking improved significantly during the 24-week duration of the study. The authors suggest that BM-MNC transplantation may offer a safe and effective strategy for treatment of peripheral ischemic disease.

An alternative strategy for potentiation of therapeutic angiogenesis in ischemic tissues involves the use of EPC as vectors for delivery of pro-angiogenic factors. The ability to culture and genetically modify these cells suggests that they are ideally suited as a substrate for cell-based therapy. Accordingly, EPC expressing angiogenic growth factors could contribute to new vessel growth by proliferating and differentiating at the site of implantation, and by secreting pro-angiogenic growth factors for the growth of pre-existing vessels. Iwaguro and colleagues recently validated this concept [59]. Using athymic mice with hindlimb ischemia, this group showed that the transplantation of murine EPC transduced *ex vivo* with an adenoviral vector expressing VEGF resulted in more efficient neovascularization and blood flow recovery than treatment with untransduced EPC. Improved neovascularization in the animals treated with VEGF-transduced EPC was attributed to enhanced proliferation and adhesion of the transplanted cells. Thus, VEGF gene transfer exerts phenotypic modulation of EPC, thereby potentiating biological properties that favor the angiogenic response.

A potential non-invasive approach for angiogenesis of ischemic myocardium in CAD involves the mobilization of EPC to the ischemic region via cytokines or conventional pharmacological therapeutic agents used in treatment of CAD, such as statins. Orlic and colleagues [258] reported recently that mobilization of bone marrow by G-CSF and SCF-1 led to decreased post-infarction mortality and functional recovery in mice with MI in association with significant regeneration and angiogenesis of the infarcted myocardium. In athymic nude mice with hindlimb ischemia, local injection of SDF-1 stimulated homing of human PB-MNC administered systemically to the ischemic muscle and stimulated vasculogenesis [239]. In patients with critical limb ischemia, VEGF gene transfer resulted in significant angiogenesis in the ischemic muscle in association with increased numbers of circulating EPC [230]. Recently, several groups showed that statin therapy increases EPC in patients with stable CAD [232, 233], suggesting that the beneficial therapeutic effect of these drugs may be mediated, at least in part, via mobilization of EPC and subsequent neovascularization of ischemic myocardium. Walter et al. (2002) showed that statin therapy accelerates re-endothelialization of balloon-injured arterial segments in rats, leading to reduction in neointimal thickening.

Endothelial cell therapy for vascular repair and bioengineering of grafts

An emerging area where cell transplantation and genetic manipulation may play a pivotal role involves repair of damaged vessels and bioengineering of prostheses and artificial organs [56–58,261,262]. For example, autologous endothelial cell transplantation may prove useful as adjunctive therapy for rapid re-endothelialization and restoration of homeostasis in blood vessels injured during revascularization procedures such as percutaneous transluminal angioplasty, stenting, atherectomy, or vein bypass grafting [261–264], or for seeding of prosthetic grafts, stents, or engineered blood vessels to create a bioactive endothelial layer [57,58, 221, 265, 266, for review see Ref. 261]. Furthermore, the cells could be genetically engineered *ex vivo* to express therapeutic genes that could impart desirable qualities to the grafts, such as an enhanced antithrombotic surface [267,268], or the capability to synthesize angiogenic, vasodilatory, or cytoprotective factors for maintenance and survival of the grafts [59,262]. We [269] and several other groups [57,58,221,263–267,270] have already demonstrated the feasibility of transplanting autologous endothelial cells to create a biosurface in ePTFE grafts and in denuded native blood vessels. We showed recently that transplantation of autologous PB-EPC results in rapid endothelialization of ePTFE graft segments and balloon-denuded carotid arteries, leading to attenuation of neointima deposition in the injured vessels [269]. Using a similar approach, Kaushal et al. [221] showed that implantation of EPC into decellularized porcine iliac vessels in turn implanted as coronary interposition grafts reconstituted a functional endothelial layer that conferred improved vasodilatory function and prolonged patency of the grafts. Using endothelial cells transduced with a RV overexpressing t-PA to seed stainless steel intravascular stents, Dicheck et al. [58] reported sustained retention of the transplanted cells to the stent surface after implantation, suggesting that this may be an option for delivery of therapeutic genes to prevent in-stent restenosis and thrombosis. Using EPC for seeding of photocured gelatine-coated metallic and microporous thin segmented polyurethane stents, Shirota et al. [265] reported comparable findings.

A less cumbersome and potentially more effective strategy to enhance re-endothelialization of damaged vessels involves the mobilization and recruitment of endogenous EPC from the bone marrow and other sources to the injured sites. Bhattacharya et al. [271] and Shi et al. [167] showed that mobilization of bone marrow by exogenous G-CSF enhances endothelialization and patency of small caliber prosthetic grafts. Using a similar strategy, we recently demonstrated that pre-treatment with G-CSF leads to accelerated re-endothelialization and concomitant reduction in neointima hyperplasia in balloon-injured carotid artery, in association with increased abundance of PB-EPC [272]. Others have shown that statin therapy [234,235] and estrogens [273] increase the number of PB-EPC and reduce neointima hyperplasia in ani-

mal models of arterial injury, suggesting that EPC mobilization and recruitment to injury sites may contribute to the vasculoprotective effects of these agents. Interestingly, Assmus and colleagues [274] reported recently that statins reduce senescence of stimulate proliferation of PB-EPC by regulating the activity of crucial cell cycle genes such as cyclins and cyclin-dependent kinase inhibitors. Thus the therapeutic potential of EPC could potentially be harnessed by non-invasive pharmacological manipulation and used to accelerate the endogenous repair mechanisms for inhibition of neointimal hyperplasia and prevention of restenosis following revascularization procedures, and to enhance vasodilatory and non-adhesive activities in atherosclerotic vessels and in prosthetic grafts.

The potential of cell transplantation for tissue engineering, however, goes beyond endothelial seeding of blood vessels and prosthetic grafts. Construction of whole artificial organs and structures capable of replicating specialized physiological function is being envisaged. Advancement in this area is largely conditioned by the development of immunocompatible biodegradable materials that could be used as scaffolds shaped to the desired configurations and to which autologous cells may be seeded to provide a biologically active surface [261]. Currently, several groups are focusing on the construction of functional blood vessels containing all the constituent cell types, with the goal of producing biological prostheses with the mechanical and biochemical properties required to withstand high pulsatile arterial pressures and respond to endogenous vasoregulatory mechanisms [275–277]. For example, Campbell and colleagues [277] used a simple and ingenious approach to produce fully functional immune-resistant vessels by introducing segments of silastic tubing into the peritoneum. The segments become cellularized with myofibroblasts, collagen matrix, and endothelial-like mesothelial cells due to the initial inflammatory reaction. Removal of the silastic scaffold leaves a biological tube with the histological architecture of native vessels.

Outstanding issues with cell-based therapy for angiogenesis and vascular repair

Although the recent pre-clinical and clinical findings regarding the therapeutic potential of cell transplantation in tissue repair and regeneration are promising, they must be considered preliminary. Further characterization of the biology of these cells and clarification of several outstanding issues are essential to future progress. The nature of the mobilizing, migratory, and homing signals for EPC and the mechanisms of differentiation and incorporation into the target tissues require identification. Multicenter controlled trials must define and standardize the optimal time and method of delivery, the subpopulation and number of cells required to achieve a sustained therapeutic benefit, and the survival of the transplanted cells. For example, the question of whether transplantation should be performed soon after infarction or after the inflammatory process has resolved remains unsettled. Bone marrow-derived cells are very sensitive to hypoxia and inflammation. A significant number of the transplanted cells die soon after implantation [278], and EPC transplanted into denuded vessels and prosthetic grafts may detach and undergo rapid turnover [269]. Strategies for improved cell adhesion and survival, particularly around the time of transplantation when the cells are most vulnerable, may need to be devised. Genetic engineering of the cells prior to grafting with vectors expressing survival genes may help reduce peri-implantation cell death and improve the long-term survival of the graft. Murasawa and colleagues [279] reported recently that genetic engineering of EPC with human telomerase reverse transcriptase (hTERT) enhances the proliferative and migratory capacity of EPC in response to VEGF stimulation due to increased basal activity of telomerase, leading to improved neovascularization of ischemic limb, whereas Zhang et al. [280] showed that survival of grafted neonatal cardiac myocytes improves greatly by adenoviral transduction of the cells with the survival gene Akt prior to transplantation.

Perspectives and future directions

The intensive investigations of the last two decades have gained recognition that the vascular endothelium play an essential physiological role in the maintenance of cardiovascular homeostasis, and it is now well established that endothelial dysfunction is a predominant feature of all major cardiovascular diseases. Indeed, the therapeutic effect of many current drug therapies used in the treatment of diseases such as hypertension, atherosclerosis, and acute coronary syndromes is attributable, at least in part, to improved endothelial function. In parallel with the unraveling of the molecular mechanisms associated with cardiovascular disease, an array of gene and cell-based strategies has evolved with potential therapeutic value for treatment of these diseases. Interestingly, Although vascular endothelium was not the primary target of genetic manipulation, the underlying therapeutic benefit of many of these experimental strategies is due, to a significant degree, to the amelioration of endothelial dysfunction. Several of these experimental therapies have transitioned into clinical trial and are now being considered for use in human patients, while several others are currently undergoing safety and feasibility evaluation in early phase trials. Notwithstanding these significant advances, we recognize the need for further developments in several aspects of cardiovascular gene and cell-based therapy. Progress in vector and delivery technologies have not kept pace with the identification of novel therapeutic targets. None of the current vectors incorporate all of the requisite features of the "ideal" vector. The development of vectors amenable to endogenous regulation and capable of conferring tissue specificity of transgene expression is essential to satisfy the safety and ethical requirements of human gene therapy. Much of this development can be accomplished using current vector platforms. Rigorous systematic evaluation of the safety and efficacy of delivery strategies and improvement of delivery devices are also essential prerequisites for human gene therapy protocols.

With regards to the use of EPC therapy for tissue repair and regeneration, there are several issues that need to be addressed. In addition to the pressing need to understand the mechanisms involved in mobilization, homing, differentiation, and survival of EPC at implantation sites, it is necessary to define and standardize the optimal conditions for therapeutic application with respect to the timing, route and method of delivery, and purity of the cells used in transplantation protocols. These issues assume particular urgency in light of the fact that progenitor cell transplantation has already moved into clinical trial. Large-scale randomized trials are essential in order to evaluate the long-term therapeutic effectiveness of cell-based treatment on mortality and morbidity. Furthermore, the long-term safety of the approach requires thorough examination amid potential concerns about late onset complications such as vascularization and growth of occult tumors, diabetes- and age-related retinopathies, or the appearance of ectopic foci in the myocardium that may lead to life-threatening arrhythmias.

Finally, the optimal genetic therapy for complex diseases such as CAD and MI may require a combination of cell transplantation and pro-angiogenic for long-term sustenance of the regenerated myocardium. Due to regulatory hurdles, such potentially synergistic combinatorial approaches seldom have been considered in the design of cardiovascular gene therapy strategies. Instead, the strategies traditionally have been developed around a single therapeutic target. We see future advances in gene and cell therapies linked to genomic research. For example, molecular phenotyping of patients utilizes genomic profiling and screening and will permit detection of disease-causing polymorphisms and the design of individualized therapies. The convergence of gene transfer technology and genomic technology will facilitate the elucidation of novel genes and may help uncover new roles for previously known genes, thereby leading to the discovery of novel therapeutic targets.

Acknowledgments

Dr. Melo is Canada Research Chair in Molecular Cardiology and a New Investigator of the Heart and Stroke Foundation of Canada and is supported by grants from the Canadian Institutes of Health Research, Heart and Stroke Foundation of Ontario, the Canadian Foundation of Innovation and the Ontario Innovation Trust. Dr. Dzau is supported by grants from the National Institutes of Health.

References

1 Rubanyi GM. The role of endothelium in cardiovascular homeostasis and diseases. *J. Cardiovasc Pharmacol* 1993; 22(Suppl):S1–S4.

2 Quyyumi AA. Endothelial function in health and disease: New insights into the genesis of cardiovascular disease. *Am J Med* 1998;105(1A):32S–39S.

3 Drexler H, Hornig B. Endothelial dysfunction in human disease. *J Mol Cell Cardiol* 1999;31:51–60.

4 Cines DB, Pollak ES, Buck CA. Endothelial cells in physiology and in the pathophysiology of vascular disorders. *Blood* 1998;91:3527–3561.

5 Asahara T, Murohara T, Sullivan A, et al. Isolation of putatitve progenitor endothelial cells for angiogenesis. *Science* 1997;275:964–967.

6 Wang J-S, Shum-Tim D, Chedrawy E, et al. The coronary delivery of marrow stromal cells for myocardial regeneration: pathophysiological and therapeutic implications. *J Thorac Cardiovasc Surg* 2001;122:699–705.

7 Khan TA, Sellke FW, Laham RJ. Gene therapy progress and prospects: therapeutic angiogenesis for limb and myocardial ischemia. *Gene Ther* 2003;10:285–291.

8 Nicklin SA, Baker AH. Tropism-modified adenoviral and adeno-associated viral vectors for gene therapy. *Curr Gene Ther* 2002;2:273–293.

9 Su EJ, Stevenson SC, Rollence M. A genetically modified adenoviral vector exhibits enhanced gene transfer of human smooth muscle cells. *J Vasc Res* 2001;38:471–478.

10 Qian HS, Channon K, Neplioueva V, et al. Improved adenoviral vector for vascular gene therapy: beneficial effects on vascular function and inflammation. *Circ Res* 2001;88: 911–917.

11 Mah C, Fraites TJ, Zolotukhin I, et al. Improved method of recombinant AAV2 delivery for systemic targeted gene therapy. *Mol Ther* 2002;6:106–112.

12 Francis SC, Raizada MK, Mangi AA, et al. Genetic targeting for cardiovascular therapeutics: are we near the summit or just beginning the climb? *Physiol Genomic* 2001; 7:79–94.

13 Isner JM. Myocardial gene therapy. *Nature* 2002;415: 234–239.

14 Stein CA. The experimental use of antisense oligonucleotides: a guide for the perplexed. *J Clin Invest* 2001; 108:641–644.

15 Akhtar S, Hughes MD, Khan A, et al. The delivery of antisense therapeutics. *Adv Drug Deliver Rev* 2000;44: 3–21.

16 Doudna JA, Cech TR. The chemical repertoire of natural ribozymes. *Nature* 2002;418:222–228.

17 Hannon GJ. RNA interference. *Nature* 2002;418:244–251.

18 Mann MJ, Dzau VJ. Therapeutic applications of transcription factor decoy oligonucleotides. *J Clin Invest* 2000; 106:1071–1075.

19 White RR, Sullenger BA, Rusconi CP. Developing aptamers into therapeutics. *J Clin Invest* 2000;106:929–934.

20 Hoppe-Seyler F, Crnkovic-Mertens I, Denk C, et al. Peptide aptamers: new tools to study protein interactions. *J Steriod Biochem Mol Biol* 2001;78:105–111.

21 Robbins PD, Ghivizzani C. Viral vectors for gene therapy. *Pharmacol Ther* 1998;80:35–47.

22 Niidome T, Huang L. Gene therapy progress and prospects: non-viral vectors. *Gene Ther* 2002;9: 1647–1652.

23 Gordon EM, Zhu NL, Forney MP, et al. Lesion-targeted injectable vectors for vascular restenosis. *Human Gene Ther* 2001;12:1277–1287.

24 Sylven C, Sarkar N, Insulander P, et al. Catheter-based transendocardial myocardial gene transfer. *J Interv Cardiol* 2002;15:7–13.

25 Prentice H, Bishopric N, Hicks MN, et al. Regulated expression of a foreign gene targeted to the ischemic myocardium. *Cardiovasc Res* 1997;35:567–574.

26 Forough R, Koyama N, Hasenstab D, et al. Overexpression of tissue inhibitor of matrix metalloproteinase-1 inhibits vascular smooth muscle cell functions *in vitro* and *in vivo*. *Circ Res* 1996;79:812–820.

27 Messina LM, Podrazik RM, Whitehill et al. Adhesion and incorporation of lacZ-transduced endothelial cells into the intact capillary wall in the rat. *Proc Natl Acad Sci USA* 1992;89:12018–12022.

28 Wright MJ, Wightman LML, Lilley C, et al. *In vivo* myocardial gene transfer: optimization, evaluation and direct comparison of gene transfer vectors. *Bas Res Cardiol* 2001;96:227–236.

29 Alexander MY, Webster KA, McDonald PH, et al. Gene transfer and models of gene therapy for the myocardium. *Clin Exp Pharmacol Physiol* 1999;26:661–668.

30 Song YK, Liu F, Chu S, et al. Characterization of cationic liposome-mediated gene transfer *in vivo* by intravenous administration. *Hum Gene Ther* 1997;8:1585–1594.

31 Li S, Huang L. Nonviral gene therapy: promises and challenges. *Gene Ther* 2000;7:31–34.

32 Herweijer H, Wolff JA. Progress and prospects: naked DNA gene transfer and therapy. *Gene Ther* 2003;10:453–458.

33 Losordo DW, Vale PR, Symes JF, et al. Gene therapy for myocardial angiogenesis. Initial clinical results with direct myocardial injection of phVEGF$_{165}$ as sole therapy for myocardial ischemia. *Circulation* 1998;98:2800–2804.

34 Dzau VJ, Mann MJ, Morishita R, et al. Fusigenic viral liposome for gene therapy in cardiovascular diseases. *Proc Natl Acad Sci USA* 1996;93:11421–11425.

35 Takeshita S, Gal D, Leclerc G, et al. Increased gene expression after liposome-mediated arterial gene transfer associated with intimal smooth muscle cell proliferation. *In vitro* and *in vivo* findings. *J Clin Invest* 19944;93:652–661.

36 Poston RS, Mann MJ, Hoyt EG, et al. Antisense oligodeoxynucleotides prevent acute cardiac allograft rejection via a novel, non-toxic, highly efficient transfection method. *Transplantation* 1999;68:825–832.

37 Mann MJ, Gibbons GH, Hutchinson H, et al. Pressure-mediated oligonucleotide transfection of rat and human cardiovascular tissues. *Proc Natl Acad Sci USA* 1999;96:6411–6416.

38 Huber P, Mann MJ, Melo LG, et al. Focused ultrasound induces localized enhancement of reporter gene expression in rabbit carotid artery. *Gen Ther* 2003;10:1600–1607.

39 Cartier R, Reszka R. Utilization of synthetic peptides containing nuclear localization signals for nonviral gene transfer. *Gen Ther* 2002;9:157–167.

40 Mah C, Byrne BJ, Flotte TR. Virus-based gene delivery systems. *Clin Pharmacokinet* 2002;41:901–911.

41 Chen D, Murphy B, Sung R, et al. Adaptive and innate immune responses to gene transfer vectors: role of cytokines and chemokines in vector function. *Gen Ther* 2003;10:991–998.

42 Steg PG, Feldman LJ, Scoazec JY, et al. Arterial gene transfer to rabbit endothelial and smooth muscle cells using percutaneous delivery of an adenoviral vector. *Circulation* 1994;90:1648–1656.

43 Turunen MP, Puhakka HL, Koponen JK, et al. Peptide-retargeted adenovirus encoding a tissue inhibitor of metalloproteinase-1 decreases restenosis after intravascular gene transfer. *Mol Ther* 2002;6:306–312.

44 Hiltunen MO, Turunen MP, Turunen A-M, et al. Biodistribution of adenoviral vector to nontarget tissues after local *in vivo* gene transfer to arterial wall using intravascular and periadventitial gene delivery methods. *FASEB J* 2000;M,14:2230–2236.

45 Newman KD, Dunn PF, Owens JW, et al. Adenovirus-mediated gene transfer into normal rabbit arteries results in prolonged vascular cell activation, inflammation and neointima hyperplasia. *J Clin Invest* 1995;96:2955–2965.

46 Channon KM, Qian HS, Youngblood SA, et al. Acute host-mediated endothelial injury after adenoviral gene transfer in normal rabbit arteries: impact on transgene expression and endothelial function. *Circ Res* 1998;82:1253–1262.

47 Hartigan-O'Connor D, Amalfitano A, Chamberlain JS (1999). Improved production of gutted adenovirus in cells expressing adenovirus preterminal protein and DNA polymerase. *J Virol* 1999;73:7835–7841.

48 Monahan PE, Samulski RJ. Adeno-associated virus vectors for gene therapy: more pros than cons? *Mol Med Today* 2000;6:433–440.

49 Maeda Y, Ikeda U, Ogasawara Y, et al. Gene transfer into vascular cells using adeno-associated virus (AAV) vectors. *Cardiovasc Res* 1997;35:514–521.

50 Rolling F, Nong Z, Pisvin S, et al. Adeno-associated virus-mediated gene transfer into rat carotid arteries. *Gene Ther* 1997;4:757–761.

51 Yan Z, Zhang Y, Duan D, et al. Trans-splicing vectors expand the utility of adeno-associated virus for gene therapy. *Proc Natl Acad Sci USA* 2000;97:6716–6721.

52 Duly G, Chernajivski Y. Recent developments in retrovirally-mediated gene transduction. *Mol Ther* 2000;2:423–434.

53 Trono D. Lentiviral vectors: turning a deadly foe into a therapeutic agent. *Gene Ther* 2000;7:20–23.

54 Skelly CL, Curi MA, Meyerson SL, et al. Prevention of restenosis by a herpes simplex virus mutant capable of

controlled long-term expression in vascular tissue *in vivo*. *Gene Ther* 2001;8:1840–1846.

55 Roks AJM, Henning RH, Buikema H, et al. Recombinant Semiliki Forest virus as a vector system for fast and selective *in vivo* gene delivery into balloon-injured rat aorta. *Gene Ther* 2002;9:95–101.

56 Parikh SA, Edelman ER. Endothelial cell delivery for cardiovascular therapy. *Adv Drug Del Rev* 2000;42:139–161.

57 Wilson JM, Birinyi LK, Salomon RN, et al. Implantation of vascular grafts lined with genetically modified endothelial cells. *Science* 1989;244:1344–1346.

58 Dicheck DA, Neville RF, Zwiebel JA, et al. Seeding of intravascular stents with genetically engineered endothelial cells. *Circulation* 1989;80:1347–1353.

59 Iwaguro H, Yamaguchi J, Kalka C, et al. Endothelial progenitor cell vascular endothelial growth factor gene transfer for vascular regeneration. *Circulation* 2002;105:732–738.

60 Chen L, Daum G, Forough R, et al. Overexpression of human endothelial nitric oxide synthase in rat vascular smooth muscle cells and in balloon-injured carotid artery. *Circ Res* 1998;82:862–870.

61 Kullo IJ, Simari RD, Schwartz RS. Vascular gene transfer. From bench to bedside. *Arterioscler Thromb Vasc Biol* 1999;19:196–207.

62 Feldman LJ, Steg G. Optimal techniques for arterial gene transfer. *Cardiovasc Res* 35:391–404.

63 Smith RC, Walsh K. Local gene delivery to the vessel wall. *Acta Physiol Scand* 2001;173:93–102.

64 Tahlil O, Brami M, Feldman LJ, et al. The Dispatch™ catheter as a delivery tool for arterial gene transfer. *Cardiovasc Res* 1997;33:181–187.

65 Feldman MD, Sun B, Koci BJ, et al. Stent-based gene therapy. *J Long Term Eff Med Implants* 2000;10:47–68.

66 Panetta CJ, Miyauchi K, Berry D, et al. A tissue-engineered stent for cell-based vascular gene transfer. *Hum Gene Ther* 2002;13:433–441.

67 Klugherz BD, Jones PL, Cui X, et al. Gene delivery from a DNA controlled-release stent in porcine coronary arteries. *Nat Biotechnol* 2000;18:1181–1184.

68 Nicklin SA, Reynolds PN, Brosnan J, et al. Analysis of cell-specific promoters for viral gene therapy targeted at the vascular endothelium. *Hypertension* 2001;38:65–70.

69 Nicklin SA, Buening H, Dishart KL, et al. Efficient and selective AAV2-mediated gene transfer directed to human vascular endothelial cells. *Mol Ther* 2001;4:174–181.

70 Schlaeger TM, Bartunkova S, Lawitts JA, et al. Uniform vascular endothelial-specific gene expression in both embryonic and adult transgenic mice. *Proc Natl Acad Sci USA* 1997;94:3058–3063.

71 Aird WC, Jahroudi N, Weiler-Guettler H, et al. Human von Willebrand gene sequences target expression to a subpopulation of endothelial cells in transgenic mice. *Proc Natl Acad Sci USA* 1995;92:4567–4571.

72 Weiler-Guettler H, Aird WC, Husain M, et al. Targeting of transgene expression to the vascular endothelium of mice by homologous recombination at the thrombomodulin locus. *Circ Res* 1996;78:180–187.

73 Jaggar RT, et al. Endothelial cell-specific expression of tumor necrosis factor-a from the KDR or E-selectin promoters following retroviral delivery. *Human Gene Ther* 1997;8:2239–2247.

74 Cowan PJ, Shinkel TA, Witort EJ, et al. Targeting gene expression to endothelial cells in transgenic mice using the human intercellular adhesion molecule 2 promoter. *Transplantation* 1996;62:155–160.

75 Mavria G, Jager U, Porter CD. Generation of a high titer retroviral vector for endothelial cell-specific gene expression *in vivo*. *Gene Ther* 2000;7:368–376.

76 Nicklin SA, Seggern DJV, Work LM, et al. Ablating adenovirus type 5 fiber-CAR binding and H1 loop insertion of the SIGYPLP peptide generate an endothelial cell selective adenovirus. *Mol Ther* 2001;4:534–542.

77 Modich U, Pugh CW, Bicknell R. Increasing endothelial cell specific expression by the use of heterologous hypoxic and cytokine-inducible enhancers. *Gene Ther* 2000;7:896–902.

78 Lum H, Roebuck KA. Oxidant stress and endothelial cell dysfunction. *Am J Physiol* 2001;280:C719–C741.

79 Gewaltig MT, Kojda G. Vasoprotection by nitric oxide: mechanisms and therapeutic potential. *Cardiovasc Res* 2002;55:250–260.

80 Gibbons GH, Dzau VJ. Molecular therapies for vascular disease. *Science* 1996;272:689–693.

81 Herttuala SY, Martin JF. Cardiovascular gene therapy. *Lancet* 2000;355:213–222.

82 Libby P. Current concepts of the pathogenesis of the acute coronary syndromes. *Circulation* 2001;104:365–372.

83 Plutzky J. Inflammatory pathways in atherosclerosis and acute coronary syndromes. *Am J Cardiol* 2001; 88(suppl):10K–15K.

84 Koning GA, Schiffelers RM, Storm G. Endothelial cells at inflammatory sites as targets for therapeutic intervention. *Endothelium* 2002;9:161–171.

85 Gianoukakis N, Thomson AW, Robbins PD. Gene therapy in transplantation. *Gene Ther* 1999;6:1499–1511.

86 Lin KF, Chao L, Chao J. Prolonged reduction of high blood pressure with human nitric oxide synthase delivery. *Hypertension* 1997;30:307–313.

87 Wang H, Katovich MJ, Gelband CH, et al. Sustained inhibition of angiotensin I converting enzyme (ACE) expression and long-term antihypertensive action by virally-mediated delivery of ACE antisense cDNA. *Circ Res* 1999;85:614–622.

88 Kibbe MR, Billiar TR, Tzeng E. Gene therapy for restenosis. *Circ Res* 2000;86:829–833.

89 Morishita R, Gibbons GH, Ellison KE, et al. A gene therapy strategy using a transcription factor decoy of the E2F

binding site inhibits smooth muscle proliferation *in vivo*. *Proc Natl Acad Sci USA* 1995;92:5855–5859.

90 Laham RJ, Simons M, Sellke F. Gene transfer for angiogenesis in coronary artery disease. *Ann Rev Med* 2001;52: 485–502.

91 Tio RA, Tkebuchava T, Scheuermann TH, et al. Intramyocardial gene therapy with naked DNA encoding vascular endothelial growth factor improves collateral flow to ischemic myocardium. *Human Gene Ther* 1999; 10:2953–2960.

92 Giordano FJ, Ping P, McKirnan MD, et al. Intracoronary gene transfer of fibroblast growth factor-5 increases blood flow and contractile function in ischemic region of the heart. *Nat Med* 1996;2:534–539.

93 Kalka C, Masuda H, Takahashi T, et al. Transplantation of *ex vivo* expanded endothelial progenitor cells for therapeutic neovascularization. *Proc Natl Acad Sci USA* 2000;97:3422–3427.

94 Quyyumi AA. Endothelial function in health and disease: new insights into the genesis of cardiovascular disease. *Am J Med* 1998;105(1A):32S–39S.

95 Bennet MR, O'Sullivan MO. Mechanisms of angioplasty and stent restenosis: implications for design of rational therapy. *Pharmacol Therapeut* 2001;91:149–166.

96 Schwartz RS. Pathophysiology of restenosis: interaction of thrombosis, hyperplasia and/or remodeling. *Am J Cardiol* 1998;81(7A):14E–17E.

97 Mach F. Toward new therapeutic strategies against neointimal formation in restenosis. *Arterioscler Thromb Vasc Biol* 2000;20:1699–1700.

98 DeYoung MB, Dichek DA. Gene therapy for restenosis. Are we ready? *Circ Res* 1998;82:306–313.

99 Tang X, Mohuczy D, Zhang CY, et al. Intravenous angiotensinogen antisense in AAV-based vector decreases hypertension. *Am J Physiol* 1999;277: H2392–H2399.

100 Kimura B, Mohuczy D, Tang X, et al. Attenuation of hypertension and heart hypertrophy by adeno-associated virus delivering angiotensin antisense. *Hypertension* 2001;37:376–380.

101 Makino N, Sugano M, Ohtsuka S, et al. Chronic antisense therapy for angiotensinogen on cardiac hypertrophy in spontaneously hypertensive rats. *Cardiovasc Res* 1999;44:543–548.

102 Zhang YC, Kimura B, Shen L, et al. New β-blocker: Prolonged reduction in high blood pressure with β1 antisense oligodeoxynucleotides. *Hypertension* 2000;35: 219–224.

103 Wang H, Katovich MJ, Gelband CH, et al. Sustained inhibition of angiotensin I converting enzyme (ACE) expression and long-term antihypertensive action by virally mediated delivery of ACE antisense cDNA. *Circ Res* 1999;85:614–622.

104 Katovich MJ, Gelband CH, Reaves P, et al. Reversal of hypertension by angiotensin II type I receptor antisense gene therapy in the adult SHR rat. *Am J Physiol* 1999; 277:H1260–H1264.

105 Martens JR, Reaves PY, Lu D, et al. Prevention of renovascular and cardiovascular pathophysiological changes in hypertension by angiotensin II type I receptor antisense gene therapy. *Proc Natl Acad Sci USA* 1998;95: 2664–2669.

106 Lin KF, Chao L, Chao J. Prolonged reduction of high blood pressure with human nitric oxide synthase delivery. *Hypertension* 1997;30:307–313.

107 Lin KF, Chao J, Chao L. Atrial natriuretic peptide gene delivery attenuates hypertension, cardiac hypertrophy and renal injury in salt-sensitive rats. *Hum Gene Ther* 1998;9:1429–1438.

108 Yoshida H, Zhang JJ, Chao L, et al. Kallikrein gene delivery attenuates myocardial infarction and apoptosis after myocardial ischemia and reperfusion. *Hypertension* 2000;35:25–31.

109 Dobrzynski E, Wang C, Chao J, et al. Adrenomedullin gene delivery attenuates hypertension, cardiac remodeling and renal injury in deoxycorticosterone acetate salt hypertensive rats. *Hypertension* 2000;36:995–1001.

110 Sabaaway HE, Zhang F, Nguyen X, et al. Human heme oxygenase-1 gene transfer lowers blood pressure and promotes growth in spontaneously hypertensive rats. *Hypertension* 2001;38:210–215.

111 Chu Y, Iida S, Lund DD, et al. Gene transfer of extracellular superoxide dismutase reduces arterial pressure in spontaneously hypertensive rats: role of heparin binding domain. *Circ Res* 2003;92:461–468.

112 Rentrop KP. Thrombi in acute coronary syndromes. Revised and revisited. *Circulation* 2000;101:1619–1626.

113 Feldman LJ, Isner JM. Gene therapy for vulnerable plaque. *J Am Coll Cardiol* 1995; 26:826–833.

114 Chowdhury JR, Grossman M, Gupta S, et al. Long-term improvement of hypercholesterolemia after *ex vivo* gene therapy in LDLR-deficient rabbits. *Science* 1991; 254:1802–1805.

115 Grossman M, Rader DJ, Muller DW, et al. A pilot study of *ex vivo* gene therapy for homozygous familial hypercholesterolaemia. *Nat Med* 1995;1:1148–1154.

116 Zsigmond E, Kobayashi K, Tzung KW, et al. Adenovirus-mediated gene transfer of human lipoprotein lipase ameliorates the hyperlipidemias associated with apolipoprotein E and LDL receptor deficiencies in mice. *Hum Gene Ther* 1997;8:1921–1933.

117 Applebaum-Bowden D, Kobayashi J, Kashyap VS, et al. Hepatic lipase gene therapy in hepatic lipase-deficient mice: adenovirus-mediated replacement of a lipolytic enzyme to the vascular endothelium. *J Clin Invest* 1996; 97:799–805.

118 Rinaldi M, Catapano AL, Parrella P, et al. Treatment of severe hypercholesterolemia in apolipoprotein E-deficient mice by intramuscular injection of plasmid DNA. *Gene Ther* 2000;7:1795–1801.

119 Oka K, Pastore L, Kim IH, et al. Long-term stable correction of low density lipoprotein receptor-deficient mice with a helper dependent adenoviral vector expressing the very low density lipoprotein receptor. *Circulation* 2001;103:1274–1281.

120 Laukkanen J, Lehtolainen P, Gough PJ, et al. Adenovirus-mediated gene transfer of a secreted form of human macrophage scavenger receptor inhibits modified low-density lipoprotein degradation and foam cell formation in macrophages. *Circulation* 2000;101:1091–1096.

121 Rader DJ, Tietge UJ. Gene therapy for dyslipidemia: clinical prospects. *Curr Atheroscler Rep* 1999;1:58–69.

122 Tangirala RK, Tsukamoto K, Chun SH, et al. Regression of atherosclerosis induced by liver-directed gene transfer of apolipoprotein A-1 in mice. *Circulation* 1999;100: 1816–1822.

123 Inoue S, Egashira K, Ni W, et al. Anti-monocyte chemoattractant protein-1 gene therapy limits progression and destabilization of established atherosclerosis in apolipoprotein E-knockout mice. *Circulation* 2002;106: 2700–2706.

124 Vassalli G, Dichek DA. Gene therapy for arterial thrombosis. *Cardiovasc Res* 1997;35:459–469.

125 Gerard RD, Collen D. Adenovirus gene therapy for hypercholesterolemia, thrombosis and restenosis. *Cardiovasc Res* 1997;35:451–458.

126 Waugh JM, Yuksel E, Li J, et al. Local overexpression of thrombomodulin for *in vivo* prevention of arterial thrombosis in a rabbit model. *Circ Res* 1999;84:84–92.

127 Dicheck DA, Anderson J, Kelly AB, et al. Enhanced antithrombotic effects of endothelial cells expressing recombinant plasminogen activators transduced with retroviral vectors. *Circulation* 1996;93:301–309.

128 Rade JJ, Schulick AH, Virmani R, et al. Local adenoviral-mediated expression of recombinant hirudin reduces neointima formation after arterial injury. *Nat Med* 1996; 3:293–298.

129 Zoldhelyi P, McNatt J, Shelat HS, et al. Thromboresistance of balloon-injured porcine carotid arteries after local gene transfer of human tissue factor pathway inhibitor. *Circulation* 2000;101:289–295.

130 Numaguchi Y, Naruse K, Harada M, et al. Prostacyclin synthase gene transfer accelerates reendothelialization and inhibits neointimal formation in rat carotid arteries after balloon injury. *Arterioscler Throm Vasc Biol* 1999;19:727–733.

131 Zoldhelyi P, McNatt J, Xu XM, et al. Prevention of arterial thrombosis by adenovirus-mediated transfer of cyclooxygenase gene. *Circulation* 1996;93:10–17.

132 von der Leyen HE, Dzau VJ. Therapeutic potential of nitric oxide synthase gene manipulation. *Circulation* 2001;103:2760–2765.

133 Channon KM, Qian HS, Neplioueva V, et al. *In vivo* gene transfer of nitric oxide synthase enhances vasomotor function in carotid arteries from normal and cholesterol fed rabbits. *Circulation* 1998;98:1905–1911.

134 Shears III LL, Kawaharada N, Tzeng E, et al. Inducible nitric oxide synthase suppresses the development of allograft atherosclerosis. *J Clin Invest* 1997;100: 2035–2042.

135 Qian H, Neplioueva V, Shetty GA, et al. Nitric oxide synthase gene therapy rapidly reduces molecule expression and inflammatory cell infiltration in carotid artery of cholesterol-fed rabbits. *Circulation* 1999;99:2979–2982.

136 Iwata A, Sai S, Nitta Y, et al. Liposome-mediated gene transfection of endothelial nitric oxide synthase reduces endothelial activation and leukocyte infiltration in transplanted hearts. *Circulation* 2001;103:2753–2759.

137 Nakane H, Miller Jr FJ, Faraci FM, et al. Gene transfer of endothelial nitric oxide synthase reduces angiotensin II-induced endothelial dysfunction. *Hypertension* 2000;35: 595–601.

138 Juan SH, Lee TS, Tseng KW, et al. Adenovirus-mediated heme oxygenase-1 gene transfer inhibits the development of atherosclerosis in apolipoprotein E-deficient mice. *Circulation* 2001;104:1519–1525.

139 Morse D, Choi AMK. Heme oxygenase-1. The "emerging molecule" has arrived. *Am J Resp Cell Mol Biol* 2002;27:8–16.

140 Zanetti M, Sato J, Jost CJ, et al. Gene transfer of manganese superoxide dismutase reverses vascular dysfunction in the absence but not in the presence of atherosclerotic plaque. *Human Gene Ther* 2001;12: 1407–1416.

141 Holmes Jr DR. State of the heart in coronary intervention. *Am J Cardiol* 2003;91(3A):50A–53A.

142 Babapulle MN, Eisenberg MJ. Coated stents for prevention of restenosis. Part I. *Circulation* 2002;106: 2734–2740.

143 Dzau VJ, Braun-Dullaeus RC, Sedding DG. Vascular proliferation and atherosclerosis: New perspectives and therapeutic strategies. *Nat Med* 2002;8:1249–1256.

144 Kim AY, Wallinsky PL, Kolodgie FD. Early loss of thrombomodulin expression impairs vein graft thromboresistance: implications for vein graft resistance. *Circ Res* 2002;90:205–212.

145 Steg PG, Tahlil O' Aubailly N, et al. Reduction of restenosis after angioplasty in an atheromatous rabbit model by suicide gene therapy. *Circulation* 1997;96: 408–411.

146 Braun-Dullaeus RD, Mann MJ, Dzau VJ. Cell cycle progression. New therapeutic target for vascular proliferative disease. *Circulation* 1998;98:82–89.

147 Morishita R, Gibbons GH, Ellison KE, et al. Single intra-luminal delivery of antisense cdc2 kinase and proliferating cell nuclear antigen oligonucleotides results in chronic inhibition of neointimal hyperplasia. *Proc Natl Acad Sci USA* 1993;90:8474–8478.

148 Morishita R, Gibbons GH, Ellison KE, et al. A gene therapy strategy using a transcription factor decoy of the E2F binding site inhibits smooth muscle proliferation *in vivo*. *Proc Natl Acad Sci* 1995;92:5855–5859.

149 Mann MJ, Whittemore AD, Donaldson MC, et al. Ex-vivo gene therapy of human vascular bypass grafts with E2F decoy: The PREVENT single-centre, randomized, controlled trial. *Lancet* 1999;354:1493–1498.

150 McCarthy M. Molecular decoy may keep bypass grafts open. *Lancet* 2001;358:1703.

151 Ehsan A, Mann MJ, Dell'Acqua G, et al. Endothelial healing in vein grafts. Proliferative burst is unimpaired by genetic therapy of neointimal disease. *Circulation* 2002;105:1686–1692.

152 Mann MJ, Gibbons GH, Tsao PS, et al. Cell cycle inhibition preserves endothelial function in genetically-engineered rabbit vein grafts. *J Clin Invest* 1997;99: 1295–1301.

153 Morishita R, Gibbons GH, Ellison KE, et al. Intimal hyperplasia after vascular injury is inhibited by antisense cdk2 kinase oligonucleotides. *J Clin Invest* 1994; 93:1458–1464.

154 Gunn J, Holt CM, Francis SE, et al. The effect of oligonucleotides to c-myb on vascular smooth muscle cell proliferation and neointima formation after porcine coronary angioplasty. *Circ Res* 1997;80:520–531.

155 Shi Y, Fard A, Galeo A, et al. Transcatheter delivery of c-myc antisense oligomers reduces neointimal formation in a porcine model of coronary artery balloon injury. *Circulation* 1994;90:944–951.

156 Chang MW, Barr E, Lu MM, et al. Adenovirus-mediated overexpression of the cyclin/cyclin dependent kinase inhibitor, p21 inhibits vascular smooth muscle proliferation and neointima formation in the rat carotid artery model of balloon angioplasty. *J Clin Invest* 1995;96: 2260–2268.

157 Chen D, Krasinski K, Sylvester A, et al. Downregulation of cyclin-dependent kinase 2 activity and cyclin A promoter activity in vascular smooth muscle cells by p27 (KIP1), an inhibitor of neointima formation in the rat carotid artery. *J Clin Invest* 1997;99:2334–2341.

158 Chang MW, Barr E, Seltzer J, et al. Cytostatic gene therapy for vascular proliferative disorders with a constitutively active form of the retinoblastoma gene product. *Science* 1995;267:518–522.

159 Yonemitsu Y, Kaneda Y, Tanaka S, et al. Transfer of wild-type p53 gene effectively inhibits vascular smooth muscle proliferation *in vitro* and *in vivo*. *Circ Res* 1998;82: 147–156.

160 Morishita R, Higaki J, Tomita N, et al. Application of transcription factor "decoy" strategy as a means of gene therapy and study of gene expression in cardiovascular disease. *Circ Res* 1998;82:1023–1028.

161 Van Belle E, Maillard L, Tio FO, et al. Accelerated endothelialization by local delivery of recombinant human vascular endothelial growth factor reduces in-stent intimal formation. *Biochem Biophys Res Commun* 1997;235:311–316.

162 Von der Leyen HE, Gibbons GH, Morishita R, et al. Gene therapy inhibiting neointimal vascular lesion: *in vivo* transfer of endothelial cell nitric oxide synthase gene. *Proc Natl Acad Sci USA* 1995;92:1137–1141.

163 Tzeng E, Shears LL, Robbins PD, et al. Vascular gene transfer of the human inducible nitric oxide synthase: characterization of activity and effects of myointimal hyperplasia. *Mol Med* 1996;2:211–215.

164 Tulis DA, Durante W, Liu X, et al. Adenovirus-mediated heme oxygenase-1 gene delivery inhibits injury-induced vascular neointima formation. *Circulation* 2001;104:2710–2715.

165 Laukkanen MO, Kivela A, Rissane T, et al. Adenovirus-mediated extracellular superoxide dismutase gene therapy reduces neointima formation in balloon-denuded rabbit aorta. *Circulation* 2002;106:1999–2003.

166 Takahashi T, Kalka C, Masuda H, et al. Ischemia- and cytokine-induced mobilization of bone-marrow-derived endothelial progenitor cells for neovascularization. *Nat Med* 1999;5:434–438.

167 Shi Q, Bhattacharya V, Hong-De, et al. Utilizing granulocyte colony-stimulating factor to enhance vascular graft endothelialization from circulating blood cells. *Ann Vasc Surg* 2002;16:314–320.

168 Fuster V, Badimon L, Badimon JJ, et al. The pathogenesis of coronary artery disease and the acute coronary syndromes (1). *N Engl J Med* 1992;326:245–250.

169 Fuster V, Badimon L, Badimon JJ, et al. The pathogenesis of coronary artery disease and the acute coronary syndromes (2). *N Engl J Med* 1992;326:310–318.

170 Boersma E, Mercado N, Poldermans D, et al. Acute myocardial infarction. *Lancet* 2003;361:847–858.

171 Jessup M, Brozena S. Heart failure. *N Engl J Med* 348;2003;2007–2018.

172 Lefer DJ, Granger DN. Oxidative stress and cardiac disease. *Am J Med* 2000;109:315–323.

173 Liao JK. Endothelium and acute coronary syndromes. *Clin Chem* 1998;44:1799–1808.

174 Kinlay S, Selwyn AP, Libby P, et al. Inflammation, the endothelium, and the acute coronary syndromes. *J Cardiovasc Pharmacol* 1998;32(Suppl 3):S62–S66.

175 Watson RDS, Chin BSP, Lip GYH. Antithrombotic therapy in acute coronary syndromes. *Brit Med J* 2002; 325:1348–1351.

176 Carden DL, Granger DN. Pathophysiology of ischaemia-reperfusion injury. *Am J Pathol* 2000;190:255–266.

177 Das UN. Free radicals, cytokines and nitric oxide in cardiac failure and myocardial infarction. *Mol Cell Biochem* 2000;215:145–152.

178 Stein EA. Identification and treatment of individuals at high risk of coronary artery disease. *Am J Med* 2002;112(8A):3S–9S.

179 Givertz MM, Colucci WS. New targets for heart failure therapy: endothelin, inflammatory cytokines, and oxidative stress. *Lancet* 1998;352(Suppl 1):S134–S138.

180 Svensson EC, Marshall DJ, Woodard K, et al. Efficient and stable transduction of cardiomyocytes after intramyocardial injection or intracoronary perfusion with recombinant adeno-associated virus vectors. *Circulation* 1999;99:201–205.

181 Melo LG, Agrawal R, Zhang L, et al. Gene therapy strategy for long term myocardial protection using adeno-associated virus-mediated delivery of heme oxygenase gene. *Circulation* 2002;105:602–607.

182 Agrawal RS, Muangman S, Melo LG, et al. Recombinant adeno-associated virus mediated antioxidant enzyme delivery as preventive gene therapy against ischemia-reperfusion injury of the rat myocardium. *Mol Ther* 2001;3:A837.

183 Li Q, Bolli R, Qiu Y, et al. Gene therapy with extracellular superoxide dismutase protects conscious rabbits against myocardial infarction. *Circulation* 2001; 103:1893–1898.

184 Chen EP, Bittner HB, Davis RD, et al. Physiological effects of extracellular superoxide dismutase transgene overexpression on myocardial function after ischemia and reperfusion injury. *J Thorac Cardiovasc Surg* 1998;115:450–458.

185 Woo YZ, Zhang JC, Vijayasarathy C, et al. Recombinant adenovirus-mediated cardiac gene transfer of superoxide dismutase and catalase attenuates postischemic contractile dysfunction. *Circulation* 1998;98(Suppl):II255–II260.

186 Zhu HL, Stewart AS, Taylor MD. Blocking free radical production via adenoviral gene transfer decreases cardiac ischemia-reperfusion injury. *Mol Ther* 2000;2:470–475.

187 Yoshida T, Watanabe M, Engelman DT, et al. Transgenic mice overexpressing glutathione peroxidase are resistant to myocardial reperfusion injury. *J Mol Cell Cardiol* 1996;28:1759–1767.

188 Suzuki K, Sawa Y, Kaneda Y. *In vivo* gene transfer of heat shock protein 70 enhances myocardial tolerance to ischemia-reperfusion injury in rat. *J Clin Invest* 1997;99:1645–1650.

189 Vander Heide RS. Increased expression of HSP27 protects canine myocytes from simulated ischemia-reperfusion injury. *Am J Physiol* 2002;282:H935–H941.

190 Chatterjee S, Stewart AS, Bish LT, et al. Viral gene transfer of the antiapoptotic factor Bcl-2 protects against chronic ischemic heart failure. *Circulation* 2002;106(Suppl):I212–I217.

191 Matsui T, Li L, Del Monte F, et al. Adenoviral gene transfer of activated phosphatidylinositol 3'-kinase and Akt inhibits apoptosis of hypoxic cardiomyocytes *in vitro*. *Circulation* 1999;100:2373–2379.

192 Brauner R, Nonoyama M, Laks H, et al. Intracoronary adenovirus-mediated transfer of immunosuppressive cytokine genes prolongs allograft survival. *J Thorac Cardiovasc Surg* 1997;114:923–933.

193 Yang Z, Cerniway RJ, Byford AM. Cardiac overexpression of A1-adenosine receptor protects intact mice against myocardial infarction. *Am J Physiol* 2002;282:H949–H955.

194 Agata J, Chao L, Chao J. Kallikrein gene delivery improves cardiac reserve and attenuates remodeling after myocardial infarction. *Hypertension* 2002;40:653–659.

195 Holly TA, Drincic A, Byun Y, et al. Caspase inhibition reduces myocyte cell death induced by myocardial ischemia and reperfusion *in vivo*. *J Mol Cell Cardiol* 1999;31:1709–1715.

196 Ueda H, Sawa Y, Matsumoto K, et al. Gene transfection of hepatocyte growth factor attenuates reperfusion injury in the heart. *Ann Thorac Surg* 1999;67:1726–1731.

197 Morishita R, Sugimoto T, Aoki M, et al. *In vivo* transfection of *cis* element "decoy" against nuclear factor κB binding sites prevents myocardial infarction. *Nat Med* 1997;3:894–899.

198 Stepkowski SM. Development of antisense oligodeoxynucleotides for transplantation. *Curr Opin Mol Ther* 2000;2:304–317.

199 Poston RS, Mann MJ, Hoyt EG, et al. Antisense oligodeoxynucleotides prevent acute cardiac allograft rejection via a novel, non-toxic, highly efficient transfection method. *Transplantation* 1999;68:825–832.

200 Herttuala SY, Alitalo K. Gene transfer as a tool to induce therapeutic vascular growth. *Nat Med* 2003;9:694–700.

201 Mack CA, Patel SA, Schwarz EA, et al. Biological bypass with the use of adenovirus-mediated transfer of the complementary deoxyribonucleic acid for vascular endothelial growth factor 121 improves myocardial perfusion and function in the ischemic porcine heart. *J Thorac Cardiovasc Surg* 1998;115:168–177.

202 Ueda H, Sawa Y, Matsumoto K, et al. Gene transfection of hepatocyte growth factor attenuates reperfusion injury in the heart. *Ann Thorac Surg* 1999;67: 1726–1731.

203 Rosengart TK, Lee LY, Patel SR, et al. Angiogenesis gene therapy: phase I assessment of direct intramyocardial administration of an adenovirus vector expressing VEGF$_{121}$ cDNA to individuals with clinically significant severe coronary artery disease. *Circulation* 1999;100:468–474.

204 Symes JF, Losordo DW, Vale PR, et al. Gene therapy with vascular endothelial growth factor for inoperable coronary artery disease. *Ann Thor Surg* 1999; 68: 830–837.

205 Hammond HK, McKirman MD. Angiogenic gene therapy for heart disease: a review of animal studies and clinical trials. *Cardiovasc Res* 2001;49:561–567.

206 Lee LY, Patel SR, Hackett NR, et al. Focal angiogen therapy using intramyocardial delivery of an adenovirus vector coding for vascular endothelial growth factor 121. *Ann Thorac Surg* 2000;69:14–24.

207 Ueno H, Li JJ, Masuda S, et al. Adenovirus-mediated expression of the secreted form of basic fibroblast growth factor (FGF-2) induces cellular proliferation and angiogenesis *in vivo*. *Arterioscler Thromb Vasc Biol* 1997;17:2453–2460.

208 Tabata H, Silver M, Isner JM. Arterial gene transfer of acidic fibroblast growth factor for therapeutic angiogenesis *in vivo*: critical role of secretion signal in use of naked DNA. *Cardiovasc Res* 1997;25:470–479.

209 Taniyama Y, Morishita R, Aoki M, et al. Angiogenesis and antifibrotic action by hepatocyte growth factor in cardiomyopathy. *Hypertension* 2002;40:47–53.

210 Aoki M, Morishita R, Taniyama Y, et al. Therapeutic angiogenesis induced by hepatocyte growth factor: potential gene therapy for ischemic diseases. *J Atheroscler Thromb* 2000;7:71–76.

211 Vale PR, Losordo DW, Milliken CE, et al. Randomized, single-blind, placebo-controlled pilot study of catheter-based myocardial gene transfer for therapeutic angiogenesis using left ventricular electromechanical mapping in patients with chronic myocardial ischemia. *Circulation* 2001;103:2138–2143.

212 Grines CL, Watkins MW, Helmer G, et al. Angiogenic gene therapy (AGENT) trial in patients with stable angina pectoris. *Circulation* 2002;105:1291–1297.

213 Losordo DW, Vale PR, Isner JM. Gene therapy for myocardial angiogenesis. *Am Heart J* 1999;138:S132–S141.

214 Bashir R, Vale PR, Isner JM, et al. Angiogenic gene therapy: pre-clinical studies and phase I clinical data. *Kidney Int* 2002;61(Suppl 1):110–114.

215 Lee RJ, Springer ML, Blanco-Bose WE, et al. VEGF gene delivery to myocardium. Deleterious effect of upregulated expression. *Circulation* 2000;102:898–901.

216 Carmeliet P. VEGF gene therapy: stimulating angiogenesis or angioma-genesis. *Nat Med* 2000;6:1102–1103.

217 Su H, Arakawa-Hoyt J, Kan YW. Adeno-associated viral vector-mediated hypoxia response element-regulated gene expression in mouse ischemic heart model. *Proc Natl Acad Sci USA* 2002;99:9480–9485.

218 Vincent KA, Shyu K-G, Luo Y, et al. Angiogenesis is induced in a rabbit model of hindlimb ischemia by naked DNA encoding an HIF-1α/VP16 hybrid transcription factor. *Circulation* 2000;102:2255–2261.

219 Rebar EJ, Huang Y, Hickey R, et al. Induction of angiogenesis in a mouse model using engineered transcription factors. *Nat Med* 2002;8:1427–1432.

220 Kawamoto A, Gwon H-C, Iwaguro H, et al. Therapeutic potential of *ex vivo* expanded endothelial progenitor cells for myocardial ischemia. *Circulation* 2001;103: 634–637.

221 Kaushal S, Amiel GE, Guleserian KJ, et al. Functional small-diameter neovessels created using endothelial progenitor cells expanded *ex vivo*. *Nature Medicine* 2001;7:1035–1040.

222 Nugent HM, Edelman ER. Tissue engineering therapy for cardiovascular disease. *Circ Res* 2003;92:1068–1078.

223 Shintani S, Murohara T, Ikeda H, et al. Augmentation of postnatal neovascularization with autologous bone marrow transplantation. *Circulation* 2001;103:897–903.

224 Hristov M, Erl W, Weber PC. Endothelial progenitor cells: mobilization, differentiation, and homing. *Arterioscler Thromb Vasc Biol* 2003;23:1185–1189.

225 Shintani S, Murohara T, Ikeda H, et al. Mobilization of endothelial progenitor cells in patients with acute myocardial infarction. *Circulation* 2001;103:2776–2779.

226 Ikenaga S, Hamano K, Nishida M, et al. Autologous bone marrow implantation induced angiogenesis and improved deteriorated exercise capacity in a rat ischemic hindlimb model. *J Surg Res* 2001;96:277–283.

227 Kocher AA, Schuster MD, Szabolcs MJ, et al. Neovascularization of ischemic myocardium by human bone-marrow-derived angioblasts prevents cardiomyocyte apoptosis, reduces remodeling and improves cardiac function. *Nat Med* 2001;7:430–436.

228 Rafii S, Lyden D. Therapeutic stem and progenitor cell transplantation for organ vascularization and regeneration. *Nat Med* 2003;9:702–712.

229 Stamm C, Westphal B, Kleine H-D, et al. Autologous bone-marrow transplantation for myocardial regeneration. *Lancet* 2003;361:45–46.

230 Kalka C, Masuda H, Takahashi T, et al. Vascular endothelial growth factor$_{165}$ gene transfer augments circulating endothelial progenitor cells in human subjects. *Circ Res* 2000;86:1198–1202.

231 Kalka C, Tehrani H, Laudernberg B, et al. Mobilization of endothelial progenitor cells following gene therapy with VEGF$_{165}$ in patients with inoperable coronary disease. *Ann Thorac Surg* 2000;70:829–834.

232 Dimmeler S, Aicher A, Vasa M, et al. HMG-CoA reductase inhibitors (statins) increase endothelial progenitor cells via the PI3-kinase/Akt pathway. *J Clin Invest* 2001;108:391–397.

233 Vasa M, Fichtlschrerer S, Adler K, et al. Increase in circulating endothelial progenitor cells by statin therapy in patients with stable coronary artery disease. *Circulation* 2001;103:2885–2890.

234 Walter DH, Rittig K, Bahlmann FH, et al. Statin therapy accelerates reendothelialization: a novel effect involving

mobilization and incorporation of bone marrow-derived endothelial progenitor cells. *Circulation* 2002; 105:3017–3024.

235 Werner N, Priller J, Laufs U, et al. Bone marrow-derived progenitor cells modulate vascular reendothelialization and neointimal formation. Effect of 3-hydroxy-3-methyl-glutaryl coenzyme A reductase inhibition. *Arterioscler Thromb Vasc Biol* 2002;22:1567–1572.

236 Boyer M, Townsend LE, Vogel LM, et al. Isolation of endothelial cells and their progenitor cells from human peripheral blood. *J Vasc Surg* 2000;31:181–189.

237 Asahara T, Masuda H, Takahashi T, et al. Bone marrow origin of endothelial progenitor cells responsible for postnatal vasculogenesis in physiological and pathological neovascularization *Circ Res* 1999;85:221–228.

238 Yamashita J, Itoh H, Hirashima M, et al. Flk1-positive cells derived from embryonic stem cells serve as vascular progenitors. *Nature* 2000;408:92–96.

239 Yamaguchi J, Kusano K, Masuo O, et al. Stromal cell-derived factor-1 effects on *ex vivo* expanded endothelial progenitor cell recruitment for ischemic neovascularization. *Circulation* 2003;107:1322–1328.

240 Lee SH, Wolf PL, Escudero R, et al. Early expression of angiogenesis factors in acute myocardial ischemia and infarction. *N Engl J Med* 2000;342:626–633.

241 Frangogiannis NG, Lindsey ML, Michael LH, et al. Resident cardiac mast cells degranulate and release pre-formed tumor necrosis factor alpha (TNF-α), initiating the cytokine cascade in experimental canine myocardial ischemia/reperfusion. *Circulation* 1998;98:699–710.

242 Woldbaek PR, Hoen IB, Christensen G, et al. Gene expression of colony-stimulating factors and stem cell factor after myocardial infarction in the mouse. *Acta Physiol Scand* 2002;173–181.

243 Rabbany SY, Heissig B, Hattori K, et al. Molecular pathways regulating mobilization of marrow-derived stem cells for tissue revascularization. *Trends Mol Med* 2003; 9:109–117.

244 Kong D, Melo LG, Mangi AA, et al. Enhanced inhibition of neointimal hyperplasia by genetically engineered endothelial progenitor cells. *Circulation* 2004;109: 1769–1775.

245 Luttun A, Carmeliet G, Carmeliet P, et al. Vascular progenitors: from biology to treatment. *Trends Cardiovasc Med* 2002;12:88–96.

246 Kawamoto A, Tkebuchava T, Yamaguchi J-I, et al. Intramyocardial transplantation of autologous endothelial progenitor cells for therapeutic neovascularization. *Circulation* 2003;107:461–468.

247 Kamihata H, Matsubara H, Nishiue T, et al. Improvement of collateral perfusion and regional function by implantation of peripheral blood mononuclear cells into ischemic hybernating myocardium. *Arterioscler Vasc Biol* 2002;22:1804–1810.

248 Kamihata H, Matsubara H, Nishiue T, et al. Implantation of bone marrow mononuclear cells into ischemic myocardium enhances collateral perfusion and regional function via side supply of angioblasts, angiogenic ligands, and cytokines. *Circulation* 2001;104:1046–1052.

249 Kobayashi T, Hamano K, Li TS, et al. Enhancement of angiogenesis by the implantation of self bone marrow cells in a rat ischemic heart model. *J Surg Res* 2000;89:189–195.

250 Fuchs S, Baffour R, Zhou YF, et al. Transendocardial delivery of autologous bone marrow enhances collateral perfusion and regional function in pigs with chronic experimental myocardial ischemia. *J Am Coll Cardiol* 2001;37:1726–1732.

251 Iba O, Matsubara H, Nozawa Y, et al. Angiogenesis by implantation of peripheral blood mononuclear cells and platelets into ischemic limbs. *Circulation* 2002; 106:2019–2025.

252 Strauer BE, Brehm M, Zeus T, et al. Repair of infarcted myocardium by autologous intracoronary mononuclear bone marrow cell transplantation in humans. *Circulation* 2002;106:1913–1918.

253 Assmus B, Schachlinger V, Teupe C, et al. Transplantation of progenitor cells and regeneration enhancement in acute myocardial infarction (TOPCARE-AMI). *Circulation* 2002;106;3009–3017.

254 Perin EC, Dohmann HFR, Borojevic R, et al. Transendocardial, autologous bone marrow cell transplantation for severe, chronic ischemic heart failure. *Circulation* 2003;107:2294–2302.

255 Tse H-F, Kwong Y-L, Chan JKF, et al. Angiogenesis in ischemic myocardium by intramyocardial autologous bone marrow mononuclear cell implantation. *Lancet* 2003;361:47–49.

256 Tateishi-Yuyama E, Matsubara H, Murohara T, et al. Therapeutic angiogenesis for patients with limb ischemia by autologous transplantation of bone-marrow cells: a pilot study and a randomised controlled trial. *Lancet* 2002;360:427–435.

257 Orlic D, Kajstura J, Chimenti S, et al. Bone marrow cells regenerate infracted myocardium. *Nature* 2001;410: 701–705.

258 Orlic D, Kajstura J, Chimenti S, et al. Mobilized bone marrow cells repair the infracted heart, improving function and survival. *Proc Natl Acad Sci USA* 2001;98: 10344–10349.

259 Jackson KA, Majka SM, Wang H, et al. Regeneration of ischemic cardiac muscle and vascular endothelium by adult stem cells. *J Clin Invest* 2001;107:1395–1402.

260 Murohara T, Ikeda H, Duan J, et al. Transplanted cord blood-derived endothelial precursor cells augmented postnatal neovascularization. *J Clin Invest* 2000;105: 1527–1536.

261 Nugent HM, Edelman ER. Tissue engineering therapy for cardiovascular disease. *Circ Res* 2003;92:1068–1078.

262 Nerem RM, Seliktar D. Vascular tissue engineering. *Ann Rev Biomed Eng* 2001;3:225–243.

263 Conte MS, Birinyi LK, Miyata T, et al. Efficient repopulation of denuded rabbit arteries with autologous genetically modified endothelial cells. *Circulation* 1994;89:2161–2169.

264 Nugent HM, Rogers C, Edelman ER. Endothelial implants inhibit intimal hyperplasia after porcine angioplasty. *Circ Res* 1999;84:384–391.

265 Shirota T, Yasui H, Shimokawa H, et al. Fabrication of endothelial progenitor cell (EPC)-seeded intravascular stent devices and *in vitro* endothelialization on hybrid vascular tissue. *Biomaterials* 2003;24:2295–2302.

266 Consigny PM. Endothelial cell seeding on prosthetic surfaces. *J Long Term Eff Med* 2000;10:79–95.

267 Dichek DA, Anderson J, Kelly AB, et al. Enhanced *in vivo* antithrombotic effects of endothelial cells expressing recombinant plasminogen activators transduced with retroviral vectors. *Circulation* 1996;93:301–309.

268 Lundell A, Kelly AB, Anderson J, et al. Reduction in vascular lesion formation by hirudin secreted from retrovirus-transduced confluent endothelial cells on vascular grafts in baboons. *Circulation* 1999;100:2018–2024.

269 Griese DP, Ehsan A, Melo LG, et al. Isolation and transplantation of autologous circulating endothelial cells into denuded vessels and prosthetic grafts: implications for cell-based vascular therapy. *Circulation* 2003;108:2710–2715.

270 Maeda M, Fukui A, Nakamura T, et al. Progenitor endothelial cells on vascular grafts: an ultrastructural study. *J Biomed Mater Res* 2000;51:55–60.

271 Bhattacharya V, Shi Q, Ishida A, et al. Administration of granulocyte colony-stimulating factor enhances endothelialization and microvessel formation in small caliber synthetic vascular grafts. *J Vasc Surg* 2000;32:116–123.

272 Kong D, Melo LG, Gnecchi M, et al. Cytokine-induced mobilization of circulating endothelial progenitor cells enhances repair on injured arteries. *Circulation* 2004;110:2039–2046.

273 Strehlow K, Werner N, Berweiler J, et al. Estrogen increases bone-marrow derived endothelial progenitor cell production and diminishes neointima formation. *Circulation* 2003;107:3059–3065.

274 Assmus B, Urbich C, Aicher A, et al. HMG-CoA reductase inhibitors reduce senescence and increase proliferation of endothelial progenitor cells via regulation of cell cycle regulatory genes. *Circ Res* 2003;92:1049–1055.

275 L'Heureux N, Paquet S, Labbe R. A completely biological tissue-engineered human blood vessel. *FASEB J* 1998;12:47–56.

276 Niklason LE, Gao J, Abbott WM. Functional arteries grown *in vitro*. *Science* 1999;284:489–493.

277 Campbell JH, Efendy JL, Campbell GR. Novel vascular graft grown within recipient's own peritoneal cavity. *Circ Res* 1999;85:1173–1178.

278 Toma C, Pittenger MF, Cahill KS, et al. Human mesenchymal stem cells differentiate to a cardiomyocyte phenotype in the adult murine heart. *Circulation* 2002;105:93–98.

279 Murasawa S, Llevadot J, Silver M, et al. Constitutive human telomerase reverse transcriptase expression enhances regenerative properties of endothelial progenitor cells. *Circulation* 2002;106:1133–1139.

280 Zhang M, Methot D, Poppa V, et al. Cardiac myocyte grafting for cardiac repair: Graft cell death and anti-death strategies. *J Mol Cell Cardiol* 2001;33:907–921.

Index

Note: page numbers in *italics* refer to figures, those in **bold** refer to tables